WITHDRAWN

TOURO COLLEGE LIBRARY
Main Campus Women's Building

Second Edition

THE NATURE

OF

STUTTERING

Charles Van Riper
Western Michigan University

TO WRITCHILDERAWNRY
Main Campus Women's Building

WAVELAND
PRESS, INC.

Prospect Heights, Illinois

Wonens Bldg   RC
              424
              .V29
              1992

For information about this book, write or call:
  Waveland Press, Inc.
  P.O. Box 400
  Prospect Heights, Illinois 60070
  (847) 634-0081

Copyright © 1982, 1971 by Prentice-Hall, Inc.
1992 reissued by Waveland Press, Inc.

ISBN 0-88133-677-7

All rights reserved. No part of this book may be reproduced, stored in a retrieval system, or transmitted in any form or by any means without permission in writing from the publisher.

Printed in the United States of America

7   6   5   4   3

11/18/97

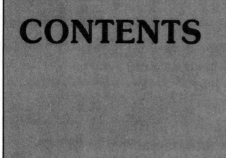

CONTENTS

4 The Onset of Stuttering   58

5 The Development of Stuttering   88

6 Phenomenology: Overt Features   111

7 Phenomenology: Covert Reactions   144

8 The Loci of Stuttering and the Adaptation Effect   177

9 The Severity of Stuttering   196

10 The Self-Concepts of Stutterers   225

15 Stuttering as the Result of Disturbed Feedback

16 Stuttering as a Disorder of Coordination

17 The Nature of Stuttering: An Attempted Synthesis

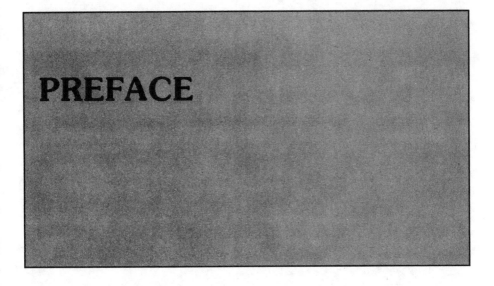

PREFACE

The original purpose in writing this book was to assemble, summarize and organize the widely scattered information concerning the nature of stuttering. In the ten years since it was first published a veritable flood of new material has become available. Two new chapters have been added, the former ones have been extensively revised, and the current concepts concerning the nature of stuttering have been presented. If we are ever to solve the problem óf stuttering we must first understand it, and if we are to understand it we should know what others have written about it.

C. Van Riper

To the ancient birch tree to whom, when I was a youth and it was a sapling, I swore an oath to find the cause and cure of the stuttering that afflicted me and so many others. Though I failed and we both have grown old I did my utmost and am content. Others will take up my quest.

THE PROBLEM AND ITS UNIVERSALITY

1

Stuttering has been called a riddle. We do not like the term because it implies a pat verbal answer and because it fails to do justice to the complexity of the disorder. Stuttering is more than a riddle. It is at least a complicated, multidimensioned jigsaw puzzle, with many pieces still missing. It is also a personal, social, and scientific problem whose equation has not yet been stated completely, a problem with many unknowns. As such it has challenged men of many lands and times to find its solution, for riddles and puzzles and problems are always viewed as being potentially soluble. These solutions have ranged all the way from Francis Bacon's prescription of hot wine to thaw a presumably frozen tongue to that of the Tlahoose Indian who required the stutterer to put his mouth to a knot hole and recite "I give my stuttering to you," as the witch doctor banged the board from the other side (Lemert, 1953) or to the modern therapist's momentary deafening of his client with masking noise.

Stuttering has probably received more attention than any other speech disorder because of the way in which it dramatically exposes many of the unpleasant sides of social living. It is the dark mirror of speech, reflecting man's frustrations in communicating with his fellows. It portrays his fears of social penalties; it reveals his shame for deviancy; it is the hallmark of man's inability to communicate with his fellows. Nuttall (1937) in his "Memoir of a Stammerer," said that anyone who could solve the problem of stuttering could solve all the important troubles of the human race.

It is difficult for those who have not possessed or been possessed by the disorder to appreciate its impact on the stutterer's self-concepts, his roles, his way of living. Once it has taken hold, after a period of insidious growth, almost every aspect of the person's existence is colored by his communicative disability. Ease in verbal communication is a vital prerequisite for more than marginal existence in any modern culture such as ours. Stuttering is not merely a speech impediment; it is an impediment

1

in social living. Lemert (1951), the sociologist, summarizes his evaluation of the stutterer as a deviant in these words: "The stutterer finds himself at a distinct loss in a culture where such a large proportion of adjustments are predominantly verbal and where competitive success in many areas depends upon the ability of the person to manipulate others through verbal controls. The stutterer simply does not possess the effective speech through which the more important roles are implemented" (p. 171). Even those who manage to cope with the disorder can do so only by continual vigilance, most stutterers feeling that they have been sentenced to endure a life of verbal hard labor. The very intermittency of the disorder compounds the problem. One of our clients said it well: "I can't get used to it. I can't get used to it. I wish I were blind or deaf or crippled. Then I'd always be that way and though it would be hard I could finally accept it. But the way it is, I talk all right for a bit and then get clobbered. I hope I can talk; I fear I can't; sometimes I can; sometimes I can't. I'm always torn." Wendell Johnson (1930) in his autobiography, puts it even more vividly: "I am a stutterer. I am not like other people. I must think differently, act differently, live differently—because I stutter. Like other stutterers, like other exiles, I have known all my life a great sorrow and a great hope together, and they have made me the kind of a person I am. An awkward tongue has molded my life" (p. 1). Stuttering is more than a verbal riddle. It can be a devastating personal problem.

It is also and perhaps primarily a puzzle, the pieces of which lie scattered on the tables of speech pathology, psychiatry, neurophysiology, genetics, and many other disciplines. At each of these tables, workers have painstakingly managed to assemble a part of the puzzle, shouting "Eureka" while ignoring the pieces of their own or other tables which fail to fit. Regretfully, but hopefully, we suspect that some of the essential pieces are not merely misplaced but still missing. Nevertheless, in this book we shall try to put together as many as we can.

STUTTERING IN FORMER TIMES

One portion of the puzzle of stuttering is concerned with its apparent universality. The disorder has evidently been with us for a long time and has existed in all the corners of the earth. Clay tablets found in Mesopotamia dating from centuries long before the birth of Christ testify to its ancient history (Van Riper, 1963, p. 306). Laotze, in China, mentions stuttering in a poem written 2500 years ago: "The greatest wisdom seems like stupidity. The greatest eloquence like stuttering." Moses has often been mentioned as having stuttered (although the original Hebrew uses a term that means "heavy mouthed or slow and sluggish of speech") but there is an old tradition that he had difficulty in enunciating the labial sounds which are rarely a problem in articulatory disorders.

> Moses, when a child, was one day taken by Pharaoh on his knee. He thereupon grasped Pharaoh's crown and placed it upon his head. The astrologers were horror-struck. "Let two braziers be brought," they counselled, "one filled with gold, the other with glowing coals, and set them before him. If he grasps the gold, it will be safer for Pharaoh to put the possible usurper to death." When

the braziers were brought, the hand of Moses was stretching out for the gold, but the angel Gabriel guided it to the coals. The child plucked out a burning coal and put it to his lips and for life remained "heavy of speech and heavy of tongue" (Hertz, 1938, Exodus 4, Footnote, pp. 10–17).

At any rate, for one reason or another, Moses protested to the Lord that his speech problem did not fit him to lead the Jews out of Egyptian captivity, and he had his brother Aaron read the ten commandments to the Israelites after he came down from the mountain, both fairly typical behaviors on the part of a stutterer. In the Koran (Surah: Taha, 25–32), we find this report: "Moses said: My Lord, relieve my mind and ease my task for me, and loose the knot from my tongue that they may understand my saying."

Whether Moses really stuttered or not we do not know, but we do know that the disorder was known to Isaiah whose verse is clear: "And the tongues of stammerers shall be ready to speak plainly" (Isaiah: 32:4). Elsewhere Isaiah speaks of "stammering lips" (30:11) and a stammering tongue (24:19).

Clark and Murray (1965) report that hieroglyphics representing the word "nit-nit" were used for stuttering in the twentieth century B.C. The ancient Greeks, too, were well acquainted with the disorder. Aristotle distinguished such a speech disorder as lisping ("the inability to master a letter") from stuttering hesitancy or phthongophobia. Demosthenes, who has been reputed to have been cured of his speech impediment by placing pebbles in his mouth and leaden plates on his chest as he climbed the mountain or orated to the surf, may really have had an articulatory problem and a weak voice instead of or in addition to stuttering. Satyrus, the actor, was his therapist—the first one of our profession unless we count the Oracle of Delphi who prescribed a change of environment (exile forever) to a stutterer named Battos, son of Polymestros.

During Roman and medieval times, handicapped persons were often known by the name of their affliction. Thus Balbus, referring to stuttering, became the surname of all members of a plebeian family named Blaesus during the Roman Republic. Similarly, a Frankish king named Ludwig the Stutterer lived and probably spoke briefly in the ninth century.

Avicenna, an Arabian poet and physician who lived from 980 to 1037 A.D., described the disorder clearly and stated its cause and treatment. Kirk (1977), an anthropologist, provides some of the early Arabic views concerning all the speech disorders, including stuttering. In Moezogothic, an early Germanic dialect, *stamm* evidently referred to stuttering, and the same term is found in Anglo-Saxon but *stommettan* was also used. At one time in northern England, *stoter* meant to stumble while *stammer* referred to stagger. In Germany the wheels of a machine were said to *stotter* when they moved jerkily. Although at present in England *stammering* is preferred to its usual synonym *stuttering*, in 1598 John Skelton composed this pretty little verse using both words:

Her tonge was verye quicke,
But she spak somewhat thicke;
Her felow did stammer and stutt
But she was a foul slut.

There are also sufficient historical figures who attest to the presence of stuttering as an old affliction of the human race. To list but a few of these we have not mentioned: Virgil, Erasmus, King Charles I and Edward VI of England, Charles Darwin, Charles Lamb, Charles Kingsley, Leigh Hunt, and Aneurin Bevan all stuttered. The references by Emerick (1966) and French (1966) have some fascinating accounts of the effect of stuttering on the lives of some of these individuals.

These are mere tidbits from a smorgasbord of historical items referring to the disorder of stuttering, and we must resist the temptation to put more on the plate than the reader can consume without indigestion. It is perhaps enough to say that stuttering has been with us throughout recorded history.

UNIVERSALITY OF STUTTERING

The universality of stuttering may also be demonstrated by its present occurrence in widely varying cultures. Although the lack of a word for stuttering can hardly be said to prove that no such disorder exists, the presence of such a term helps to corroborate its occurrence as an entity. The short list of terms referring to stuttering which we provide is illustrative, not exclusive. The disorder is so widely distributed that it is apparently found in almost all people and cultures.

Words Referring to Stuttering

European
Finnish: ankyttää
German: stottern
French: begaiement
Portuguese: gagueira
Norwegian: stamning
Italian: balbuzie
Spanish: tartamundear
Yugoslav (Slovene): jeclijati
Latvian: stostisanas
Estonian: tölpkeel
Hungarian: dadogó
Czech: koktani
Russian: zaikatsia; zaikanie
Esperanto: babuti

American Indian, etc.
Salish: sutsuts
Nanaimo: skeykulskwels
Tlahoose: ha'ak'ok
Haida: kilekwigu'ung
Chocktaw: isunash illi
Asage: the'-ce u-ba-ci-ge
Cherokee: a-da-nv-te-hi-lo-squi
Sioux: eye-hda-sna-sna; iyi-tag-tag
Eskimo: iptogetok

Pacific
Fiji: kaka
Hawaiian: uu uus

Asian
Tagalog: patalutal
Chinese (Cantonese): hau hick;
    kong'–tak–lak–kak
Japanese: domori; kitsuon
Vietnamese: su noi lap

Eastern
Persian: locknatezaban
Hebrew: gingeim
Arabic: fa faa; rattat
Hindi: khaha
Hindustani: larbaraha
Turkish: kekeke mek

African
Egyptian: tataha; tuhuhtuhuh
Ga: haamuala
Xhosa: ukuthititha
Luganda: okukunanagira
Ghana (Twi): howdodo
Nigeria (Ibo): nsu
Shangaan: manghanghamela
Somali: wùu haghaglayyá

In addition to these words for stuttering on languages throughout the world, we also provide some accounts showing its existence in widely disparate cultures.

Ernest Douglass (1953) provides the following report from a Canadian psychiatric social worker's visit to the Southhampton Island's Eskimo population:

> On Southhampton, none of the present population stutters except for the Hudson Bay Company Clerk who stutters in English but not in Eskimo. The only known cases were a father and son who are not now on the island. They spent about ten years on the island, however, and were observed by my informant at the beginning and end of that period. On both occasions their stuttering was unchanged. The father, originally seen at the age of 25 was named Okarlooktook—one who has difficulty in speaking. His symptoms consisted of the repetition of initial sounds of words, particularly the *ah* sound, facial distortions in speaking and marked head movements. The son's symptoms were essentially the same. He was described as laboring when trying to speak. The Eskimos made no attempt to treat the ailment and had no notions as to its cause except to regard it as natural since Okarlooktook apparently was a stutterer from birth. The defect didn't bother him especially. Indeed it gave him status as the comedian of the community. He had a reputation for telling jokes which he used to enhance his reputation. His stuttering was the same in all situations.

Stuttering appears to be fairly prevalent in Japan, and mention of the disorder has appeared in their literature for centuries. One of their most famous doll plays, the *Domo Mata*, tells of an artist named Domo Matahei who stuttered very severely. Despite his talent he was much penalized by his wife. She, Otoku, says to him:

> "I am sorry for you, Matahei, but you must give up your cherished desires. You have two hands with ten fingers, but it is unfortunate that you stutter." She tells Matahei that the only thing he can do to gain fame is to commit suicide, but to paint his greatest masterpiece on a stone fountain before he dies. She brings him his brushes and prepares the ink, and Matahei draws his own portrait on the stone. The Shogun who owns the fountain is enraged and cleaves the stone with his sword only to find that miraculously the portrait is also visible in the cleft, that it has penetrated the stone. And just as miraculously Matahei regains his speech. There is a touching scene in which he recites the vowels of the Japanese syllabary to convince himself that he no longer stutters. Then great rejoicings and honors and all ends well. The Domo Mata play was first performed in Osaka in 1752. Another more recent real life drama occurred in 1950 when, to the horror of all art loving and patriotic Japanese, a stutterer burned down the ancient Temple of the Golden Pavilion (Scott, 1955, p. 274).

In testimony to the universality of stuttering, we jump across the Pacific to South Africa where we find Aron (1958) describing the stuttering of Bantu and Zulu children. She concludes that "Generally it might be said that the stuttering patterns, devices, and struggle responses that are presented by our African subjects *do not differ* to any great extent from the

Figure 1. The universality of stuttering:
Zulu boy stuttering. (From Aron,
1958, by permission.)

stuttering patterns that are exhibited by European subjects" (p. 129). And she adds this interesting observation:

> Many of the click sounds that were noticed in the speech of African children were situated in the medial position in the words and presented no difficulty to the stutterers. Where the clicks appeared in the initial syllable of the word, in *no* instance was stuttering noticed on the click itself. There was either a pause before the click (usually in the case of predominantly nonvocalized stutterers); an accessory sound was used before the attempt on the word; the consonant or vowel preceding the click was repeated or prolonged; or there was no stuttering at all on the particular word including the click sound" (p. 127).

DOUBTS ABOUT UNIVERSALITY

Without further belaboring our case for the universality of stuttering by citing the many other available examples of its occurrence in widely varying cultures, we should perhaps examine the alleged exceptions. Ignoring the dubious data procured by questionnaire and correspondence in the studies by Bullen (1945) and Morgenstern (1953) in which informants claimed never to have seen a stutterer among such exotic peoples as the Patamanas of British Guiana, the Kelabits of Borneo, and the Australian aborigines, we turn to the American Indians. The Utes, Bannock and Shoshones tribes were made famous by Wendell Johnson (1944) and by his students Snidecor (1947) and Stewart (1959) who claimed that these Indians had no stuttering in part because they had no word for it. When these investigations are scrutinized carefully from the point of view of a cultural anthropologist, the possibility of methodological error seems obvious. According to Johnson (1946, p. 443), Snidecor appeared before a tribal council, demonstrated stuttering (perhaps excluding the simple repetitions of syllables or sounds because they did not fit the Iowa definition), and asked the Indians, who were "highly amused" at the white man's antics, whether they knew any member of the tribe who talked like that. They said no! (We might get the same response from a group of businessmen in Chicago depending upon the sample of stuttering exhibited.) Snidecor also reports interviewing a total of 800 members of the tribe in his two year investigation (during which he taught full time at Idaho State College) without discovering any stutterers. Had the incidence been that which is usually reported for a more stressful culture such as ours (0.7 per cent), he should have found five of them among this population. We have no description of his interviewing methods but certainly the interviews could not have been in depth. We must remember that field investigators of such Indian societies are usually met with initial suspicion and distrust. Reliable information can rarely be achieved by asking specific questions through an interpreter. Even when the investigator knows the language and has lived a long time among them, information concerning personal habits must be evoked casually and is given with extreme reluctance. To establish such rapport with 800 Indians would be most difficult. Snidecor himself says:

> The adult Indians in their own culture do not speak under pressure unless they so choose. The adult Indian faced with a critical question does not feel obligated to hurry his answer. He will frequently sit and cogitate upon the problem until he is completely ready to answer, and then his reply may be spoken with little if any substantiation for his opinion (1947, p. 494).

It would take a bold ethnologist to claim that no word for stuttering exists in a given language. Who knows all the words of a language—especially of one beginning to disappear? Moreover, the lack of a specific word for a disorder may not mean that the latter does not exist. The witch doctors of the primitive peoples on the Malay peninsula diagnosed diabetes by having their patients urinate near an anthill. If the ants went to the urine, the witch doctors put a taboo on certain sweet fruits, a fairly adequate treatment for excessive blood sugar. So far as we have been able to ascertain, the Malays have no word for diabetes. They do have two for stuttering: *peichakapan* and *gagap*. In the particular Indian tribes surveyed by Snidecor, the languages have few specific words. The phrase, not the word, is the smallest utterance. To be asked what the word for stuttering was would surely confuse such Indians. Even so, according to Liljeblad (1967), there do seem to be terms for stuttering in Bannock which are inflections of the stem *pybya-*. For example, *pybyacacadua* means "he stutters when he talks," and *ynyy-pybyanna-kaibisa-nanaka* means "he stutters so severely one can't hear him very well." There is another verb stem too which evidently refers to the tonic form of stuttering: *kycajji*. Thus *kygycajjiwynny* means "he stutters continuously."

What is more, despite Snidecor, there are also some stuttering Indians among the Bannock and Shoshone speaking peoples as reported by Liljeblad (1967), an anthropologist who has spent years among them.

The work of Stewart (1959) has often been cited as another study supporting the thesis that there exists another American Indian society, the Utes, which is entirely free from stuttering. Essentially this study provides a comparison of only 30 Cowichan (Vancouver Island) Indian households with 30 households of the Utes in terms of language, child-rearing, and other cultural activities—at best a fairly small sample. Moreover, Stewart's own protocols indicate that in two families the mother informed him that one of her children had stuttered. He justifies his selection of the Utes as his nonstuttering society in these words:

> The selection of the Ute as the "nonstuttering group" followed from reports obtained by Wendell Johnson in interviews with two physicians who stated that they had investigated the Ute community near Vernal, Utah, with relative thoroughness and had concluded that there was no stuttering within the group. Substantiation of this point, and the verification of the absence from the Ute language of a term equivalent to "stuttering" was obtained by the present investigator in communications with a Ute tribal official (p. 68).

The original statement by Johnson that the "Indians have no word for it" made an excellent title for a very important statement of his position, but we now know that American Indians do have such words or phrases and at least a few members who possess the disorder.

If we have perhaps given too much space to these investigations of the alleged nonstuttering societies, we have done so only because far too few of us have examined the meager evidence upon which the denial of the universality of stuttering has been based. Perhaps this quotation from Kluckhohn (1954), the noted anthropologist, may serve also to help set things straight:

> However, the fact that I have been unable to find a single unequivocal case of the complete absence of stuttering among a people suggests that biological or idiosyncratic life history factors can be productive of stuttering in all cultures. On the other hand, impressive differences in degree of incidence suggests that cultural influences are operative. The matter needs much more careful and systematic examination . . . (p. 944).

The apparent universality of stuttering must hold some clue as to its nature. If the disorder is to be considered a neurosis, it must be one shared by many diverse cultures with many different value systems. It would have to be based upon conflicts common to all human beings. Stein (1949) has presented some interesting speculations concerning stuttering as a disorder which can be understood as a regression to atavistic behaviors such as the primitive clicks which were alleged to be common in the infancy of human speech and also as a regression to the babbling and sucking movements which all persons of every race employ during the first years of life. In this latter connection, he writes: "The stammerer unconsciously wishes to remain a suckling. The patient, owing to anxiety, unconsciously reverts to the suckling stage and so replaces consonants with clicks." Others, notably the psychoanalysts, have used similar explanations which, with some stretching, seem to account in some small way for the universality of stuttering.

If stuttering is to be viewed only as learned behavior, the necessary antecedents and consequences should also be common to all races and times if the universality of the disorder is to be explained. If it is a problem due to excessive parental concern or high standards and parental misdiagnosis, these concerns and standards must be common to all cultures. If it is established and maintained by secondary gains or other reinforcements, these too must be present in all people. Doubtless a case can be made for such an explanation but no one has yet made it.

Finally, if stuttering is viewed as a coordinative disorder, one in which the intricate timing of simultaneous and successive muscular contractions required for fluent utterance tends to become disrupted under stress, its universality should not surprise us. The automatic control of the motor sequences of speech is universal and so is stress. It would indeed be astonishing, when we consider the intricacies of the servosystem which monitors speaking, if stuttering disruptions did not occur.

BIBLIOGRAPHY

ANDREWS, G. AND M. HARRIS. 1964.   *The syndrome of stuttering.* London: Heinemann.

ARON, M. 1958.   An investigation of the nature and incidence of stuttering among a Bantu group of school-going children. Masters thesis, University of Witwatersrand, South Africa.

BULLEN, A. K. 1945.   A cross cultural approach to the problem of stuttering. *Child Development* 16: 1–87.

CLARK, R. M. AND F. M. MURRAY. 1965.   Alterations in self concept: a barometer of progress in individuals undergoing therapy for stuttering. In *New directions in stuttering,* ed. D. E. Barbara. Springfield, Ill.: Thomas.

CLIFFORD, S. 1965.   Stuttering in South Dakota indians. *Central States Speech Association Journal* 16: 59–60.

DOUGLASS, E. 1953.   Personal communication.

EMERICK. L. 1966.   Bibliotherapy for stutterers: four case studies. *Quarterly Journal of Speech* 52: 74–79.

FRENCH, P. 1966.   The stammerer as hero. *The Encounter* 27: 67–75.

GREENE, J. S. 1946.   Hope for the stutterer. *Hygeia* 24: 120–21.

GUSTAFSON, C. G. 1944.   A talisman and a convalescence. *Quarterly Journal of Speech* 30: 465–71.

HERTZ, J. H. 1938.   *The Pentateuch and the Haftorahs.* London: Soncino Press.

JOHNSON, W. 1946.   *People in quandaries.* New York: Harper.

——. 1944.   The Indians have no word for it: stuttering in adults. *Quarterly Journal of Speech Disorders* 30: 330–37; 456–65.

——. 1930.   *Because I stutter.* New York: Appleton-Century-Crofts.

KIRK, L. 1977.   Stuttering and quasi-stuttering in Ga. In *The problem of stuttering: theory and therapy,* ed. R. W. Rieber. New York: Elsevier.

KLUCKHOHN, C. 1954.   Culture and personality. In *Handbook of Social Psychology,* ed. G. Lindzey. Cambridge, Mass.: Addison-Wesley.

LEMERT, E. M. 1951. *Social pathology*. New York: McGraw-Hill.

———. 1953. Some Indians who stutter. *Journal of Speech and Hearing Disorders* 18: 168–74.

LILJEBLAD, S. 1967. The Indians have a word for it. Paper read to Nevada State Speech Association, May 6, 1967.

MORGENSTERN, J. J. 1953. Psychological and social factors in children's stammering. Doctoral dissertation, University of Edinburgh.

———. 1956. Socio-economic factors in stuttering. *Journal of Speech Disorders* 21: 25–33.

NUTTALL, W. 1937. The memoir of a stammerer. *Psyche* 17: 151–84.

RIEBER, R. W. 1977. *The problem of stuttering: theory and therapy*. New York: Elsevier.

SAPIR, E. 1915. *Abnormal types of speech in the Nootka*. Ottawa, Canada: Dept. Mines. Geological Survey Memoir 62, Anthropological Series.

SCOTT, A. C. 1955. *The Kabuki theatre of Japan*. London: Allen and Unwin.

SKELTON, J. 1598. *Elynour Rummynge*.

SNIDECOR, J. C. 1947. Why the Indian does not stutter. *Quarterly Journal of Speech* 33: 493–95.

STEIN, L. 1949. *The infancy of speech and the speech of infancy*. London: Methuen.

STEWART, J. L. 1959. Problem of stuttering in certain North American Indian societies. *Journal of Speech and Hearing Disorders*, Monograph Supplement 6: 1–87.

VAN RIPER, C. 1963. *Speech correction: principles and methods*. 4th ed. Englewood Cliffs, N.J.: Prentice-Hall.

WALEY, A., trans. 1927. *Laotze: the way and the power*. London: Allen and Unwin.

STUTTERING
its definition

2

DEFINITIONS

Many very good minds have attempted definitions of stuttering, but the variability among them makes clear that this complex and variable disorder is hard to delimit. Some of its complex behaviors always seem able to evade capture. Some of the definitions are merely statements of the authors' points of view with respect to the cause or nature of the disorder. To cite some examples we present such statements as these: "Stuttering is a psychoneurosis caused by the persistence into later life of early pregenital oral nursing, oral sadistic, and anal sadistic components (Coriat, 1943)." "Stuttering is a psychological difficulty and should be diagnosed and described as well as treated as a morbidity of social consciousness, a hypersensitivity of social attitude, a pathological social response (Fletcher, 1943, p. 33)." "Stuttering is a symptom in a psychopathological condition classified as a pregenital conversion neurosis (Glauber, 1958, p. 78)." "Stuttering is an evaluational disorder. It is what results when normal nonfluency is evaluated as something to be feared and avoided; it is, outwardly, what the stutterer does in an attempt to avoid nonfluency (Johnson, 1946, p. 452)."

Some definitions are so broad that they fail to provide proper limitations, something a good definition always tries to do. For example: "Stuttering is a deviation in the ongoing fluency of speech, an inability to maintain the connected rhythms of speech." "Stuttering is a disorder of rhythm." Such definitions would suggest that there are no normal speakers—unless the word *deviation* is further characterized. We all deviate at times from perfection in fluency. Normal speech is far from being connected; many studies have shown that frequent breaks occur in verbal continuity. Goldman-Eisler (1967), for example, found that 30 per cent of her speakers' talking time was spent in filled or unfilled pauses. Normal fluency does not mean uninterrupted flow.

Conversely, there are definitions which are so restrictive that they exclude many persons who would be commonly called or would call themselves stutterers. Wendell Johnson preferred to restrict *stuttering* to designate the speech of only those individuals who were showing "anticipatory hypertonic avoidance reactions" due to misevaluations of normal disfluencies. This definition by exclusion was most convenient in supporting his semantogenic theory, but Johnson was never quite able to persuade all of us, or even most of us, that we must never use the label of stuttering except in his restricted sense. Brutten and Shoemaker (1967, p. 61) also use what seems to us to be an unduly restrictive definition. They say: "Stuttering is that form of fluency failure that results from conditioned negative emotion." Their provision that every moment of stuttering must involve negative emotion does not seem to fit the facts—as we shall see later in this text. Theorists often take care of the exceptions to their theory by defining them out of existence.

Other definitions are frankly descriptive lists of behaviors, overt or covert, shown by different stutterers. Such catalog descriptions are always incomplete, and all stutterers do not show all the behaviors listed. Finally there are the definitions consisting of descriptions of phenomena which seek to identify the essential speech characteristics that differentiate stuttering behavior from other phenomena with which it could be confused. These try to describe the behaviors common to all stutterers, and to indicate the kinds of accessory behaviors shown only by some. Wingate's definition will illustrate this:

> The term "stuttering" means: I. (a) Disruption in the fluency of verbal expression, which is (b) characterized by involuntary, audible or silent, repetitions or prolongations in the utterance of short speech elements, namely: sounds, syllables, and words of one syllable. These disruptions (c) usually occur frequently or are marked in character and (d) are not readily controllable. II. Sometimes the disruptions are (e) accompanied by accessory activities involving the speech apparatus, related or unrelated body structures, or stereotyped speech utterances. These activities give the appearance of being speech-related struggle. III. Also, there are not infrequently (f) indications or report of the presence of an emotional state, ranging from a general condition of "excitement" or "tension" to more specific emotions of a negative nature such as fear, embarrassment, irritation, or the like. (g) The immediate source of stuttering is some incoordination expressed in the peripheral speech mechanism; the ultimate cause is presently unknown and may be complex or compound (Wingate, 1964, p. 498).

The differential diagnosis of stuttering from normal disfluency is not at all difficult when the disorder is severe or in its advanced stages. Diagnostic difficulty arises mainly when the disorder is very mild or in its earliest stages of development. This is to be expected. Hearing loss, asthma, allergies, a hundred other of the ills that plague the human race are hard to identify in their incipient stages or minor manifestations. Just because stuttering is occasionally difficult to distinguish from normal disfluency in its early or minor forms (and we must remember that stutterers also have normal disfluencies) we need not deny that stuttering exists as an entity. The insistence of millions of stutterers and their listeners that there is something wrong with the way they talk is difficult to disregard.

STUTTERING AS BEHAVIOR

What are the basic behaviors that stutterers show which distinguish them from normal speakers? This simple question has bedevilled many workers in the field of speech pathology although, as Robert West (1957) said long ago, "Everyone but the expert knows what stuttering is." One of the difficulties is that stuttering behaviors are notoriously variable, not only from one stutterer to another but even in the same stutterer at different times and on different words. Another problem is that normal speakers *occasionally* may demonstrate some of the same behaviors.

Not all of the interruptions to the forward flow of speech are signs of stuttering. Fortunately, it is possible to inhale occasionally without being referred to the speech clinic. We can repeat words and phrases, pause silently, scratch our heads, lick our lips, utter "ah's" and "ums" and interrupt the continuity of our speech in a hundred ways without causing our listeners to raise an eyebrow or bulge an eyeball. Such interrupting behaviors do not seem to play an important role in the diagnosis of the disorder of stuttering. According to Mahl (1956) syllabic repetitions accounted for only six per cent of all the varieties of fluency breaks shown by normal speakers. McClay and Osgood (1959) analyzed the spontaneous speech of speakers at a conference to determine the kinds of repetitions shown. Repetitions of whole words constituted 71 per cent; repetitions of phrases, 17 per cent; and "part word repetitions" only 12 per cent. Soderberg (1967) analyzed the speech of some stutterers in the same way and found that the proportion was reversed, that 63 per cent were part word repetitions.

This finding, which has been corroborated by numerous other researchers, makes it clear that the stutterer is not merely a disfluent speaker. He is disfluent but the interruptions in the forward flow of his speech are primarily due to disruptions in the utterance of sounds, syllables and words. Wendell Johnson tried to equate all types of disfluencies with stuttering although his own research showed clearly that his stutterers showed a preponderance of part-word repetitions whereas his normal speakers did not (Johnson, 1955). Broken or repeated phrases or sentences are not the hallmark of stuttering; it is the broken word that characterizes the majority of the stutterer's difficulty. Stuttering interruptions to the forward flow of speech are primarily intra-morphemic; normal disfluencies are primarily supra-morphemic.

Since Wingate (1964) has reviewed most of the literature, we shall consider only a few of the studies which support these statements.

In one of the first studies Voelker (1944) compared the fluency breaks of stutterers with those of normal speaking children. They differed only in that the stutterers had significantly more prolongations of sounds and more repetitions of syllables and words. Wyrick (1949) showed that syllabic repetitions comprised only an insignificant fraction of the total number of disfluencies shown by normal speakers. In the study mentioned frequently, Williams and Kent (1958) reported that "syllable repetition and prolongation of sounds were more consistently responded to as stuttered interruptions" than were interjections, word or phrase repetitions, or revisions. Boehmler (1958) in a very careful investigation found that sound and syllable repetitions were judged to be moments of stuttering significantly more often than were word repetitions, phrase repetitions, or other types of disfluency and that this held true for naive as well as professional judges. Although stressing the overlap between his normal and stuttering groups, Johnson (1961) showed conclusively in another study that "of all the types of disfluency, part word repetitions are more likely to be classified by listeners, at least in our general culture, as 'stuttering' and that certain other kinds of disfluency, most notably perhaps interjections, revisions, and phrase repetitions, are more commonly considered as 'normal' disfluencies." McDearmon (1968) showed the same finding in his reanalysis of Johnson's *Onset of Stuttering* data (1959). Young (1961) demonstrated that "the types of speech disfluency that appear to be associated with ratings of severity of stuttering are syllable or sound repetitions, sound prolongations, broken words, and words involving apparently unusual stress or tension."

This was corroborated by Schiavetti (1975) who found that disfluencies that break words or delay their utterance are judged as being more severe than those which leave the integration of whole words intact. Floyd and Perkins (1974) had public school teachers judge eighteen samples of different kinds of disfluencies. Those with syllable repetitions were most often called stutterers. Huffman and Perkins (1974) investigated the syllabic disfluencies of children. The normal speakers had only 1.2 per cent whereas the stutterers had 9.8 per cent. Bjerkan (1979) in Norway in an intensive study of the spontaneous speech of 110 nursery school children found only two children who showed a significant amount of broken words and these were the only children regarded by their parents and teachers as being stutterers. In contrast, in the 37,800 words spoken by the other normal speaking 108 children, only four instances of word fragmentation were found. All in all, it seems evident that the motor patterns of *words* rather than phrases or sentences are what are disrupted in stutterers and that it is this which makes them disfluent.

MOLAR VERSUS MOLECULAR IDENTIFICATIONS

One of the major contributions of the decade of the seventies was the recognition that it was necessary to specify the exact characteristics of the behaviors generally lumped together under the label of a *moment of stuttering*. In earlier research, the clinician or experimenter had the stutterer read a passage and underlined on a corresponding passage those words on which "moments of stuttering" apparently occurred. They were using "molar" identifications, gross categories. Those "moments of stuttering" could include anything from a pause or interjection or a repeated word or phrase to a facial grimace. This wastebasket phrase, in addition to its other limitations, presented great practical difficulties in locating the nuclei of stuttering. For example, if a stutterer said "It's a-a-a-a a fine day," was he stuttering four times on the article *a* or was he simply inserting an interjection to postpone the utterance of the word *fine*? If he said "It's a a fine, a fine, it's a fine day," how many moments of stuttering did he have and where were they located? Brutten (1975) makes this pertinent statement:

> It is no easy matter to discriminate the behavioral characteristics of stuttering and to distinguish them from those of normal speech and from other forms of fluency failure. The use of *moments* made it possible to temporarily skirt these essential distinctions. Moments are so molar—relate to units so large—that stuttering behaviors were thought likely to be caught in the net even though they were not specified. But moments masked more than they revealed. Their behavioral elements were never fully described (p. 201).

Accordingly, Webster (1966) suggested that a "molecular" approach be instituted to clarify what occurs in these moments of stuttering, and that we must specify just what occurs, thereby defining the term *stuttering* more precisely. That there is substantial justification for a more refined analysis was shown by Hood (1969) who found that within some 2,908 moments of stuttering there were 4,395 specific types of disfluency, and by Zenner (1971) who similarly discovered 4,804 "molecular" events in 2,775 molar "moments of stuttering." As Hood (1974) states:

> What the stutterer does at any point of time is in part the behavioral consequence of what he has already done. The stuttering behaviors that we observe are the culmination of certain tensing, speeding, avoiding, postponing, holding back, struggling or escaping behaviors that have already occurred (p. 25).

They may not always enumerate all the specific kinds of stuttering behaviors when counting stutterings or locating the words on which stuttering occurs. If they do not, the authors count and locate only those which fall within specified categories. That is, they count as stuttered words only those on which part-word repetitions or prolongations of a sound or articulatory posture, etc., were found. We propose, therefore, our own definition of a stuttering behavior: *Stuttering occurs when the forward flow of speech is interrupted by a motorically disrupted sound, syllable, or word or by the speaker's reactions thereto.*

The latter part of this definition is essential because many of the avoidance and struggle behaviors also interrupt the forward flow of

d   ʜκiα   ʃ   κd   d   dα ʜ   ℓκℓ   ʜF   α
And I come from Springville Ohio and the town's all got about five thousand

           dα   ɪ́   ad ɪ́   ʜ́ d
people and it's all got a bowling alley and all there's a building that makes,

ʟd κ ɪ́ ʟ   dα   d   ɪ́   α   ɪ́ F
It m..It's the world's largest ah caster maker and it's called ah Corbets.

           ᴊʜ   ʟd   d   α.   dd
And then there's a well I got one brother and that's it.   I live..... *

Analysis of Specific Disruption Form-Types within Moments of Stuttering:

Audible-Vocalized Disruptions

a.	part-word reps. H̶I̶T̶ ///	Total 8
b.	word repetitions	Total 0
c.	multiple word reps.	Total 0
d.	sound prolongations H̶I̶T̶ H̶I̶T̶ ////	Total 14

Total 22

Audible-Nonvocalized Disruptions

e.	part-word reps.	Total 0
f.	sound prolongations ///	Total 3

Total 3

Inaudible-Nonvocalized Disruptions

g.	hard contacts	Total 0
h.	silent fixations H̶I̶T̶	Total 5

Total 5

Avoidance-Escape Behaviors

i.	vocalized pauses and starters H̶I̶T̶ ///	Total 8
j.	Silent pauses /	Total 1
k.	Broken words, word postures and recoils ////	Total 4
l.	substitutions and circumlocutions ///	Total 3

Total 16

Total of All Disruption Form-Types   46

*Nonmeaningful words are crossed out. Underlined portions of transcript represent molar moments of stuttering. Letters above underlined words represent specific disruption form-types from molecular analysis.

Figure 2. The molecular analysis of stuttering. (From Hood, 1974, by permission.)

speech. Iterations, (the use of 'uh-uh' or 'um' or 'er'), are often used by both normal speakers and stutterers. However, when they are used as a response to the anticipation of difficulty in producing an integrated sound, syllable, or word, they are avoidance stuttering behaviors. Hegde and Hartman (1979) showed that when simulated speech samples contained more than 20 per cent of schwa interjections, the listeners tended to label them stuttering. Tense pauses have also been included in the molecular analysis of stuttering, and when these are responses to the anticipation of broken sounds, syllables, and words, they too are stuttering behaviors. Circumlocutions, gasps, head jerks, and all the other behaviors that represent struggle or avoidance may similarly be included in the category of stuttering behaviors when they are responses to the *anticipation* or *experience of disrupted sounds, syllables or words.*

THE CORE OF STUTTERING

It is even possible that the lowest common denominator of stuttering is the motorically disrupted *phoneme*, for if the synergies of respiration, phonation, and articulation required for the production of a sound are mistimed, then the syllable and the word will also be disrupted. Indeed, we are tempted to define a stuttering behavior as a temporally distorted sound and the speaker's reactions thereto, but the necessary research has not yet been done. We do have some indications that this may be the case. Zimmermann (1980) showed that stutterers had time lags, aberrant postures, and asynchronies in the production of sounds and syllables—even when these were spoken fluently—and that these were more evident when stuttering occurred. Fibiger (1977) found co-contractions of antagonistic articulatory muscle groups occurring at the moment of stuttering, and Freeman (1979) showed that similar behaviors were present in the laryngeal muscles.

Agnello (1966) and Stromsta (1965) found acoustic differences in the phonemes produced during stuttering which indicated a lack of the appropriate juncture formants necessary for the coarticulation needed to produce a syllable or word. Other studies (Agnello, Wingate and Wendell, 1974; Hillman and Gilbert, 1977) discovered time lags in voice onset and voice termination times. Differences in oral air pressure and air flow in the production of the stutterer's sounds and syllables have also been revealed. We shall review these researches later (Chapter 16), but it is sufficient now merely to mention them in support of the possibility that the core of stuttering might lie in a temporally disrupted phoneme, that is, that its respiratory, phonatory, and articulatory motor components are not properly synchronized.

STUTTERING AS A DISORDER

Thus far we have been discussing the *behaviors* which characterize stuttered speech but there is an important difference between stuttering as behavior and stuttering as a disorder. The latter demands an evaluative judgment on the part of a listener.

TYPE B/65 SONAGRAM ® KAY ELEMETRICS CO. PINE BROOK. N. J.

ðʌ   ðʌ   ðɪs

Figure 3. Sonogram of repetitive stuttering on the word "this." Note sudden vocal arrests of phonation on the first two abortive attempts.

Semantics of the Term Stuttering

Some of the difficulty in defining stuttering results from the way the term is used. When we use the verb *to stutter* or the phrase *a moment of stuttering* we refer to certain kinds of behaviors. When we use the noun *stuttering* categorically we designate a disorder. When we employ the word *stutterer* we refer to a role or special kind of deviant. Two early investigations, one by Voelker (1942) and the other by Villareal (1945), explored the semantics of the terms referring to stuttering by asking a large number of *normal* speakers these questions and getting these positive replies:

		Voelker	*Villareal*
1.	Have you ever had a stuttering defect in speech?	10.4%	14.0%
2.	Have you ever been called a stutterer?	4.2	6.7
3.	Have you ever been said to have been stuttering?	30.2	29.1
4.	Have you ever thought you had the habit of stuttering?	1.0	1.8
5.	Have you ever thought you have spoken stutteringly?	72.9	76.0
6.	Have you ever called yourself a stutterer?	6.3	9.9

Sander (1963) found similar evidence that the terms *stuttering* and *stutterer* may refer to quite different patterns of behavior. He says:

Many listeners by their usage seemed to feel that it was clearly possible to "stutter" without being a "stutterer." Listeners responded: "I don't think he stuttered enough to be called a 'stutterer,'" "He stuttered because he couldn't find the word he wanted."

In another study Sander (1965, p. 26) provides some examples of the variant usages:

In terms of their language behavior, the responses of the listeners in this study might be grouped on a continuum beginning with "He repeated," or "He hesitated" (relatively descriptive terms), passing first to "He stuttered" (less descriptive), then to "There was evidence of a speech impediment" (something removed from the behavior heard), and finally to "He has a speech defect" (a "thing"-like quality possessed by the speaker), or "He seemed to be a stutterer" (a personification of the behavior).

Gateley (1967) found much the same distinctions when he had listeners diagnose the tape recording of a mild stutterer: "Of eighty-three subjects who noted that the speaker 'stuttered' or exhibited 'stuttering' only thirty-five judged him to be a 'stutterer.'"

The term *disorder* to many people implies a disease. It may well be, however, that the medical model does not fit the problem of stuttering in all of its varieties. Strong cases have been made for viewing it merely as a group of learned maladaptive responses. In this text we see stuttering as a disorder the same way we see reading disability as a disorder.

19

A single cough has little significance; frequent spells of coughing may indicate emphysema, tuberculosis, or other disorders. A few sneezes are part of normal living; continual sneezing may mean hay fever or even a brain tumor. The characteristics of the cough or sneeze are scrutinized by the physician in determining if a true disorder is present. Also the conditions under which coughing or sneezing occur may help determine the diagnosis. We use these analogies to introduce the concept of stuttering as a disorder. Stuttering behaviors, broken words, constitute a disorder when they are diagnosed as such by the speaker or by his listeners based upon the scrutiny of their frequency, their characteristics, and the conditions under which they occur.

As a disorder, stuttering is identified by a process of differential diagnosis. The speech must appear to be outside the norms of the culture for speech production. It must also be differentiated from other forms of speech deviancy.

Stuttering is primarily a disorder of the temporal aspects of speech, not of the articulatory, phonatory, or symbolic features. Anyone who has known many stutterers will of course recognize that some of them show abnormalities in the way they articulate or phonate a given sound or syllable. We have watched severe stutterers attempt a vowel with the mouth tightly closed, or a labial plosive with the jaws agape; we have heard them prolong a sound with a fire-siren kind of inflection; we have seen them apparently unable to produce voice. But these are not features common to all stutterers nor are they always characteristic of the single stutterer who occasionally demonstrates them. The essential feature that distinguishes a stutterer from a person with an articulatory disability is the former individual's apparent inability to perform the motor sequencing of a given sound or syllable or word at the proper moments in time. Speech is patterned in time, both motorically and acoustically; the movements, the sounds, the syllables must occur in a prescribed sequence. When this sequencing of word utterance is noticeably disrupted in a certain way and evaluated as undesirable, the person is said to possess the disorder of stuttering.

The term *disorder* implies that it is somehow unpleasant and undesirable. Any stutterer or anyone who has talked with one for some time will agree that this is true. But we have very little research bearing directly upon this feature. Perrin (1954) using a sociometric technique showed that speech defects in general tended to create isolates when school children were asked to choose partners. Giolas and Williams (1958) created three tapes of the same story, one spoken normally, one with a number of interjections ('um's' and 'ah's') and the third with the same number of stutterings. Second grade children were asked to tell which of the storytellers they would desire as their teacher. The results were not unexpected: the children chose the normal speaker first, the interjectionist second, and the stutterer third. Culatta and Sloan (1977) had two groups of elementary school children listen to the tape of a woman telling a story twice. One of the narrations were spoken normally; the other included frequent repetitions and prolongations. Al the children preferred the fluent narration.

These and other researches, as well as the testimony of stutterers and their listeners, indicate that stuttering as a disorder is evaluated unfavorably in our culture and in that of many others.

Indeed, as we shall see in Chapter 10 on the self-concepts of stutterers, certain cultural sterotypes about stuttering as a disorder are prevalent. Here we cite only the work of two researchers to make the point. Woods and Williams (1976) found that both classroom teachers and speech clinicians generally believed that the stutterer was a rather submissive, nonassertive person who was tense, insecure, and fearful. The same sterotype was demonstrated by Turnbaugh, Guitar and Hoffman (1979) who showed that even trained speech clinicians tended to attribute negative personality traits to stutterers, and the more severe the stuttering, the more negative were the judgments.

THE ROLE OF FREQUENCY IN EVALUATION

In making the diagnosis as to whether or not a person is a stutterer, that is, has the disorder of stuttering, the frequency of his stuttering behaviors is probably one of the major factors. All of us speak stutteringly at times, occasionally repeating a syllable, or showing a silent fixation of an articulatory posture. What identifies a speaker as a stutterer is that he shows *too many* disrupted sounds, syllables, and words or reacts to them by obvious struggle or avoidance. A single syllabic repetition in a hundred words has very little stimulus value; fifty of them would be noticed by any listener.

This relationship of frequency to diagnosis has been demonstrated by Sander's (1963) research. He contrived recorded speech samples having different amounts of single-unit (Sa-Saturday) and double-unit syllabic repetitions and submitted one of these to each of 240 college students who had to describe the speech, tell whether it should be considered defective, and to decide whether the speaker was a stutterer. In essence, Sander found that the more single-unit syllabic repetitions there were in a sample, the more frequently that sample was judged as being stuttering or the speech of a stutterer. Also fewer double syllable repetitions than single syllable repetitions yielded a stuttering diagnosis.

As we mentioned earlier, according to Sapir (1915) the language of the Nootka Indians was so full of syllabic repetitions that, according to Indians of other tribes, they were all said to be stutterers. (If so, the Nootkan who failed to use reduplicated syllables often enough would probably be noticed and evaluated by his fellow tribesmen as having a speech defect!) Standards of fluency vary not only in different cultures but even within the same culture. All stuttering yardsticks are not of the same length. We Americans use a longer one for children than we do for adults. Wendell Johnson felt that the Bannock and Shoshone Indians had no yardsticks at all. Some mothers have greater tolerances for their children's broken words than other mothers. Some children seem to be able to tolerate fewer of these morphemic interruptions than other children can. Nevertheless, despite the variations in normative criteria, a speaker must keep his broken words within the frequency limits of his listeners or be noticed and judged as having the disorder of stuttering.

OTHER CRITERIA OF STUTTERING AS A DISORDER

Listeners also make their judgments as to whether or not a person is a stutterer on criteria other than the frequency with which stuttering behaviors occur. The duration of prolonged sounds or silent articulatory postures and the length of the interruptions due to repetitions, iterations, or revisions may also cause the listener to identify the speaker as a deviant.

To our knowledge there is no research bearing directly on the duration of the internal word gaps or the prolongations of a sound or articulatory posture as related to diagnosis. All we have are the many researches which indicate that it takes a stutterer longer to read a given passage than it takes a normal speaker to do so. The wide variations in reading and speaking rate among normal speakers makes such talking-time measures rather useless when trying to decide whether a specific person has or does not have the disorder of stuttering. However, it is quite possible to measure the durations of prolonged phonemes and morphemic gaps and we hope that future researchers will do so. Our own pilot investigations have shown that 100 per cent of our listeners noticed any sound which was prolonged more than three seconds and 50 per cent of them recognized as abnormal any sound prolonged longer than two seconds. Silent pauses within the word boundaries are recognized even more easily. A silent gap of even one fifth of a second within a fractured word is enough to indicate abnormality. Silent pauses just prior to word initiation have less stimulus value (need to be longer to be recognized as abnormal) unless they are accompanied by the assumption of a visible articulatory posture. The presence of tremors or contortions or other accessory behaviors lead, of course, to immediate recognition. In general, we think we are safe in saying that the longer the duration of a sound or silent gap, the more likely it will be that a diagnosis of stuttering will be made. Any speaker who would hold the /n/ in the word *no* for 20 seconds, as some of our stutterers have done, even though it occurred only once in a thousand words, would immediately be suspected of having something wrong with him.

There are other ways in which words are temporally disrupted which provoke listeners to make (or corroborate) a tentative diagnosis of stuttering. The tempo of multiple syllabic repetitions is also important. We need to known how much faster or slower they occur than the ordinary rate of syllabic emission. If every time the speaker repeats a syllable, he does it three times faster than he emits the other syllables of his normal speech, that syllable will stand out like a third thumb. We have all known stutterers whose speech motors race in this way. However, the converse also seems to be true. If the speaker says a syllable, pauses, says it again, pauses deliberately and then says the word, most listeners would feel that he is having trouble getting that word out. This sort of behavior shows up mostly in the confirmed stutterers of the interiorized variety described by Freund (1935) and Douglass and Quarrington (1952), stutterers who often are otherwise very successful in hiding their disorder. Another clue indicating that the person either has, or is in danger of acquiring the disorder of stuttering is found in the irregularity of the syllabic repetitions. The few syllabic repetitions which normal speakers show not only occur at the same tempo as the rest of their syllables, but they occur evenly, regularly. When we find a person repeating syllables jerkily rather than smoothly, we tend to diagnose abnormality. This is only our clinical impression for the research is still to be done.

Another feature that may distinguish the syllabic repetitions of stutterers from those of normal speakers is the perceived presence of the schwa vowel. Stuttering repetitions often have it; normal repetitions do not. We say "perceived" because although the listener hears the stutterer saying "Suh-suh-suh-soap" instead of the normal "So-so-soap" the research (Allen, Peters, and Williams, 1975; Freeman, Borden, and Dorman, 1976) seems to show that the perception of the neutral schwa vowel is due to the fact that the standard vowel is suddenly interrupted and is too brief for recognition. The presence of the perceived schwa in the syllabic repetitions may also be due to a failure in coarticulation. Stromsta (1965) analyzed the spectrograms of children's repetitions and found that when they showed anomalies in coarticulation and sudden interruptions in voice or airflow, they were still stuttering ten years later. In contrast, those children whose spectrograms did not show these coarticulation failures nor sudden arrests of phonation in their repetitions recovered spontaneously and were no longer stuttering.

Our definition of a stuttering behavior also included the avoidance and struggle responses to disrupted sounds, syllables, and words for they too may interrupt the forward flow of speech. In the identification of stuttering as a disorder these accessory reactions play a very important role. Facial contortions, body jerks, tremors of the lips, tongue thrusts, and all the other gross behavioral abnormalities shown by severe stutterers yield an immediate diagnosis of deviancy. Often it is the severity of stuttering behaviors rather than their frequency which identifies the stutterer.

Also we find many avoidance behaviors, inappropriate to the normal act of speaking, such as verbal circumlocutions, stallers, and unusual interjections or substitutions of odd synonyms. These are viewed by the listener as efforts to avoid the anticipated fluency break. When they occur frequently enough or last long enough or are bizarre enough, they too lead to the diagnosis of stuttering. All these bits of information go into the listener's computer and the read-out is deviancy when their assemblage exceeds that listener's norms for fluency.

Finally, listeners may make their judgment of stuttering as a disorder on clues indicating that the speaker is feeling frustration or fear or embarrassment at the moment that the disrupted sounds, syllables, and words are shown. To give but one example, if a speaker averts his eyes or flushes every time he shows a broken word, his listener will tend to evaluate him as a stutterer.

DIAGNOSING STUTTERING IN CHILDREN

When stuttering behaviors occur frequently and are severe, the clinician has little difficulty in recognizing that a disorder exists. More advanced stutterers, by their struggle or avoidance reactions and emotionality, show that they know they have a serious fluency problem. However, in young children the differential diagnosis is more difficult. Bloodstein (1970, 1975) proposed in his *continuity hypothesis* that no distinction can be made solely on the basis of the stuttering behaviors we have described since normal speaking children show them too occasionally, and that stuttering as a problem begins when the child evaluates these breaks in fluency as unpleasant and begins to show fear, avoidance, and struggle reactions. The continuity hypothesis, reminiscent but not identical with Wendell Johnson's (1955) position, insists that stuttering behaviors and normal disfluencies differ only in degree. Bloodstein's view has not gained wide acceptance, however, perhaps because clinicians have become increasingly aware of the inadvisability of ignoring what Walle (1976) has termed the "danger signs" of incipient stuttering. As Adams writes:

> Often speech clinicians are asked to evaluate nonfluent children and to determine if the youngsters' fluency failures reflect the presence of an incipient stuttering problem or are merely innocuous developments, irregularities that are likely to diminish in time. In attempting to make this important discrimination, therapists must avoid two major and rather obvious errors. First, they would not want to inappropriately identify the child as a stutterer, since that might contribute to the development of a fluency disorder where one does not really exist at the time of the diagnosis. Second, clinicians would not want to incorrectly judge a beginning stutterer as being normally nonfluent, since this would lead to the child being withheld from therapy experiences that he actually needed (Adams, 1977, p. 141).

In the first edition of this text (Van Riper, 1971), we offered a set of guidelines for the differential diagnosis of stuttering versus normal disfluency in young children. While they still must be considered tentative, incomplete, and unsubstantiated by research, we hope that their inclusion here may stimulate the latter. (See Table 2.1.)

It is perhaps fortunate that we have run out of letters of the alphabet in creating the items of our guidelines. This list, formidable as it is, can hardly be said to be complete and we are not happy with the quality of the items nor with their lack of quantification. They are just the best indications known to those who daily confront these problems. One of the gross

TABLE 2.1   Guidelines for Differentiating Normal from Abnormal Disfluency

BEHAVIOR	STUTTERING	NORMAL DISFLUENCY
Syllable Repetitions:		
a. Frequency per word	More than two	Less than two
b. Frequency per 100 words	More than two	Less than two
c. Tempo	Faster than normal	Normal tempo
d. Regularity	Irregular	Regular
e. Schwa vowel	Often present	Absent or rare
f. Airflow	Often interrupted	Rarely interrupted
g. Vocal tension	Often apparent	Absent
Prolongations:		
h. Duration	Longer than one second	Less than one second
i. Frequency	More than one per 100 words	Less than one per 100 words
j. Regularity	Uneven or interrupted	Smooth
k. Tension	Important when present	Absent
l. When voiced (sonant)	May show rise in pitch	No pitch rise
m. When unvoiced (surd)	Interrupted airflow	Airflow present
n. Termination	Sudden	Gradual
Gaps (silent pauses):		
o. Within the word boundary	May be present	Absent
p. Prior to speech attempt	Unusually long	Not marked
q. After the disfluency	May be present	Absent
Phonation:		
r. Inflections	Restricted; monotone	Normal
s. Phonatory arrest	May be present	Absent
t. Vocal fry	May be present	Usually absent
Articulating Postures:		
u. Appropriateness	May be inappropriate	Appropriate
Reaction to Stress:		
v. Type	More broken words	Normal disfluencies
Evidence of awareness:		
w. Phonemic consistency	May be present	Absent
x. Frustration	May be present	Absent
y. Postponements (stallers)	May be present	Absent
z. Eye contact	May waver	Normal

deficiencies is the lack of item weights. Obviously, all these items are not equal in differentiating value. The author has his own system for weighting the item probabilities, but we will not give it the presumed validity of appearing in these pages. Let each person devise his own item weights until we have the research we need so badly. We must do the best we can with what we have available to us.

Perhaps stimulated by our guidelines, we have two contributions from the literature that should be mentioned. The first, by Cooper (1973), is an article describing a *Chronicity Check List* devised to help clinicians predict whether or not a disfluent child would "outgrow" or spontaneously recover from his incipient stuttering. The second of these contributions is an illuminating account of how Adams (1977) performs his differential diagnosis. A direct quotation from this article will make clear the procedure:

> In attempting to differentiate the incipient stutterer from the normal nonfluent child the author has proceeded in the following way. During that portion of the diagnostic session that is spent with the youngster, an effort is made to secure a 300–500 word sample of the child's conversational speech. From this sample, the examiner extracts (1) the total number of words spoken; (2) the total number of nonfluencies exhibited; (3) the ratio of number of nonfluencies per 100 words uttered; (4) the number of part word repetitions and sound prolongations among all the fluency failures noted; (5) the number of part word repetitions and sound prolongations that seem to be marked by the abnormal stoppage of voice or airflow; (6) the number of times a unit is iterated in each part word repetition; and (7) the number of part word repetitions in which the schwa appears (Adams, 1977, p. 144).

OTHER PROBLEMS IN DIFFERENTIAL DIAGNOSIS

While the major diagnostic problem faced by speech clinicians is the differentiation of stuttering from normal disfluency there are some other disorders which should be recognized as having symptoms which more or less resemble stuttering. Three of the most common of these, though the clinician will encounter them rarely, are palilalia, dysphatic disfluency, and cluttering.

Palilalia

Another disorder in which the speech is characterized by repetition is palilalia. It is easily differentiated from stuttering, not only because it is associated with neurological diseases such as Parkinsonism, pseudobulbar palsy, Alzheimer's disease, and other such problems, but because the repetitions are of whole words, phrases or sentences. The perseverative repetitions of these supra-morphemic units usually get faster and faster and the intelligibility of speech worsens as the articulation becomes slurred. In simple tasks such as naming objects sometimes no repetitions are heard, but with more complex utterances they are. Upon demand, the patient seems to be unable to stop the repeating once it begins. Illustrative cases have been presented by Helm and Butler (1980), Allan (1970) and Boller, Albert, and Denes (1975).

Dysphatic Stuttering

Stuttering-like behaviors have also been found in patients who have suffered a cerebrovascular insult and developed dysphasia. Many patients become very disfluent (after the stroke or other cause of the brain disorder) when they experience difficulty in word finding or word utterance or sequencing. Apraxia creates breaks in the smooth flow of speech and the patient responds with pauses, static positioning of the articulators, or repetitions of all types. Most of the latter represent perseverative repetitions of whole words and phrases but sound and syllable repetitions also occur, though more rarely. Deal and Darley (1972) analyzed the disfluency errors of patients with apraxia and found that 13 per cent of them were repetitions and prolongations similar to those of stutterers, but they occurred mainly on the longer words and did not disappear under masking noise. Caplan (1972) found that though there were repetitions and prolongations, interjections (the use of "uh, uh," etc.) were the major features of the broken speech. She also found differences from stuttering in that their loci were different and that the disfluencies increased rather than decreased when repeated trials were requested.

Cluttering

Another disorder of fluency, cluttering, deserves consideration. A precise definition of cluttering has proved even more difficult than that for stuttering for, as usually envisaged, its symptomatology includes far more than the disordered fluency which is only one of its characteristics. The clutterer is said to show deficits or abnormality also in symbolic language development and formulation, in articulation, and in phonatory characteristics as well as in fluency. Other language functions such as reading, writing, and formulating are impaired. Since the present text is dedicated to stuttering and because cluttering has been described very adequately by other authors, notably Freund, Arnold, Luchsinger, and Weiss* we shall refer the reader to their writings and get on with our own.

BIBLIOGRAPHY

ADAMS, M. R. 1977.   A clinical strategy for differentiating the normal nonfluent child and the incipient stutterer. *Journal of Fluency Disorders* 2: 141–48.

———. 1978.   Further analysis of stuttering as a phonetic transition defect. *Journal of Fluency Disorders* 3: 365–71.

——— AND P. HAYDEN. 1976.   The ability of stutterers and nonstutterers to initiate and terminate phonation during the production of an isolated vowel. *Journal of Speech and Hearing Research* 19: 290–96.

AGNELLO, J. 1974.   Laryngeal and articulatory dynamics of disfluency interpreted within a vocal tract model. In *Vocal tract dynamics and fluency*, eds. M. Webster and L. Furst, pp. 40–69. New York: Speech and Hearing Institute of New York.

AGNELLO, J., M. E. WINGATE, AND M. WENDELL. 1974.   Voice onset and voice termination times of child and adult stutterers. *Journal of the Acoustical Society of America* 56: 362.

AINSWORTH, S. 1939.   Empathic breathing of auditors while listening to stuttered speech. *Journal of Speech Disorders* 4: 149–56.

* See the following selected references: Freund, H., "Studies in the Inter-relationship between Stuttering and Cluttering," *Folia Phoniatrica*, IV (1952), 146–68; Luchsinger, R., and G. E. Arnold, *Voice-Speech-Language.* Belmont, California: Wadsworth, 1965; and Weiss, D. A., *Cluttering.* Englewood Cliffs, N.J.: Prentice-Hall, 1964.

ALLAN, C. M. 1970.   Treatment of non-fluent speech resulting from neurological diseases—treatment of dysarthria. *British Journal of Disorders of Communication* V: 3–5.

ALLEN, G., R. PETERS, AND C. WILLIAMS. 1975.   Spectrographic study of fluent and stuttered speech. Convention Address, ASHA.

AREND, R., L. HANDZEL, AND B. WEISS. 1962.   Dysphatic stuttering. *Folia Phoniatrica* 14: 55–62.

BEASELEY, B. 1870.   *Stammering: its treatment.* London: Hamilton.

BJERKAN, B. 1980.   Word fragmentation and repetitions in the spontaneous speech of 2–6 year old children. *Journal of Fluency Disorders* 5: 137–48.

BLOODSTEIN, O. 1970.   Stuttering and normal nonfluency: a continuity hypothesis. *British Journal of Disorders of Communication* 5: 30–39.

———. 1975.   Stuttering as tension and fragmentation. In *Stuttering: a second symposium,* ed. J. Eisenson. New York: Harper and Row.

———, J. ALPER, AND P. ZISK. 1965.   Stuttering as an outgrowth of normal disfluency. In *New directions in stuttering: theory and practice,* ed. D. E. Barbara. Springfield, Ill.: Thomas.

BOEHMLER, R. M. 1958.   Listener responses to nonfluencies. *Journal of Speech and Hearing Research* 1: 132–41.

BOLLER, F., M. ALBERT, AND F. DENES. 1975.   Palilalia. *British Journal of Disorders of Communication* 10: 92–97.

BRUTTEN, G. J. 1975.   Stuttering: topography, assessment and behavior change strategies. In *Stuttering: a second symposium,* ed. J. Eisenson. New York: Harper and Row.

BRUTTEN, G. J. AND D. J. SHOEMAKER. 1967.   *The modification of stuttering.* Englewood Cliffs, N.J.: Prentice-Hall.

CAPLAN, L. 1972.   An investigation of some aspects of stuttering-like speech in adult aphasic subjects. *Journal of South Africa Speech and Hearing Association* 19: 52–66.

COOPER, E. B. 1973.   Development of a stuttering chronicity prediction checklist. *Journal of Speech and Hearing Disorders* 5: 215–23.

CORIAT, I. H. 1943.   Psychoanalytic concept of stammering. *Nervous Child* 2: 167–71.

CULATTA, R. AND A. SLOAN. 1977. The acquisition of the label 'stuttering' by primary level school children. *Journal of Fluency Disorders* 2: 19–34.

CULLINAN, W. L. AND E. M. PRATHER. 1968.   Reliability of live ratings of the speech of stutterers. *Perceptual and Motor Skills* 27: 403–9.

DEAL, J. L. AND F. L. DARLEY. 1972.   The influence of linguistic and situational variables on phonemic accuracy in apraxia in speech. *Journal of Speech and Hearing Research* 15: 639–53.

DEHIRSCH, K. AND W. LANGFORD. 1950.   Clinical notes on stuttering and cluttering in young children. *Pediatrics* 5: 934–40.

DOUGLASS, E. AND B. QUARRINGTON. 1952.   Differentiation of interiorized and exteriorized secondary stuttering. *Journal of Speech and Hearing Disorders* 17: 377–85.

DRASEKE, J. 1921.   Ueber mitbewegungen bei gesunden. *Deutsche Zeitschrift für Nervenheilkunde* 64: 340–46.

EMERICK, L. 1960.   Extensional definition and attitude toward stuttering. *Journal of Speech and Hearing Research* 3: 181–86.

FIBIGER, S. 1977.   Quantitative electromyographic evaluation of stuttering severity by means of describing the course of muscle activity in the lip-articulatory muscles in connection with labial stop consonants. *Proceedings XVII Congress of Logopedics and Phoniatrics.* Interlaken, 1–14.

FLETCHER, J. M. 1943.   A predisposing cause of stuttering. *Quarterly Journal of Speech* 29: 480–83.

FLOYD, S. AND W. H. PERKINS. 1974.   Early syllable disfluency in stutterers and nonstutterers: A preliminary report. *Journal of Communication Disorders,* 7: 279–82.

FREEMAN, F. J. 1979.   Phonation in stuttering: a review of current research. *Journal of Fluency Disorders* 4: 79–89.

———. 1974.   Fluency and phonation. In *Vocal Tract Dynamics and Dysfluency,* eds. M. Webster and L. Furst. New York: Speech and Hearing Institute of New York.

———, C. BORDEN, AND M. DORMAN. 1976.   Laryngeal stuttering: combined physiological and acoustic studies. Convention Paper, ASHA.

FREUND, H. 1966.   *Psychopathology and the problems of stuttering.* Springfield, Ill.: Thomas.

———. 1935.   Ueber inneres stottern. *Zeitschrift Ohrenheilkunde* 69: 146–48.

FROESCHELS, E. 1943.   Pathology and therapy of stuttering. *Nervous Child* 2: 148–61.

———. 1913–14.   Zur pathologie des stotterns. *Arch f. Exper. u. Kleine Phonet.* 1: 372–80.

GATELEY, W. G. 1967.   Anxiety and tension in stuttering. Convention Paper, ASHA.

GIOLAS, T. G. AND D. E. WILLIAMS. 1958.   Children's reactions to nonfluencies in adult speech. *Journal of Speech and Hearing Research* 1: 86–93.

GLAUBER, I. P. 1958.   The psychoanalysis of stuttering. In *Stuttering: a symposium,* ed. J. Eisenson, pp. 71–120. New York: Harper.

GOLDMAN-EISLER, F. 1967.   Sequential temporal patterns and cognitive processes in speech. *Language and Speech* 10: 131–40.

HAHN, E. 1943.   *Stuttering: significant theories and therapies.* Stanford: Stanford University Press.

HALL, W. W. 1869.   *The guide board.* London: D. E. Fisk.

HEGDE, M. N. AND D. E. HARTMAN. 1979.   Factors affecting judgments of fluency: 2-word repetitions. *Journal of Fluency Disorders* 4: 13–22.

HELM, N. A. AND R. B. BUTLER. 1980.   Neurogenic acquired stuttering. *Journal of Fluency Disorders* 5: 219–79.

HILLMAN, R. E. AND H. H. GILBERT. 1977.   Voice onset time for voiceless stop consonants in the fluent reading of stutterers and nonstutterers. *Journal of the Acoustical Society of America* 61: 610–11.

HOOD, S. B. 1969.   Investigation of the effect of communicative stress on audible, inaudible and avoidance-escape components of stuttering. Doctoral dissertation, University of Wisconsin.

———. 1974.   Clinical assessment of the moment of stuttering. *Journal of Fluency Disorders* 1: 22–34.

HUFFMAN, E. S. AND W. H. PERKINS. 1974.   Disfluency characteristics identified by listeners as "stuttering" and "stutterer." *Journal of Communication Disorders* 7: 89–96.

JOHNSON, W. 1946. *People in quandaries*. New York: Harper.

————. 1955. *Stuttering in children and adults*. Minneapolis: University of Minnesota Press.

————. 1959. *The onset of stuttering*. Minneapolis: University of Minnesota Press.

————, S. F. BROWN, J. F. CURTIS, C. W. EDNEY, AND J. KEASTER. 1952. *Speech handicapped school children*. New York: Harper.

LUCHSINGER, R. AND G. E. ARNOLD. 1965. *Voice—speech—language*. Belmont, Cal.: Wadsworth.

MAHL, G. 1956. Disturbances and silences in the patient's speech in psychotherapy. *Journal of Abnormal Social Psychology* 53: 1–15.

McCLAY, H. AND E. I. OSGOOD. 1959. Hesitation phenomena in spontaneous English speech. *Word* 15: 19–44.

McDEARMON, J. R. 1968. Primary stuttering at the onset of the stuttering: a reexamination of data. *Journal of Speech and Hearing Research* 11: 631–37.

MINIFEE, F. D. AND H. S. COOKER. 1964. A disfluency index. *Journal of Speech and Hearing Disorders* 29: 189–93.

MYSAK, E. D. 1960. Servo theory and stuttering. *Journal of Speech and Hearing Disorders* 25: 188–95.

PERRIN, E. H. 1954. Social position of the speech defective child. *Journal of Speech and Hearing Disorders* 19: 250–52.

RILEY, G. D. AND J. RILEY. 1979. A component model for diagnosing and treating children who stutter. *Journal of Fluency Disorders* 4: 179–93.

ROSENBERG, S. AND J. CURTIS. 1954. The effect of stuttering on the behavior of the listener. *Journal of Abnormal Social Psychology* 49: 355–61.

SANDER, E. K. 1963. Frequency of syllable repetition and stutter judgments. *Journal of Speech and Hearing Research* 6: 19–30.

————. 1963. Assessing cultural speech fluency expectations. *ASHA* 5: 619–21.

————. 1965. Comments on investigating listener reactions to speech disfluency. *Journal of Speech and Hearing Disorders* 30: 159–65.

————. 1963. Frequency of syllable repetition and 'stutterer' judgments. *Journal of Speech and Hearing Disorders* 28: 19–30.

SAPIR, E. 1915. *Abnormal types of speech in Nootka*. Ottawa, Canada: Dept. Mines. Geological Survey Memoir 62, Anthropological Series.

SCHAEF, R. AND J. MATTHEWS. 1954. A first step in the evaluation of stuttering therapy. *Journal of Speech and Hearing Disorders* 19: 467–73.

SCHIAVETTI, N. 1975. Judgments of stuttering severity as a function of type and locus of disfluency. *Folia Phoniatrica* 27: 26–37.

SCRIPTURE, E. W. 1923. *Stuttering and Lisping*. New York: Macmillan.

SODERBERG, G. A. 1967. Linguistic factors in stuttering. *Journal of Speech and Hearing Research* 10: 801–10.

STEIN, L. 1942. *Speech and Voice*. London: Methuen.

STROMSTA, C. 1965. A spectrographic study of dysfluencies labeled as stuttering by parents. *De Therapia Vocis et Loquellae* 1: 317–20.

TRAVIS, L. E. 1957. The unspeakable feelings of people with special reference to stuttering. In *Handbook of speech pathology*, ed. L. E. Travis. Englewood Cliffs, N.J.: Prentice-Hall.

TURNBAUGH, K. R., B. E. GUITAR, AND P. R. HOFFMAN. 1979. Speech clinicians' attribution of personality traits as a function of stuttering severity. *Journal of Speech and Hearing Research* 22: 37–45.

VAN RIPER, C. 1971.   *The Nature of Stuttering*. Englewood Cliffs, N.J.: Prentice-Hall.

———. 1937.   The influence of empathic response on frequency of stuttering. *Psychological Monographs* 49: 224–36.

VILLAREAL, J. J. 1945.   Semantic aspects of stuttering in nonstutterers: additional data. *Quarterly Journal of Speech* 31: 477–79.

VOELKER, C. H. 1944.   A preliminary investigation for a normative study of fluency; a clinical index to the severity of stuttering. *American Journal of Orthopsychiatry* 14: 285–94.

———. 1942.   On the semantic aspects of stuttering in nonstutterers. *Quarterly Journal of Speech* 28: 78–80.

WALLE, E. 1976.   *The Prevention of Stuttering* (Film). Memphis: Speech Foundation of America.

WEBSTER, L. M. 1966.   An audio-visual exploration of the stuttering moment. Masters thesis, Southern Illinois University.

——— AND G. J. BRUTTEN. 1972.   An audio-visual analysis of the stuttering moment. *Behavior Therapy* 3: 555–60.

WEST, R. 1957.   *The Rehabilitation of Speech*. New York: Harper.

WILLIAMS, D. E. AND L. KENT. 1958.   Listeners' evaluations of speech interruptions. *Journal of Speech and Hearing Research* 1: 124–36.

WINGATE, M. E. 1976.   *Stuttering theory and treatment*. New York: Irvington-Wiley.

———. 1964.   A standard definition of stuttering. *Journal of Speech and Hearing Disorders* 29: 484–89.

WOODS, C. L. 1978.   Does the stigma shape the stutterer?" *Journal of Communication Disorders* 11: 483–7.

——— AND D. E. WILLIAMS. 1976.   Traits attributed to stuttering and normally fluent males. *Journal of Speech and Hearing Research* 10: 267–78.

WYLLIE, J. 1894.   *The disorders of speech*. Edinburgh: Oliver and Boyd.

WYRICK, D. R. 1949.   A study of normal non-fluency in conversation. Masters thesis, University of Missouri.

YOUNG, M. A. 1964.   Identification of stutterers from recorded samples of their 'fluent' speech. *Journal of Speech and Hearing Research* 7: 291–303.

———. 1961.   Predicting ratings of severity of stuttering. *Journal of Speech and Hearing Disorders* Monograph Supplement 7: 31–54.

ZENNER, A. A. 1971.   A molecular analysis of stuttering behaviors during massed oral readings of the same material. Doctoral dissertation, Syracuse University.

ZIMMERMANN, G. 1980.   Articulatory behaviors associated with stuttering: a cine-fluorographic analysis. *Journal of Speech and Hearing Research* 22: 108–21.

THE PREVALENCE AND INCIDENCE OF STUTTERING

3

One of the neglected pieces of the stuttering puzzle is its incidence. How many stutterers are there in the general population? How many of us have passed through a period of stuttering and have recovered? Are there subpopulations, special groups, in which the disorder is found very frequently or others in which it appears rarely? Is the incidence of stuttering declining? The answers to these questions may contribute to the solution of its mystery.

Unfortunately, the extensive literature on the subject is not very illuminating. We have critically surveyed most of it and we find so many omissions of criteria, such vague descriptions of survey procedures, and so obviously inadequate samplings that any conclusions seem premature. The curious thing about these studies of incidence, however, is that the magical number of one per cent seems to occur over and over again, most of the incidence figures seeming to cluster about this value. We also find higher incidences reported for the younger age groups and, without exception, more males are reported as having the disorder than females.

There are many hazards lying in wait for the investigator who concerns himself with a study of the incidence of stuttering. First of these is the matter of definition. As we saw in the preceding chapter, definitions vary widely, especially when incipient stuttering is considered. The differential diagnosis of abnormal from normal disfluency is not always easily accomplished. Moreover, as Voelker (1942) pointed out long ago, and others have since, the same people who feel that they have spoken "stutteringly" or have "stuttered" are very insistent that they have never been "stutterers." Another difficulty is that the disorder is intermittent. In the early stages of its development, temporary remissions seem to be the rule rather than the exception. Some young stutterers are certain to be missed because their stuttering appears in waves. Moreover, we now have enough solid evidence (Sheehan and Martyn, 1966; Dickson, 1969) that self-recovery is more common than had formerly been believed. It is clear that some individuals would have been classified as stutterers at one age but not at another. This is an important point in differentiating between the concepts of incidence and prevalence. True incidence figures will always be higher than the prevalence ones reported in cross-sectional studies.

INCIDENCE VERSUS PREVALENCE

There are only two ways of estimating the true incidence of stuttering and both have been used. The first (and probably the least valid) is by using retrospective reports from parents or ex-stutterers themselves. Typically, a large population of parents is given a questionnaire, or college students are asked if their children or if they themselves have ever experienced the disorder of stuttering during their lifetimes. The resulting percentages of affirmative answers are then used as incidence figures. As we have mentioned earlier, there are many sources of error in such studies.

The other way to determine the true incidence of stuttering is to sample a large population of children and to follow them up over the course of many years. Only such longitudinal studies can determine the actual incidence of the disorder and they are very hard to do.

To our knowledge, only one careful longitudinal study bearing on the true incidence of stuttering has yet been performed. It was carried out in the city of Newcastle-on-Tyne in England and has been reported by Morley (1957) and by Andrews and Harris (1964). It shows both the onset of stuttering and its remission or disappearance in about 1,000 children followed from birth through age 15. Most of the cases of stuttering began before the age of five, and no new cases were discovered after the age of 11. About a third of the stuttering children seemed to pass through a period of marked nonfluency (developmental stuttering) between 2–4 years; another third (the "benign stutterers") began to stutter rather later (mean age of onset 7.5 years) and the stuttering in this group, as in the first group, lasted an average of only two years. The final third of the stuttering children began to stutter between the ages of 3–6 years and continued to stutter thereafter.

The important contribution made by this longitudinal research is that it permits us, for the first time, to compare total incidence figures with the prevalence of stuttering at certain ages. The incidence, that is the percentage of children who went through a period of stuttering which lasted six months or more, was three per cent. If children who passed through a period of stuttering which lasted less than six months are added to this group, then the total incidence was 4.5 per cent. In contrast, the prevalence figures (how many were stuttering each year) shows a variation from 0.5 per cent at the age of three, reaching a maximum of 1.6 per cent at the age of eight, and stablizing at 1.1 per cent at age 12.

Studies of Prevalence

Most of our information on the number of stutterers comes from cross-sectional surveys of school children. The methods used vary from investigator to investigator. Some used questionnaires; some used referrals only; a few personally examined each child, although we rarely know how extensively or thoroughly. All of them contain sources of error. Different age ranges are covered in different studies. One of the first surveys in this country was conducted by Wallin (1916), who sent questionnaires to school principals, and he reported that 0.7 per cent of 89,000 school children stuttered. Two years later, Carrie (1918) surveyed all the school children in Hamburg, Germany, and found a prevalence of 0.84 per cent. He also reported two earlier surveys, one in the Berlin parochial schools in 1886 in which 1.0 per cent of 155,000 school children stuttered and another in Amsterdam, Holland, in 1910 where 1.19 per cent of the Dutch children stuttered. All of these were studies in which questionnaires were sent to teachers. Perhaps the most ambitious of these questionnaire surveys was that reported in the first White House Conference Report of 1931 where the results of 44 questionnaire surveys of children and youths (ages 5–21) were pooled to yield a population of 3,800,000 of whom 1.2 per cent were said to be stuttering.

We have three reports of prevalence in which children were examined individually. The first of these was performed by Voelker (1943) who, with his assistants, claimed to have screened a total of 101,020 individuals, 50 per cent of whom were under 19 years of age. His article is difficult to evaluate but he reported an incidence of 1.87 per cent of dysrhythmia and, from his other writings, the term refers to stuttering. The second study, by Mills and Streit (1942), seems well designed and carefully performed. They personally interviewed 4,685 children in the first through sixth grades of the Hartford, Connecticut, public schools. The screening was done carefully: "Each child was tested in an individual conference and by at least two examiners. Occasionally a third examiner was called in on a case. These conferences were held in the school building during regular school hours in order to keep the situation as familiar to the child as possible. All children old enough to read were tested in both reading and spontaneous speech." Mills and Streit found an overall average "incidence" (prevalence) of 1.5 per cent. When their population was broken down by grades, 2.7 per cent stuttered in grades 1–3 as compared to 1.1 per cent in grades 4–6.

The third study is the National Speech and Hearing Survey (Hull and Timmons, 1969). Mobile units with trained examiners sampled school populations in many areas throughout the United States with provision being made for reliability checks. Preliminary results indicate that the prevalence of stuttering was 0.8 per cent in a sample of 38,000 elementary school children.

Some Questionnaire Studies

American

Root (1952): school children in grades 1–8; 1.2%
Burdin (1940): 3,600 children in grades 1–4; 1.2% (averaged)
Louttit and Halls (1937): 200,000 American Indian school children; 0.77%

Schindler (1955): examined school records of 23,000 Iowa school children; 0.55%

Dickson (1971): 4,025 elementary school children; 1%

Gillespie and Cooper (1973): 5,054 junior and senior high school children; 2.1%

Foreign

McAllister (1937): 21,000 English children aged 5–18; 1.0%

Morgenstern (1956): 35,000 Scottish school children; 1.02%

Schreiber (1955): 18,000 German school children; 1.0%

Chrysanthis (1947): 1,100 Cypriot school children; 1.85%

Watzl (1924): 136,000 Viennese school children; 0.6%

Seeman (1959): 26,000 school children in Prague; 0.55%

Katsovakaia (1960): preschool children of the Ukraine, Russia; 1.5%

Aron (1962): 6,500 African school children; 1.26%

Toyoda (1959): 140,000 Japanese school children; 0.82%

Ozawa (1960): 7,600 Japanese school children; 0.9%

Petkov and Iosifov (1960): 45,000 Bulgarian school children; 1.7%

Brestovici (1976): 578 Jugoslav elementary school children; 1.9%

SPONTANEOUS RECOVERY

The major reason for the distinction between incidence and prevalence figures is that many, perhaps a majority, of children who begin to stutter eventually become fluent. They "pass through" a period of pronounced disfluency marked by the presence of the usual stuttering behaviors and then spontaneously recover. The term *spontaneous* must not be understood to mean sudden, for usually the transition to normal speech is gradual. What it really seems to signify is that the recovery seems to take place without treatment. In any event, true incidence figures must include those persons who at one time in their lives were considered by themselves and others to be stutterers.

The research on spontaneous recovery in stutterers is even less clear cut than that on general incidence and prevalence. This is probably because most of it is based upon retrospective reports, that is, presently normal speaking adults were asked if they had ever gone through a period of stuttering or had ever been a stutterer. The possibility of error in such accounts is very evident as Young (1975) has pointed out, yet there seems to be no doubt that a subtantial number of children who begin to stutter show spontaneous recovery. A summary of most of the studies follows:

Some Studies of Spontaneous Recovery

Milisen and Johnson (1936): Observation of children; 40%

Bryngelson (1938): Observation of children; 80%

Froeschels (1948): Observation of children; 80%

Andrews and Harris (1964): Observation of children; 94%
Dostalova and Dosuzkov (1965): Observation of children; 17.8%
Sheehan and Martyn (1970): Retrospective interview—college; 80%
Cooper (1972): Retrospective Interview—Junior and Senior high school; 36%
Panelli, McFarlane, and Shipley (1978): Observation of children; 80%

AGE OF SPONTANEOUS RECOVERY

When do children who stutter "outgrow their stuttering"? This question is important to our knowledge of prevalence since any cross-sectional study of the number of stutterers in a population will be affected by its answer. The research that is based upon actual observation of children seems to show that most of the recovery occurs in the preschool or elementary school years [Andrews and Harris (1964); Johnson (1959); Panelli *et al.* (1978)]. This also seems to be borne out by parental reports (Glasner and Rosenthal (1957); Dickson (1971)). However, the retrospective research by Wingate (1964), Shearer and Williams (1965), and Martyn and Sheehan (1971) turned up a number of individuals who claimed to have overcome their stuttering during adolescence or later without or despite therapy. Our impression, after surveying all these studies, is that most of the spontaneous recovery takes place early in childhood but that a few persons do recover later.

Were it not for the few studies we have of stuttering prevalence in adults such as that of Morley (1952) who found, in screening 33,000 college students at the University of Michigan, that one per cent of them still stuttered, we would expect that the number of stutterers would gradually decrease in the adult years either as the result of successful therapy or spontaneous recovery. A marked decrease in stuttering incidence during the adult years has indeed been shown by Shames and Beams (1956) who sent questionnaires to clergymen asking them how many stutterers they had among their parishioners and their ages. As the authors make clear, however, the sources of error in such a study are so great as to leave the matter in much doubt. We do know that some stutterers continue to stutter until they die—Somerset Maugham, the novelist, for one. We also know that a very few individuals do begin to stutter in adulthood as cited in the articles by Froeschels (1919), Kingdon-Ward (1941), Arnold (1948), and Wallen (1961), usually as the result of traumatic experiences. Nevertheless, in summary, we feel that the literature, miserable as most of it is, indicates clearly that the total *incidence* of stuttering probably amounts conservatively to about 4 per cent of the general population, and that its *prevalence* is highest in preschool years declining thereafter to an unstable value of less than 1 per cent.

If we are to understand the basic nature of stuttering we must somehow account for these incidence and prevalence figures and for spontaneous recovery. Of the three major explanations that have been offered: that it is a neurosis, or a learned bad habit, or a disorder of motor coordination, the latter would seem to fit the facts better than the others.

INCIDENCE IN OTHER CULTURES

As we have seen, the statistics on incidence and prevalence of stuttering in our own culture leave much to be desired, but when we look for some valid estimates of the number of stutterers in other societies, the available data is appallingly meager and its validity seems questionable. Lemert's (1953) investigation of the Salish Indian tribes on Vancouver Island gives us a prevalence figure of 1.9 per cent. Stewart (1960) found only .02 per cent in another Indian population presumably similar in child rearing practices and culture. In another field investigation using informants, Lemert (1962) reported his impression that there were more stutterers among the Japanese than among the Polynesians, attributing the difference to the beliefs held concerning the nature of the problem, and the amount of compliance demanded by the two societies. The Polynesians believe that "stutterers are born that way and nothing can be done about it" whereas the Japanese feel that the disorder "can and should be corrected." Moreover, there are fewer time pressures and conformity demands among the Hawaiian and Samoan peoples than among the Japanese. Besides these investigations by anthropologists using informants, we find in Japanese literature several professional surveys of the prevalence of stuttering among elementary school children, yielding prevalence figures ranging from 0.8 to 1.0 per cent.

Perhaps the more a society resembles our own, the more likely it is to have the same prevalence of stuttering. Both Lemert (1953) and Stewart (1960) seem to attribute the alleged greater prevalence of stuttering among the Kwakiutl and Cowichan tribes than among the Utes and Shoshones in part to the greater competitiveness of the former societies and the resulting social pressures on the children. In the same vein, Aron (1962) found a prevalence of 1.26 per cent among Bantu school children in South Africa and attributed it to the fact that urban African children are subjected to many of the same stresses and speech conformity pressures that exist in the general European–American culture.

The prevalence of stuttering in a subculture, such as that of the blacks in the southern states of our country, might be expected to differ from that in the main culture. Several such studies have been made. Carson and Kantner (1945) report that in the schools of Baton Rouge, Louisiana, the prevalence of stuttering among white children was 1.1 per cent, whereas that of black children was 60 per cent higher. Neely (1960), however, who carefully studied the parochial elementary schools in the New Orleans area found no significant differences in prevalence between white and black children. We also have some figures for black children in northern cities where presumably the factor of upward mobility pressure might be expected to be present. Waddle (1934) personally tested 1,582 children in segregated schools of Topeka, Kansas, finding that a ratio of 1.7/1 existed, with black stutterers in the majority, and Pritchett (1966) reported a similar ratio of 1.3/1 for the east St. Louis schools. The results of these investigations indicate no major support for the commonly held belief that stuttering is much more common among blacks as a race of subculture.

The prevalence of stuttering is doubtless affected by many factors, and one of those frequently cited is that of socio-economic status. It has been felt that families striving for greater status place demands on their children for excellence in speech as well as for other attributes. Also, there are many investigations, such as McCarthy's (1954), indicating that children from the lower socio-economic levels are retarded in language development, using shorter and less mature sentence forms than those of children from the upper strata of our society. Morgenstern (1956), whose study is perhaps best known in this respect, found higher percentages of stutterers in the families of semiskilled laborers than in those of middle or upper-class families. Andrews and Harris (1964), however, found little evidence to support the belief that stuttering appears more frequently in subgroups concerned with upward social mobility.

PREVALENCE OF STUTTERING
AMONG THE MENTALLY RETARDED

An intriguing facet of the problem of stuttering is that it seems to be much more prevalent among the mentally retarded than in the general population. Moreover, it is apparently found much more frequently in mongoloids than in nonmongoloid retarded individuals. If stuttering is basically a neurosis it is difficult to see why these increases in prevalence occur. Most mongoloids that we have known have been fairly happy persons, far from neurotic by nature. We would expect, if stuttering is a neurosis, that the incidence among the more severely retarded would be less than among those mildly impaired. Just the opposite seems to be true. And why, if stuttering is basically learned behavior, do we find such a high prevalence in children who find learning most difficult? Surely those who are less mentally retarded than the others should show more stuttering if this is true. Mongoloid children show organicity in many ways. Is their high prevalence of stuttering a reflection of neurological deficits which make the sequential timing of speech movements unusually difficult?

Although the research is fairly consistent in showing these trends, it is not definitive beyond question. One of the basic problems is that of definition and differential diagnosis. Is the disorder that they show stuttering or cluttering? Do they falter because of their admitted difficulty in finding and manipulating the symbols of speech? Is their stuttering or cluttering merely a reaction to language deficit? The incidence of all types of speech defects is very high among the mentally retarded. It might be merely that the temporal dimension of speech is affected equally with those of articulation, voice, or symbolization.

With Wendell Johnson's definiton of stuttering as something that exists only after the person begins to react with fear and struggle to his "normal" repetitions and prolongations, then few of the severely impaired mentally retarded could be said to stutter. Most of them have short memories and little foresight. They anticipate contingencies with difficulty. With such a definition—which we feel is unduly restrictive and useful more to defend a theory than to describe the disorder—one would probably be forced to conclude that few mongoloids do stutter and that most of the mentally retarded do not either. However, if we view stuttering as a developmental disorder which usually begins with an excessive amount of repetitions and prolongations of syllables, sounds, or words and which then progresses through a series of gradual phases of reactivity until fear and frustration predominate, the mentally retarded do show an unusual amount of the earlier signs of stuttering. Typically, they have rather simple disfluencies. We rarely see the complicated patterns of avoidance behavior so characteristic of the advanced stutterer with normal intelligence. The disorder tends also to be more episodic as it does in the beginning stutterer. We find some mildly feared speaking situations but little word or phonemic fears. In our experience, the consistency in terms of stuttered words is low, and adaptation is less marked. Most of the time they do not seem to be aware that they have stuttered or are stuttering. They are often frustrated in trying to communicate, primarily because of word-finding and coding difficulties, but they do not seem to feel frustrated because they cannot utter a given word when they try to. We have heard a mongoloid child repeat the first syllable of his name 18 times without showing any signs of frustration.

Lerman, Powers, and Rigrodsky (1965) studied a group of 14 retardate stutterers in the Mansfield State Training School, and have this to say about their characteristics:

> The stutterers involved in this study reflected stuttering behavior which closely paralleled the early stages of development of stuttering in normal children. Although the most obvious difference was the lack of chronic avoidance and apprehension, it should be emphasized that fear of the speech act can occur. The observation of the continual use of syllable repetition in contrast to whole word repetitions may suggest that other factors are contributing to the etiological and continuing aspects of this disorder (p. 32).

Except for automatisms which they have overlearned, such as saying "Thank you" or "Good morning," much of the speech of the severely mentally retarded, when it appears at all (and often they speak only under great urging or need) shows many forms of hesitant behavior. They begin to say something and then forget where they are going or where they have been. Not all of them do this of course, but those that do also show many other breaks in fluency besides stuttering. The mispronunciations and misarticulations cause listeners to show that they are not comprehending, and this too may interrupt speech flow. It is a difficult diagnostic problem. Perhaps the best we can say is that they seem to be speaking "stutteringly" or "clutteringly."

As has been indicated, several of the writers on the subject insist that what mentally retarded children show is "cluttering." If we accept Weiss' (1964) position that all stuttering begins as cluttering (which we do not) then the problem of differential diagnosis presents no problem—many of these children clutter. They show the accompanying language deficits, the misarticulations, the reversals, the lack of fear or awareness that characterizes cluttering. We do not find the tachylalia, the hurried bursts of rapid speech, the swift revisions of whole phrases seen in most clutterers. And we have found tonic stuttering with occasional tremors in a minority of these children.

We do find a preponderance of fluency breaks on the syllable and sound. If stuttering represents the final common path of a group of related disorders, a syndrome, one of which arises in cluttering and language disability, then this is the type of stuttering that the mentally retarded show.

Cabanas (1954) analyzed the speech patterns of 50 mongoloids and felt that their characteristic repetitions and distorted sounds resembled cluttering more than stuttering. However, both Preus (1972) and Bonfanti and Culatta (1977) provide data which indicates that many mental retardates, including the mongoloids, show the essential behaviors characteristic of stuttering as well as cluttering.

One prevalence study which attempted to differentiate between the stutterers and clutterers was done by Preus (1972). Carefully done, it showed the following percentages in a group of 47 persons with Down's Syndrome (mongolism): 27 per cent "pure stutterers," 12 per cent "pure clutterers," 19 per cent in which both cluttering and stuttering were found, and the rest had normal speech so far as fluency was concerned. Some of the stutterers showed associated struggle behaviors in addition to their part word repetitions and prolongations but none seemed concerned about their speech. Keane (1970) reported a stuttering prevalence of 10 per cent. Otto and Yairi (1974) analyzed the kinds of disfluencies shown by individuals with Down's Syndrome and found that the disfluencies were those most characteristic of stutterers.

Prevalence figures for stuttering in the mentally retarded population have varied widely from one research to another. We summarize them in Table 3.1.

In evaluating these sparse investigations, we should keep in mind the caution of Zisk and Bialer (1967):

Published reports leave unclear the exact nature of the problem, thus making it exceedingly difficult to speculate as to possible causes. Further research should aim at providing precise definitions and objective criteria of the behavior under consideration.

If this further research corroborates the trend of the research we now possess, this higher prevalence of stuttering among mental retardates and especially the mongoloids would seem to point to some deficiency in the

TABLE 3.1 Prevalence of Stuttering Among the Mentally Retarded.

RESEARCH	TYPE OF POPULATION	PREVALENCE
Gottsleben (1955)	General retardates	14%
	Mongoloids	33%
Schlanger and Gottsleben (1957)	General retardates	17%
	Mongoloids	45%
Edson (1964)	Mongoloids	39%
Schubert (1966)	General retardates	8%
	Mongoloids	15%
Schaeffer and Shearer (1968)	General retardates	7%
Preus (1972)	Mongoloids	60%
Chapman, A.H. (1973)	General Retardates	2.5%

* These percentages include both stuttering and cluttering. In contrast to the high prevalence figures reported in the above studies, Sheehan, Martyn, and Kilburn (1968) found only one stutterer among 216 retardates in a California state institution.

motor control of the learned coordinations needed for normal speech rather than to neurotic or conditioned fear responses.

THE SEX RATIO

One of the most interesting findings concerning the prevalence of stuttering is the complete agreement (reached by all the investigators of the subject in all lands) that males show more stuttering than females. The preponderance is not minor. Though different researchers have given different ratios, most of them range about the figure of three or four to one. Why should so many more males than females stutter?

Immediately we confront a conflict situation which we shall meet many times in our study of stuttering: the differing points of view with respect to the nature and etiology of the disorder, namely that stuttering has a constitutional basis, that it is a learned behavior, or that it is a neurosis. And there is also the composite view that stuttering is a syndrome in which each of these may play a part and any one of them may create a homogeneous subpopulation, or combine with the others to form a multiple-faceted disorder, a position expounded in the present text.

Despite long search, we have been unable to find a study or report which shows that there are more female than male stutterers. The converse is consistently found. Unfortunately, as with the studies of general incidence, the true proportion is in some doubt for several reasons. Besides the inadequacy of survey methods, most of the investigations of the sex ratio in stuttering fail to take into account the ratios of total male to female populations from which the samples were obtained. Also, several authors have held that the proportion of males to females tends to increase with age. However, the male/female sex ratio of college stutterers who reportedly had recovered from stuttering reported in Sheehan and Martyn's study (1967) was about five to one rather than the reverse, and Mills and Streit's (1942) careful survey showed no change with grade placement. In spite of all the limitations of the investigations, however, we cannot doubt that the sex ratio exists and must have some significance. A summary of some of the results of various studies follows:

Studies Reporting Sex-Ratio in Stutterers

McDowell: 2.9/1 (1928); White House Conference: 3.9/1 (1931); Brown: 4/1 (1932); Louttit and Halls: 3.8/1 (1936); Wepman: 4.4/1 (1939); Mills and Streit: 5/1 (1942); Schindler: 2.8/1 (1955); Morley: 4.3/1 in college students (1952); Morgenstern: 4.4/1 (1956); McCallien: 2.1/1 Ga-speaking African children (1956); Aron: 3.2/1 Bantu school children (1962); Daskalov: 3.1/1 Bulgarian clinic cases (1962); Hirschberg: 5/1 Hungarian clinic cases (1965); Dickson: 2/1 American school children (1969); Hull and Timmons: 3.1/1 (National Survey, 1969); McMahon: 4/1 Canadian school children (1969); Andrews and Harris: 2.5/1 British school children (1964); Sato: 4.5/1 Japanese nursery school children (1961); Williams, Silverman, and Kools: 4/1 young clinic cases (1968); Barbaix and Snepps: 5/1 Belgian children and adults (1974); Kidd, Kidd, and Records: 2.93/1 First degree relatives of stutterers (1978).

In view of the remarkable unanimity of these reports, it is evident that a real sex difference may exist in the incidence of stuttering. The most carefully performed of all these studies, Kidd, Kidd, and Records (1978) examined possible sources of error. They say:

> Possible causes of the unequal sex ratio include various ascertainment biases, incomplete reporting, social role differences, X-linked inheritance, or a combination of environmental and genetic elements. Each of these has been examined against data collected in a large family study of stuttering, and all but one have been eliminated. Only the gene-environmental interaction hypothesis can be supported by the data. Statistical analysis confirms that the sex effect in stuttering is real.

Why Do More Males Than Females Stutter?

One of the common explanations for the sex ratio is that many other types of deviancy show a similarly larger number of males, Chorea, asthma, convulsions, tetany, and epilepsy are only some of the spasmodic disorders which could be so cited. Baldness, cleft palate, and spinal bifida are just a few of many other disorders where males outnumber females. There appear to be more birth injuries and more illnesses among boys than girls. This point of view unfortunately does not tell us much that is useful, especially since the reported sex ratios for stuttering are far greater than for most of these other problems. Perhaps more explanatory, if not entirely convincing, is the belief held by Cobb and Cole (1939) and Karlin (1947) and others that there are more male stutterers because speech is learned during a period when the myelinization of the cortical areas subserving speech and language in male children is delayed when compared to that of female children. The difficulty with this theory is that no one has shown why or how this delay produces stuttering intermittently or why only a few of the many male children are so affected. So far as we have been able to ascertain, no one has done comparative autopsy studies of child stutterers and nonstutterers, either male or female. One little hint of another explanation for the sex ratio comes from DeSantis (1959). He found unusual endocrine changes in 16 of 20 male stutterers, primarily those of hypogonadins. Unfortunately no control group was employed.

A fair case has been made for the sex ratio in terms of learning theory. Since speech is learned, and almost all the research indicates that girls are more advanced in speech and language during the early years, equally disrupting pressures applied to boys and girls of the same age should presumably produce more disfluency in the boy child than in the girl. That this might possibly be true is indicated by Mahaffey and Stromsta's (1965) and Bachrach's (1964) research showing that delayed auditory feedback evidently disrupted the fluency of males more than females even at the college level. Different critical delay times required to produce maximal disruption have also been reported, the females requiring the longer delay times to create broken speech.

Another explanation of the sex ratio is that parents tend to penalize or react unfavorably to normal disfluencies in the speech of their boys more than they do to those in girls. Or that our culture does! The tests of this explanation have been negative. Bloodstein and Smith (1945) found that college students did not make more diagnoses of stuttering for samples of sexually ambiguous speech recordings when told that they were made by boys rather than girls. Mysak (1959) in a similar study with adolescent boys and girls found no significant differences in the tendency to diagnose stuttering in terms of sex identification. Quite apart from this scanty research we find it hard to believe that parents would be likely to be more tolerant of marked disfluency in their daughters than in their sons, since the gift of speech has certainly been highly prized by the fairer if not fainter sex.

Again, in terms of learning theory, if boys generally show more disfluencies of all types than girls, perhaps the sex ratio could be explained in terms of contingent punishment or reward. Unfortunately for this possibility, the research of Johnson (1959) and Kools and Berryman (1971) found no significant sex differences in the total disfluences or any special kinds of disfluency in normal speaking children.

One of the explanations which has never been particularly convincing to us is the one by Schuell (1946, 1947) that stuttering is due to the differential cultural treatment of the sexes in childhood. More boys are said to stutter because they are subjected to more parental pressures for excellence in speech and in social behavior at a time when they are linguistically more immature than girls. More parental pride is invested in them; more demands for conformity are brought to bear upon them. Schuell's explanation for the sex ratio has been widely quoted in the literature, but the actual evidence on which her wide reaching conclusions were based leaves much to be desired. She simply questioned 161 boys and 142 normal speaking girls about parental practices regarding praise and punishment. These subjects were taken from the fifth to seventh grades—far later than the age at which stuttering generally begins. Her questions seem inappropriately designed to elicit significant information regarding communicative pressures, and no reliability check was made. More boys than girls reported being punished for being noisy, quarreling, spending money, staying out late, being bad, procrastinating, having poor manners, and not helping with the housework. These items hardly seem pertinent to the age levels when stuttering usually has its onset. Moreover, we find it hard to believe that three or four times as much differential social pressure is focused directly on the prosody of male children to produce the sex ratio. One test of Schuell's position would be to discover a culture where boys and girls are treated very much alike during their speech-learning years. This has been reported by Eisenson (1966), who found the usual sex ratio of stuttering in the kibbutz colonies of Israel, where children are separated from their parents for most of their waking hours and both sexes are treated in the same way. Many other cultures which vary widely from our own in child-rearing practices such as the African Bantus (Aron, 1962) show the same sex ratio.

Those who believe stuttering to be a primary neurosis usually find the sex ratio very difficult to explain. It has been attributed in Freudian theory to the greater conflicts a male child has with his ever-present mother as an Oedipal love object than girls experience with their absent fathers, or to castration fears, or to great inhibitions in oral-anal smearing. In most of the non-Freudian presentations of stuttering as a neurosis, the sex ratio is ignored, perhaps because no other recognized neurosis has its onset so early or shows such a high proportion of males.

In conclusion, it would seem that the sex ratio must in some way reflect a less stable neuromuscular control system for speech in the male at least during the early years of life. The temporal organization of his speech, as well as its vocabulary, articulation, and other aspects, may be less mature than that of the female at this time and accordingly more vulnerable to disruption. We see no need to explain everything in terms of environmental or neurotic influences. Even as the male has a constitutional predisposition to have a phallus, it is perhaps possible that he also has a minor one to have an unstable system for coordinating sequential speech in his early years.

FAMILIAL INCIDENCE

We do not feel it appropriate at this point to discuss the hereditary factor in stuttering since we are considering problems of incidence and not etiology. Our question is only whether or not there is a higher incidence or prevalence of stuttering in the families of stutterers than in the families of nonstutterers—quite apart from its mode of transmission or correlation. Most of the pertinent studies indicate that the incidence is much higher in the families of stutterers. Unfortunately, many of the investigations speak of family incidence rather than actual incidence. Wepman (1939), for example, found that 68 per cent of the families of stutterers had some other members who stuttered while only 15.6 per cent of the families of nonstutterers had such members. To know the actual incidence figures we must know how many members of the families there were and for what generations. Johnson (1961) similarly reports that in the 44 families of his stuttering subjects, 37 other members had stuttered whereas in a comparable group of nonstutterers' families only eight had stuttered. Nevertheless, we can conclude that the familial incidence of stuttering is apparently higher than in the general population, as demonstrated by the following studies: Boome and Richardson (1931): 34 per cent of 522 stutterers had a family history of stuttering; West, Nelson, and Berry (1939) report an incidence of 3 per cent in families of stutterers as compared to 0.5 per cent for the relatives of the controls; Meyer (1945): ten times more stutterers in families of stutterers; Jameson (1955): 36 per cent of 69 stutterers; Mussafia (1964): 39 per cent of 241 stutterers had other stutterers in their families; Andrews and Harris (1964) found 30 per cent of their stutterers to have relatives who stuttered as compared with .02 per cent for the controls; Martyn and Sheehan (1968) found a 30 per cent reported incidence of stuttering in the families of college students still stuttering as compared to 7.2 per cent for those who had once stuttered but recovered. Cooper (1972) found that 29 per cent of 177 stutterers showed a familial history of stuttering.

That this reported high incidence of stuttering in the families of stutterers is not confined within the border of our own country is found in the studies by Daskalov (1962) in Russia (32 per cent); Kamiyama (1967) in Japan (20 per cent); Fritzell (1976) in Sweden (47 per cent); and Petrak (1977) in Russia (58 per cent).

Most of the above studies leave much to be desired in terms of methodology. However, we have some very carefully done research by Kidd and his colleagues (1976, 1977, 1978, 1980) which supports these general findings. Table 3.2 summarizes some of their results.

If, as Kidd and his co-workers maintain, this heightened familial incidence is due to the interaction between heredity and environmental influences, what are the latter? One suggestion, made by Sheehan and Martyn (1967), is that the stuttering parents of stutterers become more concerned about the normal disfluencies of their children and, as Johnson

TABLE 3.2   Frequency of Stuttering Among First Degree Relatives of Adult Stutterers (from Kidd, Heimbuch and Records, 1980)

	MALE PROBANDS	FEMALE PROBANDS
Fathers	52/293 = .178 ± .022	21/103 = .204 ± .040
Mothers	14/293 = .048 ± .012	12/103 = .117 ± .032
Brothers	71/360 = .197 ± .021	24/106 = .226 ± .041
Sisters	12/288 = .042 ± .012	17/139 = .122 ± .028
Sons	26/118 = .220 ± 0.38	19/53 = .359 ± .066
Daughters	11/119 = .092 ± 0.26	8/46 = .174 ± .056

The frequencies are given with their binomial standard errors. As in all tables, stuttering is considered as "ever stuttered." The slightly increased frequencies for sons and daughters are not statistically significant but may reflect a slight loss of very mild cases from the other categories because past episodes have been forgotten.

had maintained earlier, tend to label and react to them as stuttering. Perkins (1971) puts it another way: "Parents of stutterers, being sensitive to the problem, become 'bird watchers,' scanning each other's family tree for signs of stutterers roosting there; more stutterers are found because more looking is done" (p. 316).

While this may be possible, we must not forget that the high incidence of stuttering in the families of stutterers also indicates that some hereditary factor may also be present. Perhaps it is an inherited susceptibility to breakdown in the synchronizing of motoric speech.

TWINNING

Among the subgroups in which a high incidence of stuttering has been reported are twins. Most of the evidence seems to show that it is higher in monozygotic twins than in dizygotic twins. Where stuttering occurred in one monozygotic twin it also occurred in the other twin 9 out of 10 times, but when stuttering occurred in one dizygotic twin, it occurred in the other one only one out of 15 times (Nelson, Hunter, and Walter, 1945). When stuttering occurs through several generations in twins, they tend to be fraternal. The onset of stuttering also seems to be earlier for this population. The "incidence" figures for stuttering in twins varies widely from study to study, ranging from 1.9 per cent (Graf, 1955) to 24 per cent (Nelson, Hunter, and Walter, 1945). Most of the studies report higher prevalence figures than those of Graf. Perhaps the explanation for the higher incidence is merely that these twins are usually delayed in speech and fail to organize their motor patterns early enough to avoid social pressures.

THE BRAIN-INJURED

Stuttering has been alleged to have a high rate of incidence among the brain-injured. Disregarding, for the moment, those individuals said to show minimal brain damage and concentrating on the more grossly impaired, we find higher proportions of stutterers in the cerebral-palsied population as cited by Palmer and Osborn (1938) and Rutherford (1938), both reporting twice as many stutterers in this group as among normal speakers. In a later study using a control group, Rutherford (1946) corroborated this higher incidence. Although stuttering has been viewed by some workers, notably West (1958), as a form of epilepsy and by others as an epileptic equivalent, about all we really know is that the incidence of the disorder in the epileptic population is apparently high. Gens (1951) found a stuttering prevalence of 3.2 per cent among the 1,252 epileptics in a state hospital in Michigan, and Harrison (1947) on a smaller sample found an even higher percentage.

In the text by Becker, Vlassova, Asatiani, and Hev (1977), there is a report of a study of 152 stutterers in the Soviet Union of whom 41 per cent showed residual signs of brain injury. This figure seems very high. Böhme (1977) reversed the process and surveyed 802 cases of brain-injured children in Germany, finding that 155 (19.3 per cent) were stutterers. This incidence, of course, is much higher than occurs in the general population. Böhme also states that 8 of 35 brain damaged, forceps-delivered children were stutterers.

Many individual case reports of stuttering behavior accompanying aphasia and other disorders resulting from brain injury occur in the literature but we have found none that provide appropriate information for incidence or prevalence studies. If future research corroborates these tentative findings, the higher incidence in the brain-injured population would support the position that the coordinative and monitoring aspects of speech are what become impaired to produce stuttering. An alternative explanation might be that the brain-injured are more emotionally disturbed as a result of their disabilities.

THE DEAF

There exists a fairly unanimous opinion that the incidence of stuttering in the congenitally deaf is very low though most of the research has been based upon questionnaire surveys of schools for the deaf. It has also frequently been stated that no stuttering ever occurs among this population but Backus (1938) found six totally deaf (not all congenitally) stutterers in questionnaire reports from 206 schools for the deaf with a population of 13,691. Harms and Malone (1939) found eight totally deaf stutterers in a population of 14,458 individuals in oral schools for the deaf and hard of hearing, also by questionnaire, and Voelker and Voelker (1937) and others have reported a few case studies which indicate that, though very rare, stuttering can occur among the congenitally deaf. The task of identifying stuttering in these individuals is not an easy one primarily because of the limited and distorted speech and other difficulties in communication. Sternberg (1946) attributes the low incidence to the fact that the deaf scan more carefully, speak more slowly and controllably, and have less social pressure.

Brannon (1966) points out that the deaf person speaks more slowly than the non-deaf because he prolongs his syllables. This is of some interest because the marked reduction in stuttering found in many stutterers when speaking under delayed auditory feedback may be due to their use of longer syllable durations. One interesting study by Silverman and Silverman (1972) reports the results of a questionnaire sent to schools for the deaf asking if any non-oral behavior akin to stuttering behaviors were shown by members of this population. Thirteen of those who responded reported seeing "repetitions of signs, repetition of initial letters in finger spelling, hesitations in finger spelling, interjections, and extra movements." So perhaps, in their manual communication, some deaf individuals show behaviors equivalent to stuttering.

It is difficult to account for the low incidence of stuttering in the deaf in terms of neurosis or learning theory or as a disorder of motor coordination. One possibility is that the lack of hearing precludes any interference from aberrations or conflicts in feedback from the air-conducted or bone-conducted sound of their voices.

THE DIABETIC

A very low incidence of stuttering in diabetics has also been frequently reported in the literature. West (1943) says, "The thirteenth part of our puzzle is one, the significance of which is particularly obscure, that no diabetic has been reported as stuttering." West speculated that the high blood sugar levels characteristic of diabetics inhibited the minor convulsions of the pyknolepsy which he felt constituted the basis of stuttering. If there were no diabetic stutterers, then such a hypothesis could be seriously considered. Hamre and Emerick (1967) reviewed the literature on pyknolepsy and concluded that West's use of the term and concept was in error. West's belief in the absence of stuttering among diabetics seems to have been based upon a master's thesis by Schuster (1936), in which more than a thousand case histories of diabetes mellitus were examined at the Wisconsin General Hospital at Madison. In all of these histories Schuster found no mention of stuttering and, when he interviewed two staff physicians, they said they had never known a diabetic stutterer. This is hardly impressive evidence. In view of the probability that hospital records of diabetics would not necessarily include a mention of stuttering even if present, the validity of this finding is to say the least, questionable. Later, another master's thesis at the same university was done by Boldon (1955) who questioned a larger number of physicians and did turn up some diabetic stutterers. We personally have examined five diabetic stutterers so we know they do exist. The incidence of stuttering among diabetics as compared to the general population remains a problem for future investigation. Again, a once promising path into the mystery becomes obscured.

INCIDENCE AMONG PSYCHOTICS

In the search for some clues as to the nature of stuttering, the hunt has even been extended into the back wards of mental hospitals. If stuttering is a character neurosis, and if a neurosis is a defense against repressed instinctual urges seeking expression, then once the individual really became psychotic, he should stop stuttering. Or, if he were basically psychotic rather than neurotic, he just should not stutter. So runs the involved reasoning. Accordingly, Barbara (1946) surveyed 7,000 psychotic patients at the Central Islip State Hospital in New York and found an incidence of only 0.28 per cent. This low incidence might be said to lend some mild support for the neurotic theory of stuttering. Pitrelli (1948) found no stutterers among 300 psychotic females though three of them had stuttered prior to the advent of the psychosis. This, he felt, indicated the nature of stuttering as a neurotic defense against psychosis. This meager evidence was evaluated by Freund (1955) in the light of his own survey of another mental institution in which the incidence of stuttering was not lower than that usually found but higher (3.2 per cent). He also showed that the incidence of stuttering among institutionalized neurotics was approximately the same (4 per cent). Among our own successful cases we have never had one stutterer who became psychotic once he became fluent.

IS THE INCIDENCE OF STUTTERING DECLINING?

To one who has worked in the field of stuttering for many years, it appears that the incidence of stuttering has been declining in the last 30 years. Milisen (1963) also holds this opinion. When the author of this text began to practice in 1934, the high schools seemed full of stutterers and there were many adult stutterers to be encountered everywhere. This does not seem to be true today. We still have adult stutterers seeking our services but most of them come from afar. The skeptical may attribute this to the clinical failures of the public school clinicians which cause the stutterer to lose all hope of being helped, and so do not seek it. Sheehan and Martyn (1970) support this view. They found that a group of university students who had previously stuttered but recovered did not attribute that recovery to effective public school therapy. It is quite possible, however, that if the incidence of stuttering has declined it may be due to the marked changes in the attitude of society toward the stutterer, and to the parent and teacher education contributed by the public school clinicians.

Only a few decades ago, stuttering was viewed as a bad, dirty habit to be broken by punishment or by will power. The whole field of rehabilitation had hardly made an impact. Speech therapy has drastically revised these old attitudes and practices. Stuttering is now viewed as a clinical problem. Information regarding prevention and treatment is widely available and so is therapy. All these influences must have had some impact.

Unfortunately, we have little research upon this important matter. Van Horn (1966), who conducted individual screening of all children prior to school entrance, reports that the prevalence percentage of stutterers who were found in Kalamazoo in 1962–1965 had decreased a fourth from those discovered in the same schools using the same screening methods that had been found in 1941–1944. Also we have Black's report (1966) of the percentage of stuttering-in the total caseloads of public school speech therapists in Illinois. In 1950–1951 7.4 per cent of the total caseload in Illinois were stutterers; in 1964–1965 the percentage was only 3.2 per cent. This, of course, does not reflect the prevalence of stuttering in the general population, merely the number of stutterers being enrolled in

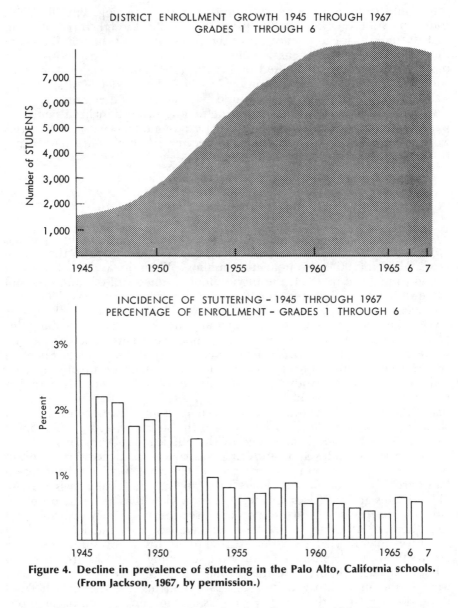

Figure 4. Decline in prevalence of stuttering in the Palo Alto, California schools.
(From Jackson, 1967, by permission.)

speech therapy. Nevertheless, a reduction by one half in 15 years must reflect some sort of change.

Dean and Brown (1977) examined the state records of stutterers enrolled in the public schools between 1964 and 1973 but found no decline in the incidence of stuttering within this time period. Jackson (1967), using a longer time period (Fig. 4) showed a marked decline between 1945 and 1955 but a lesser decline thereafter. Let us hope it will continue.

BIBLIOGRAPHY

ANDREWS, G., AND M. HARRIS. 1964. *The syndrome of stuttering.* London: Heinemann.

ARNOLD, G. E. 1948. *Die traumatischen und konstitutionellen störungen der stimme und sprache.* Vienna: Urban and Schwarzenberg.

ARON, M. 1962. Nature and incidence of stuttering among a Bantu group of school going children. *Journal of Speech and Hearing Disorders* 27: 116–28.

BACHRACH, D. L. 1964. Sex differences in reactions to delayed auditory feedback. *Perceptual Motor Skills* 19: 81–82.

BACKUS, O. 1938. Incidence of stuttering among the deaf. *Annals of Otology, Rhinology and Laryngology* 47: 632–35.

BAR, A. 1968. Investigating stuttering in a special culture. *Journal of Speech and Hearing Disorders* 33: 94–95.

BARBAIX, M. AND R. SNEPPS. 1974. Stammering and therapy: an attempt at a mechanographic study of the facial musculatures of stammerers. *Le Langage et l'homme* 25: 30–34.

BARBARA, D. A. 1946. A psychosomatic approach to the problem of stuttering in psychotics. *American Journal of Psychiatry* 103: 188–95.

BECKER, K. F., N. A. VLASSOVA, N. M. ASATIANI, AND W. HEV. 1977. *Stottern.* Berlin: V.E.B. Verlag Volk and Gesundheit.

BERRY, M. F. AND J. EISENSON. 1956. *Speech disorders.* New York: Appleton-Century-Crofts.

BLACK, M. E. 1966. *Annual Report to Superintendent of Schools, State of Illinois.* Springfield, Ill.

BLOODSTEIN, O. AND M. SMITH. 1954. A study of diagnosis of stuttering with special references to the sex ratio. *Journal of Speech and Hearing Disorders* 19: 459–66.

BLUEMEL, C. S. 1913. *Stammering and cognate defects of speech.* New York: Stechert.

BÖHME, G. 1977. *Das stotter-syndrome: aetiologi, diagnose and therapie.* Bern: Verlag Hans Huber.

BOLDON, A. T. 1955. The coexistence of, and certain relationships between diabetes and stuttering. Masters thesis, University of Wisconsin.

BONFANTI, B. H. AND R. CULATTA. 1977. An analysis of the fluency patterns of institutionalized retarded adults. *Journal of Fluency Disorders* 2: 117–28.

BOOME, E. J. AND M. A. RICHARDSON. 1931. *The nature and treatment of stammering.* London: Methuen.

BRANNON, J. B. 1966. The speech production and spoken language of the deaf. *Language and Speech* 9: 127–36.

BRESTOVICI, B. 1976. Speech of children in elementary school. *Defektologie* 8: 54–60.

BROWN, F. W. 1932. Stuttering: its neurophysiological bases and probable causation. *American Journal of Orthopsychiatry* 2: 363–76.

BRYNGELSON, B. 1938. Prognosis of stuttering. *Journal of Speech Disorders* 3: 121–23.

BURDIN, L. G. 1940. A survey of speech defectives in the Indianapolis public schools. *Journal of Speech Disorders* 5: 247–58.

CABANAS, R. 1954. Some findings in speech and voice therapy among the mentally retarded. *Folia Phoniatrica* 6: 34–37.

CARRIE, W. 1918. Statistik über sprachgebrechliche schulkinder in den Hamburger volkschulen. *Monatsschrift für Ohrenheilkunde* 52: 178–87.

CARSON, C. AND C. E. KANTER. 1945. Incidence of stuttering among white and colored school children. *Southern Speech Journal* 10: 57–59.

CHAPMAN, A. H. 1973. Nature of stuttering in a mentally retarded population. *American Journal of Mental Deficiency* 78: 153–57.

CHRYSANTHIS, K. 1947. Letter to the editor. *Lancet* 252: 270.

COBB, S. AND E. M. COLE. 1939. Stuttering. *Physiological Review* 19: 49–62.

COOPER, E. B. 1972. Recovery from stuttering in a junior and senior high school population. *Journal of Speech and Hearing Disorders* 15: 632–38.

DASKALOV, D. D. 1962. On the problem of basic principles and methods of prevention and treatment of stammering. *Zhurnal Nevropatologii i Psikhiatrii imeni S. S. Korsakova* 53: 1047–52.

DEAN, C. R. AND R. A. BROWN. 1977. A more recent look at the prevalence of stuttering in the United States. *Journal of Fluency Disorders* 2: 157–66.

DE SANTIS, M. 1959. Endocrine research into cases of stammering. *Valsalva* 35: 328–33.

DICKSON, S. 1971. Incipient stuttering and spontaneous remission of stuttered speech. *Journal of Communication Disorders* 4: 99–110.

DOSTALOVA, N. AND T. DOSUZKOV. 1965. Uber die drei hauptformen des neurotischen stotterns. *De Therapie et Loquellae* 1: 273–76.

DUNLAP, K. 1944. Stammering: its nature, etiology and therapy. *Journal of Comparative Psychology* 37: 187–202.

EDSON, S. K. 1964. The incidence of certain types of nonfluencies among a group of institutionalized mongoloid and non-mongoloid children. Masters thesis, University of Kansas.

EISENSON, J. 1966. Observations of the incidence of stuttering in a special culture. *ASHA* 5: 391–94.

FORCHHAMMER, E. 1955. Speech defectives in the schools for the mentally retarded in the Danish isles. *Nordisk Tideskrift for Tale og Stemme* 15: 171–74.

FREUND, H. 1955. Psychosis and stuttering. *Journal of Nervous and Mental Diseases* 122: 161–72.

FRITZELL, B. 1974. The prognosis of stuttering in school children. *Proceedings of the XVI International Congress of Logopedics and Phoniatrics.* Interlaken: Karger, 128–131.

FROESCHELS, E. 1919. Die sprachärztliche therapie in kriege III das stottern. *Monastsschrift für Ohrenheilkunde* 53.

———. 1948. *Twentieth Century Speech and Voice Correction.* New York: Philosophical Library.

GENS, G. W. 1951. The speech pathologist looks at the mentally deficient child. *Training School Bulletin* 48: 19–27.

GILLESPIE, S. K. AND E. B. COOPER. 1973. Prevalence of speech problems in junior and senior high schools. *Journal of Speech and Hearing Research* 16: 739–43.

GIOLAS, T. G. AND D. E. WILLIAMS. 1958. Children's reactions to nonfluencies in adult speech. *Journal of Speech and Hearing Research* 1: 86–93.

GLASNER, P. J. AND D. ROSENTHAL. 1957. Parental diagnosis of stuttering in young children. *Journal of Speech Disorders* 22: 288–95.

GOLDMAN, R. 1965. The effects of cultural patterns on the sex ratio in stuttering. *ASHA* 7: 371.

GOTTSLEBEN, R. H. 1955. The incidence of stuttering in a group of mongoloids. *Training School Bulletin* 51: 209–18.

GRAF, O. I. 1955. Incidence of stuttering among twins. In *Stuttering in Children and Adults*, ed. W. Johnson. Minneapolis: University of Minnesota Press.

HAMRE, C. E. AND M. E. WINGATE. 1967. Pyknolepsy and stuttering. *Quarterly Journal of Speech* 53: 374–77.

HARMS, H. A. AND J. Y. MALONE. 1939. The relationship of hearing acuity to stammering. *Journal of Speech Disorders* 4: 363–70.

HARRISON, H. S. 1947. A study of the speech of sixty institutionalized epileptics. Masters thesis, Louisiana State University.

HIRSCHBERG, J. 1965. Stuttering. *Orvosi Hetilap* 106: 780–84.

HULL F. M. 1969. National speech and hearing survey—a preliminary report. Convention address, ASHA.

―――― AND R. J. TIMMONS. 1969. *National Speech and Hearing Survey*. U. S. Office of Education, Project No. 5-0978; Grant No. 32-15-0050-5010.

HUNT, J. 1967. *Stammering and stuttering: their nature and treatment*. Reprinted, New York: Hafner.

JACKSON, R. M. 1967. Stuttering report. Convention address, California Speech and Hearing Association.

JAMESON, A. M. 1955. Stammering in children. *Speech* (London) 19: 60–67.

JOHNSON, W. 1959. *The Onset of Stuttering*. Minneapolis: University of Minnesota Press.

JONES, E. 1959. *Free Associations: Memoirs of a Psychoanalyst*. New York: Basic Books.

KAMIYAMA, A. 1957. *Handbook for the study of stuttering*. Tokyo: Kongo-Shupan.

KARLIN, I. W. 1947. Psychosomatic theory of stuttering. *Journal of Speech Disorders* 12: 319–22.

KATSOVAKAIA, I. 1960. The problem of children's stuttering. *Proceedings Third Session Institute of Defektologi*: 13334.

KEANE, V. C. 1970. An investigation of disfluent speech behavior in Down's syndrome. Masters thesis, University of Oregon.

KIDD, K. K. 1980. Genetic models of stuttering. *Journal of Fluency Disorders* 5: 187–202.

――――. 1977. A genetic perspective on stuttering. *Journal of Fluency Disorders* 2: 259–69.

――――, J. R. KIDD AND M. A. RECORDS. 1978. The possible causes of the sex ratio in stuttering and its implications. *Journal of Fluency Disorders* 3: 13–23.

KINGDON-WARD, W. 1941. *Stammering*. London: Hamilton.

KOOLS, J. A. AND J. D. BERRYMAN. 1971. Differences in disfluency behavior between male and female nonstuttering children. *Journal of Speech and Hearing Research* 14: 125–31.

LEMERT, E. M. 1953. Some Indians who stutter. *Journal of Speech and Hearing Disorders* 18: 168–74.

――――. 1962. Stuttering and social structure in two pacific societies. *Journal of Speech and Hearing Disorders* 27: 3–10.

LENNON, E. J. 1962. *Le bégaiement: therapeutiques modernes*. Paris: Dion and Cie.

LERMAN, J. W., G. R. POWERS, AND S. RIGRODSKY. 1965. Stuttering patterns observed in a sample of mentally retarded individuals. *Training School Bulletin* 62: 27–32.

LOUTTIT, C. M. AND E. C. HALLS. 1936. Survey of speech defects among public school children of Indiana. *Journal of Speech Disorders* 1: 73–80.

MAHAFFEY, R. B. AND C. STROMSTA. 1965. The effects of auditory feedback as a function of frequency, intensity, time and sex. *De Therapia Vocis et Loquellae* 2: 233–35.

MARTYN, M. M. AND J. SHEEHAN. 1968. Onset of stuttering and recovery. *Behavior Research and Therapy* 6: 295–307.

MCALLISTER, A. M. 1937. *Clinical Studies in Speech Pathology*. London: U. London Press.

MCCALLIEN, C. 1956. Problems of speech defect in the Accra district. *Speech* (London) 20: 15–18.

MCCARTHY, D. 1954. Language disorders and parent-child relationships. *Journal of Speech and Hearing Disorders* 19: 514–23.

MCDOWELL, E. 1928. *Educational and emotional adjustment of stuttering children*. Columbia University Teachers College Contributions to Education, No. 314.

MCMAHON, E. M. 1969. *Report of the three year survey to assess speech and hearing needs in British Columbia, 1962–1964*.

METRAUX, R. W. 1950. Speech profiles of the pre-school child. *Journal of Speech Disorders* 15: 33–36.

MEYER, B. C. 1945. Psychosomatic aspects of stuttering. *Journal of Nervous and Mental Diseases* 101: 127–57.

MILISEN, R. 1963. The public schools in a site for speech and hearing. *Speech Teacher* 12: 1–9.

———— AND W. JOHNSON. 1936. A comparative study of stutterers, former stutterers and normal speakers whose handedness has been changed. *Archives Speech* 1: 61–86.

MILLS, A. AND H. STREIT. 1942. Report of a speech survey in Holyoke, Mass. *Journal of Speech Disorders* 7: 161–67.

MORGENSTERN, J. J. 1956. Socio-economic factors in stuttering. *Journal of Speech and Hearing Disorders* 21: 25–33.

MORLEY, D. E. 1952. A ten year survey of speech disorders among university students. *Journal of Speech Disorders* 17: 25–31.

MORLEY, M. 1957. *The development and disorders of speech in childhood*. Edinburgh: Livingstone.

MUSSAFIA, M. 1964. The role of heredity in language disorders. *Folia Phoniatrica* 16: 228–38.

MYSAK, E. D. 1959. Diagnosis of stuttering as made by adolescent boys and girls. *Journal of Speech and Hearing Disorders* 24: 29–33.

NEELEY, M. M. 1960. An investigation of the incidence of stuttering among elementary school children in the parochial schools of Orleans parish. Masters thesis, Tulane University.

NELSON, S. E., N. HUNTER, AND M. WALTER. 1945. Stuttering in twin types. *Journal of Speech Disorders* 10: 335–43.

OTTO, F. M. AND C. YAIRI. 1974. Speech disfluencies in Down's syndrome and in normally intelligent subjects. *Journal of Fluency Disorders* 1: 26–32.

OZAWA, Y. 1960. Studies of misarticulation in Wakayama district. *Journal of Medicine: University of Osaka* 5: 319.

PALMER, M. AND C. OSBORN. 1938. One thousand consecutive cases of speech defects. *Transactions Kansas Academy of Science* 41: 16–27.

PANELLI, C. A., S. C. McFALANE, AND K. G. SHIPLEY. 1978. Implications of evaluating and intervening wth incipient stutterers. *Journal of Fluency Disorders* 3: 41–50.

PERKINS, E. 1977. *Speech pathology: an applied behavioral science.* St. Louis: C. V. Mosby.

PETKOV, D. AND I. IOSITOV. 1960. Our experience in treatment of stuttering in a speech rehabilitation colony. *Zhurnal Neuropatologii e Psychiatrii imeni S. S. Korsakova* 11: 903–4.

PETRAK, H. 1977. Zur Umerziehung Stotternden Kinder Innerhalb des Logogadischen Prozesses an einer Sprachheilschule. In *Stottern,* eds. Becker, K. P., Vlassova, N. A., N. M. Asatiani, L. I. Beljakova and W. Rey. V. E. B. Verlag Volkund Gesundheit.

PITRELLI, F. R. 1948. Psychosomatic and Rorschach aspects of stuttering. *Psychiatric Quarterly* 22: 176–94.

PREUS, A. 1973. Stuttering in Down's syndrome. In *Neurolinguistic Approaches to Stuttering,* eds. Y. LeBrun and R. Hoops. The Hague: Mouton.

PRICHETT, M. 1966. The role of the east St. Louis schools: a study of the effectiveness of the multi-approach in stuttering therapy. *Proceedings Illinois Speech Association,* November, 1966.

ROOT, A. R. 1925. A survey of speech defectives in the public elementary schools of South Dakota. *Elementary School Journal* 26: 531–41.

RUTHERFORD, B. 1946. A comparative study of loudness, pitch, rate, rhythm and quality of the speech of children handicapped by cerebral palsy. *Journal of Speech Disorders* 9: 263–71.

——. 1938. Speech reeducation for the birth injured. *Journal of Speech Disorders* 3: 199–206.

SCHAEFFER, M. L. AND W. M. SHEARER. 1968. A survey of mentally retarded stutterers. *Mental Retardation* 6: 44–5.

SCHINDLER, M. D. 1955. The educational adjustments of stuttering and nonstuttering children. In *Stuttering in Children and Adults,* ed. W. Johnson. Minneapolis: University of Minnesota Press.

SCHLANGER, B. B. 1953. Speech examination of a group of institutionalized mentally handicapped children. *Journal of Speech and Hearing Disorders* 18: 339–49.

—— AND R. H. GOTTSLEBEN. 1957. Analysis of speech defects among the institutionalized mentally retarded. *Journal of Speech and Hearing Disorders* 22: 98–103.

SCHREIBER, W. 1955. Die Medizin in Dienst der Sprachheilfürsorge. *Psychological Abstracts* 29: 255 (abstract).

SCHUBERT, O. W. 1966. The incidence rate of stuttering in a matched group of institutionalized mentally retarded. Convention address, American Association on Mental Deficiency, Chicago.

SCHUELL, H. 1946–47. Sex differences in relation to stuttering. *Journal of Speech Disorders* 11 (1946), 277–98; 12 (1947), 23–38.

SCHUSTER, G. 1936.   Diabetes mellitus and epilepsy viewed from the standpoint of dysphemia. Masters thesis, University of Wisconsin.

SEEMAN, M. 1959.   *Sprachstörungen bei Kindern.* Marhold: Halle-Saale.

SHAMES, G. H. AND H. L. BEAMS. 1956.   Incidence of stuttering in older age groups. *Journal of Speech and Hearing Disorders* 21: 313–16.

SHEARER, W. M. AND J. D. WILLIAMS. 1965.   Self-recovery from stuttering. *Journal of Speech and Hearing Disorders* 30: 288–90.

SHEEHAN, J. AND M. M. MARTYN. 1967.   Spontaneous recovery from stuttering. *Journal of Speech and Hearing Research* 10: 121–35.

———. 1970.   Stuttering and its disappearance. *Journal of Speech and Hearing Research* 13: 379–89.

———, AND K. L. KILBURN. 1968.   Speech disorders in retardation. *American Journal of Mental Deficiency* 73: 251–56.

SILVERMAN, F. H. AND E. M. SILVERMAN. 1972.   Stutter-like behavior in the manual communication of the deaf. *Perceptual and Motor Skills* 33: 45–6.

STASSI, J. 1961.   Disfluency of normal speakers and reinforcement. *Journal of Speech and Hearing Research* 4: 358–61.

STERNBERG, M. L. 1946.   Auditory factors in stuttering. Masters thesis, State University of Iowa.

STEWART, J. L. 1960.   The problem of stuttering in certain North American Indian societies. *Journal of Speech and Hearing Disorders,* Monograph Supplement No. 6: 1–87.

TOYODA, B. 1959.   A statistical report. *Clinical Paediatrica* 12: 788.

VAN HORN, H. 1966.   Comparative incidence of stuttering after twenty years. *Western Michigan University Journal of Speech Therapy* 3: 6–7.

VOELKER, C. H. 1944.   A preliminary investigation for a normative study of fluency: a critical index to the severity of stuttering. *American Journal of Orthopsychiatry* 14: 285–94.

———. 1943.   Incidence of pathologic speech behavior in the general American population. *Archives of Otolaryngology* 38: 113–21.

———. 1942.   On the semantic aspects of stuttering in nonstutterers. *Quarterly Journal of Speech* 28: 78–80.

VOELKER, E. AND C. VOELKER. 1937.   Spasmophemia in dyslalia cophotica—case report. *Annals of Otology, Rhinology and Laryngology.*

WADDLE, E. 1934.   A comparison of speech defectives among colored and white children. Masters thesis, University of Iowa.

WALLEN, V. 1961.   Primary stuttering in a 28-year-old adult. *Journal of Speech and Hearing Disorders* 26: 394–95.

WATZL, I. 1924.   Statistiches Erhebungen über das Vorkommen von Sprachstörungen in den Wiener Schulen. *Proceedings First International Congress of Logopedics and Phoniatrics,* Vienna.

WEISS, D. A. 1964.   *Cluttering.* Englewood Cliffs, N.J.: Prentice-Hall.

WEPMAN, J. M. 1939.   Familial incidence in stammering. *Journal of Speech Disorders* 4: 199–204.

WEST, R. 1958.   An agnostic's speculations about stuttering. In *Stuttering: A Symposium.* New York: Harper.

———. 1943.   The pathology of stuttering. *Nervous Child* 2: 96–106.

WEST, R., S. NELSON, AND M. BERRY. 1939.   The heredity of stuttering. *Quarterly Journal of Speech* 25: 23–30.

WHITE HOUSE CONFERENCE ON CHILD HEALTH AND PROTECTION. 1931.   Section 3: *Special Education: The Handicapped and the Gifted.* New York: Century.

WILLIAMS, C. Y. 1964.   Parental attitudes and maternal rejection of stuttering children among southern negroes. Masters thesis, Ohio University.

WILLIAMS, D., F. SILVERMAN, AND J. KOOLS. 1968.   Disfluency behavior of elementary school stutterers and nonstutterers. *Journal of Speech and Hearing Research* 11: 622–30.

WINGATE, M. E. 1964.   Recovery from stuttering. *Journal of Speech and Hearing Disorders* 29: 312–21.

YOUNG, M. A. 1975. Onset, prevalence and recovery from stuttering. *Journal of Speech and Hearing Disorders* 40: 49–58.

ZISK, P. K. AND J. BIALER. 1967.   Speech and language problems in mongolism: a review of the literature. *Journal of Speech and Hearing Disorders* 32: 228–41.

THE ONSET
OF STUTTERING

4

In the ten years since this text was first published, very little new information about the onset of stuttering has become available, and this we have included. It is very difficult to procure valid information about when stuttering begins or its nature at its incipience. Most parents are vague in their accounts, and the self reports of stutterers often are either hearsay or reflect only an early experience in which they became highly aware of their difficulty. Again we meet the problem of the definition of stuttering as behavior and as a disorder. Many laymen, as Young (1976) has pointed out, find it difficult to distinguish between stuttering and normal disfluency. Finally, any testimony about onset by parents or by the stutterer himself is usually given long after the event and may therefore be suspect. Nevertheless, we shall summarize what is known about the onset of stuttering.

AGE OF ONSET

One of the few solid bits of information we have about stuttering is that it usually begins in childhood. Very rarely we do find a person whose disorder clearly began during adulthood, although when we do there is always some suspicion or even evidence to indicate that the adult stuttering was a recurrence of a problem which had shown itself much earlier in the person's life. Those who view stuttering merely as a neurosis find this early onset rather difficult to explain. Neuroses may begin at any age, but most of them first show themselves later than the preschool years. With great consistency, stuttering begins early in the person's life.

Some of the evidence for this belief comes from clinical observations and surveys and some from research. While we always prefer the latter to the former, the unanimity of statements made by clinicians from many different countries has some value. We will review just a few of these.

Japanese writers report the following onset data. Otsuki (1958): 55 per cent of 331 stutterers began before five years, 93 per cent before ten years; Shiraiwa (1958): 70 per cent of 70 stutterers began before age six; Fujita (1964): 40 percent of 80 stutterers began between ages two and three years. Other Japanese writers give similar results: Takagi (1962): most stutterers begin at two and three years, a few after six years; Toyoda (1967): onset usually between two and three years.

Ohashi (1976) provides the following summary of the reported onset of stuttering in 44 Japanese children referred to the speech clinic of the Kyoto University Hospital:

Age of Onset:	2	3	4	5	6	7	8	9	10	11	12
No. of Cases:	19	12	6	4	0	1	2	0	0	0	0

In Africa, McCallien (1956) reports that 66 per cent of 138 children began to stutter prior to school entrance. Aron (1958) interviewed parents of African and European school children and found the average age of onset to be three years, four months, for the African, and four years, ten months, for the European stutterers.

In France, de Ajuriaguerra (1958) and his co-workers found 51 cases with onset prior to seven years and 33 cases who began later than this time. Radol'skii (1965) reports in a Russian publication that of 125 stuttering children, stuttering first appeared in 116 of them between the ages of two through five, and only in nine did it have a later onset. Seeman (1959) found that 66 per cent of the first signs of stuttering occurred in children between the ages of three through six at the time the child is mastering sentence structuring. Fritzell (1963) found that the disorder usually begins between two through four years in Sweden. Jameson (1955) intensively studied 69 English children and found that most had begun to stutter before age four. Two of the more extensive studies are by Daskalov (1962) in Bulgaria and by Hirschberg (1965) in Hungary. Daskalov gives this data on age of onset for 655 stutterers: two years—13 per cent; four years—13 per cent; five years—13 per cent; six years—9 per cent; seven years—14 per cent; eight years—12 per cent; nine years—3 per cent; ten years—1 per cent; 11 years—1.5 per cent; 12 years—2 per cent; 13 years—2 per cent. Hirschberg's data (p. 782) may be best presented in the form of a graph. See Figure 5.

From Norway we have the ages of onset of stuttering for 98 stutterers: 37 began to stutter between the ages of 2–3 years; 35 between 4–5; 13 between 6–7; 9 between 8–9 and the remaining 4 after ten years of age (Preus, 1981).

In Great Britain, the longitudinal studies reported by Morley (1957) and by Andrews and Harris (1964) provide us with some of our best information concerning the age of onset. The Andrews and Harris'

Age of the Stutterers at Onset

Figure 5. Age of stutterers at onset. (From Hirschberg, 1965.)

findings may be summarized as follows:

Age in years:	3	4	5	6	7	8	9
Number of children:							
Morley (1957)	1	20	12	2	2	—	—
Andrews and Harris (1964)	6	34	15	11	10	3	1

Morley also reports ages of onset for another population of 249 stutterers (p. 348) in which the same pattern of early onset was demonstrated.

The two major American investigations of the onset of stuttering were reported by Johnson (1959) and by Darley (1955), both based on intensive interviewing of parents. Earlier, Johnson (1955) found that the median age of onset was three years for 46 children. He writes:

> It is to be underscored perhaps that in three-fourths of the cases the difficulty began at or before the age of three years, two months, and that in half the cases it began sometime within an eight-months period between the ages of two years, six months, and three years, two months. The modal age of onset found in this study is somewhat earlier than that given by most writers in the field. The most important reason for the discrepancy would appear to be the fact that in the present study the case histories were obtained relatively soon after onset while memories were presumably comparatively fresh (p. 63).

Darley (1955) interviewed the mothers and fathers of his 50 stuttering children separately, hoping thereby to have some check on the validity of the information procured. The median age of onset reported by the mothers was three years, seven months (onset range = 1 yr. 3 mos.–9 yrs.); and by the fathers (onset range: 18–132 months); the median age of reported onset was four years, seven months.

While this discrepancy in parental reports is hardly sufficient to make us doubt the overwhelming consensus that most stuttering begins in the preschool years, it should also make us very cautious in evaluating a reported age of onset when it is provided by an adult stutterer. Darley's and Johnson's subjects were the parents of stutterers, not the stutterers themselves, and the interviewing was done only a relatively short time after the onset of stuttering had occurred. Despite this, the parental replies were often vague and very inconsistent. Aron (1958) compared the age of onset reported by the stutterers themselves with what the stutterers said their parents had told them and with the parents' actual statements. She found huge discrepancies. Most importantly, the stutterers themselves tended to place the age of onset much later than the parents did. We must remember this when considering the validity of onset data given in such questionnaire studies as that by Martyn and Sheehan (1968) in which adult college stutterers and former stutterers served as the subjects. The difficulty of recall, the lack of precise definition, the absence of written records, all these factors militate against placing complete confidence in such testimony.

Even more susceptible to error are parental answers to questionnaires administered long after the reported onset. They forget, they guess, they confuse normal disfluency with stuttering. Discounting for probable error, about the only reasonable conclusion is that stuttering has its usual onset at about the age of three and that perhaps those who recover spontaneously start to stutter a bit later than those who continue.

TIME LAPSE BETWEEN ONSET OF SPEECH AND ONSET OF STUTTERING

In what proportion of stutterers does the onset of stuttering coincide with the onset of speech? This question is of more than casual importance. For example, Bluemel (1957) distinguished between *stuttering* as "unorganized speech" and *stammering* as "disorganized speech." Are there different kinds of stutterers—those who never attained normal fluency and those who once had it but lost it? Are the so-called "recovered stutterers" those who are recovering or convalescing from an episode of stuttering or are they discovering a fluency they never possessed? Should therapy be structured around learning or unlearning? If stuttering has a strong organic component, should not the disorder become evident as soon as connected speech appears? These are just a few of the reasons why we need to know more about the relationship between the onset of speech and the onset of stuttering.

Unfortunately our data on this important matter leave much to be desired, again primarily because of the difficulty in getting reliable information concerning the onset of both speech and stuttering. Johnson (1955) writes:

> Because of differences among parents in their extensional definitions of "word" and "sentence" and because of parental pride, as well as the relative difficulty of recall in the absence of written records, information of this kind is difficult to obtain with a high degree of precision by the interview method. We simply recognized the operation of these factors and did what we could to counteract their influence by careful interviewing (pp. 47–48).

Darley and Winitz (1961), in their extensive review of the literature concerning age of first words, have added:

> In summary, it would seem that the use of operational definitions of the first word have been so consistently different from investigator to investigator as to

be an important source of error in the reported age of appearance of the first word. Coupled with it are other sources of error: the inadequacy of parental records; the fallibility of parents' memory; parents' "wishful hearing," "optimism," and pride; and the infrequency and meagerness of sampling of infants' vocalizations by observers other than parents (p. 283).

We thus have two major sources of error: the dating of stuttering onset and the dating of speech onset. Moreover, if the onset of speech is considered to occur not with the first words but instead with the first connected speech, even more vagueness and inaccuracy in parental testimony is to be expected. All we can do, therefore, is to cite what research we do possess and keep our fingers crossed in interpreting it.

Most of the meager information we have deals with the percentages of stutterers who reportedly have stuttered since the beginning of speech. Thus Berry (1938) found that 72 per cent of 500 stutterers began to stutter within the first year after onset of speech. Aron (1958) interviewed parents of 16 stuttering children and found nine of them who said the stuttering had coincided with the first speech. Of Morley's (1957) 249 stutterers, 50 claimed never to have had a period entirely free from stuttering. Andrews and Harris (1964) showed that the severe stutterers (at age ten) in general had an earlier onset of stuttering than milder stutterers. At that age, only nine per cent of the mild stutterers had stuttered since the beginning of speech while 33 per cent of the severe stutterers had always stuttered. Most of the stutterers in their population, however, had experienced a period of fluent speech before beginning to stutter.

The Iowa studies also demonstrate that the stuttering appeared only after normal fluency had been achieved. Johnson (1955) gives his findings as follows:

> If we consider the ages at which first words were spoken, the extent of the interval between first spoken words and the onset of stuttering ranged from six months to eight years. The median interval was 23 months, the 25th percentile fell at 17 months, and the 75th percentile at 32 months. The extent of the interval between the first speaking of sentences and the onset of stuttering ranged from minus ten months to plus seven years and seven months (91 months). That is, in one case the onset of stuttering was reported to have occurred ten months before the child began to speak sentences. In two other cases the onset of stuttering occurred four months and two months, respectively, before sentences were spoken. In all other cases the speaking of sentences occurred before the child was regarded as a stutterer. The median interval was 13 months, the 25th percentile fell at seven months, and the 75th percentile at 24 months (p. 63).

Darley (1955) also provides data on the interval between the age of first speaking sentences and the onset of stuttering. Using the mothers' estimates, he found that the interval ranged from a minus twelve months (that is, that the child stuttered when in the one-word sentence stage) to 66 months, with a median interval of one and a half years between the first sentences and the first stutterings. Darley points up the significance of this finding in the following words:

> A theory of stuttering that posits any type of constitutional difference which somehow predisposes certain children to stutter must account for the apparently normal speech behavior manifested during this interval (p. 135).

We must remember, however, that other research has shown that some children do begin to stutter from the onset of consecutive speech or at least that the diagnosis was made at that time. Stuttering behaviors— temporally disrupted words—may occur very early but not be diagnosed as a disorder until later.

We have analyzed the case records of 114 children whom we saw personally and whose parents we interviewed within six months after the time of this diagnosis. Five of these we saw on the day of onset and nine within a week, and we felt fairly certain that the diagnosis was justified. Of the 61 cases, all were seen within three weeks after onset. The age-range of onset was from two years, one month to nine years, three months; the median age of onset was three years, one month.

IS THE ONSET OF STUTTERING SUDDEN OR GRADUAL?

This is a very difficult question to answer, posing as it does the problem of definition and differential diagnosis from normal disfluency. As we shall see, there are many anecdotal accounts and case reports of stuttering occurring very suddenly after a specific incident, but a search of the literature and a survey of our own cases indicates that in the large majority of instances, stuttering begins gradually. Levina (1968) states:

> Our [Russian] studies have confirmed that stammering usually begins at ages three to four. In almost all cases of stammering among children it sets in gradually, beginning with slightly interrupted speech similar to the physiological difficulties accompanying the transition to phraseological speech (p. 28).

De Ajuriaguerra (1958) and his colleagues intensively studied 51 stutterers in France, reporting that 44 of them showed a gradual onset while 15 others showed a sudden one. Three of the latter began to stutter after a period of mutism. Morley (1957) found a sudden onset in only three of 37 children in her longitudinal research. She says:

> In most of the children, however, the onset was gradual, beginning with a slight degree of occasional hesitant speech: and the age of onset, as reported to us, is probably the age at which the mother first became aware of the child's difficulty. Many more children than the 37 mentioned may have passed through a period of hesitant speech, accepted by the mother as "a normal and transient stage in speech development," (pp. 41–42).

Preus (1981) reports that 76 per cent of his 98 Norwegian stutterers were said to have begun to stutter gradually and the rest suddenly. In this country, Berlin (1954) found that 69 per cent of his subjects showed a gradual onset. All these findings about the gradual onset of stuttering are difficult to evaluate. How gradually does any parent become aware that his or her child is having difficulty speaking? Parents look back and remember that their child had perhaps shown other broken words at one time or another, that he had repeated syllables and spoken "stutteringly" on occasion. Perhaps this is what they mean when they say the disorder developed gradually. The diagnosis itself probably always begins with a sentence such as this "Isn't Johnny beginning to stutter?" Then there follows a period of observation and checking until negation or confirmation is achieved. Since this too takes time, the impression is gained that the disorder is developing gradually when perhaps it is only the diagnosis which is gradual.

In this discussion we are not opposing the idea that stuttering behaviors probably show a gradual increase in frequency, duration, and a number of other significant features until they evoke a diagnosis of disorder. We think that this is what usually happens, though not in all cases. We are merely saying that there is a built-in bias in favor of the concept of gradual onset and that this bias must be considered in any theory which bases itself partly upon this matter. Bloodstein, Alper, and Zisk (1965), for example, hold that stuttering is an exacerbation and outgrowth of normal non-fluency. If the onset of stuttering is universally gradual in nature, this should support their position. Also, if there are different types of stutterers, perhaps those whose stuttering started very suddenly (and we are pretty sure that some of them do have this sort of onset) comprise a different subpopulation within the syndrome. Again we need more and better research bearing directly on this facet of the problem. In our own observations of 114 children whom we personally were able to see within six months of reported onset, we found that in only 11 of these individuals were we fairly certain that the stuttering occurred very suddenly. One of them was the author's own daughter.

THE ONSET OF STUTTERING IN ADULTS

Although, as we have seen, the onset of stuttering in adulthood is comparatively rare, it does seem to occur occasionally, and when it does it appears suddenly. The literature is not extensive, and much of it consists of general observations such as the following one from Freund (1966):

> Hysterical stuttering tends to have its onset later in life than the other types. It may occur in adulthood. Bizarre and hysterical forms of stuttering were observed by us and others after shell shock, head trauma, or the first parachute descents. It tends to begin suddenly rather than gradually, and these stutterers or their parents report that it began during or following trauma or cumulative stress. Histories of complete mutism as the initiating feature are not uncommon (pp. 139–40).

All of the adults who suddenly develop stuttering behaviors, however, are not hysterics. Glaser (1936) reports the onset of stuttering after injections of epinephrine were used subsequent to removal of ovaries. Eisenson (1947) and many other authors mention stuttering resulting from strokes. Head injuries, war-time or otherwise, have produced many accounts in which stuttering followed the trauma as has been reported by Kingdon-Ward (1941), Fahy, Irving, and Millac (1967) and Peacher and Harris (1946). Mochizuki (1962) tells of two adult men, aged 25 and 56, who developed stuttering as a result of the great shock caused by the atomic bomb at Hiroshima. Hirschfield (1916) found frequent instances of sudden onset of stuttering following shell explosions. Froeschels (1917) described in detail a case study of a traumatic war stutterer who began with clonic repetitions of syllables then progressed to tonic prolongations as he endeavored to cope with his frustration. In another publication, Froeschels (1916) declares that it is possible to tell the difference between traumatic and developmental stuttering by an analysis of the symptoms. Traumatic stutterers do not show starters or breathing abnormalities or inappropriate speech postures; developmental stutterers do. Wallen (1961) described an adult stutterer whose speech remained repetitive:

> He first came to the attention of the medical staff when he reported in for "sick call" one morning. He was visibly disturbed—trembling, crying, and stuttering severely. . . He stated that he had been overworking for several months, having little time to spend with his family.
>
> On admission to the hospital his speech was characterized by rapid repetitions of initial syllables of words and prolongations of vowels, especially the vowel /æ/. The disfluency was pronounced at the beginning of sentences and tapered to fluency at the end.
>
> Testing indicated that he was basically a passive-dependent person with introversion tendencies who used repression and withdrawal as primary ego defense mechanisms.
>
> Several days later [after his admittance to the hospital] the acute signs of trembling, crying, and stuttering abated and disappeared. It was noted that the patient had a mild tendency to stutter automatically and without any evidence of anxiety. He would say, for example, "I-I-I didn't like the long hours. It looks like—looks like I'll be here for a while, I never minded the re-re-re-responsibility." He denied ever being aware of any speech problem until his present hospitalization (p. 394).

As we remarked earlier, one must evaluate such accounts of adult onset of stuttering with some caution. When carefully investigated, some of them turned out to be interiorized stutterers who, under great stress, could no longer hide their disorder. Others were stutterers in their youth who recovered, and the adult onset often has all the features characteristic of ordinary relapse. Klinger (1963) reported three cases of adult onset, all of whom "showed psychiatric or neurologic signs." However, later on he found that although all three men had stated that they had not had any history of stuttering prior to examination, one of them turned out to have the notation of "speech defect" on his Army induction records and another turned out to be a "pathological liar" (Klinger, 1966). The third case was well documented and the onset of stuttering at 43 years of age was evidently genuine. We have gone over our own case records and have found seven individuals who we are fairly certain did develop their stuttering for the first time in adulthood. Three of these were highly neurotic, one was psychotic, and the other three began to stutter suddenly and severely after head injuries. Though there was no sign of aphasia in the latter three cases, all had experienced mutism for some hours after regaining consciousness. We also had 17 other cases who reported adult onset of the disorder but for whom we were able to find earlier evidence of stuttering in their childhood. It seems surprising to us that more adult neurotics do not assume the symptomatic picture of stuttering. Stuttering is highly visible; it is easily simulated; it should serve as an excellent defense against a wide variety of intolerable realities; it can beget sympathetic consideration as well as penalty; it has its secondary gains. If it is a neurosis, why then does it appear so rarely in adulthood?

SPEECH CHARACTERISTICS AT ONSET

How do children first begin to stutter? What kind of speech behaviors do they show at the time when parents first decide that a child is having an abnormal amount of disrupted fluency? What is the child doing that impels parents to diagnose stuttering? The answers to these questions are vitally important to most theories. An impressive amount of opinion— and a little research—indicates that usually the first sign of the disorder to be diagnosed as stuttering is an excessive amount of repetitive speech, primarily of repeated syllables. Less commonly, but also of diagnostic importance, are the prolongations of silent articulatory postures (blockages) or of voiced sounds.

Hoepfner (1911) was one of the first authors to describe syllabic repetitions as the earliest features of stuttering. He attributed them to some neurological deficit in the organization of the motor sequencing of words. Froeschels, in a long series of publications in both German and English, also insisted that the first signs of stuttering at onset consisted of iterations (syllable and word repetitions.) Unlike Hoepfner, Froeschels viewed these repetitions as a normal phase of speech development due mainly to wordfinding difficulties under communicative stress. He writes:

> The opinion that frequent iterations are the usual start of stuttering is based upon statistics on 800 cases. They consisted partly of patients which when seen by the writer did not show any signs of stuttering other than iterations, and partly of cases with other signs of stuttering whose case history revealed that the first signs of speech trouble were exclusively word- or syllable-repetitions. In order to avoid any suggestive question, the patients and/or their parents were not asked what the signs were. Only if a description of the initial state was given spontaneously was it considered a reliable scientific fact. These spontaneously delivered reports described *without a single exception iterations as the first sign of the speech trouble* (Froeschels, 1952, p. 221).

In another publication, Froeschels (1943) said that in 700 stutterers he had only found one case with a "tonic" beginning, that is, where it began with a tensed fixation or prolongation although he mentions that H. Gutzmann, Jr., had claimed that occasionally the first sign of stuttering was tonic (with pressure) rather than repetitive. Many of the statements in the literature referring to the type of stuttering behavior at onset are just such statements so that their validity is difficult to assess.

In Wendell Johnson's (1959) monumental study of the onset of stuttering, the majority of the children labeled as stutterers by their parents showed a preponderance of simple easy repetitions but 35 per cent also showed some evidence of tension. Martyn and Sheehan (1968) concluded from their retrospective research that stuttering tended to begin with syllable repetitions in those who later recovered whereas those whose stuttering began with complete stoppages continued to stutter. This was corroborated by Dickson (1971).

CASE STUDIES

We also have a fair number of individual case reports such as those by Wyatt (1969), Solomon (1933), Gondaira (1960) and Schmeer (1966). In each of these reports, one child who had begun to stutter was examined and studied intensively very soon after onset. We have read most of these case reports and find it difficult, even in the best of them, to do the kind of differential diagnosis outlined in a preceding chapter. To provide a sample, let us give our translation from the German of Schmeer's account.

> On January 28th, 1965, Andreas was aged 4 years and 4 months. As usual, once a week that winter, he was fetched from kindergarten which he had attended since the end of May, 1964, by his grandmother with whom he was to have dinner, spend the afternoon and night, and from where he would return to kindergarten the next morning.
>
> The grandmother phoned me that evening and told me that Andreas had started repeating the initial syllables of his words when speaking. When she had bathed him he had been very excited and had threatened to lock her up in a prison and shoot her with a gun: Bang! Bang! etc. . . . She had never seen the child like this before; he had always been quite well behaved and responsive to her attempts to teach him good manners. When the next day Andreas was fetched from the kindergarten by his mother, he stuttered quite obviously, repeating his initial syllables as many as 16 times. I was alarmed because I feared that Andreas would develop the same speech impediment affecting his father and three other relatives on his father's side . . . (p. 46).

These detailed case reports, of course, should not be ignored. They are a far cry from such casual observations as Fogerty's (1930): "A tramp looked in the window and frightened the twins. One began to stammer three weeks later" or Greene's (1924): "One child began to stutter at the sudden opening of an automatic umbrella; another when he fell off the sofa on his head." The better case reports are very detailed and careful observations and in some instances are those of the author's own child as in the case of Nana reported by the speech pathologist Wyatt (1969). In this sense they are probably more valid than data procured by interviewing parents, especially when the questioning is done months after onset. Unfortunately, the reports still lack enough analytical precision in description to enable us to be certain just what speech behaviors did occur. Generally, however, they indicate that the main feature of the speech at stuttering onset seems to be the presence of an excessive number of syllabic repetitions. Wyatt describes it thusly:

> These compulsive repetitions must be differentiated clearly from developmental repetitions. The linguistic units repeated under the influence of frustration or anxiety are no longer representative of the child's normal stage of language development; they are different in kind from developmental repetitions. Compulsive repetitions do not serve as building blocks in the construction of larger syntactic units. The child is no longer able to shift freely back and forth between simpler and more advanced language patterns. An example of compulsive repetition is *I-I-I wa-wa-want to, to, to, th-th-throw the c-c-clay away* (p. 87).

Not all the authors of these anecdotal studies of the onset of stuttering report this feature of compulsivity, but most of those that we have examined mention frequent syllabic repetitions, usually with many of them occurring in the same word.

INTERVIEW DATA

Taylor (1937) compiled the data procured by 12 interviewers of parents of 47 children who had begun to stutter a few weeks or months before. The interviewers had also observed the children speaking. Of the 47 children, 85 per cent exhibited only repetitions at onset; 6 per cent had sound stoppages, and 2 per cent showed prolongations. Also, of the total number, 8 per cent showed some forcings and struggle, 6 per cent accompanied their stuttering with abnormal co-movements of head and limbs, and 6 per cent seemed to have been aware of the difficulty immediately.

The most extensive interview studies of the nature of stuttering at onset were performed by Johnson (1955, 1959) and his students. These have been quoted often as supporting the proposition that the kind of speech shown by stutterers at onset is indistinguishable from normal disfluency, a belief which Johnson sought to foster since it supported his semantogenic theory. For example, he repeatedly (and, in our opinion, unjustifiably) lumped together repetitions of phrases and whole words with the syllabic repetitions to conclude that "the same kinds of nonfluency were reported" by the parents of stutterers and nonstutterers. Nevertheless, when these studies are rigorously examined, as they have been both by us and by McDearmon (1968), they show clearly that *syllabic* repetitions in the main and, to a less extent, prolongations of sounds, were the dominating features which distinguished the behaviors diagnosed by parents of stutterers as stutterings from those noticed by parents of nonstuttering children as being normal nonfluencies. Tucked away in Johnson's formidable monograph (p. 229) is his own recognition of this finding:

> There were interesting group differences with reference to the various kinds of repetition. Sound or syllable repetitions were reported for significantly more experimental group children, phrase repetitions were reported for significantly more control group children, and there was not a significant group difference for word repetitions.

In his reanalysis of Johnson's data McDearmon (1968) gives this summary:

> (1) Among experimentals, children labeled as stutterers by at least one parent, at least 63 per cent at onset of stuttering evidenced primary stuttering (simple repetitions and prolongations of sound and syllables), and at least 28 per cent evidenced only normal nonfluencies (repetitions of words and phrases, and other interruptions common in children), as indicated by parents' responses to one question. (2) This primary stuttering was much more frequent, and normal nonfluency much less frequent, in experimentals at onset of stuttering than in controls; and these differences were statistically significant. (3) Slight tension was the only secondary reaction indicated in more than 15 per cent of the experimentals at onset, according to parents' responses to other questions (p. 637).

While the study did not specifically consider speech at onset, in his cross-sectional study of stuttering, Bloodstein (1960) showed that among the youngest of his cases, the 30 children aged two and four years, repetitions and prolongations were the characteristic features in 75 per cent of these children. Forty per cent showed occasional hard contacts and 33 per cent had other associated symptoms. He reports that the repetitions "are most often reported by parents as the earliest noticed symptoms of the disorder." And further:

> The word and syllable repetitions described above are referred to as stuttering for several reasons. (1) They were in most cases both far more frequent and far more prolonged than the repetitions usually observed in the speech of young children. (2) In many cases, including some of the mildest who were brought for examination, the parents' and the author's evaluation of the repetitions as abnormal was apparently shared by relatives, friends, or neighbors who had referred to them as "stuttering." (3) Even in cases in which it might have been possible, by a somewhat liberal interpretation of speech adequacy, to regard the repetitions as not wholly or essentially different from those of normal children, there was often a past history of unquestionable stuttering which served to destroy the illusion of a completely typical child with normal nonfluency (p. 221).

During the years 1934–36, the author held a research appointment with the Department of Child Welfare at the University of Iowa, and his

TABLE 4.1 Behavior at Onset of Stuttering

	OBSERVED	REPORTED BY PARENT AT ONSET
Sound and syllable repetitions:*		
("s-s-s-some;" "to-to-today")	49	53
Single syllable word repetitions:		
("can-can-can-can")	43	50
Prolonged sounds:†	17	11
Prolonged articulatory postures†		
Without tension:	12	3
With tension:	9	7
Broken words:	4	0
(medial gaps: "v——ery")		
Evidence of awareness:	9	5

* In this tabulation, we refer to syllabic or word repetitions which occurred more than three times on a single word.

† Duration had to exceed two seconds to be counted.

Note: As is evident from this table, some children showed several of these behaviors. Our data regrettably are incomplete as to repetition rate, regularity, airflow, and other features.

project was to discover the cause of stuttering. We advertised in newspapers and on the radio for information concerning children who had just begun to stutter and, when we heard of them, we went directly to their homes to interview their parents and associates and to observe the children carefully. Although the material was never published, the 30 case studies we obtained served as the basis for a continuing interest in the onset of stuttering, and we have since augmented the data considerably. Of the 61 cases reported in Table 4.1, nine were seen within a week of reported onset and the others within three weeks. The kinds of behaviors shown were observed by the author.

In reviewing all this information, it is obvious that much more needs to be done before we can be sure what actually happens at the onset of stuttering. We regret that the longitudinal studies reported by Morley (1957) and Andrews and Harris (1964) provide no data on this important matter and we hope that any future longitudinal study will do so.

CONDITIONS AT ONSET

In this section we invade a never-never land in which much of our information is suspect. The parents of stutterers, the stutterers themselves, even our casual acquaintances always ask the age old question: "What is the cause of stuttering?" When we temporize and answer that there seems to be no one cause and that stuttering is probably the end result of many forces both external and internal, both past and present, our questioners, if they do not immediately judge speech pathology to be a benighted profession, tend to ask: "Then under what conditions does it arise? What sets it off?" These too are very difficult for us to answer unhesitatingly and without stammering a little. Our own study of the literature and our long clinical experience, in which we tried very hard to come to some definite conclusions about the matter, have not yielded us any real assurance. Indeed we envy those writers of the past and present who seem so certain about the causes of stuttering. Witness this quotation from Stein (1942):

> One of my patients had a purely tonic stammer due to an extremely short frenulum which made the articulation of all dental sounds impossible. The disorder with all its anxiety and inferiority symptoms disappeared after the tongue had been freed by cutting the frenulum (p. 110).

Though the pudding has apparent therapeutic proof, we still find it difficult to swallow the alleged etiology.

We are also duly impressed but not convinced by the authoritarian statements of presumed causes which certain writers have been able to identify in their series of cases. For example, the Russian, Katsovskaia (1962), states flatly that the causes of stuttering in 200 children were found in 35 per cent of the cases to be due to psychic shocks; 27.5 per cent to the sequellae of illnesses affecting the brain; 26 per cent to delayed speech and language; 4.5 per cent to imitation; and 2 per cent to forcing a premature development of speech. We also have some doubts about the Hungarian investigation in which Hirschberg (1965) summarizes his findings as follows:

Infection	11 cases
Tonsillar hypertrophy	67
Change-over of left-handed children	38
School conflicts	5
Unfavorable family background, deficient education	43
Imitation	7
Frightened by animals	23
Other psychic trauma	13
Falls, being beaten	18
Bilingualism	2

Hirschberg does qualify these results with the following statement: "We must stress that we have not been able to determine in all cases of stuttering the circumstances which were directly responsible for the stuttering or the speech neurosis." Nor have we—even for those we investigated in depth! We found some of the same circumstances (bad tonsils!) which Hirschberg mentioned but we were never sure that they were either predisposing or precipitating causes of the stuttering. All we could say was that they might have contributed.

But we must not confine these examples to the area behind the Iron Curtain for it is not hard to find many of the same ilk on our own side. Thus McAllister (1958) in England reports an etiological investigation of

139 cases of stuttering, and classifies them into four groups according to "possible causes": (1) 13.6 per cent had some abnormality in structure or functioning [sic!] of the speech organs; (2) 6.5 per cent were left-handed; (3) 5.7 per cent were due to imitation; and (4) 75 per cent had emotional conflicts and complexes of many varieties.

SOURCES OF ERROR

These figures were probably obtained by scrutinizing a series of casefolders for information obtained by interviewing either the stutterers themselves or their parents. Many years have elapsed since the disorder began and truth is always diluted by time. Moreover, the alleged circumstances surrounding onset, when reported by the stutterer himself, may merely be those that occurred at the time when he became highly aware of his speech disability. Since this awareness usually occurs in situations of emotional stress, he will report that the disorder began under these emotional conditions. Whenever possible, we have tried to determine if the person showed a history of stuttering prior to the alleged emotional shock, illness, or other such reported causal experiences. The following may illustrate:

> A 16-year-old stutterer was brought to us by his mother with a clear history of onset at the age of eight years. Both the mother and the boy remembered the incident vividly. The boy was on his way home in the early darkness of a winter evening and stumbled across the body of a dead man on the sidewalk in front of the boy's home. (They had the newspaper clipping to prove it.) The boy rushed into the house, opened his mouth to speak, and was unable to do so for some minutes despite repeated attempts. His stuttering dated from this time, so they said, and it was interesting that his major stuttering behavior was this same wide gaping mouth. The mother was absolutely convinced that the boy had been completely fluent previously. Nevertheless, we were able to find school records, and to get the testimony of his first grade teacher who remembered the boy because of his speech difficulty. It was clearly established that he had been stuttering fairly frequently and severely, though repetitively, before the incident.

This and many other similar discrepancies have taught us to evaluate with some skepticism such reports when they come to us long after onset. This is not to say that stuttering may not emerge originally from such dramatic events. We have found enough instances which we could corroborate to know that at times the disorder does arise in such an emotional context, but we are no longer naive enough to accept such testimony at face value. Parents and stutterers also are so frequently asked what caused the disorder that they have had to come up with some answer, usually one which absolves them of any responsibility. If there happens to be another child in the block who stutters, then they tell us he caught it by imitation; if the little stutterer happened to be ill prior to onset, then the cause was the illness; if he had a stuttering great aunt whom he had never met, then he inherited the disorder. And so on! Irwin and Duffy (195 same point of view:

> It is natural for parents to look for some condition or exper.. account for the onset of stuttering—a physical injury, an emotional upset, a severe illness, or the appearance of a stuttering child in the neighborhood. That a severe illness might retard speech development and account for a period of nonfluency is quite possible. However, it is difficult to establish that such dramatic events are basic to the onset of stuttering. In fact, it often happens that children whose stuttering is attributed to such dramatic experience had shown hesitations, repetitions, and prolongations in their speech long before such events occurred (p. 49).

With these cautions in mind, let us review the literature on the subject of the "precipitating causes" of stuttering.

Shocks and Fright

The older literature is filled with accounts of stuttering beginning after a shock or frightening experience.

According to Luchsinger and Arnold (1965), Gutzmann, in 1900, found 14 per cent of his stutterers reporting the onset as being due to frightening events and these authors add: "In most cases minor physical or emotional mishaps are incriminated: a dog barked suddenly; a rooster flew onto the child's shoulder; or the child stumbled over a carpet in a department store (p. 745)." Makuen (1914) reported that 28 per cent of his 1,000 stutterers suffered shocks or frights prior to onset.

Illness

Illnesses, also, have been mentioned often as precipitating causes of stuttering. It is highly probable that some of the illnesses which most children contract during the years when the disorder usually begins will inevitably precede its onset. Whether or not they have a causal rather than a correlative relationship is not so evident. We can be fairly certain, however, that if stuttering did appear subsequent to some illness, the parents would be prone to view it as the essential cause if only to relieve themselves of any responsibility they may feel. One mother we interviewed was very sure that her son's suffering followed a siege of scarlet fever, but in the hospital records we found that the illness had preceded her dating of the onset of stuttering by 11 months! Nevertheless, throughout the literature we find repeatedly the reference to illness as contributing to the onset of the disorder.

The causal relationship of illness to onset of stuttering is certainly not a simple one. Gutzmann (1939) found that in almost 10 per cent of his cases the stuttering followed severe attacks of infectious diseases and even intestinal infestation with worms. Berry (1938) surveyed the medical histories of stuttering children and concluded that two groups of illnesses appeared with greater frequency in stutterers than they did in normal speakers. The first group consisted of severe respiratory infections,

.neumatic fever, scarlet fever, whooping cough, bronchitis, and pneumonia; the second group consisted of encephalitis, epilepsy, and convulsions. West, Nelson, and Berry (1939) reported that "from 16 to 20 per cent" of their stutterers began to stutter immediately upon recovery from one of these diseases. Again we wonder about the validity of the word "immediately," and we hunger to understand how these diseases actually triggered the stuttering if indeed they really did so. Perhaps a reasonable explanation may be found in this quotation from Luchsinger and Arnold (1965):

> The causative influence of infections or worm infestation should not be construed to represent a specific neurological damage. What is important is the general debilitation and the reduction of physical and mental resistance. Following such a breakdown of psychophysical well-being, stuttering may develop as a psychic reaction. To what extent such illnesses may alter the reactivity of the infant brain is beyond our comprehension at the present time (p. 745).

The pertinence of these remarks may be applied to Goda's (1961) account of stuttering following spinal meningitis. A seven-year-old boy had normal speech until an attack of spinal meningitis resulted in a right hemiplegia. Many of the physical activities he had formerly enjoyed were then denied him, and he had to remain an extra year in the second grade. He spoke without difficulty on his return to school, but two months later he began to stutter and with increasing severity. Was it the spinal meningitis which triggered the stuttering or the other consequences of the disease?

Fortunately we have two experiments concerned with illness and onset in which control groups were used. Johnson (1959) found no significant differences in the number of illnesses as reported by parents of stuttering and nonstuttering children fairly soon after onset, and Andrews and Harris (1964) reported that their 80 pairs of stuttering and nonstuttering children showed almost identical histories of illness. There the matter should rest in peace until some future investigator in this morbid boneyard unearths some better evidence.

Imitation

As we have shown previously, the onset of stuttering has been ascribed by many writers as due to the child's imitation of some other person's stuttering. We often confront this belief in clinical practice. Many of our own stutterers have claimed that their disorder began this way. As we have seen in the studies by Van Riper (1937) and Ainsworth (1939), a listener tends to empathize with the stutterer. Many children use a kind of mockery which is not always vindictive but rather an attempt to perceive unusual behaviors. They limp when they see a lame person. They imitate a facial tic. It is their way of trying to understand what the behavior must be like. It seems logical that some children who, for other reasons, are on the verge of stuttering anyway, will develop stuttering through imitation.

Parents might also find such an etiology highly convenient in absolving themselves of guilt.

The earlier literature stressed imitation as a causative factor much more than we do today. Thus Mygind (1898) found that in 13 per cent of his stutterers, usually those who had other stuttering family members, imitation was the important precipitating cause. The belief is still prevalent. In Japan, Otsuki (1958) claimed that imitation was a significant causal factor in 70 per cent of his cases, which is by far the highest guess we have discovered. Most contemporary authors place imitation as the precipitating cause in from 4 per cent (Katsovskaia, 1962) to 12 per cent (Froeschels, 1943). We suspect that Froeschels, in claiming this latter percentage, may have been involved in justifying his belief that those stutterers who show *prolongations of sounds or postures without the usual concomitant pressure or tension* must have acquired their disorder through imitation. This belief is an interesting hypothesis as yet unsupported by objective physiological research. Froeschels tells us that whenever he saw this particular behavior (which he called pseudotoni) he was able through questioning to elicit the fact that the stutterer had been in close association with some other stutterer. Although generally, the old emphasis on imitation as an essential and common cause of stuttering seems to have faded, nevertheless, we still occasionally find such case reports as that by Soufi (1960) appearing in our own journals. Soufi tells of a boy named Ricky who, previously denied much companionship, moved to an aunt's home in which the youngest boy stuttered severely.

> After ten days in this environment, Ricky stuttered in exactly the same manner as his cousin. After about two weeks of the stuttering, Ricky's mother informed him that he did not need to keep talking that way just because his cousin did. Ricky cried and said, "That's the only way I know how to say it" (p. 411).

For many years we have sought evidence for imitation as a precipitant of the onset of stuttering in every case we examined. Though we have never counted up the cases we saw in those years, they constitute a substantial number. We tried to trace every account of imitation as a source of stuttering and only in one single stuttering child do we feel fairly confident that the disorder was triggered in this way. In many cases, when we compared the stuttering behaviors of our case with those of the person he was said to have imitated (a playmate or the father), we found the stuttering patterns substantially dissimilar. These also were children whom we examined soon after onset and before other changes might have occurred. In the one case where we did feel imitation might have served as a trigger, there was a very close identification of the child with a very beloved playmate and we remembered what Blanton and Blanton (1936) said long ago: "A child might imitate dozens of stutterers and never have any difficulty in a real sense unless he selected some one *with whom he was under a compulsion to identify himself* (p. 99)." In most instances of alleged imitation that we investigated, the contact and association had been so minimal and transient that even had the behaviors shown some resemblance, which they did not, it was difficult to see how they could have been connected causally.

If imitation were a substantial factor in precipitating or creating stuttering, we should expect that each member of a pair of twins would be prone to stutter. In none of our own collection of eight pairs of twins did both individuals stutter. Although the incidence of stuttering among twins seems to be higher than that among singletons, the appearance of the disorder in both members of the pairs is surprisingly rare. Graf (1955) found that in only three of her 18 pairs of twins did both individuals stutter. In the other 15 pairs, which included six presumably identical pairs, only one of the two twins stuttered. Surely, if imitation were as potent a precipitating factor as it has been said to be, we should have expected a greater concordance of stuttering. In this connection Brodnitz (1951) reports that the two identical twins whom he studied stuttered in completely different ways.

Again, if imitation were a strong precipitating factor, one might expect that because of the greater contact, younger siblings would be more likely to stutter than older ones, and that siblings in general would show a fairly high incidence of stuttering. Our own unpublished data do not corroborate these assumptions. The only large scale study of the problem was done 43 years ago by Nadoleczny (1938) who reported that there were ten times more nonstuttering siblings in the families of his stutterers than there were stuttering siblings. In summary, we conclude that imitation is not a very important factor in the onset of stuttering.

Conflict

More than any other etiological factor, emotional conflict has been blamed as the source of stuttering. We find this belief running throughout the literature, and it is certainly held by most of the parents of the young stutterers we have interviewed. Without prejudging the validity of the belief, we should point out that few lives are free from conflict and that most children at the typical age of onset are having a difficult time reconciling their urges and impulses with the demands for conformity that adults are then requiring. Some coincidence of the onset of stuttering with some conflict seems inevitable just because the child lives in a state of rather continual conflict at this period. As Sheehan (1958) has shown, conflicts involving ambivalence (approach-avoidance tendencies) may occur on many levels. At the word level, for example, the child is caught between conflicting urges to say a certain word or not to say it. In an old article, Dunlap (1917) illustrates such a conflict by attributing stuttering to the boy's approach-avoidance urges to say forbidden or dirty words. He says:

> The boy, in constant fear lest one of his obscene terms may slip out in the wrong company, and having experienced this dangerous tendency of words to go astray, soon comes to hesitate over every word which begins in the same way as do these dangerous words; and as the hesitation becomes a more and more

fixed and noticeable habit, it extends to other types of words also. . . . The peculiar feature of stuttering, the repetition of the syllable many times, is a result of the usual method of checking the utterance of a word (p. 46).

There are many other such conflicts at the word level: trying to say unfamiliar words; trying to say the right word without being sure which one is right (Froeschels' word-finding difficulties); having to utter the unspeakable, the unacceptable word, and so on. These conflicts are not unknown even to adults; certainly they occur in young children. Our question however is this: Does stuttering begin in such word conflicts?

Conflicts can also arise at the situation-level. The onset of stuttering in four of our cases was said by the parents to have occurred when the child was asked to talk on the telephone for the first time. In these instances, the stuttering seemed to be localized only in the telephoning situation for some days before it spread to other types of communication. Another child whom we observed shortly after onset surprisingly showed a concentration of stuttering when speaking to his puppy or to some of his stuffed animals. We could not believe the parents when they told us this, but it was true. They said they had first noticed the stuttering shortly after the boy had called the puppy to him and had been knocked down by the dog. We report this reluctantly, hating to contribute any more to the fantastic folklore of the disorder, but we are pretty sure that this is what happened. Is it possible that the motor patterning of words can be so disrupted by such situation conflicts that the disorder of stuttering could result?

Conflicts of course can occur on the relationship level, and it is here that we find more testimony than for any other type of approach-avoidance conflict. It seems to us that disturbed personal relationships are alleged by parents as the cause of stuttering onset more often than any other factor. Again, however, we must be cautious in evaluating such testimony. Such disturbed relationships probably occur very frequently in the homes of nonstuttering children too at one time or another. They also probably occurred earlier in the child's home many times before the actual onset occurred. Their concurrence with the time of onset may therefore be no more than accidental. Nevertheless, the innumerable accounts reported in the literature and in our own clinical practice demand that we consider them seriously.

First let us consider some representative case reports. Solomon (1933) tells of a conflict which involved a sibling, an older brother:

> For more than a half year, since the younger child had been getting more and more active, the older one had been doing his utmost to dominate him, interfere with his free activity, play, and decisions, make him pattern after him and be obedient to his wishes. He took joy in teasing B. as much as possible. He would repeatedly call him into his room and then abruptly put him out and shut the door on him. He would offer him some toy and then purposely take it away from him. He would display his possessions to B. but at the same moment caution the latter not to touch them or would dare him to do so. He would go into B.'s room when B. was playing there alone, and begin to boss him around. He would frighten B., ridicule him, call him baby and sissy. The

younger boy, although resenting the other's annoying tendencies as much as he could, also took his older brother as his hero and patterned after him to his best ability. "Ralph does this or says this and that" was his frequent remark. The parents, although not showing favoritism, had for some time done their best to control the situation diplomatically and prevent undue domination of and repression of the younger by the older son. Finally, about a month before the onset of the stuttering, the mother had independently entered upon a persistent, vigorous and unremitting campaign to stop, once and for all, the misbehavior of the older child, so that there followed almost constant quarrelling and tense scenes, whenever the older boy was at home at the same time as his mother and younger brother, the former now annoying the latter even more than before as revenge against the mother who was pursuing him most of the time. At supper, when the whole family ate together, and conversation flew thick and fast, B. was especially excited. B. was the center about which the conflict raged.

> After this had been going on for a month or more, B. began to stutter occasionally with repetition of initial consonants. This took place almost exclusively in the presence of the older boy, mainly when the latter teased him, or interfered with his play, or put him out of his room. When not excited and when his brother was not at home, there was no stuttering. One day, while at supper, with the conversation lively, B. asked for an object, seemed unable to recall its name, pointed to it and then went into a definite block. This was repeated several times during the meal, B. getting red in the face and appearing embarrassed when blocked. Thereafter occasional speech blocks as well as repetition occurred during the day when not at meals. Within a week of the onset of speech block the case was intensively studied with the unearthing of the above data (p. 40).

Many of the reported conflicts are between parents and child as one might expect at this time of growing independence and assessing limits of freedom. Usually, the mother-child relationship is cited as the basic problem, but the fathers are also occasionally implicated. Maslow and Mittelmann (1941) for example tell of a boy who was continually rejected by his father and who found it impossible to speak to him without stuttering, a behavior which further enraged the father. The boy showed no stuttering in speaking to his mother or to other children or to anyone else. Despert (1943), Baurand and Striglioni (1968), and many other authors feel that a disturbed mother-child relationship is very potent in precipitating stuttering. One illustration from Harle (1946) may suffice:

> Patty was referred to the clinic at the age of three and a half by her mother who was concerned about the child's stuttering. This symptom had started three months earlier following a spanking administered by the mother after the child had run into the street and narrowly missed being run over by a car. Shortly afterward the stuttering had cleared up but a few weeks later, after a second spanking for running into the street, she again began to stutter (p. 156).

Regrettably mothers must do most of the spanking in our culture, and many children have been so punished without setting off any stuttering. In Harle's case, however, as the rest of her article makes clear, a profoundly disturbed mother-child relationship was indeed present.

Perhaps the most eloquent and convincing evidence for disturbed family relationships being productive of stuttering has been contributed by Wyatt (1969). Her series of case studies, including that of her own child, strongly supports her developmental crisis theory of stuttering. Briefly, her position is that stuttering arises when a child finds difficulty in communicating with a significant adult, especially at a critical time of developmental stress or crisis. One excerpt from her book, which is well worth reading by all students of the disorder, is as follows:

> The onset of Nana's stuttering occurred at a time when her mother, because of acute illness, had become inaccessible to the child. Nana consequently experienced a break in a previously well-established speech chain. This disruption coincided with a critical period in Nana's language development, the change from mere naming to the learning of grammatical speech patterns (p. 93).

Of course, many children experience such crises without developing stuttering, and we do not have an adequate explanation which would tell us why some do and some don't. It is at least tenable that the motor sequencing of speech breaks down when communication is overloaded by stress of any kind and certainly the kinds of interpersonal conflicts we have been describing do constitute an important stress. Glasner (1949) showed that many young stutterers demonstrated other behaviors unrelated to stuttering which appeared to be consequences of emotional overloading. He studied 70 young stutterers under five years of age and says:

> All of the children studied had exhibited some degree of emotional manifestation other than stuttering. Fifty-four per cent were characterized as "feeding problems." Twenty-seven per cent were enuretic. Twenty per cent had exaggerated sibling jealousy, nail-biting, encopresis, masturbation, emotional vomiting, and numerous others. It is realized, of course, that the "normal" child is a fiction, not a reality, but these children apparently had more than their share of behavior symptoms (p. 137).

Glasner's observations were made some time after the onset of stuttering and could therefore be effects of the disorder rather than reflections of its etiology in terms of emotional conflict, a supposition which seems supported by his comments about how the children reacted when speaking. Nevertheless, many of the children whom we studied shortly after onset showed evidence of greater emotionality than we would expect to find in the ordinary child. This clinical impression we have refused to dignify by citing any percentage figures because we had no controls. Johnson's (1959) data and that obtained by Andrews and Harris (1964) show no significant differences in the amount of emotional conflicts between the stuttering children and their normally speaking controls. Nevertheless, we have studied individual cases in which stuttering did seem triggered by such conflicts, and it is difficult for us to ignore these experiences.

Communicative Conflicts

Although it is hard to separate communicative from emotional conflicts, since no one can really tell how much emotion may have been generated in any communicative interaction, we often find accounts of stuttering beginning under such circumstances. This quotation from Duncan (1949) will illustrate:

> When I was four years old my mother took a job and put me in a day nursery. . . . We had moved to an apartment at about that time which was located on the top floor and we were required to walk up five flights of stairs to get up to it. One of my habits was to run up the five flights and upon getting into the house I would try to speak while out of breath. This is the first time I can remember "stumbling" in my speech (p. 258).

Or this from Rand, Sweeny, and Vincent (1962):

> Laughing at the child's cute accent or his imperfect pronunciation is particularly dangerous since children are unable to discriminate kinds of laughter and do not always know the laughter of indulgent amusement from that of mockery. . . . Self-consciousness or fear of ridicule as a rule produces one of two results: either it discourages effort and tends to produce silence or it provides one of the commonest causes of stuttering (p. 192).

Woolf (1957) tells of a boy who had been unduly precocious in speech and had received much praise for it. The stuttering began when the parents and an older sister gave him tongue-twisters and other difficult sentences to say. Schuell (1949) provides an example which we have found frequently in parental reports: "Sarah's trouble is that she never gets a chance to say anything. The rest of us talk all the time and she can't get anyone to listen to what she wants to say (p. 253)."

In determining the circumstances surrounding the onset of stuttering, we have our greatest trouble with those children who seem to have started to stutter very early or at the same time that they began to speak phrases and sentences. Even when the reported onset of both speech and stuttering is as late as six and seven years, the parents of these children are so concerned about the delay in acquiring any speech at all or adequate articulation or intelligibility that they tend to ignore any stuttering which may accompany the speech. Most of those we have seen at onset were children receiving therapy for delayed speech and language either in our clinic or from other clinicians. The cluttering component in these cases is often evident, and it is difficult to tell when the stuttering emerges from it. However, it is quite apparent that these children have a great burden placed upon their communicative efforts. They must acquire vocabulary, proper grammatical structures, and perfect articulation as well as some fluency. Watching such older children struggle to learn to talk, we can see how very young children may have had some of the same difficulties, but it is very difficult to pinpoint them. One of the factors contributing to the onset of stuttering in these cases seems surprisingly to be the parents' delight in the newly attained speech. Often they overpraise and overencourage the child once he begins to talk and demand more and more verbal facility. Many times we have been able to eliminate the stuttering merely by reducing these parental expectations and demands. In the same connection we occasionally find an onset of stuttering being reported as due to overcorrection of articulatory errors, but most of these turn out to have had a previous history of marked disfluency or stuttering.

Except for many researches that show various kinds of disfluencies in the speech of children when they are learning to talk, we have little hard evidence that stuttering has its onset in the difficulties of language learning. Soderberg (1967) reported that grammatical and lexical uncertainty tended to precipitate stuttering behaviors in young children. Bloodstein (1974) hypothesized that difficulties in mastering the syntactic rules of our language characterized the beginning stutterer, that is, that the fragmenting of speech occurs not so much within the word but rather in the organization of phrases and sentences. Murray and Reed (1977) administered two language tests to seven preschool stutterers and matched controls, finding significant differences in language mastery on one test but not on the other. Hall (1977) found that some language disordered children suddenly became very disfluent as the result of language therapy and provides two illustrative case reports.

In this connection we also should call attention to the French and Russian literature, much of which attributes stuttering to a failure to learn the rhythmic and temporal organization of language. In the view of these workers, young children must learn to master prosody as well as all of the other aspects of language, and some children find it so difficult that they begin to hesitate and stutter. Accordingly, such stuttering children are routinely given special training not only in the sequential organization of successive words in phrases and sentences but also in the "sounding-out" of individual words. A summary of this literature may be found in Van Riper's *The Treatment of Stuttering* (1973, pp. 383–87).

By its sheer length, the previous discussion may have led the reader to believe that it is usually possible to identify one or another of the circumstances surrounding the onset of stuttering as being a significant cause. Nothing could be further from the truth. In the great majority of the children we have carefully studied soon after onset, we were unable to state with any certainty (or even with some feeling of probability) what precipitated the stuttering. In most instances there simply were no apparent conflicts, no illnesses, no opportunity to imitate, no shocks or frightening experiences. Stuttering seemed to begin under quite normal conditions of living and communicating. We cannot, of course, be sure of this. Who can look within the inner world of a child? All we can say is that usually we could not account for the onset of stuttering in terms of the conditions surrounding it. In only a fraction of our cases do we feel we identified the circumstances that might have been precipitating. If this is a confession of incompetence, then at least we are in good company—as the following quotation from Wendell Johnson (1959) would indicate:

> ... the conditions reportedly associated with the "first" stuttering of the experimental group children were, in general, the same as those associated with the "first" nonfluencies which the control group parents said they observed in the speech of their children. The major conclusion would seem that, generally speaking, the problem of stuttering was found to develop under quite ordinary circumstances (p. 131).

SUMMARY

The basic conclusions from this survey of the literature on the onset of stuttering are these: Stuttering usually begins in the preschool years and only rarely in adults. While some children are said to have begun to stutter at the time they first learned to speak, most of them begin a year or two later. The first stuttering behaviors shown are usually easy repetitions of syllables or sounds but some individuals show complete blockings and tension. The disorder usually begins gradually rather than suddenly but instances of sudden onset do occur. While fright, shock, or other trauma are reported to have taken place just before onset in a few individuals, these factors are not generally present. Imitation and illness or conflict are not common conditions at the time stuttering begins.

Of the three major explanations of the nature of stuttering, the neurotic theory would have difficulty in accounting for these findings; the view that stuttering is a learned, habitual way of speaking could possibly explain some but not all of this information; and, in our opinion, the most reasonable explanation is that which attributes stuttering to the difficulty some children are bound to experience in mastering the synchronized timing of the motor coordinations required for speech. We invite the reader to consider this material and make his own judgment—as we have made ours.

BIBLIOGRAPHY

AIKINS, A. 1925. Casting out the stuttering devil. *Journal of Abnormal Social Psychology* 18: 137–52.

AINSWORTH, S. 1939. Studies in the psychology of stuttering XII. Empathic breathing of auditors while listening to stuttering speech. *Journal of Speech Disorders* 4: 149–56.

AJURIAGUERRA, J. R. DE, DIAKINE, H. DE GOBINEAU, S. NARLIAN, AND M. STAMBAK. 1958 Le Bégaiement. *Presse Mèdicale* 66: 953–56.

ANDREWS, G. 1965. The nature of stuttering. *Journal Australian College of Speech Therapists* 15: 6–15.

——— AND M. HARRIS. 1964. *The syndrome of stuttering*. London: Heinemann.

ARNOLD, G. E. 1948. *Die traumatischen und konstitutionellen Störungen der Stimme und Sprache*. Vienna: Urban and Schwarzenberg.

ARON, M. L. 1958. An investigation of the nature and incidence of stuttering among a Bantu group of school children. Doctoral dissertation, University of Witwatersrand, South Africa.

———. 1962. Nature and incidence of stuttering among a Bantu group of school going children. *Journal of Speech and Hearing Disorders* 27: 116–28.

BABA, K. 1952. A cured case of infantile stuttering. *Japanese Journal Otology* 55: 51–52.

BARBARA, D. A. 1959. Stuttering. In *American Handbook of Psychiatry*, ed. S. Arieti. Vol. I. New York: Basic Books.

BAURAND, G. AND L. STRIGLIONI. 1968. Importance du facteur parental dans le symptome bégaiement. *Journal Française O. R. L.* 17: 209–16.

BECKER, K. P., N. A. VLASSOVA, N. M. ASATIANI, AND W. HEV. 1977. *Stottern.* Berlin: V.E.B. Verlag Volk and Gesundheit.

BERLIN, A. J. 1954. An exploratory attempt to isolate types of stuttering. Doctoral dissertation, Northwestern University.

BERRY, M. F. 1938. Developmental history of stuttering children. *Journal of Pediatrics* 12: 209–17.

BLANTON, S. AND M. G. BLANTON. 1936. *For stutterers.* New York: Appleton.

BLOODSTEIN, O. 1975. Stuttering as tension and fragmentation. In *Stuttering: A Second Symposium,* ed. J. Eisenson. New York: Harper and Row.

———. 1974. The rules of early stuttering. *Journal of Speech and Hearing Disorders* 39: 379–94.

———. 1960. The development of stuttering. *Journal of Speech and Hearing Disorders* 25: 219–37; 366–76.

———, J. ALPER, AND P. ZISK. 1965. Stuttering as an outgrowth of normal disfluency. In *New Directions in Stuttering: Theory and Practice,* ed. D. A. Barbara. Springfield, Ill.: Thomas.

BLUEMEL, C. S. 1913. *Stammering and cognate defects of speech,* Vol. I. New York: Stechert.

———. 1957. *The riddle of stuttering.* Danville, Ill.: Interstate.

BOOME, E. J. AND M. A. RICHARDSON, 1932. *The nature and treatment of stuttering.* New York: Dutton.

BREUR, J. AND S. FREUD. 1955. *Studies on hysteria.* London: Hogarth Press.

BRODNITZ, F. S. 1951. Stuttering of different types in identical twins. *Journal of Speech and Hearing Disorders* 16: 334–36.

DALTON, P. AND W. J. HARDCASTLE. 1977. *Disorders of fluency.* London: Edward Arnold.

DARLEY, F. L. 1955. The relationship of parental attitudes and adjustments to the development of stuttering. In *Stuttering in Children and Adults,* ed. W. Johnson. Minneapolis: University of Minnesota Press.

DARLEY, F. L. AND H. WINITZ. 1961. Age of first word: review of research. *Journal of Speech and Hearing Disorders* 26: 272–90.

DASKALOV, D. D. 1962. Basic principles and methods of prevention and treatment of stuttering. *Nevropatologii i Psikhiatrii imeni S. S. Korsakova* 62: 1047–52.

DE HIRSCH, K. AND W. S. LANGFORD. 1950. Clinical note on stuttering and cluttering in young children. *Pediatrics* 5: 934–40.

DENHARDT, R. 1890. *Das Stottern: Eine Psychose.* Leipzig.

DESPERT, J. L. 1943. Stuttering in children. *Nervous Child* 2: 79–207.

Dickson, S. 1971. Incipient stuttering and spontaneous remission of stuttered speech. *Journal of Communication Disorders* 4: 99–110.

Duncan, M. H. 1949. Home adjustment of stutterers and non-stutterers. *Journal of Speech Disorders* 14: 195–98.

Dunlap, K. 1944. Stammering: its nature, etiology and therapy. *Journal of Comparative Psychology* 37: 187–202.

———. 1917. The stuttering boy. *Journal of Abnormal Psychology* 12: 44–48.

Eisenson, J. 1947. Aphasics: observations and tentative conclusions. *Journal of Speech Disorders* 12: 290–92.

Fahy, T. J., M. H. Irving, and P. Millac. 1967. Severe head injuries. *Lancet* 272: 475–79.

Fletcher, J. M. 1928. *The problem of stuttering*. New York: Longmans Green.

Fogerty, E. 1930. *Stammering*. New York: Dutton.

Freund, H. 1966. *Psychopathology and the problems of stuttering*. Springfield, Ill.: Thomas.

Fritzell, B. 1963. On stuttering and on studies of stuttering in Marburg. *Svenska Lakartidningen* 60: 3396–3405.

Froeschels, E. 1919. Die spracharztliche therapie im kriege. 3. Das Stottern, *Monatsschrift für Ohrenheilkunde* 53: 161–90.

———. 1943. Pathology and therapy of stuttering. *Nervous Child* 2: 148–61.

———. 1952. The significance of symptomatology for the understanding of the essence of stuttering. *Folia Phoniatrica* 4: 217–30.

———. 1916. Zur Differentialdiagnose zwischen frischem, traumatischem, und veraltetem Stottern. *Med. Klin.* 12: 694–96.

———. 1917. Zur Frage der Entstehung des tonischen Stotterns und zur Frage der Wirkungslosigkeit der elektrischen Stromes in der meisten Fallen von Stottern. *Med. Klin.* 13: 448–50.

Fujita, K. et al. 1964. The diagnostic statistics of 80 cases of stutterers. *Japanese Journal Otorhinolaryngology* 67: 343. Abstract No. 297 in G. Kamiyama, *Handbook for the study of stuttering*. Tokyo: Kongo-Shupan.

Gertsmann, J. and P. Schilder. 1921. Studien über Bewegungstörungen über die typenextrapyramidaler pseudobulbar Paralyse. *Zeitschrift für Neurologie und Psychiatrie* 79: 350–54.

Glasner, P. J. 1949. Personality characteristics and emotional problems in stutterers under the age of five. *Journal of Speech and Hearing Disorders* 14: 135–38.

Glaser, E. M. 1936. Possible relationship between stuttering and endocrine malfunctioning. *Journal of Speech Disorders* 1: 81–89.

Goda, S. 1961. Stuttering manifestations following spinal meningitis. *Journal of Speech and Hearing Disorders* 26: 392–93.

Gondaira, T. 1960. A case study of a boy with stuttering and physical malformation. *Japanese Journal of Child Psychology* 1: 340–50.

Graf, O. I. 1955. Incidence of stuttering among twins. In *Stuttering in Children and Adults*, ed. W. Johnson. Minneapolis: University of Minnesota Press.

Greene, J. S. 1924. Your child's speech. *Hygeia* 2: 11–12.

Guillaume, J., G. Mazars, and Y. Mazars. 1957. Epileptic mediation in certain types of stammering. *Revue Neurologique* 96: 59–62.

Gutzmann, H. 1939. Erbbiologische, soziologische und organische Faktoren die Sprachstörungen begunstigen. *Archive für Stimmheilkunde* 3: 133–36.

HALL, P. K. 1977.   The occurrence of disfluencies in language-disordered school age children. *Journal of Speech and Hearing Disorders* 42: 364–69.

HARLE, M. 1946.   Dynamic interpretation and treatment of acute stuttering in a young child. *American Journal of Orthopsychiatry* 15: 156–62.

HASTINGS, I. 1966.   A case of stammer and tongue thrusting. *Speech Pathology, Diagnosis, Theory and Practice*. Edinburgh: Livingstone.

HIRSCHBERG, J. 1965.   Stuttering. *Orvosi. Hetilap* 106: 780–84.

HOEPFNER, T. 1911–12.   Stottern-als assoziative Aphasie. *Zeitschrift für Pathopsychologie* 1:448–552.

IRWIN, J. AND J. K. DUFFY. 1955.   *Speech and hearing hurdles*. Columbus, Ohio: School and College Service.

JAMESON, A. M. 1955.   Stammering in children—some factors in prognosis. *Speech* (London) 19: 60–67.

JOHNSON, W. 1955.   A study of the onset and development of stuttering. In *Stuttering in Children and Adults*, ed. W. Johnson. Minneapolis: University of Minnesota Press.

———. 1959.   *The onset of stuttering*. Minneapolis: University of Minnesota Press.

KAMIYAMA, A. 1967.   *Handbook for the study of stuttering*. Tokyo: Kongo-Shupan.

KANNER, L. 1942.   *Child psychiatry*. Springfield, Ill.: Thomas.

KASTEIN, S. 1947.   The chewing method of treating stuttering. *Journal of Speech Disorders* 12: 195–98.

KATSOVSKAIA, I. I. K. 1962.   The problem of children's stuttering. *Deafness, Speech and Hearing Abstracts* 2: 296.

KINGDON-WARD, W. 1941.   *Stammering*. London: Hamilton.

KLINGER, H. 1963.   The onset of stuttering in adults: a presentation of three cases. *ASHA* 5: 782 (Abstract).

———. 1966.   Personal communication.

KOPP, H. 1942–43. The relationship of stuttering to motor disturbance. *Nervous Child* 2: 107–16.

LEVINA, R. Y. 1968.   Study and treatment of stammering among children. *Journal of Learning Disabilities* 2: 24–30.

LUCHSINGER, R. AND G. E. ARNOLD. 1965.   *Voice—speech—language*. Belmont, Cal.: Wadsworth.

MAKUEN, G. H. 1914.   A study of 1,000 cases of stammering with special reference to the etiology and treatment of the affection. *Therapeutic Gazette* 38: 385–90.

MARTYN, M. M. AND J. SHEEHAN. 1968.   Onset of stuttering and recovery. *Behavior Research and Therapy* 6: 295–307.

MASLOW, A. H. AND B. MITTELMANN. 1941.   *Principles of abnormal psychology: the dynamics of psychic illness*. New York: Harper.

MCALLISTER, A. H. 1937.   *Clinical studies in speech therapy*. London: University London Press.

———. 1958.   The problem of stammering. *Speech Pathology and Therapy* (London) 1: 3–8.

MCCALLIEN, C. 1956.   Problems of speech defect in the Accra district. *Speech* (London) 20: 15–18.

MCDEARMON, J. R. 1968.   Primary stuttering at the onset of stuttering: a re-examination of the data. *Journal of Speech and Hearing Research* 11: 631–37.

MOCHIZUSKI, S. 1962. Personal communication.

MORLEY, M. E. 1957. *The development and disorders of speech in childhood.* Edinburgh: Livingstone.

MURRAY, N. L. AND C. G. REED. 1977. Language abilities of preschool stuttering children. *Journal of Fluency Disorders* 2: 171–6.

MYGIND, H. 1898. Über die Ursachen des Stotterns. *Archive für Laryngologie und Rhinologie* 8: 294–307.

NADOLECZNY, M. (1938), quoted in R. LUCHSINGER, AND G. E. ARNOLD. 1965. *Voice—speech—language.* Belmont, Cal.: Wadsworth.

NELSON, S. E., N. HUNTER, AND M. WALTER. 1945. Stuttering in twin types. *Journal of Speech Disorders* 10: 335–43.

OHASHI, Y. 1977. Development of stuttering in children: a cross-sectional study. *Japanese Journal of Child Psychiatry* 17: 57–68.

——. 1976. Development of stuttering in children with onset at 2.6–3.6 years. *Practica Otologica Kyoto* 69: 825–32.

ORCHINIK, C. W. 1958. On tickling and stuttering. *Psychoanalysis and Psychoanalytic Review* 44: 25–29.

OTSUKI, H. 1958. Study on stuttering: statistical observations. *Otorhinolaryngology Clinic* 5: 1150–51.

PEACHER, W. C. AND W. E. HARRIS. 1946. Speech disorders in World War II: stuttering. *Journal of Speech Disorders* 11: 303–8.

PREUS, A. 1981. *Attempts at identifying subgroups of stutterers.* Oslo: University of Oslo Press.

RAND, W., M. E. SWEENY, AND E. L. VINCENT. 1962. *Growth and development of the young child.* 3rd Ed., Philadelphia: Sanders.

RAZDOL'SKII, V. A. 1965. State of speech of stammerers when alone. *Zhurnal Nevropatologii i Psikhiatrii imeni S. S. Korsakova* 65: 1717–20.

ROZHDESTVENSKAYA, G. G. 1974. The role of psychogenic trauma in the development of stuttering and the characteristics of neurotic reactions in those states. *Zhurnal Nevropatologii i Psikhiatrii imeni S. S. Korsakova* 74: 569–74.

SCHACHTER, M. 1967. Aphémie suivie de bégaiement d'origine psychodramatique chez une fillette de quatre ans. *Acta Paedopsychiatrica* 34: 1–32.

SCHMEER, G. 1966. Zur genese des stotterns. *Praxis Kinderpsychologie* 15: 45–50.

SCHUELL, H. 1949. Working with parents of stuttering children. *Journal of Speech Disorders* 14: 251–54.

SCRIPTURE, E. W. 1912. *Stuttering and lisping.* New York: Macmillan.

SEEMAN, M. 1959. *Sprachstörungen bei Kindern.* Marhold: Halle-Saale.

SHAMES, G. AND C. SHERRICK. 1963. A discussion of nonfluency and stuttering as operant behavior. *Journal of Speech and Hearing Disorders* 28: 3–18.

SHEEHAN, J. 1958. Conflict theory of stuttering. In *Stuttering: A Symposium,* ed. J. Eisenson. New York: Harper.

SHIRAIWA, T. 1958. Study of the cause of stuttering. Abstract No. 185. In G. Kamiyama, *Handbook for the study of stuttering.* Tokyo: Kongo-Shupan, 1967.

SMITH, L. G. 1921. Speech defect resulting from ether shock. *Pedagogical Seminary* 27: 308–12.

SODERBERG, G. A. 1967. Linguistic factors in stuttering. *Journal of Speech and Hearing Research* 10: 801–10.

SOLOMON, M. 1933.   Incipient stuttering in a preschool child at half years. *Proceedings American Speech Correction Association* 3:

SOUFI, A. 1960.   One month stutterer. *Journal of Speech and Hear* 411.

SSIKORSKI, I. A. 1891.   *Über das Stottern*. Berlin: Hirschwald.

STEIN, L. 1942.   *Speech and voice*. London: Methuen.

TAKAGI, S., et al. 1962.   The characteristic of young stutterers and their follow up study. Abstract No. 272. In G. Kamiyama, *Handbook for the study of stuttering*. Japan: Kongo-Shupan.

TAYLOR, G. L. 1937.   An observational study of the nature of stuttering at its onset. Masters thesis, State University of Iowa.

TOYODA, B. 1965.   Stuttering of infants. *Voice and Language Medicine* 6: 14–15, Abstract No. 328. IN G. Kamiyama, *Handbook for the study of stuttering*. Tokyo: Kongo-Shupan, 1967.

TREITEL, L. 1894.   Störungen der Lautfolge: Stottern. Excerpts from this work are found in M. V. Jones, Leonard Treitel on stuttering, *Journal of Speech and Hearing Disorders* 13: 19–22.

VAN RIPER, C. 1937.   The Influence of Empathic Response on Frequency of Stuttering. *Psychological Monographs* 49: 244–46.

———. 1971.   *The nature of stuttering*. (First Edition), Englewood Cliffs, N.J.: Prentice-Hall.

———. 1973.   *The treatment of stuttering*. Englewood Cliffs, N.J.: Prentice-Hall.

VAN THAL, J. 1950.   The relationship between war conditions and defects of voice and speech. *Folia Phoniatrica* 2: 165–67.

VLASOVA, N. A. 1962.   Prevention and treatment of children's stuttering in U.S.S.R. *Ceskoslovenska Otolaryngologie* 11: 30–32.

———. 1965.   Late follow-up analysis of some cases of recurrent stuttering. *Zhurnal Neuropatologii i Psikiatrii imeni S. S. Korsakova* 65: 750–51.

WALLEN, V. 1961.   Primary stuttering in a twenty-eight-year-old adult. *Journal of Speech and Hearing Disorders* 26: 394.

WEST, R. 1943.   The pathology of stuttering. *Nervous Child* 2: 96–106.

———, S. NELSON, AND M. BERRY. 1937.   The heredity of stuttering. *Quarterly Journal of Speech* 25: 23–30.

WOOLF, G. 1967.   The assessment of stuttering as struggle, avoidance and expectancy. *British Journal of Disorders of Communication* 2: 158–71.

WYATT, G. L. 1969. *Language Learning and Communication Disorders in Children*. New York: Free Press.

YOUNG, M. A. 1975. Onset, prevalence and recovery from stuttering. *Journal of Speech and Hearing Disorders* 40: 49–58.

THE DEVELOPMENT OF STUTTERING

5

Most observers agree that stuttering behaviors often change, growing more abnormal with the passage of time. Although a large number of beginning stutterers (perhaps as high as 80 per cent) show the disorder only for a short time and then regain or acquire normal fluency, this chapter is mainly concerned with those who continue to stutter. When it persists, stuttering rarely continues to present the same picture shown at onset, new behaviors replacing or joining the original ones. In the confirmed stutterer there is an incredible variety of contorted, tense struggling and morbid emotional reactions bearing little resemblance to the earlier stuttering. These bizarre new behaviors seem meaningless unless considered in the light of their developmental history. Much of the mystery and confusion that befogs our understanding of stuttering results from our failure to realize how it grows. Stuttering theories often conflict with one another because they have been based on the nature of the disorder after it has already made its morbid growth. Because stuttering develops differently in different people, our research, which has been done mostly with the adult population, has often added to the confusion.

Several of the older writers have commented on the fact that stuttering changes its appearance with the years. The anonymous author of *The Irrationale of Speech*, quoted by Hunt (1861), says:

> . . .the stammer may take very different forms from year to year; and the boy who began to stammer with the lip may go on to stammer with the tongue, then with the jaw, and last and worst of all, with the breath; and in after life try to rid himself of one abuse by trying in alternation all the other three (p. 187).

Potter (1882) is more explicit. He writes:

> At first there is noticed a halt on some syllable beginning with an explosive consonant, followed by anxiety and a condition of expectancy on the part of the

person affected for the next difficult syllable, producing a mental search for a synonym of easier pronunciation, resulting in a halting, irregular hesitation in speech, an outré manner of expressing the ideas. Soon another difficult syllable is encountered, for which a synonym cannot be found, the embarrassement of the sufferer is increased, spasms of the various organs of articulation occur more frequently;—now of the lips, affecting the labial sounds; then of the tongue, affecting the dental consonants; the articulating organs seeming as if temporarily glued together in some cases, in others as though alternately attracted to and repelled from each other. As embarrassment increases, the spasms become more violent, until in severe cases a general spasmodic condition of the muscles of articulation, phonation, and respiration ensues, with even tetanic rigidity of some groups; the patient's voice becomes lost, he gasps for breath with a nearly empty lung, and silence alone brings temporary relief to the general distress of body and mind (p. 81).

In his first book, *Stammering and Cognate Defects of Speech,* Bluemel (1913) recognized these changes. He differentiated between "pure stammering" and "secondary or physical stammering," the latter being characterized by learned fears and learned motor behaviors. In later works (1932, 1935, 1940) he developed further his concept of stuttering as a learned habit based on conditioned inhibition and his terms "primary" and "secondary" stuttering are still used by many to indicate the changing nature of the disorder. In Europe, Hoepfner (1912) sketched the course of stuttering development, but the most detailed exposition of how the disorder grows was provided by Emil Froeschels (1964). He showed, in a series of publications, that stuttering follows a fairly consistent course of development. Here, in outline form, is the first part of Froeschels' sequence:

Steps in the Development of Stuttering
(*After Froeschels*)

  I. Syllable and word repetition; normal tempo; no tension. Child's reaction: stops and tries again.
 II. Syllable and word repetition; normal tempo; no tension. Reaction: child continues until word is uttered.
III. Syllable and word repetition; normal tempo; some tension. Child still stops and begins again.
 IV. Syllable and word repetition; faster tempo than normal; tension. Reaction: child stops and begins again.
  V. Syllable and word repetition; faster tempo than normal; increased tension. Child continues until word is uttered.
 VI. Syllable and word repetition; slower than normal tempo; marked tension. Child now may stop and try again consciously and deliberately or may hurriedly continue until word is uttered.
VII. Prolongation of a sound or articulatory posture; slower tempo than normal; marked tension. Child will stop and try again or struggle until word is emitted.

In Froeschels' (1955) own words:

If the tonic (pressure) component is dominant, abnormal breathing will result, for the openings through which the breath should escape are temporarily blocked. In the state of primary clonus (repetition) no breathing difficulty is present. Another consequence of the tonic component is accompanying movements, such as grimaces, clenched fists, etc. At later stages, and in exceptional cases at an early stage, all sorts of accompanying movements develop, such as stamping of the foot, looking to one side or up and down, as well as the so-called embolophrasias. Embolophrasias are sounds, sound combinations, or words used as starters in moments of speech difficulties (p. 113).

Froeschels says that the overt features of stuttering in this advanced stage are so variable that in 16,000 cases he never found two alike. He also goes on to describe a terminal phase which he calls "concealed stuttering" wherein the stutterer develops various tricks and strategies for hiding his speech difficulty. Concealed stuttering "is almost universal in the development of stuttering in Europe, but relatively rare in the United States" (Froeschels, 1942, p. 86). He believes that all genuine stuttering tends to follow this sequential pattern and, when it does not, he attributes the exceptions to imitation or hysteria or to faulty therapy.

Bloodstein (1960) tried to delineate the developmental course of stuttering. In a series of three articles he summarized his clinical observations of 418 stutterers, aged 2 to 16 years. His findings were based solely on the first interview of the parent and the first examination of the child. In interpreting his result and conclusions, we must bear in mind that Bloodstein's study was not longitudinal. It does not tell us anything about how the stuttering behaviors changed in an individual child. Instead it was cross-sectional, based on groups at different age levels without regard to the length of time the individuals had had the disorder. Thus, the six-year-old group might include some who had just begun to stutter and some who had been stuttering for several years. At best this is a crude way of gathering developmental data, and the results must be interpreted very cautiously, as the author himself admits. It is surprising, then, that gross developmental trends were indeed revealed. Table 5.1 shows the data from Bloodstein's study (1960, p. 220).

Bloodstein's findings are difficult to interpret. If we assume that most of his subjects had begun to stutter at two to five years of age (which is what our review of the onset research seems to indicate), then certainly gross changes in stuttering behaviors have occurred. The stuttering patterns change from simple to complex and grow in severity in each consecutive age group. Making the same assumption, it appears that hard contacts and struggle and avoidance reactions gradually increase as children continue to stutter, and that their fluent periods diminish. (Bloodstein's anticipation data is especially suspect since his criterion for anticipation was the consistency effect, and later research has shown that the same consistency of hesitations and nonfluencies occurs in normal speakers who certainly are not afraid of stuttering.) What Bloodstein really found is that stuttering does not remain static, that it changes with time. On the basis of these data, Bloodstein also discerns four phases of stuttering development, and he gives profiles of each. In illustrating the profile of a Phase III stutterer Bloodstein cites the following case:

TABLE 5.1. Percentage of Subjects Exhibiting Each of Various Features of Stuttering Behavior at Age Levels from 2 to 16. Numbers in Parentheses Indicate the Number of Subjects on Which the Percentage was Based Where this Differs from the Total Number (N) in the Age Group.

	AGE LEVEL						
	2–3 N-30 %	4–5 N-74 %	6–7 N-79 %	8–9 N-60 %	10–11 N-79 %	12–13 N-47 %	14–15–16 N-49 %
Slow, easy repetitions	30	34	28	37	30	9	8
Easy repetition or prolongation as sole symptoms of stuttering	43	32	18	18	11	4	4
Hard contacts	40	32	44	45	53	51	53
Associated symptoms	33	39	57	58	57	64	65
Fluent periods	47	45	27	10	10	9	00
Difficult stituations			27 (15)	67 (27)	71 (56)	75 (40)	72 (39)
Difficult words or sounds				82 (17)	62 (45)	72(32)	73 (33)
Anticipation				38 (26)	45 (51)	62 (37)	71 (41)
Word substitution				48 (23)	65 (48)	66 (32)	83 (36)
Avoidance of speech	00	5	11	17	28	40	45

P.M., aged 10–3, exhibits severe hard contacts, preformations, long pauses, frowning, and sharp exhalations. He has more difficulty at school than in any other situation. He reports some anticipations and difficult words and sounds, but no substitutions. He does not avoid speaking, frequently volunteers to recite in class, and is a "talker" by reputation (p. 374).

Ohashi (1976) studied 30 stuttering Japanese children and observed the stuttering behaviors according to the lapse of time after onset. She analyzed the stuttering behaviors in terms of repetitions, prolongations, complete blockings, accessory secondary behaviors, awareness, emotional difficulties, and situational avoidance reactions. Essentially she found that the shorter the lapse between onset and diagnostic examination, the more the behaviors were monosymptomatic and that they primarily consisted of repetitions and prolongations. Overt features of stuttering preceded the development of such covert reactions as awareness and fear as the disorder developed. Frustration because of being unable to speak fluently seemed to be more important than listener penalty or reaction. The suddent arrest of speech seemed to create the child's first awareness, and anticipation, anxiety, and other negative emotions followed in that sequence. However, Ohashi did not find discrete stages that her stutterers passed through.

STAGES OF STUTTERING

In the foregoing discussion we have indicated that there may be something wrong with the whole concept of stages of stuttering. Are there really any Phase I, II, III, or IV stutterers? Or for that matter, what validity is there in Bluemel's primary and secondary kinds of stuttering or in Van Riper's

(1963) primary, transitional, and secondary stages, or any of the other developmental categories which have been spread over so many pages of print? We must confess that we have never been very comfortable with the criteria for our own developmental stages. Too many of our cases resisted placement in any of them. In preparing this book, the miserable task of going through 30 years of case folders and a mountain of clinical notes to see what developmental data we could uncover has at least opened our eyes to our error. Seduced by Bluemel's concepts of primary and secondary stuttering, which were attractive because they described the marked differences between beginning and advanced stutterers, we first accepted these two kinds of stuttering, then added a third, called transitional stuttering, to accomodate those who fit neither category. Finally, in 1963, we added a fourth stage between primary and transitional. It was sheer folly. Carried to the extreme, we could have had an infinite number of minimally differentiated categories. In clinical practice, we had often found the distinctions difficult to use. Some children never showed any primary stuttering; some never became secondary. Also, a child could be a secondary stutterer one day, a transitional stutterer the next, and within a week be a primary stutterer or even a normal speaker. Or he could run the gamut back and forth within a single day. Bloodstein's four developmental phases of stuttering (based on averaging behaviors in terms of chronological age), suffer from the same limitations.

That we are not alone in our unhappiness with "stages" of stuttering development is demonstrated by this quotation from Wingate (1976, p. 67): "We should abandon the use of words with special and biasing connotations such as 'primary,' 'secondary,' 'phase,' 'stage,' and the like and instead stay closer to direct and verifiable observations."

The inadequacy of all this sectioning and categorizing now seems quite clear, and when adequate longitudinal data are available the concept of phases or stages will probably be completely discarded. This does not mean that the beginning stutterer should be treated in the same way we would treat him after he has learned to struggle or avoid. It means that our treatment should fit his needs as shown by his current behaviors, including their history; it should not be a prescribed treatment appropriate only to the child's classification in a developmental category. Human beings have a way of slipping through the meshes of all categories. We are tired of wielding empty nets.

NEED FOR LONGITUDINAL STUDIES

We urgently need longitudinal, not cross-sectional, research if we are to know how stuttering changes with time. It is difficult to do, and the money and time needed seem almost prohibitive. It will probably require a dedicated investigator or team of investigators working for years to assemble the necessary information. But it must be done.

We have only a few longitudinal studies of stuttering. The first of these was done in England and has been reported by Morley (1957) and by

Andrews and Harris (1964). Although important data was gathered about other features of the disorder, they did not attempt to study the changes in stuttering behaviors with age. They did find that many of the children who began to stutter early did recover and that those who persisted often became more severe.

Over a period of ten years Björn Fritzell (1974) studied 91 Swedish children who stuttered. He examined and checked them every two years, in terms of Bloodstein's four stages. Unfortunately, he reports only on data procured in the final examinations. These showed that 42 of the 91 who had been stuttering at the time of the first contact were then speaking normally; 21 of them (Stage 2) knew that they stuttered but did not care, and spoke freely; 25 (Stage 3) were concerned, irritated, and frustrated by their stuttering, and had some word and situation fears or were occasionally reluctant to speak. Only two (Stage 4) stutterers were seriously handicapped and avoiding words and opportunities to talk. Unfortunately, this preliminary report does not describe the changes in the actual stuttering behaviors shown at each of the two year periods.

The next sections of this chapter contain our observations of individual cases in a longitudinal way. These findings do not fulfill the requirements of objective research. We could not see all of the subjects routinely at specified intervals. The number of contacts, though they were many, varied from stutterer to stutterer. At times our clinical notes were too sketchy. The early observations were made before tapes were available, and even afterward we found that recordings have an astonishing ability to disappear from the files. How much contamination was produced by therapy we do not know, but certainly it had some influence. We tried to help all the subjects. We counselled their parents, and we worked directly or indirectly with all of them. The 44 stutterers whom we were able to follow from onset to adolescence or adulthood thus represent clinical failures, and it is on this small population that the conclusions are mainly based. It is our impression, however, that many other stutterers, for whom we succeeded in arresting the development of the disorder, or who did so themselves, showed similar developmental patterns. Maybe we have again deluded ourselves in thinking that we have found some common paths down which children stumble to lose themselves in the dark swamp of stuttering. In essence, we think the course of stuttering is often oscillatory, and there are at least four tracks the stutterers may follow in development.

THE OSCILLATORY COURSE OF DEVELOPMENT

One of the weaknesses in the concept of progressive stages of development is that it implies that the course of the disorder is linear, that it moves consistently forward toward greater severity and morbidity. Many authors have noted the prevalence of remissions in young stutterers. For a week or months or even longer the stuttering disappears, only to return again at a later time. An examination of our records, not only of the 44 stutterers we were able to follow from onset to maturity, but also of several hundred others with whom we had contact for only three or four years, demonstrated to our satisfaction that the development of stuttering is usually oscillatory. Only when it reached its final form did we find any stability of behavior.

In most instances, the younger the stutterer, the more he tended to oscillate from one level of severity to another. Periods characterized by many syllabic repetitions on many words alternated with other periods as long as a week or month when only two or three such repetitions occurred per day. Later in development, when frustration reactions with facial contortions and struggle appeared, they would persist for weeks and then give way to the earlier, simpler stuttering pattern. Developmentally the severity of stuttering seems to see-saw back and forth. Sometimes on the backswing, the stutterer may become completely fluent for days. We have watched children develop situation fears and avoidances, then lose them in succeeding weeks. Vivid awareness of their speech difficulties will be followed by long periods when no sign of awareness can be detected.

These swings are very important to the diagnostician. He must make sure that what he is observing in the examination situation is a representative sample for the period. He must also try to get an idea of the *range* of stuttering behaviors. We always try to assess not only the average or most characteristic kinds of behavior shown by the child, but also (through parental interview or repeated examinations) the extremes of greatest and least severity, its furthest and nearest points on the developmental schedule. We want to know, for example, if the child has any extended periods when the stuttering appears only as unforced, normally timed syllabic repetitions of if he is ever fluent for sustained periods.

It has been our clinical observation that these extreme points on the range of stuttering behaviors can provide very important information in terms of both diagnosis and prognosis, as will become evident in the following sections.

DIFFERENT TRACKS OF DEVELOPMENT

An examination of 300 case folders of stutterers we first saw in childhood (including the 44 on whom we had sufficient longitudinal observations) revealed certain common patterns of progressive change. Despite the oscillation, the general course of the disorder in those who continued to stutter for some years showed a series of features that seemed to follow each other in a definite sequence. In this search we were not looking for types of stutterers or etiological factors—we were trying to find out how stuttering changed with the passage of time. At first, we found the same sequence occurring so often we thought there was only one track, but as we hunted for exceptions it became fairly clear that there were instead several tracks. All but 3 of our 44 cases and all but 69 of the 300 fell into four major courses of development. Not all of the individuals in any one track followed its sequence exactly in every detail, and of course the sample may not be representative. So, it is only our opinion that in general the disorder developed with fair consistency according to one of four major sequential patterns. Despite initial doubt and continued skepticism we became convinced that the course of stuttering was not after all a random wandering in the wasteland. Selah!

Track I

Track I was by far the most common. Of the 44 stutterers in our best sample, 21 showed this developmental sequence and 141 of the other children followed it at least part of the way. It went like this. Stuttering first appeared, after a period of normally fluent speech, between 30 and 50 months, though actual age of onset was difficult to establish since it began gradually. Several remissions occurred for periods of a week or longer within the first two years after onset. In fact, Track I stutterers showed the greatest amount of oscillation in development. Their swings are more frequent and more extensive than those of the children on the other tracks. They are less consistent, sometimes showing a behavior characteristic of the most advanced forms of stuttering, then in a day or two returning to the simplest of syllabic repetitions or even quite normal speech. Track I stutterers have more complete remissions and for longer periods of time than those of the other groups. Also, most of the stutterers who spontaneously recover or who profit most swiftly from therapy have shown this course of development.

The behaviors of Track I stutterers consisted of frequent syllabic repetitions (without the schwa), uttered at the same tempo as the normally spoken syllables. They were multiple repetitions, averaging about three per word and rarely exceeding five per word. They were effortless, and so far as we could tell the child showed no signs of awareness. They occurred most frequently on the first word spoken after a pause or on the most meaningful word of the sentence. The single-syllabled words were repeated as wholes but polysyllabic words were not. Often the repetitions occurred in volleys or clusters which in turn were followed by considerable normal fluency. The stutterings constituted only a small but very noticeable fraction of the total speech output. When the children were fluent, they were very fluent. Luper and Mulder (1964) give their version of these features as follows:

> Incipient stuttering fluctuates considerably. Periods of days, weeks, and months may go by without the appearance of an unusual amount of stuttering. Sometimes the stuttering is reported to disappear completely before reappearing. More rarely, instances of periods of a year or more of fluency may be reported. Gradually (and the periods of time necessary for these changes to occur varies considerably) the periods of fluency become shorter and shorter and the presence of stuttering is noted more than its absence. It is noteworthy that at the onset of stuttering the disorder is essentially episodic—shifting to essentially chronic and finally to chronic insofar as observable periods of fluency are concerned (p. 21).

Next the tempo changes as the disorder develops. The repetitive syllables become irregular and are often spoken more rapidly than other fluent syllables. An occasional schwa is heard. The number of repetitions per syllable increases, first in terms of their range and then in terms of their average. The percentage, or number of stutterings per 100 or 1,000 words, increases. To the listener they seem compulsive. Freund (1966) expresses the latter impression well:

> The repetitions here are not used for the purpose of filling in a gap but for the purpose of overcoming a hindrance which, as it were, towers within the syllable itself, between its articulatory closure phase and phonation. These forms of intrasyllabic, struggling repetitions become quickly compulsive, fixed, and conditioned (p. 72).

Further development is marked by an occasional prolongation of a voiced continuant sound. At first they appear largely at the conclusion of the repetitions and upon the first sound of the word that is then spoken, but later they may be heard earlier in the stream of repetitions. Following this, some children demonstrate prolongations of the vowels within the syllables. We hate to see any of this development, and we regard these vowel prolongations as a definite danger signal. We have seen too many children react to them with awareness and frustration which often leads them to produce a rise in pitch resembling a fire siren on the prolonged vowel.

In most of these children, as the disorder grows, the prolongations move forward, from the final repeated syllable of a series to the initial syllable. Very soon thereafter prolongations tend to become increasingly predominant behaviors (though syllabic repetitions may occur sporadically throughout life in a confirmed stutterer.) Tension and forcings then make their appearance, first on the voiced and then on the silent prolongations of an articulatory posture during these prolongations, and we find the stuttering tremor showing itself for the first time. It is in this phase that many of the children begin to show concern. The frustrating awareness manifests itself initially as surprise, almost shock. The child may stop talking abruptly, look at his listener helplessly or angrily or even say, "I can't talk." They may cry or strike out at their listener.

As we have also discovered, Bloodstein (1960) found that these behaviors can occur very early in life:

> Of the nine two-year-old subjects, four were said to have reacted to repetitions or other types of blockage by exclaiming, "I can't talk," by crying, or by looking down and blushing. In one case, seen three weeks after reported onset, the child was said to have become "so annoyed" by his repetitions that he hit himself on the mouth and stopped talking for three days (p. 233).

Despite these comments and reactions, this awareness seldom lasts very long. In a few days the disorder has again reversed its course and no signs of frustration can be detected. The stuttering is still very intermittent with remarkably long periods of completely fluent speech, but when the volleys occur they last longer. One can also witness the growth of these prolon-

gations in time. At first very short, their durations increase depe,
upon the communicative stress and other factors to be described late,

Next, surges of tension appear and with them signs of obvious strug,
as the child seeks to interrupt his closures and fixations. Facial contortions,
jaw jerks, co-movements of the limbs are seen in various combinations,
much of the behavior almost appearing random and unstereotyped. The
tension, first located in the lips or jaws, overflows to adjacent structures.
The child is now highly aware of his difficulty, greatly frustrated by it,
and doing his utmost to interrupt it so that he can continue to communicate.
Stein (1942) puts it this way:

> His deliberate efforts have brought the stammerer "out of the frying pan into
> the fire." He is now quite convinced that speaking is hard work, and is puzzled
> about how other people are able to master it. He now follows the rule which we
> all follow when our motor attempts are not successful: we think we have not
> made enough effort (p. 121).

As the child makes an effort to overcome what he senses as the obstacles
in his speaking, he shows various kinds of struggle behavior. Some of
them are signals to himself, devices to aid in timing the next attempt or
to help force out the word. But they are often simply the result of
spreading tension. When these behaviors appear, the parents react with
surprise and horror, reactions which the child notices soon enough, and
which in turn create even greater struggling or lead, as we shall see, to
anticipation, expectancy, and fear. Remember the oscillatory course of the
disorder. We have seen extreme behaviors of this sort disappear a few
days later so that the child is stuttering effortlessly again. We recognize
their danger of course. As the swings move further forward, the changes
are less that the back swings will return within the range of normal fluency.
But our concern deepens when we see signs of fear.

In quicksand, the more you struggle the deeper you sink, and the child
soon finds himself in a quagmire of fear. Fear is the anticipation of
unpleasantness, and once the child has repeatedly experienced the frustrations of interrupted communication, he comes to expect it when certain
stimuli that were associated with the experience earlier now present
themselves again. Many of the young stutterers we have studied show their
first fears on words rather than situations—but this may be due to our
active intervention to keep the child's associates from penalizing him for
the stuttering. In all the children who showed situation fears before word
fears, the child's associates, parents or siblings, had somehow called the
stuttering to his attention, had shown their anxiety and concern, or had
mocked or punished him. Where we were able to prevent this, the word
fears came first.

What are these fears and what are their nuclei? It is always difficult to
determine. In their play-talk commentary, one of the older children told
us of invisible little green men who squirted glue in his mouth; another
said that something squeezed in his tongue tight when he wasn't looking;
still others, simply that some words were just too hard to say and that they

could see them coming. One little girl would whisper something with her mouth onto a piece of paper and then erase it hard. She said it was a "trouble word." One boy insisted that some words wanted to go down when they should come up, and he often squatted when struggling with his stuttering. Most of the children cannot tell you. The clinician, however, will not find it difficult to identify the signs of fear. There are pauses before the utterance or before the word. The rate of speech suddenly slows, becomes hesitant. Words are tackled gingerly, almost pre-tasted for danger. The breathing is altered with jerky over-inhalations, it is held before vocalization, or it becomes very shallow. The voice loses its flexibility of intonation. And you can see the fear on the child's face and in the suddent immobility of his body posture.

Once fear arises, avoidance follows. Synonyms are used and stallers, rituals of timing, or disguise behaviors. The loci of stuttering become more consistent. We have watched the spread of these fears in many children. The earliest gradient of generalization seems to be phonemic rather than semantic. The fear of /p/ words spreads to /b/ words, then to the other bilabials, then to labiodentals. Even advanced stutterers are often able to use synonyms with some success, which probably reflects this same observation. Other verbal features are scanned for danger signals: the length of the word, its familiarity, its position, its propositionality. All or any of these can become cues.

Situation fears show a similar pattern of growth by generalization. When a given listener, whether it be parent or playmate, reacts to the child's stutterings punishingly, other listeners become able to generate fear depending on how much they resemble the punisher. We have watched fear spread from its origin in reaction to the impatient mother of a favorite playmate to other older women, and then to the child's own mother. We have seen the stuttering child who formerly played freely with all the children in the block gradually restrict his play space and partners until finally he would play only with a little sister in his own yard. The first situational fears tend to be fears of people rather than of the conditions of communication. Later we find them precipitated by cues associated with communicative experiences such as talking at the dinner table, answering questions, making requests. One child showed his first situational fear in the family car after having been shouted at by his father for an especially severe moment of stuttering. Afterward, he was not afraid of speaking to his father in any situation other than while being transported, even when his mother did the driving. We have been unable to discern any common patterns in the growth of these sound, word, and situation fears except that the process of stimulus generalization makes itself evident, and that avoidance increases their intensity. The fears grow and the fears spread, but each child develops his own unique constellation depending on the specific circumstances under which he has experienced communicative frustration or punishment.

In the final phases of the disorder's development, which we shall describe with more detail in a succeeding chapter, a series of important changes occur. Patterns of stuttering behavior, both overt and covert, become stabilized and stereotyped. The stuttering child acquires the self-concept and role of a "stutterer" with all the evil these entail. Personality changes may occur; defenses are set up. The disorder becomes an integral part of his existence.

Track II

The analysis of our records also revealed another fairly common developmental route. Of the 44 stutterers whom we were able to study until they reached maturity, 11 showed Track II development as did 31 others on whom we have less complete records. One of the marked differences between these children and those of Track I is that the fluency disruptions began much earlier in speech development. Most, though not all, of these children also showed retarded speech development and did not use phrases or sentences until they were from three to six years of age. What is distinctive is that the disorder appeared when they began to talk consecutively. In those whom we observed, and from the parental reports of those we did not, it seems clear that these children had no previous history of sustained normal fluency. The onset of stuttering came with the onset of connected speech. We are pretty sure of this since six of the 11 persons mentioned above began to stutter (or clutter?) while they were receiving help for delayed speech and language in our own clinic, and we have had more than a few reports from other speech therapists who saw "stuttering" develop before their eyes in the children they were trying to teach to talk.

These then are the children who have been able to comprehend the long involved sentences of others for some time before they themselves could communicate verbally. For some time, even years, they have used gestures, a few single words, or jargon to make their wants known. As they break free from their shackles, their urge to communicate creates an exorbitant demand on their small store of available expressive symbols. The speech is very unorganized. Arranging, sorting, sequencing according to dimly perceived, standard syntactical patterns, these children need more than the usual amount of time and do not usually get it. They need simple models and much patience from their listeners and when these are not forthcoming, breaks in fluency appear. We find some of the same picture in aphasics as they began to regain their speech.

The literature has many accounts of this sort of onset. In Hungary, Hirschberg (1965) writes:

> In our own series of patients, we found in 48 cases, that is, in nearly one third of all the patients examined, a delayed speech development. This agrees with the figures reported by Borel-Maisonny, who found late development of speech in 58 per cent of her stutterers (p. 783).

Andrews and Harris (1964) noted that the children who were severely delayed in speech at the age of three and four began to stutter as they became intelligible. Dostalova and Dosuzkov (1965) classified them as

TOURO COLLEGE LIBRARY

belonging to a group they called "Balbuties Tarda" and stated that they had the poorest prognosis. De Parrel (1965) echoes a long French tradition of ascribing stuttering onset to the delayed beginning of true speech. Some children do seem to start stuttering in this way.

The early behaviors in Track II are not exactly the same as those of Track I. There are the same syllabic repetitions, but from the beginning they are hurried and irregular, and whole words of one syllable constitute the greater proportion of these early repetitions. Later on this changes. There are more silent gaps, more hesitations, than in Track I. More stumbling occurs, more abortive beginnings, more revisions, more interjections. Before they speak these children often hold their breath, then blurt. They seem to be searching for words. There are more back-ups, more retrials, more changes in direction. Articulation errors are prevalent. This is the unorganized speech described so clearly by Bluemel (1957); it is the early cluttering-like speech delineated by Weiss (1964).

The children on this track seem relatively free from frustration. Their tolerance of fluency breaks seems to be very great, perhaps because so many of them have never known what it feels like to talk without stuttering. Moreover, awareness, fear, struggle, and avoidance develop much more slowly than in Track I. Track II children do not seem to listen to themselves. It is conceivable that this auditory imperceptiveness to their own speech was one of the factors which produced the original delay. They may have skipped the stage of self-listening which most children go through before they learn to monitor their utterance primarily by proprioception. Perhaps their inattention to their own fluency breaks results from the fact that they often have many other problems too, problems of coordination, musicality, articulation, language, and general organization. We have followed some of these children from onset to adulthood and marvelled to see how they filter out the junk in their speech.

This track also differs from Track I in that these children rarely show prolongations and fixations. They repeat long strings of syllables or words, often very swiftly and compulsively, but they rarely hold a sound or articulatory posture during the early development of the disorder. Occasionally on the first word of a sentence or phrase (especially if it begins with a vowel) they silently preform the vowel, holding back in preparation for the verbal rush to follow, but this seems different from the tremor-infused prolongations of Track I. These children are often tremor-free for a long time. They also have fewer complete blockings of the airway at the lips or palate or in the larynx than other stutterers in the later stages of development.

There are also characteristic differences in the development of fears in these children. Situation fears come first, and for many they remain the only ones. Phonemic fears are at best vague and unreliable. They are not intense, not phobic. The children on Track II do not show the complexity, the spread, or the intensity of logophobia so characteristic of other stutterers. When they have word fears, the cues that precipitate them are word length or unfamiliarity rather than particular sounds associated with frustration or penalty.

TOURO COLLEGE LIBRARY

Track II children seldom exhibit grotesque facial or body movements, even late in the disorder's development, perhaps because they have so few prolongations or fixations. Since Track II children rarely have complete blockage, they have little need for the timing or releasing jerks or associated movements which create so much abnormality in others. What they do show, in the more severe cases, are long series of repetitions of syllables and whole words, often produced so compulsively as to render their speech completely unintelligible. These "runaway" behaviors (so labelled by older members of Track II) are difficult to describe in words. The person begins a syllable, and it seems to recycle perservatively like some normal speakers on the delayed feedback apparatus. The syllabic repetitions are very fast, often accelerating throughout their duration, and arhythmic. They are also often accompanied by a rise in pitch. Once caught in these oscillations, the Track II stutterer seems unable to terminate them until the exhalation is finished. We have seen some even yelp or shout in the effort to interrupt the compulsive oscillatory yapping. During these spasmodic experiences, the eyes of these stutterers often seem fixed and glazed, but they are highly aware that something devastating is happening to them. Older ones have told us that when they get started on one of these "runaways," they can't stop. Interestingly enough, for those in the terminal phase of Track II, even after many of these experiences, although they have a few word or sound fears, it is the experience itself or the situation in which it occurred which is most dreaded. Only a very few of the children of Track II, however, reach this traumatic destination; most of them terminate in speech that is mildly stuttered but mainly cluttered.

It might be objected that what we have been describing is not stuttering but cluttering. The early patterns shown by these children could certainly be viewed as cluttering, but later on they certainly show all the characteristics of true stuttering. The problems of differential diagnosis are difficult, and almost all authorities agree that stuttering may emerge from cluttering and that both disorders may coexist in the same individual. The individuals in Track II end up as stutterers. They do not become fluent when they try to talk slowly and carefully. They eventually become aware of their disordered speech (especially on the "runaway" repetitions) and they develop some rare but real situation and phonemic fears. They talk in torrents. They use avoidance tricks and consider themselves stutterers. Some cluttering component is probably present since, when their stuttering decreases as a result of therapy, they speak more clutteringly than before. Without arguing the diagnosis, we can say that some stutterers show this pattern of disorder development. De Hirsch and Langford (1950) make the following comment on the Track II type:

> There is another smaller group who have similar symptoms but at a later age. Many of these children start talking late. . . . Frequently their motor speech patterns are so poor that their speech is practically unintelligible. . . . Investigation of the family background of these children frequently reveals a history of language difficulty. . . . The speech of these children closely resembles a type of disturbance seen at all ages and known as cluttering (p. 936).

Preus (1981), relying upon parental reports, found a group of his stutterers who showed the characteristics of development we have described for Track II. They did not develop much anxiety or struggle; the major stuttering behaviors were repetitions and prolongations.

Track III

We would like to illustrate the third route of stuttering development with a brief case presentation.

B.J., a boy of five years, was walking with his father down a residential street one evening when a dog rushed out from a yard and bit him so severely he had to be hospitalized for two weeks and given the painful series of rabies shots. He had been speaking at the time he was bitten. Until this incident, the boy had been very fluent, but in the hospital and thereafter his speech was marked by spasmodic inhalations prior to all utterance. Laryngeal closures with marked tension initiated all speech attempts after all pauses. We had known the child before the trauma and visited him while still in the hospital. Despite all we could do, this child developed a very severe stuttering problem, and it has persisted now for over 20 years. Its symptomatology has changed little, though the laryngeal blockings with their preceding inhalations do not occur after *every* pause as formerly. They show themselves only under various kinds of communicative stress, in reciting, in talking to authority figures, etc. The normal speech is completely fluent. B.J. has word and phonemic fears, the vowels being especially dreaded. He has developed a variety of avoidance behaviors, primarily of postponement, but they fail him more often than they help. The stuttering behavior is remarkably consistent and stereotyped and monosymptomatic. He has had psychotherapy and speech therapy for years and still stutters in the same way he began.

Only 5 of the 44 persons we studied longitudinally and on whom we had sufficient data fit the pattern of this track, but we were able to discern the same patterning in 13 other cases whom we were able to treat successfully before they reached the terminal behaviors. Few of the stutterers in Track III provide as clear a history of the circumstances surrounding onset as that of B.J. Usually all we know is that the disorder started very suddenly and that it began with an apparent inability to speak or to continue speaking. Most parents cannot account for this sudden appearance of what they call "blocking," but some attribute it to frightening experiences, shocks, sudden changes in environment, and a host of other causes most of which when investigated appear to have little pertinence. Since this section is not concerned with etiology but only with how stuttering develops, we want to stress the initial behavior rather than the presumed conditions under which it arose. Vague as these parents often are about the "causes," they are very specific about what made them aware that the child was having trouble. "He opened his mouth and tried to talk but nothing came out." "It was like he couldn't get any sound out." "She would try and try again to get started but wasn't able to." "It really wasn't like stuttering. She didn't repeat over and over; she just tried to talk and couldn't. Now she repeats, but not at first. She was stuck that's all."

All of the children in this group had spoken quite fluently for some years, and the age of onset is usually later than in Track I. Most of them begin stuttering during the years from five to nine, although we have found the same pattern occasionally in a child as young as two years and also in adults. The stuttering is at first consistently confined to the beginning of an utterance after a pause, and once the sentence or phrase is under way no further difficulty is experienced until another and different utterance is begun. The basic initial behavior is fixation not oscillation; it is tonic, not clonic. The first articulatory posture is held and prolonged. It is accompanied by tension and struggle almost from the first. The closure is primarily at the level of the larynx. Breathing abnormalities appear very soon and often become stereotyped rituals of attack. An intermittent vocal fry can be heard during the struggle for phonation.

These children develop awareness and frustration almost immediately. Struggling and forcing also appear very soon. Tremors show up in the tensed musculature. Often the child will cry helplessly or attack the listener or stop talking for long periods. Regressions in social behavior patterns ensue: enuresis, thumb-sucking, other long-outgrown forms of infantile behavior. We have seen the eyes cross during the struggle. An overflow of tension results in facial contortions and associated limb movements. The child may finally shout the word with which he has attempted to begin his utterance. All of this behavior develops very suddenly and swiftly although it may completely and dramatically disappear for a considerable period only to show up again in a slightly different form. But in far too many, the disorder grows like a brushfire. From the frustration and the struggle and the great concern shown by the child's associates—a concern that is most difficult to conceal since it seems so merited—the fears and avoidance arise. No one who has witnessed the malignant growth of this behavior can doubt the traumatic experience felt by the child.

As the child progresses along Track III the silent fixations at the level of the larynx spread to the lips and the tongue. We have noticed in the few of these children with whom we would work directly that multiple occlusions of the airway occurred. First, after a quick intake of breath, the larynx was raised up under the hyoid, and the vocal folds were tightly adducted as in startle. Then abdominal pressure was suddenly increased in an effort to break the blockade. This was the elementary pattern of behavior that took place during the abortive attempt to speak. Next we noticed that other structures were also beginning to occlude the airways. First the lips were closed, then the tongue was pressed against the palate. In the longest moments of this kind of stuttering, all three closures occurred simultaneously. Most of the children showed only one closure during any one moment of stuttering. We found generally, however, that within a few weeks prolongations of vowels and the continuant consonants would make their appearance and that then there was a sudden decrease in the number of the old silent laryngeal closures. It seemed almost as though the child was able to substitute this other type of prolonged fixation. As proportionately more prolonged /s/, /f/, /m/, /n/, and other phonemes appeared, the pronounced struggle behaviors also decreased and the child seemed less frustrated. He began to talk more again.

Next in the development of stuttering in this group of children, syllabic repetitions appear for the first time in substantial quantity. There is some repetitive behavior in the early behavior, but it is more retrial than clonic repetition. In other words, the child would get so stuck, he had to stop completely and then try again. This is quite different from the automatic syllabic bouncing of the Track I children. In the Track III children, the repetitions follow the prolongations, and often each repetition begins with a slight prolongation of the first sound (tonoclonus). It seems as if the child is trying to find the proper integration of the initial syllable of the word. One of the characteristic features distinguishing this group is the relative rareness of their stuttering on the later syllables of a polysyllabic word, even upon a syllable carrying the primary accent. They simply have trouble getting started! Evidently this phase presents a favorable opportunity for the reacquisition of fluency since we have noted that a good many of the children who do recover, do so at this stage of development.

Those who do not are swept over the falls of fear and into the whirlpool of chronic stuttering. They present the most morbid picture of any of the three groups of children we have described. Their fears are stronger; their patterns of stuttering behavior more complex. Avoidance is very marked. They scan approaching situations and prospective utterances with greater anxiety. They become very severe stutterers, often of the interiorized type described by Freund (1934) and by Douglass and Quarrington (1952).

Track IV

The onset of the disorder in these children is usually later than for those of the other tracks. As in the children of Track III, stuttering begins suddenly and after several years of fluency. The initial behavior, however, is different. From the first it seems highly stereotyped, almost deliberate and contrived. The child seems very aware of it from the first and even more aware of its impact on the listener, whom he watches carefully. He is testing, testing, testing. Often he may smile slightly.

In some of these children the first behaviors are repetitions of whole words or phrases rather than syllables, although they soon change to include the latter. The initial word or phrase is repeated many more times than is usual in normal nonfluency. The inflection and intonation patterns are demanding, insisting. The child begins a sentence with "I-YI-YI-YI-YI-I-I-I" or "Mommy-mommy-mommy-mommy-mommy" or "When can, when can, when can, when can, when can, when can I go?" A bit later that some child will be saying, "Whe-whe-when-when-wh-wh-when-when can I go?" The lengthy repetition of words already spoken normally is a continuously characteristic feature of this group. Even in the advanced stages these children sometimes say a word or phrase correctly, then stop and say it again with pronounced nonfluency. They return to the utterance to stutter upon it.

There are some, who seem to belong to this group, who show no repetitions at all. The first behaviors are gaps and pauses accompaniéd by stereotyped postures and activities such as sobbing, grunting, biting, or tongue or lip protrusions. The jaws may be opened widely and retching noises made. Whimpering sounds accompanied by tremulous movements of the lower lip may fill the pauses.

One of the children we studied intensively was brought to us by his anxious mother because he had suddenly begun to interrupt his fluency with successive inhalations until his chest was greatly distended. He would hold this thoracic posture for some moments, sometimes until he staggered. We learned that early in infancy the boy had done a lot of breath-holding in moments of frustration. It was plainly evident that he was using the behavior to control his mother and we did what we could through referral to a child psychiatrist to solve the problem, but in vain. We have watched the disorder develop over the years and at present this person, now an adult, would be classified as a severe stutterer by anyone. Other reactions have joined the initial respiratory behavior, but the latter still dominates the symptom picture. He is infantile, neurotic, controlling still.

One of the major distinguishing characteristics of Track IV is that the behavior changes very little over the years. The frequency of stutterings may increase, but the basic patterns seem very stable. Most of the other stutterers we have described pass through many phases and finally develop a repertoire of different avoidance or release reactions. Those on this track, however, tend to be monosymptomatic. Moreover, they develop few avoidance tricks; the disguise and masking behaviors are conspicuous by their absence. Interruptor behaviors are few. These children offer you their stuttering openly. They watch you as you react to it. And they are rarely emotional about it. As adults, they talk a lot about their tragic speech handicap, but somatic evidence of stress is not impressive. GSR recordings show little disturbance even when pronounced speech interference is demonstrated. When they are fluent, they are very, very fluent. When they are not, their behavior is stereotyped, almost symbolic, and there is that small, brave smile. These stutterers suffer less than their listeners. One can sense the controlling, punishing, wheedling, exploitative urges behind the behavior. Only four of our 44 children fit the pattern we have outlined as characteristic of this track and only five others of our larger population seemed to show the described onset and development. It is our impression that those who begin to stutter in adulthood are more likely to portray these behaviors than children. And the adults show very few changes once they begin to stutter this way. They continue to stutter much the same way they began.

Other Courses of Development

We have described four of the common courses of stuttering development, and the first two are by far the most common. Some stutterers we have studied do not follow any of these tracks; some shift intermittently from one to another at different times. We could not fit three of our smaller group and 69 of our larger group into any track. Remember also that these are just observations, the gleanings of 35 hectic years. Until we have careful longitudinal studies of large groups of stutterers, studies which present very great difficulties in design and administration, we must rely on such clinical observations or on the information we get from cross-sectional studies. Table 5.2 and Table 5.3 summarize these four courses of development.

TABLE 5.2. Tracks of Development at Onset

TRACK I	TRACK II
Begins 2½ to 4 years.	Often late. At time of first sentences.
Previously fluent.	Never very fluent.
Gradual onset.	Gradual onset.
Cylic.	Steady.
Long remissions.	No remissions.
Good articulations.	Poor articulation.
Normal rate.	Fast; spurts.
Syllabic repetitions.	Gaps, revisions, syllable, and word repetitions.
No tension; unforced.	No tension.
No tremors.	No tremors.
Loci: First words, function words.	Loci: First words; long words; scattered throughout sentence; content words.
Variable pattern.	Variable pattern.
Normal speech is well integrated.	Broken speech with hesitation and gaps even when no disfluency.
No awareness.	No awareness.
No frustration.	No frustration.
No fears; willing to talk.	No fears; willing to talk.

TRACK III	TRACK IV
Any age after child has consecutive speech.	Late, usually after four years.
Previously fluent.	Previously fluent.
Sudden onset, often after trauma.	Sudden onset.
Steady.	Erratic.
Few short remissions.	No remissions.
Normal articulation.	Normal articulation.
Slow, careful rate.	Normal rate.
Unvoiced prolongations.	Unusual behaviors (see text).
Laryngeal blockings.	
Much tension.	Variable tension.
Tremors.	Few tremors.
Beginning of utterance after pauses primary.	First words; rarely on function words; content words especially.
Consistent pattern.	Consistent pattern.
Normal speech is very fluent.	Normal speech is very fluent.
Highly aware.	Highly aware.
Much frustration.	No frustration.
Fears speaking; situation and word fears.	No evidence of fear; willing to talk.

TABLE 5.3. Developmental Characteristics

TRACK I	TRACK II
Repetitions of syllables increase in frequency and speed and become irregular.	Behaviors remain the same but the speed increases; their number also increases.
Then:	
Repetition of syllables begin to end in prolongations.	Little change in form.
Then:	
Prolongations show increased tension, tremors, struggle. Evidence of frustration.	Little change; little awareness; little frustration.
Then:	
Overflow of tension; facial contortions; retrials; speech output decreases; signs of concern	Duration of nonfluencies increases; more syllabic repetitions; little awareness.
Then:	
Word fears and avoidance occur. Fears of certain sounds arise. Then situation fears develop. Repetitions and prolongations turn into silent fixations with struggle (blocking). Poor eye contact and tricks to disguise the difficulty are observed. Shows hesitancy, embarrassment.	Occasional fears of situations, not of words or sounds. Long strings of syllabic repetitions at fast speed are added to other behaviors. Some fears of situations. Good eye contact. No disguise. Output of speech increases. Little avoidance. Primarily repetitive. Unorganized.

TRACK III	TRACK IV
An increase in the frequency but the behavior at first changes little. Signs of frustration.	The number of instances increases, and they are shown in more situations.
Then:	
More retrials are seen; lip protrusions, and tongue fixations appear; prolongations of initial sounds.	Little change in form; monosymptomatic and symbolic.
Then:	
Tremors; struggling; facial contortions; jaw jerk, gasping; marked frustration.	Little change.
Then:	
Interruptor devices become prominent; rate slows; more hesitancy; more refusals to talk.	Little change in type but duration and visibility increase; no interruptors or new forcings; increased output of speech.
Then:	
Intense fears of words and sounds; many avoidances; patterns change in form and grow more bizarre; much overflow; output of speech decreases; will cease trying to talk. Poor eye contact; the normal speech becomes hesitant. Nonvocalized blockings are frequent. Primary tonic blocks with multiple closures.	Very few avoidance or release behaviors. Not much evidence of word fears. Few consistent loci. Very aware of stuttering. Stutters very openly. Good eye contact. Little variability in the stuttering behavior. Normal speech very fluent. Talks a lot. Consisten pattern; few silent blockings. Either tonic or clonic.

At the time that we provided the account of how stuttering develops in terms of different tracks, we hoped that others would soon make this information obsolete, but ten years have elapsed and little more has been done. The only exception is found in the investigation of Ohashi (1973) who studied the longitudinal development of stuttering in only eleven children, observing them at monthly intervals. Major findings were these: Stuttering changed its appearance similarly to that described in Van Riper's Tracks I and II; repetitions constituted the earliest stuttering behaviors and grew more complex and abnormal with lapse of time; the appearance of prolongations or complete blockings represented a further stage in the development of the disorder; avoidance and awareness reactions had not appeared by the time the study was completed—40 months from the first interviews; and the frequency of stuttering occurrence was not representative of the severity of individual moments of stuttering.

Again may we state our hope that someone will do a long term longitudinal study of the development of stuttering. Except for our understanding of the nature of the core of stuttering, no matter is so urgent as this. To cite just two of the several implications of this information, Preus (1981) felt that the stutterers in Tracks I and II represent two different types of stuttering and Heidemann and Schönfelder (1976) recommend parent counseling for Track I stutterers, parent counseling and speech therapy for Track II stutterers, and parent counseling and psychotherapy for Tracks III and IV stutterers. In any event, we need better longitudinal studies than those we now possess.

SUMMARY

To summarize all this information, we can say that there is clear evidence that the behaviors that characterize stuttering change as the disorder persists. The majority of stutterers, but not all, begin with repetitions of sounds and syllables or with prolongations but most of them develop additional struggle and avoidance reactions as time passes, and as fear, frustration, and embarrassment are experienced. Not all stutterers show the same pattern of development, however, and we have offered the suggestion (with some questionable evidence to support it) that four tracks of development may be discerned. The need for long-term longitudinal studies has been emphasized.

Again, of the three major theories concerning the nature of stuttering, the neurotic theory does not seem to be congruent with this information. It is obvious, however, that learning theory could explain the changes in the form of the stuttering behaviors and their increasing severity. The view that the core behavior of stuttering may be the result of motor coordination difficulties in timing the synergies involved is compatible with this information, but it is evident that many of the accessory behaviors are learned.

BIBLIOGRAPHY

ANDREWS, G. AND M. HARRIS. 1964. *The syndrome of stuttering*. London: Heinemann.

BLOODSTEIN, O. 1960–61. Development of stuttering. *Journal of Speech and Hearing Disorders* 25: 219–37; 366–76; 26: 67–82.

BLUEMEL, C. S. 1932. Primary and secondary stammering. *Quarterly Journal of Speech* 18: 187–200.

———. 1940. Stammering and inhibition. *Journal of Speech Disorders* 5: 305–8.

———. 1957. *The riddle of stuttering*. Danville, Ill.: Interstate.

———. 1935. *Stammering and allied disorders*. New York: Macmillan.

———. 1913. *Stammering and cognate defects of speech*, Vol. I. New York: Stecher.

DE HIRSCH, K. AND W. S. LANGFORD. 1950. Clinical note on stuttering and cluttering in young children. *Pediatrics* 5: 934–40.

DE PARREL, S. 1965. *Speech Disorders*. Oxford: Pergamon.

DOSTALOVA, N. AND T. DOSUKOV. 1965. Uber die drei Hauptformen des neurotische Stotterns. *De Therapia Vocis et Loquellae* 1: 273–76.

DOUGLASS, E. AND B. QUARRINGTON. 1952. Differentiation of interiorized and exteriorized secondary stuttering. *Journal of Speech and Hearing Disorders* 17: 377–85.

FREUND, H. 1966. *Psychopathology and the problems of stuttering*. Springfield, Ill.: Thomas.

FRITZELL, B. 1974. The prognosis of stuttering in school-age children. A ten year longitudinal study. *Proceedings of the XVI Congress of Logopedics and Phoniatrics*. Interlaken: Basel: Karger, 128–31.

FROESCHELS, E. 1955. Core of stuttering. *Acta Otolaryngologica* 45: 115–19.

———. 1943. Pathology and therapy of stuttering. *Nervous Child* 2: 146–61.

———. 1940–64. *Selected papers (1940–1964)*. Amsterdam: North-Holland, 1964.

———. 1943. Survey of the early literature on stuttering, chiefly european. *Nervous Child* 2: 86–95.

———. 1952. The significance of symptomatology for the understanding of the essence of stuttering. *Folia Phoniatrica* 4: 217–30.

GLASNER, P. J. 1949. Personality characteristics and emotional problems of stutterers under the age of five. *Journal of Speech and Hearing Disorders* 14: 135–38.

HEIDEMANN, B. AND T. SCHÖNFELDER. 1976. Stuttering in children and adolescents. *Der Nervenarzt* 47: 287–94.

HIRSCHBERG, J. 1965. Stuttering. (Hungarian text) *Orvosi Hetilap* 106: 780–84.

HOEPFNER, T. 1912. Stottern-als assoziative Aphasie. *Zeitschrift für Pathopsychologie* 1: 448–553.

HUNT, J. 1861. *Stammering and stuttering, their nature and treatment* (Original Edition). Reprinted New York: Hafner, 1967.

JOHNSON, W. 1959. *The onset of stuttering*. Minneapolis: University of Minnesota Press.

KNUDSEN, R. 1948. Personal communication.

LUPER, H. L. AND R. L. MULDER. 1964. *Stuttering therapy for children*. Englewood Cliffs, N.J.: Prentice-Hall.

MORLEY, M. 1957. *The development and disorders of speech in childhood*. Edinburgh: Livingstone.

OHASHI, Y. 1973.   The development of stuttering in children. *Japanese Journal of Child Psychiatry* 14: 142–66.

―――. 1976.   Development of stuttering in children with onset at 2.6–3.6 years. *Practica Otologica Kyoto* 19: 825–38.

―――. 1977.   The development of stuttering in children: a cross sectional study. *Japanese Journal of Child Psychiatry* 17: 57–68.

ORTON, S. T. 1937.   *Reading, writing and speech problems in childhood.* New York: Norton.

PELLMAN, C. 1947.   *Overcoming stammering.* New York: Beechurst.

POTTER, S. O. L. 1882.   *Speech and its defects.* Philadelphia: Blakeston.

PREUS, A. 1981.   *Attempts at identifying subgroups of stutterers.* Oslo: University of Oslo Press.

ROBINSON, F. B. 1964.   *An introduction to stuttering.* Englewood Cliffs, N.J.: Prentice-Hall.

ROMAN, K. G. 1959.   Handwriting and speech. *Logos* 2: 29–39.

STEIN, L. 1942.   *Speech and voice.* London: Methuen.

VAN RIPER, C. 1963.   *Speech correction: principles and methods* (4th Edition). Englewood Cliffs, N.J.: Prentice-Hall.

VLASOVA, N. A. 1962.   Prevention and treatment of stuttering in children in the U.S.S.R. *Ceskoslovenska Otolaryngologie* 11: 30–32.

WEISS, D. A. 1964.   *Cluttering.* Englewood Cliffs, N.J.: Prentice-Hall.

―――. 1960.   Therapy for cluttering. *Folia Phoniatrica* 12: 216–28.

WINGATE, M. E., 1976. *Stuttering: theory and therapy.* New York: Irvington-Wiley.

WYLLIE, J. 1894.   *The disorders of speech.* Edinburgh: Oliver and Boyd.

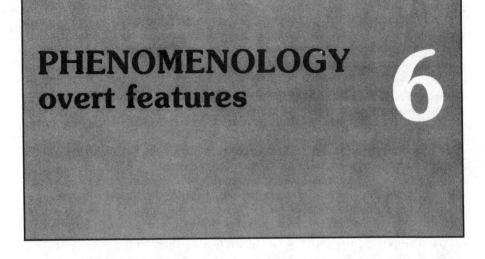

PHENOMENOLOGY
overt features

6

This chapter describes the features of stuttering in its full fledged form. Having discarded the phrase "secondary stuttering" for reasons mentioned earlier, adjectives such as "advanced" or "confirmed" will be used to refer to fully developed stuttering. Wyllie (1894) gives a vivid description of stuttering in its morbid maturity.

> He (the stutterer) closes the oral canal at one or other of the closing points, according to the nature of the letter to be articulated, and this he does as well as a man who possesses the faculty of speech could do it; instead, however, of allowing the vowel to follow without delay, he presses his lips, or his tongue and teeth, or his tongue and palate, more firmly together than is necessary; the explosive escape of the air does not take place, the other muscles of the face and those of the glottis and even the muscles of the neck become spasmodically affected like those of articulation; gesticulatory movements are made, the abdomen is retracted, the head is drawn backward, and the larynx is drawn forcibly upward, until finally he works himself into a state of frightful agitation; his heart beats forcibly, his face becomes red and blue, his body is bedewed with perspiration, and he may present the appearance of a complete maniac* (pp. 21–22).

VARIABILITY

Not all confirmed stutterers show so severe a disorder, but anyone who has worked with more than a few adult cases will recognize the picture as

---

* Wyllie evidently translated this from an earlier article by Kussmaul in Ziemssen's Medical Encyclopedia (1877). We are glad to help the venerable German's words reverberate a little longer.

a familiar one. And this is only one of many such portraits in the rogue's gallery of stuttering. The newcomer to this gallery is often both appalled and bewildered by the variegated display. How can all these behaviors constitute one disorder? Why does the stutterer do what he does when trying to talk? One young man stopped suddenly in the middle of one of his contorted struggles, grinned at us, and then blurted with complete fluency, "The trouble with stuttering is that it just doesn't make any sense." We hope this chapter will help make overt stuttering behaviors more comprehensible.

In most stutterers, the early behavior is primarily syllabic repetitions and prolongations of a sound or articulatory posture (see Chapter 5). But people react to the frustration and penalties that follow these behaviors in many different ways. There are literally thousands of possible reactions that can be used to escape, avoid, or disguise the inability to say a word. We have reports of identical twins who stuttered differently. Most adult stutterers pass through a whole series of different reaction patterns before they develop the final set which is as unique as their fingerprints. At four years of age, the stutterer may have only syllabic repetitions; at five, postural fixations. By his 11th birthday he could be retching and gasping; by his 16th, his speech may also be punctuated by long pauses. When he is 30, all of these behaviors may be in his stuttering repertoire, and there may also be some head-jerks. But some of these behaviors may also be suddenly discarded or replaced by others less abnormal. We knew one man, at the age of 70, who stopped the struggling and avoiding of many years and began to stutter easily and with the syllabic repetition of his childhood. He told us he was too tired and too old to stutter so hard any longer.

At any age, a stutterer shows some variety. Those who are mono-symptomatic are very rare, and they are the kind Freund (1966) calls hysterical. Most advanced stutterers have more than one behavior in their repertoire, and some have so many that at times of great stress they hardly know which one to use. Different kinds of behaviors may be used when stuttering on words beginning with vowel sounds than when stuttering on words beginning with stop consonants. A stutterer who used a nasal snorting noise to interrupt a long tremorous fixation on the first sound of the word "take" never showed this behavior when stuttering on the word "ache." Instead he had an intermittent vocal fry or a rise in pitch. One stutterer used a quick inhalatory vocalization to release himself from hypertensed laryngeal closures on voiced CV or VC syllables, but never used it on syllables beginning with an unvoiced consonant. These different responses seem to have no reason for existing until we note that the nasal snort may at least initiate airflow, that vocal fry cannot be produced with true or ventricular vocal fold occlusion and so on. Many of the strange behaviors shown by stutterers seem to have some method in their madness when they are viewed as attempts to search for the integrations that will make the utterance of the word possible. If we look only at the variability itself, the picture is indeed confusing.

HIERARCHIES OF STUTTERING BEHAVIORS

When the advanced stutterer's overt behaviors are closely scrutinized, it becomes apparent that they are arranged in a sort of hierarchy. Some of the responses in the stutterer's armamentarium (as Robert West might have called it) are fairly inconspicuous. Saying "ah" to postpone the speech attempt, or to interrupt prolongation, belongs in this category. So might a single licking of the lips or a sudden inhalation. If the fear is weak, these inconspicuous reactions are the only ones used, but, as the fear of frustration become more intense, more conspicuous behaviors are called into play. The stutterer now struggles more visibly; his gasping, grunting, and other sounds (such as the vocal fry) become more audible. The tongue now comes out all the way. Stutterers in an extreme panic of helplessness sometimes run through their entire repertoire several times, finally ending with large trunk movements almost seizure-like in their severity. Bluemel (1957) gives an example:

When asked a direct question such as his age, the young man sniffs loudly several times through his nose, then he sucks in his checks and exhausts the breath from his lungs. Meanwhile his face becomes suffused. He bends his head forward and blinks his eyelids vigorously. He opens his mouth, whereupon the jaw and facial muscles engage in violent "spasm." His head pulls over to the left; and the entire body, especially the left side of the body, becomes rigid. Finally, after violent and prolonged effort, the patient suddenly speaks rapidly and fluently on almost exhausted breath (pp. 47–48).

Why does the stutterer use one behavior first or second or third? How does the sequence develop? We have been able to watch this aspect of the disorder develop in only a few cases, but it is our impression that there are two factors determining the sequence of the various behaviors. First, the final hierarchy often reflects the order in which the coping behaviors were acquired. Those the stutterer adopted first are those that occur first in the sequence; those developed last are the final ones to be tried out as he struggles to utter the word. Second, the behaviors may occur in the order of their social visibility or listener wince-value. Thus the stutterer may use the least conspicuous coping behavior first. If this fails, he uses one that is just a bit more visible or abnormal, and so on until finally he gives up trying to hide his difficulty. It is then that he shows his most bizarre struggle. Gottlober (1953) gives this description:

[The substitution of synonyms] works but soon he fears the word he is using for substitution, and it is not long before he runs out of synonyms. Then the "starters" begin, sounds or acts which he thinks will help him begin talking. He snaps his fingers, stamps his feet, clenches his fists, screws up his face or whistles. Each trick has its few moments of effectiveness and then helps no more. But he continues to use them just the same and the ritual that precedes even a single word may take from a few moments to more than a minute to complete (p. 87).

STUTTERING AS INTEGRATED BEHAVIOR

To the naive observer, this incredible variety of stuttering behaviors appears chaotic, spasmodic, and random. When a stutterer's abnormal behaviors are scrutinized carefully, however, they are found to be highly organized, well integrated, almost stereotyped patterns. The breathing abnormalities of such a stutterer as he stutters *on the same word* at different times are remarkably similar (Van Riper, 1936). Sonographic, electromyographic, and sound pressure recordings also show highly consistent features. Each confirmed stutterer acquires his own unique *set* of stuttering behaviors.

We do not wish to imply that this means that stutterers show the same behaviors on *all* the words or sounds on which they stutter. Prins and Lohr (1968) showed clearly that such a consistency does not occur. They usually stutter differently on words beginning with a vowel than they do on those beginning with a stop plosive or a fricative but when we examine many samples of stuttering on the same sound or word, we find the behaviors remarkably similar. When differences do occur, they reflect different grades of the hierarchal set of behaviors in his stuttering repertoire. The research of Prins and Lohr (1968) has been erroneously interpreted as showing that patterns of stuttering behaviors unique to the individual do not occur but unfortunately they did not examine the similarities shown on specific words or sounds. Hutchinson (1975) found that unique aerodynamic profiles of airflow and intraoral air pressure were consistently used by individual stutterers during their stuttering episodes.

Many writers have described these unique stuttering patterns of behavior and we provide only a few of them:

> An adult of our acquaintance suddenly would look as though she were about to pray as she talked. Both palms would be placed together in front of her, pressed together tightly, then a word or phrase would be produced as she suddenly pulled them apart. . . . Another moved her feet around as she talked. If she were standing, it would at times look like she were about to perform a soft-shoe routine (Robinson, 1964, p. 6–7).

> . . . Some patients for example, will repeatedly jerk the head backwards or forwards; others will preface speech with violent movements of the arms or legs; others again will exhibit facial twitchings, eye-blinking, or clenching of the jaw (Boome and Richardson, 1932, p. 42).

> The act of stuttering is often accompanied by various associated movements. Most commonly involved are: wrinkling of the forehead, frowning, blinking, pressing the eyelids together tightly, and many other forms of grimacing appear as soon as the child makes an effort to speak. The head may be thrown backwards. Swallowing movements may occur. The patient may jerk the extremities, or clench his fists or stamp his feet (Kanner, 1942, p. 314).

Perhaps we get the impression that these stuttering behaviors are spasmodic and random because they are so patently maladaptive. Why show anyone close his lips tightly in order to say a word beginning with a vowel? Or open his jaws for one beginning with an /m/? Why should anyone gasp and jump and jerk trying to say *Good morning*? Why interject a prolonged zzzzz or squeeze one's eyes shut? Surely all this is not only maladaptive behavior; it must also be random. But it is not. The patterns occur too consistently. They are not a complete breakdown; they do not have the chaotic characteristics of panic behavior. Instead they are highly integrated responses, and when their history of development is examined, they appear to be the habituated descendants of instrumental acts that were once highly meaningful. Most of these responses, as Van Riper (1937) pointed out long ago, were originally used to postpone, avoid, or time the dreaded speech attempt, or to disguise, interrupt, or escape from the stuttering so as to avoid penalty.

Not all of the contortions, grimaces, retrials, rituals, and forcings of the developed stutterer have their origins in conscious and deliberate attempts to cope with the core behavior. Some of them are learned almost by chance. They may have coincided with release from tremor or with utterance. If, for example, a stutterer jerked his head, and if, just as he did so, he also said the word on which he had been stuttering, the utterance itself would reinforce the head-jerk. At that moment, there would be some relief from specific anxiety or at least from frustration. What is more important, the head-jerk would be followed by communication. He could continue. The head-jerk also terminates any phonemic, word, or situation fear. All these events are powerfully rewarding. A pigeon can be taught to continuously rotate clockwise by shaping its movements with reinforcement. The stutterer may also find himself doing some oddball things that seem unrelated to speech. In acquiring many motor skills, learning to play golf for example, certain inappropriate movements or limb or head postures may become fixed because they occasionally preceded a fair wallop of the ball. These behaviors are difficult to unlearn and become more so as they are practiced.

CORE BEHAVIORS

Repetitions

Thus far we have been describing the general features of stuttering in the confirmed stutterer. Now we turn to the specific behaviors and we begin with the basic ones.

According to Sheehan (1974), who made a phonetic analysis of 500 stutterings provided by twenty adult stutterers, sound and syllable and word repetitions were found in all of their speech samples. All of the *word* repetitions occurred on short words of one syllable and therefore could also be included under the category of syllable repetitions. The sound repetitions might also be considered syllabic too because even the unvoiced plosive consonants such as /k/ or /t/ require a puff of exploded air to be identified. In any event, Sheehan found that repetitions occurred on 66 per cent of the 500 stutterings, and that none of his stutterers failed to show them.

Let us look more closely at these syllabic repetitions. First, we note that they can vary in number. We once counted 19 successive repetitions of the syllable /su/ in the word *sooner* before the stutterer gave up and took a new breath, then 13 more repetitions before the word was finally uttered. This, of course, is unusual. Ordinarily according to Sheehan, the number of repeated syllables range from one to three.

Next we observe that these syllabic repetitions may vary in rate, not only among different stutterers but in a single individual at different times. In younger beginning stutterers the repetitions tend to occur at the syllabic rate of their fluent speech but as the disorder progresses, they become much faster. In some stutterers the rate of syllabic repetitions during stuttering is even swifter than they can repeat the same syllables voluntarily, almost as though an automatic recycling mechanism has taken control. The experience is similar to the repetitions felt by normal speakers under delayed auditory feedback. Stutterers have a phrase for these; they call them their "runaway stutterings." They also feel they cannot stop them until they have run their course. This may or may not be true but that is what they tell us.

On the other hand we find some stutterers who repeat very slowly with long pauses between the syllables. This tends to occur more often on single-syllable words and usually indicates a deliberate attempt to reintegrate a broken word or it indicates the anticipation of further difficulty. Janssen and Kraaimant (1977), in their factorial study of molecular behaviors in stuttering, found that these *slow* repetitions belonged to the factor that represented "avoidance-postponement" whereas fast repetitions had their best fit in the factor that included prolongations, struggle behaviors, and general severity.

The regularity or rhythmicity of these repetitions also changes as the disorder continues to develop. At first, they are fairly regular but with the development of awareness and tension, they become irregular and arhythmic, often occurring in bursts or volleys. When we find a confirmed stutterer who, for example, always repeats a syllable three times and very regularly, we tend to suspect pseudo-stuttering or neurosis. Very few stutterers show this pattern however.

We are also interested in the terminal features of these repetitions. Although each of the repetitions, in turn, often seems to end abruptly, with a sudden interruption to the airflow or phonation*, rarely is there any real pause between them (unless they are of the slow postponement type.) Instead, the stutterer recoils instantly into the initial posture of the next syllabic repetition, a posture which is usually invested with tense tremor

---

* However, as Adams (1975) has shown, when a repeated syllable begins with an unvoiced sound as in "p-p-peach," the airflow may continue as the sound is repeated. Repeated CV syllables beginning with voiced sounds often have that first sound unvoiced as in "p-p-p-back."

Spectrographic analysis of the vowels of the syllabic repetitions has demonstrated that they often do not contain the necessary transitional formants for the co-articulation required to produce the syllable or word (Stromsta, 1965; Agnello, 1975; Adams, 1978). When a stutterer produces a syllable that fails to contain the necessary motor and acoustic features to effect a transition to the rest of the word, he seems to try again and again until he utters one that does have these features. Only then does the stuttering stop and the attempted word is completed. This repetition of sounds and syllables seems to be an automatic searching, hunting process, perhaps cybernetic in nature.

When we listen to these syllabic repetitions of stutterers we observe that often the vowel does not seem to be the one appropriate to the utterance of the syllable or word. Instead it resembles the schwa vowel /ə/. They seem to say suh-suh-soap, not so-so-soap. Frick (1965) attributes this to a failure in coarticulation due to a faulty motor plan for the entire word. However, the matter may not be that simple. Freeman (1976) found, in a single subject, that although the repetitions sounded as though they contained the schwa vowel, spectrographic analysis revealed that it was a misperception, due to the appropriate vowel being uttered very briefly. Montgomery and Cooke (1976), using acoustic analysis, found that the true schwa vowel occurred in only 25 per cent of the repeated syllables. Allen, Peters, and Williams (1975) reported that repetitions heard as containing the schwa were usually very brief and weak renditions of the proper vowel. We believe the best reconciliation of these views is to conclude that some of the repeated syllables do contain the schwa and reflect a failure in coarticulation whereas the others, those showing brief bursts of the appropriate vowel, reflect a failure in the synchronization of the musculatures of respiration, phonation, and articulation necessary to produce the correct sound. Either one of these could trigger the sudden arrest and recoil. Hill (1942, 1954) demonstrated clearly that repetitive behaviors ensued when serial motor activities are suddenly interrupted and blocked. We speculate that the cause of the interruption is that the cybernetic sensors detect error in the output and so recycling occurs. Again, to repeat ourselves, we feel that the error is either the production of a sound that lacks the necessary coarticulation features, or of a sound that is disrupted because of the mistiming of its respiratory, articulatory, or phonatory component movements. Once more it seems as though the "atomic" core of stuttering may lie in a disrupted, distorted phoneme and that the repetitions are reactions thereto.

Prolongations

Besides repetitions, another set of behaviors seems to be demonstrated by all confirmed stutterers. These have usually been called *prolongations*, although perhaps the term *fixations* might be more descriptive. They are the distinctive characteristics of what was formerly called *tonic* as opposed to *clonic* (repetitive) stuttering. The stutterer's speech flow is disrupted by moments of static positioning which do not occur to any significant extent in fluent speech which is continuous. He may produce the word *man* with a prolonged /m/ sound (mmmmmmmmman) or the word *boy* by assuming the lip posture for the /b/ and holding it too long in that fixed position. Prolongations may be silent as well as audible.

How long do these prolongations have to last to be perceived as abnormal? Not very long! Most of us speak at a rate of from 200 to 300 syllables per minute, which gives an average syllabic duration of from 0.4 to 0.5 seconds. In Figure 6 we have a graph showing the durations of the prolongations found in the speech of Sheehan's (1974) stutterers. On the average, they last longer than the entire syllable does and some prolongations have been known to have had durations of several minutes. Since normal utterance is characterized by continuous movement, even slight prolongations of a sound or posture can be conspicuous, especially if they occur frequently.

Developmentally, prolongations seem to develop later than repetitions in the great majority of stutterers. Beginning or incipient stutterers may not show any prolongations at all, but as the disorder grows, the speech of most stutterers is interrupted by them. In the same "moment of stuttering" they may co-exist with repetitions, as the old terms *clonotonus* and *tonoclonus* indicate. A stutterer may begin a word with syllabic repetitions and then terminate the stuttering with a prolongation. At other times he or she may show the reverse sequence. The proportion varies

Figure 6. Length of prolongations occurring in 500 instances of stuttering. (From Sheehan, 1974, by permission.)

from stutterer to stutterer, but usually prolongations, as we have said, seem to increase as the disorder progresses.

Let us examine these prolongations more closely. In terms of their phonetic features, it is obvious that the vowels and continuant consonants are more easily prolonged than the plosives, and so we find that most of the audible prolongations are found on these sounds. Similarly most of the *silent* fixations of an articulatory posture occur on CV or CVC syllables when they begin with a plosive. Moreover, when the first sound is a voiced consonant such as /b/, /d/, or /g/, no voicing is heard and often the prolonged silent posture is interrupted by short bursts of their cognates /p/, /t/, and /k/ before the syllable is finally spoken. It should also be noted, however, that even when the syllable begins with a voiced consonant, fricative, or vowel, stutterers frequently start it with a tense, fixed, and silent posture. The so-called "interiorized stutterer" is especially prone to use these silent prolongations but almost any stutterer who fears the public display of his stuttering may use silent prolongations rather than audible ones.

When these prolongations are closely observed it becomes apparent that they are rarely smooth. Instead one finds fluctuations in loudness, tension, air flow, and even pitch. They appear unstable. Often toward the termination of the prolonged sound or silent posture these variations become more prominent, almost as though the speaker were searching for the transitional movements he requires to be able to move forward. Pseudo-stuttering can be distinguished from real stuttering by these features alone.

How do the prolongations begin? Sometimes they are preceded by little silent rehearsal movements of the articulators, almost as though the stutterer were tasting his anticipated syllable or word to see if stuttering is imminent. Often the particular muscle groups required for the production of the syllable are suffused with tension. An illustration of this is found in Freeman and Ushijima's (1975) electromyographic recording of the superior longitudinal muscle of the tongue which raises its tip. In Figure 7, long before the tip was raised for the prolonged sound /l/ in the word *lllllllless*, the recording showed activity in this muscle.

Also, prior to the vocalized prolongation of the /l/, there was activity in *both* the adductor posterior cricoarytenoid and its antagonist, the vocalis, and this joint activity persisted during the prolongation. Then, just before it ended, the posterior cricoarytenoid relaxed. As Freeman and Ushijima pointed out, "the abductor-adductor reciprocity, so characteristic of fluent utterance, is disrupted in stuttering utterance. The most common pattern occurring during moments of stuttering is simultaneous, presumably antagonistic, abductor-adductor activity." This feature of stuttering has also been demonstrated by the research of Zimmermann (1980) and others.

Why do stutterers show prolongations in their speech? We are not sure how this vital question should be answered but there are several possibilities. Since prolongations usually appear later in the development of the

Figure 7. Comparison of abductor-adductor patterns in stuttered and fluent (right) utterances of the word "less" (PCA: Posterior Cricoarytenoid; VOC: Vocalis, medial portion of the Thyroarytenoid; SL: Superior Longitudinalis, intrinsic tongue muscle). (From Freeman and Ushijima, 1975, by permission.)

disorder following the earlier repetitions, they may reflect the stutterer's attempt to prevent those repetitions because of the frustration or penalties they generate. If one prolongs, one doesn't repeat. Or, the prolongation serves as a time gaining device to permit the proper transitional movements to be programmed into the motor pattern of the syllable and word, that is, to allow time for proper synchonization or coarticulation to be planned. Or, the stutterer prolongs because he is afraid that if he stops he may not be able to get the airflow or voice started again. Or, he perseverates as a way of preventing sudden arrest of airflow or phonation. Or, he prolongs so he can hold his listener. Or, on a more esoteric level, he is simply caught in the static middle of an approach-avoidance conflict (Sheehan, 1958). Or, as Hill (1942) showed, when a series of movements has been automatized, and one of those movements is blocked, the preceding one is repeated or prolonged. Perhaps the servosystem senses that when a stutterer fails to round his lips anticipatorily as he produces the /s/ sound in the word *suit*, it automatically blocks forward progress in the sound sequence and prolongation of the /s/ ensues. None of these explanations is completely satisfactory either considered singly or in combination. All we can really say is that a prolongation indicates that something has gone wrong with the timing of the simultaneous or sequential muscular contractions that usually produce a fluent syllable or word.

Blockages

Confirmed stutterers tell us that they don't mind their repetitions and prolongations half as much as they do their "blocks." They insist that often they cannot get started speaking, that something seems to be interfering with airflow or phonation. They feel "stuck." Do these moments of being unable to produce speech constitute a third kind of basic behaviors like repetitions or prolongations? We do not believe so. We feel that they belong under the category of prolongations, that they reflect the silent and prolonged fixations of articulatory or laryngeal postures. Certainly they are very common, and in some stutterers they comprise the major part of the speech deviation. Researchers and observers have recorded them as "tense pauses" and certainly these gaps in the forward flow of speech are overtly observable.

If one carefully scrutinizes these blockages, it is immediately apparent that the stutterer has closed off his airway. The closure may be produced by pressing the lips together, or by the tongue being pressed firmly against the teeth or roof of the mouth, or by closing the false or true vocal folds. Fujita (1966) observed tight closure of the glottis and even partial closure of the pharyngeal cavity in the films of these hard blockings in stutterers. Ushijima et al. (1969) showed films of ventricular closures and also epiglottic closures during stuttering. Tight lip and lingualveolar constrictions were found by Zimmermann (1980), and Hutchinson (1975) showed that prolonged silent blocks on the stop consonant syllables, produced by constriction of the tongue or lips, were characterized by strong increases in interoral air pressure. Gautheron, Liorzon, and Vallancien (1973) provide glottographic recordings showing that tight and complete closure of the vocal folds (the glottal stop) occurred in 60 per cent of the stutterings.

There are also times when the airway may be plugged by multiple occlusions simultaneously at any of these sites. Simultaneously the lips may be closed tightly, the tongue pressed against the roof of the mouth, and the true and false vocal folds adducted. We have tried to determine, in these multiple blockades, whether or not certain closures are released before others. Generally, it is our impression that the laryngeal constriction is the last to be released, while that produced by the tongue is the first.* Some writers (Kenyon, 1943 and Schwartz, 1974) have stated that complete closure in these silent blocks is always at the level of the larynx but we have seen many stutterers who leaked air or snorted through the nose while keeping their lips pressed tightly together.

Also, we have seen stutterers who characteristically occluded the airway at a site that had nothing to do with the usual place of articulation. A "kissing stutterer" began most of her inaudible prolongations of silent postures of most of her sounds by protruding her lips and squeezing them tightly, then releasing this gesture with a sucking noise. Even when the

---

* We have also been fascinated to observe that some stutterers, in the course of a long silent block, will finally release themselves from the blockade at one site only to plug the airway at another.

syllable begins with a vowel, the lips or tongue may produce complete closures of the airway in some stutterers.

When the stutterer says he feels "stuck" and cannot even utter a sound we can be pretty sure that one of the closures is in the larynx. Van Riper (1974) has called this the *ablauf* problem, using a term coined by Fernau-Horn in Germany. Essentially the synchronization of the timing of laryngeal and articulatory or respiratory movements seems to be impaired. Certainly, the tight laryngeal closures prevent airflow or phonation. However, it is also possible that, at these times, the vocal folds may not be adducted but that the inability to produce voice or airflow is due to the excessive supraglottal pressure caused by closures of the lips and tongue. Agnello and Wingate (1971) and others have found that when the closures of the lips or tongue occur, the supraglottal air pressure increases markedly even if the glottis is open and that this by itself may impede phonation or airflow.

These blockings or closures are some of the most important phenomena in the multifaceted disorder of advanced stuttering. The stutterer senses such a closure very vividly. For a moment he feels impotent, out of control. The normal speaker may be able to share the experience by imagining a sudden inability to lift his hand or move a finger on command. Stutterers speak of having their lips glued together, of the tongue being cemented to the roof of the mouth. They say that something seems stuck in their throat. It is a deeply threatening experience, and the stutterer reacts to it with panic and frustration, with struggle and forcing, or by recoil and reattempt. Over 50 years ago Makuen (1914) said it this way: "To be suddenly stricken dumb when one is in full possession of his faculties is an alarming predicament and even a few repetitions of this will very naturally arouse an overpowering fear in the affected individual." (p. 386)

ACCESSORY OR SECONDARY STUTTERING BEHAVIORS

Thus far we have been describing the basic behaviors of stuttering, the repetitions and prolongations that are the hallmark of the disorder. All stutterers show these. But now we seek to describe the behaviors that vary from stutterer to stutterer. Essentially we feel that they are learned and habituated reactions to the *experience* or *fear* of having repetitions and prolongations. One stutterer responds in one way to these basic difficulties that impede the forward flow of speech; another responds differently. They are accessory* because they are not basic; they are secondary because they occur later in the developmental sequence. However we name them, they often constitute the major share of the burden of stuttering so far as its abnormality and severity are concerned.

The variety of these accessory or secondary behaviors is almost incre-

---

* The term *accessory* to describe these behaviors was first used by Wingate (1964) in his article "A Standard Definition of Stuttering."

dible. We have observed stutterers who pant, gasp, or try to speak on inhaled air. Some have fainted from holding their breath too long. During their abnormal utterances we have seen stutterers raise their larynges into a tense swallowing posture. We have heard them gag and retch. Some squeeze or blink their eyes, or contract or flare their nostrils. The tongue may protrude or the lips form a snout. There are stutterers who have bitten their tongues or lips until they bled. Jaw jerks, head jerks, even sudden body jerks may occur. Some stutterers tap their feet or kick when in the throes of their hard blockings. Several of our clients have waltzed across the room, attempting the word on each third beat. A few snort or sniff compulsively.

One of the stutterers pounded her side until it was black and blue. Often there are sudden, almost spasmodic, movements of the hand or arm or head. We worked with one stutterer who uttered sudden barking noises that started slowly then accelerated while the pitch of his voice rose in an appalling crescendo. We have heard others who inserted interminable interjections of meaningless syllables, words and phrases before the words they feared. And we have known some stutterers who just stopped everything and remained tense and immobile for long moments, their faces blank masks. This catalog of abnormal overt behaviors is far from complete for there are many others that could be mentioned. It does illustrate however that severe stuttering can be a very serious problem, and that we must not think of it only in terms of repetitions and prolongations.

Bewildering as the variety of secondary reactions seems to be, they can be understood if one begins to sort them into two classes of responses (1) those that are reactions to the experience of the basic behaviors, and (2) those that are responses to the fear of them.

TENSION AND TREMOR

When the child becomes aware of his basic stuttering behaviors as frustrating or unacceptable to others, tension appears in the speech musculatures involved in the repetitions and fixations. In severe stutterers this tension sometimes spreads widely even into the arms and legs. Often it spreads to the nose to produce wrinkling or flaring of the nostrils. One can almost see it radiate from an initial focus in the lips, tongue, or throat. Prins and Lohr (1968) found tension spreading to produce eye closings. This tension may also be responsible for repetitions turning into prolongations. Most certainly it plays an important part in creating the closures of the airway. The stutterer tells us he is "trying to break the block by forcing," and that at times a sudden surge of tension does seem to effect release.

But the most important effects of tension are the tremors that it produces and maintains. We have previously referred to tremors that accompany the prolongations and the closures of advanced stuttering and we wish to stress their importance here. No other feature of the disorder contributes as much to the stutterer's feeling of helplessness or being out of control as do these tremors, yet they have been generally ignored by researchers and clinicians.

The stuttering tremor is basically a physiological tremor according to Platt and Basili (1973) but its amplitude is much greater than the invisible rhythmic contractions that normally maintain a muscle in a state of readiness to react. Its frequency lies within the normal range of the physiological tremor (8–10 Hz.) and like physiological tremor, it is produced by the *simultaneous* contraction of opposing and antagonistic muscles or muscle groups.

There seems to be no doubt that these amplified tremors occur in confirmed stutterers. They have been found in the lips, tongue, and jaw musculatures (Prins and Lohr, 1968; Fibiger, 1972; Platt and Basili, 1973; Zimmermann, 1980). They have also been shown to occur in the laryngeal musculatures (Chevrie-Muller, 1963; Fibiger, 1972; Freeman, 1976; and Conture, 1977). Schilling (1960) also found rapid clonic movements, probably tremors, in the breathing apparatus, especially the diaphragm. The co-contraction of abductor and adductor muscle groups have been demonstrated in most of these studies.

Tremors can occur simultaneously at the sites of all of the usual closures or at only one of them depending upon the amount of tension. Fibiger (1971) found that when tremor activity appears in the facial muscles, phonation either stops or it becomes weaker. The probable reason for this very important finding is not that facial tremor may be inhibiting phonation directly but that the laryngeal muscles may also be thrown into tremor at the same time. Tremors have long been known to spread from one muscle group to another as the tension increases.

Under certain conditions all of us experience the high-amplitude tremors so characteristic of stuttering but not in the speech musculatures. After extreme exertion our legs and arms may tremble obviously and this trembling represents our physiological tremors being magnified. The same behavior is shown in fright and extreme cold. It has been demonstrated that under stress our adrenal glands secrete large amounts of adrenalin into the bloodstream and according to Foley, Marsden, and Owen (1967), this always raises the amplitude of the physiological tremor*. It is also possible for most of us to produce large amplitude tremors voluntarily in our legs and arms by highly tensing the antagonistic muscles simultaneously and then making a sudden ballistic movement or producing an extra surge of tension. Platt and Basili (1973) showed that normal speakers, when simulating stuttering, could produce tremors by the isometric contraction of the jaw muscles which appeared identical with the tremors shown by stutterers speaking the same words. This indicates perhaps that stuttering tremors could be conditioned to certain word or phonetic cues. Whether this is true has not yet been demonstrated by the research.

What usually seems to happen is that tremors begin when the stutterer

---

* Edgren, Leanderson, and Levi (1969) found that in stressful speaking situations, stutterers show an increase of 300 per cent in the excretion of adrenalin.

Figure 8. EMG recordings from antagonistic muscle groups during stuttering. (Courtesy of Rolf Leanderson and A. Persson, Karolinska sjukhiset, Sweden.)

creates a fixed closure, invests its antagonistic musculatures with tension, and then suddenly produces an increase of air pressure behind or below the closure. At the moment this increase occurs, the antagonistic musculatures become suffused with a sudden burst of further tension and the stuttering tremor comes into being. Then it persists until interrupted by a sudden movement of the abductor muscles (a movement which is out of phase with the frequency of the tremor) or, alternatively, when the heightened air pressure subsides, or the adductor muscles relax.

It is interesting that many techniques employed in therapy for stuttering seem expressly designed to prevent these tremors. The common use of relaxation, speaking on a sigh, gentle onsets or loose contacts, and very slow speaking rates tend to prevent not only the closures and the tension but also the sudden co-contractions of antagonistic muscle groups.

Tremors are most easily observed during the longer prolongations or fixations but they also may accompany fast syllabic repetitions. Often the initial consonant of the final repeated syllable is invested with tremor just before the word is uttered. Also, as we shall see, severe stutterers often begin to tremor even before the word is actually attempted.

These tremors affect the stutterer strongly. They make him feel helpless. He cannot understand why they persist or how they begin or are maintained. They violate the integrity of the self for they are sensed as being involuntary. The stutterer feels that he has lost control. Robinson (1964) puts it this way:

> The tremors cause a child to feel literally blocked in his efforts to talk. Feelings of frustration change to fear. Fear may change to panic. Escape is sought in any possible way. Unfortunately, the very devices that release the tremor and free the child to talk serve only to complicate his problem (p. 62).

REACTIONS TO PERSEVERATION

When the repetitions, fixations, and tremors last too long and the stutterer feels frustration from his inability to continue, he reacts in several ways to terminate them. Often he simply stops and tries again to say the sound, syllable, or word on which he experiences difficulty, sometimes returning to the beginning of the phrase or sentence. However, this strategy is often unsuccessful and he finds himself again in the throes of another prolonged repetition, fixation, or tremor.

We have studied carefully what occurs during these perseverations, and what changes occur that seem eventually to lead to their release and the utterance of the word. Usually some variation occurs. The syllabic repetitions may slow down or gradually come to contain the necessary coarticulation features. The stutterer may begin with several repetitions containing the schwa vowel or sudden arrests of phonation, then utter the succeeding syllables with better approximations to the vowel. Or they end less abruptly with slower termination times.

Repositioning of the articulators often occur in both repetitive and prolonged sounds or syllables. Prins and Lohr (1968), for example, found many instances of right and left deviations of the jaws and lips occurring before release. Zimmermann (1980) discovered consistent repositioning of the lips, jaw, and tongue during both repetitions and prolongations just before the word was spoken. The postures of the jaw and lip and tongue often are changed to approximate the standard or the rest position. Hutchinson (1975) reported that similar variations occurred in the intraoral pressure peaks during repetitions and that they gradually approximated the normal pressures as the moment of release occurred. He termed this "the normalization effect." Adams (1975) suggested that the perseveration of repetitions and prolongations may have some utility as a means for gaining time so that the stutterer may make the motor modifications needed to produce the appropriate transition into the word.

The same variations and changes also occur in the larynx as well as in the articulators during long repetitions and prolongations. The tense closures of the antagonistic musculatures governing the glottis show changes as the time of release approaches. Freeman (1975) stated that the successful termination of a block was "found to coincide with a marked drop in either adductor or abductor activity" which would of course alter the co-contracting needed to maintain a laryngeal tremor. There is also some evidence that the stutterer makes changes in the site of the laryngeal closure. The glottal closure may be supplemented by ventricular fold adduction, and even by the tuberculum of the epiglottis making contact with the adducted arytenoids when the larynx is raised almost into the position for swallowing. We have seen several severe "swallowing stutterers" who showed the latter pattern. During long laryngeal blocks, stutterers may shift their tension loci back and forth from one to another of these sites before returning to the glottal closure and relaxing one of the adductors enough to permit air flow and phonation.

VOCAL FRY

A very common response to tense laryngeal closure or tremor is the use of the vocal fry register. Short bursts of vocal fry can often be heard on VC syllables as in "a . . . a . . . apple" and almost always they follow a glottal stop or brief tense tremor in the laryngeal muscles. The fry also occurs to end blocking on voiced consonant sounds when the articulatory posture is assumed but no air flow is evident.

In our view the vocal fry represents a shift away from tense glottal fixation. Blocked by the closure produced by the simultaneous contraction of the abductor-adductor muscles, the stutterer tries to make a change in positioning. Allen and Hollien (1972) demonstrated that the vocal folds are thicker in the fry register and that the ventricular folds seem to be pressed down upon them. McGlone and Shipp (1971) state that during vocal fry there are also differences in the action of the thyroarytenoid and cricothyroid musculatures, the former showing higher than normal activity and the latter lower activity. What this represents is a change, a variation in the way that phonation is produced and the stutterer, feeling that he cannot produce voice in the usual manner, resorts to a different approach. Some stutterers show a similar variation when they try to break out of their laryngeal closures by shifting to the falsetto. Long ago, Scripture (1923) trained his stutterers to use the "octave twist" when they felt stuck in the production of their vowel sounds and we have seen stutterers who reacted to laryngeal closures and tremors by large upward shifts in the pitch of the voice. Even young stutterers show this siren-effect. Changes in intensity, mainly resorting to a very weak phonation, are also frequently observed.

We wish to emphasize that these reactions to the perseverating prolongations and repetitions are not deliberate or voluntary. Rarely is the stutterer consciously aware of the mechanics involved or how they represent progressive approximations to the required normal utterance. All he knows is that something happens that releases him from his stuttering. Tragically he does not know how they accomplish the final integration or how their variations finally create the necessary conditions for phonation and air flow. Instead, he attributes the release to his blind struggling.*

INTERRUPTOR REACTIONS

Many of the most bizarre behaviors found in severe stutterers are those we have chosen to call interruptor devices. They are attempts to overcome blockings. Most of them are sudden—head and body jerks, foot or hand movements, inhalations, facial grimaces, nasal snorts. There is an incredible variety of interruptors, but most stutterers use only a few, trying first one then another, or repeatedly using the same one in the hope that finally the closure will be broken.

We cannot stress too strongly the importance of closures and interruptor devices because far too much has been written about avoidance as the dominant characteristic of stuttering. Stuttering often includes avoidance as a response to anticipated unpleasantness, but escape responses are a much more important feature. When the stutterer's forward progress is blocked by a closure, the unpleasantness is already under way, and he needs to escape from it as quickly as possible. It is both psychologically and semantically unwise to stretch the term avoidance to include these escape reactions. Wendell Johnson loved a paradox, and when he defined stuttering as the stutterer's attempts to avoid stuttering or disfluency, he

---

* In his youth the author fell into the hands of a psychologist who told him that his stuttering was due to the tense closure of his throat, and who trained him to lift his head to relax this area. Several times this deliberate head lifting did seem to terminate his hard laryngeal blocks Or at least the head lifting happened at about the time the release occurred. When the head lifting failed to end the closures, the author would try it again, and then again, and soon the behavior seemed to become completely involuntary. Certainly it became a characteristic feature of his stuttering. So compulsive were they that once, when sitting on a bench by a window, his head jerks shattered the panes behind him and it cost him $2.35 to get it fixed.

beclouded the issue. A closure is a closure is a closure! Closures are devastatingly unpleasant, and most stutterers want to get out of them as quickly as possible. The ways they learn to do so contribute much to the abnormality of the problem. More practically, the therapist will find that escape behaviors are much more easily extinguished than avoidance reactions but that they demand different therapeutic procedures, an observation which may throw some light on the curious finding that many of the most grotesque and severe stutterers respond more favorably and quickly to therapy than milder stutterers who have fewer actual stutterings but more avoidance.

Whether they arise by chance association or by deliberate intent, these interruptor reactions create much of the confirmed stutterer's overt abnormality. The sudden gasps, the body jerks, the attempt to speak on inhalation, the sudden abdominal thrusts and many other grotesque reactions seem to be first learned as attempts to escape from the clutch of the basic behaviors that last too long. To the casual observer these interruptor reactions appear spasmodic and random but they are not. We feel they are operantly conditioned responses to the experience of the basic behaviors.

SPEAKING ON COMPLEMENTAL AIR

Another reaction to prolonged laryngeal closures or tremors is the use of complemental air. We often find stutterers who interrupt their fixations by exhaling almost all of their tidal air and making the speech attempt only when it is markedly reduced. One stutterer said, "At the end of my breath my vocal cords must relax because they know they have to open or I die." That this is a reflexive response which causes a reduction of adductor activity and an opening of the glottis, seems very tenable. At any rate, we often see this sudden extreme exhalation following a tight laryngeal closure and preceeding a new attempt to speak. The low subglottal and intraoral pressures produced by speaking on complemental air seem to reduce the tension of the constrictions located in or above the larynx. A strong relationship exists between the amount of muscle activity at a closure site and the amount of air pressure behind it. Stutterers try to blow the corks out of their speech bottles but the harder they blow, the tighter they squeeze in that cork. By speaking on complemental air, they prevent this situation and so occasionally find release.

GASPS AND SPEECH ON INHALATION

Among some of the most severe secondary behaviors shown by confirmed stutterers are the sudden gaspings that seem to be used to interrupt the closures of the airway. There are the so-called "sniffing stutterers" who seek to open the laryngeal closures by inhaling air through their noses, and the "sucking stutterers" who inhale through the mouth, thus opening lip and tongue closures. Occasionally these gasps are successful in momentarily opening the airway long enough to enable the stutterer to produce airflow and sound, but far too often they fail, and so the stutterer must gasp or sniff again. When these behaviors become conditioned to the experience of closure or tremor, the severity of stuttering increases greatly. Some clinicians have encouraged the use of strong inhalation as a means of preventing stuttering but we feel this is very unwise. We have seen gasping stutterers become hyperventilated by their compulsive gasping.

Some stutterers even seek to overcome their blockages by resorting to speech on inhalation and this too can occasionally be successful. Some old therapists used to recommend "drawback phonation" as a major part of their therapy. Unfortunately the speech produced thereby is so weak and abnormal that few stutterers will use the technique and a few of them manage to close off the airway so that even inhalation is impossible. We have had some stutterers who fainted and fell to the floor when doing this.

OVERT REACTIONS TO THE FEAR OF STUTTERING

Most of the behaviors we have been describing have been reactions to the *experience* of repetitions, prolongations, and closures. While much of the stutterer's abnormality can be attributed to these frustration responses, there is a substantial amount that stems from the fears that stutterers develop as the result of that frustration and the listener penalties they soon experience. Basically, the group of behaviors we are about to describe are avoidances. The stutterer tries to avoid the interruptions produced by the basic behaviors and their abnormal accompanying reactions.

Again, since different stutterers develop different avoidance behaviors, it is necessary to make an attempt to categorize them. This unfortunately creates some problems because, though the behaviors themselves are overt, the dynamics are not. We cannot be sure that a stutterer is being truthful when he claims that he is putting off or postponing saying a word by repeating the preceding phrase because he has found that gaining time sometimes prevents him from stuttering. Practically, we just accept the inference that he is exhibiting a postponement behavior and so that is what we call it. Hood (1974) found that clinician agreement in identifying such inferential behaviors was unanimous 80 per cent of the time. We shall therefore put them into the following major categories: avoidances, postponements, starters, and disguise reactions.

AVOIDANCE BEHAVIOR

No description of stuttering behavior would be complete without a discussion of the behaviors stutterers use to avoid the experience of fractured fluency. After a long history of communicative frustration and social penalty most confirmed stutterers will try almost anything that will prevent stuttering from occurring. They scan approaching speech situations and certain words with an alertness almost inconceivable to the normal speaker. Their radars are constantly revolving. They devise and revise strategies; they marshall alternative modes of avoidance to be used if the one selected fails; they assess the probability of unpleasant listener response; they estimate their own tendency to block. In their heads, the computers of probability whirr.

The most successful avoider, however, eventually finds this incredible burden of vigilant scanning so unbearable that the volleys of stuttering that occur sooner or later (even despite all his stratagems) are almost a relief. When the stutterer has successfully used some device or reaction which enables him to speak with no apparent difficulty, his fears do not subside. Indeed they are increased, for he reasons that this time he was not only alert but lucky. He knows that the avoidance tricks or rituals have not always "worked." Just because he has escaped the experience or revelation of his abnormality doesn't mean he can decrease his alertness. He walks a jungle path of communication where many enemies and hazards lurk. If this description seems unbelievable to the normal speakers who read it, we doubt that it will to the stutterer who is a chronic avoider.

As one stutterer said, "Stuttering is like the mythical hoop snake. If you run after it, it flees; but if you run away it chases you." The tragedy of chronic avoidance is that it causes the situational and phonemic fears to spiral. Flight from stuttering makes it all the more frightful. It provides no opportunity to test reality. The expectation of approaching misery often is exaggerated, and successful avoidance corroborates the exaggeration. Perhaps it is for this reason that avoidance conditioned responses are so difficult to extinguish.

It is interesting that the more severely a person stutters, the less he resorts to avoidances. This happens because the severe stutterer soon discovers that he is stuttering even on the stallers, postponement tricks, starting phrases, synonyms, or circumlocutions that he uses to avoid feared words. Milder stutterers have more avoidances because they have more fluency and a better chance to hide their abnormality. Often, however, they have more intense word fears than the severe stutterer, probably because of their chronic avoidance. We worked for a year with one woman of 35 who claimed that she had really stuttered only once, and that at the age of 17. We never heard her actually stutter in all that time, but we have never known a case to have such tortured, almost unintelligible speech because of her panicky substitutions and circumlocutions. We have never seen word phobias of such intensity. She carried a heavy burden.

Types of avoidance behavior. Since the basic purpose of avoidance behavior is to prevent stuttering from occurring there are several behaviors that are fairly common. First there is *refusal behavior.* The stutterer refuses to enter communicative situations in which he expects to stutter, or he refuses to attempt certain feared words. Here too there is alert scanning, a frantic estimation of probabilities, a search for ways to prevent stuttering from happening. In our intensive work with thousands of stutterers we have been continually amazed at the lengths to which these people will go to avoid exposing their abnormality or experiencing frustration. They have had the telephones removed from their houses; they had sold their homes and changed their addresses; one even legally changed his name. Many stutterers feign stupidity in school to avoid reciting; others feign deafness so they can write out what they have to say. A few stutterers simply stop speaking when they sense a feared word coming, leaving the sentence unfinished, thus inviting other listener penalty. Bluemel (1957) has a good passage:

> The chronic stage of stammering is usually marked by speech avoidance and aversion. The stammerer avoids difficult words, and he attempts to escape menacing situations. He is obsessed in his attitude toward his speech difficulties, and he lives his anxieties in retrospect and in anticipation.
>
> The stammerer dodges not only words; he dodges people and situations. He will cross the street or turn the corner rather than face the necessity for conversation. In scanning a menu he will look for words that he can say, and when he gives his order it represents a choice of words and not a choice of foods. Often the stammerer maneuvers a conversation so that difficult words will fall to his partner's questions instead of his own statements, and not infrequently the stammerer remains silent rather than face the struggle with speech (p. 59).

Most frequent of all the refusal behaviors are those involving substitution and circumlocution, the use of synonyms, or alternative coding of the thought. Some stutterers develop very large vocabularies as a result of habitual substitution, and their speech is so tortuous and strangely imprecise that a listener must work hard to comprehend its meaning. One of our cases told us of a telegram he had to send by phone. He wanted to say "Returning noon Friday by plane. Please meet me." This is what the wire finally read: "I'll be on airplane coming home day after tomorrow about lunchtime. Hope you will be able to have car for me there." The message cost him three times as much, and despite all this avoidance he said he stuttered on more words and more severely than he would have if he had kept to the essential information. Despite this insight no real learning occurred, for as he told of the experience he was constantly revising, substituting, and garbling his account of what had happened. In contrast, other stutterers, especially those for whom the frequency of stuttering is very high, develop a sort of telegraphic speech. Talking is such hard work that they speak as tersely as possible. We have seen a stutterer so fatigued by the terrific struggle accompanying each word of a sentence that at the end of it he was on the verge of physical collapse. We have watched little children stop talking and cry helplessly and, oddly, silently. Several of our cases of voluntary mutism and spastic dysphonia began with refusal behavior related to stuttering.

Using odd ways of speaking. Stutterers also adopt other strategies for avoiding stuttering by altering the way they speak. Some may resort to a sing-song or metronomic type of utterance or chant their words. Others speak very rapidly, running their words together. One of our clients adopted a foreign accent and when this failed, a drawling dialect. Another nasalized all his vowels; still another employed a very loud, pompous manner of speech when he feared he might stutter. We have even had a few clients who spoke in a falsetto, many who used a monotone, and a few others who used a bass voice full of vocal fry. All of them told us that they had less stuttering when they first used these odd ways of talking but that later "the tricks wore out" and no longer helped. We suspect that these strategies owe their temporary effectiveness to distraction.

POSTPONEMENT

Most confirmed stutterers learn that the probability of abnormality or frustration can occasionally be lessened by delaying the speech attempt. There are several possible explanations for this, the most plausible being that fear seldom has a steady state. It fluctuates in time, rising and falling in intensity, flaring suddenly, then subsiding a bit. Stutterers tell us that if they can time the speech attempt at the very instant that the fear is decreasing—in the trough of the wave, so to speak—they sometimes say the word normally or at least better than they had originally anticipated.

We have done some unpublished research in which we made polygraphic recordings of the respiration of stutterers attempting single words following a signal by the experimenter. When the signal to speak was given at the moment when the anticipated stuttering had come to the end of its rehearsal, as indicated by the polygraph, fewer moments of overt stuttering occurred and they were of shorter duration than when the signal to speak was given at the beginning of the rehearsal behavior. It may be that stutterers use postponement reactions because they try to time the moment of speech attempt to coincide with the moment of maximum reactive inhibition. It is very difficult to do, but even if it succeeds only once in a while it may provide the intermittent reinforcement necessary for maintenance. Wendell Johnson (1930) describes his own early stuttering in these words:

> . . . words embedded in a sentence sometimes offer less difficulty than words, even the same words, at the beginning of a sentence. Knowing this, I frequently back up, so to speak, and take a running start at sounds on which I expect to encounter difficulty in order to permit the articulatory and vocal momentum to carry me over (pp. 115–116).

Stutterers use many different strategies to gain time without being conspicuous. Many postponements resemble the same behaviors used by normal speakers when confronted by uncertainty in formulation, or listener loss. All of us filibuster at times, using "ahs," "ums," "ers"; facial and hand gestures; repeating previously spoken phrases or words; inserting communication-holding phrases such as "What I mean is . . . ," "Let me see . . . ," "and uh, and uh"; or other interjections whose major function is to maintain verbal momentum and to prevent silent gaps. We use them to ward off interruption by others, to maintain our hold on the listener's ear. They are signals that we have not finished sending our message.

By deliberately using postponement mechanisms that closely resemble those used by nonstutterers, the stutterer gains more time to wait for the fear to ebb or for the covert rehearsal behavior to be completed than he could get by using silence alone. Filled time, as many experiments have shown, is perceived as shorter than empty time by both the speaker and the listener. In addition, silence, as Sheehan (1958) and others have made clear, is often threatening, especially in our highly garrulous and swiftpaced culture. Silence may even hint of impotence or death for the more morbid souls. Some stutterers postpone silently without moving a muscle for interminable lengths of time, then suddenly blurt out the word. These interiorized nonvocalized stutterers are as hard on the therapist as they are on their other listeners. One of ours resembled the peasant mentioned by the Latin poet Horace who came to the bank of a river and waited for it to run by. Most stutterers are not so interiorized nor so tolerant of silence. They fill their communicative gaps with some sort of overt audible or visible behavior.

Occasionally we find postponement behaviors that are extremely complex. One of our stutterers had developed a stereotyped hierarchy of postponement reactions to the anticipation of stuttering on a feared word which ran as follows. First, he licked his lips; then he said "ah"; then he said, "Well . . ."; then he looked upward with furrowed brow as if thinking; then he coughed; finally he yawned. If the fear was intense all six behaviors occurred, and always in that order. If it were mild, perhaps only the first, or the first and second of these reactions would precede the speech attempt. Van Riper and Milisen (1939) found that stutterers can successfully predict the crude duration of their stuttering. This stutterer was so good at it that he seldom showed any overt blocking. He only postponed, apparently using the ritualistic disguise behavior as a stuttering equivalent. After each component of the sequence he made a sort of predictive assessment of the probability of stuttering were he to make the speech attempt at that instant. He said he never gave himself the benefit of the doubt; he tried to say the word only when he was certain he wouldn't stutter. We asked him what happened when he had exhausted his repertoire but still felt uncertain, and he answered that he went back to the first item of his postponement hierarchy, licking his lips, and started over. His behavior corroborated this account.

Not all stutterers are as fortunate, if that is the appropriate term, in using postponement to prevent overt stuttering. Despite their tricks, the inevitable moment comes when speech is mandatory, when they can postpone no longer. The stuttering that then occurs is often more severe than if the postponement had not been used. Why then does the stutterer continue to use his stallers? There may be many reasons. Careful observation and interview will reveal what reasons motivate a particular stutterer. Here are a few reasons, listed in random order. The stutterer postpones:

1. To give him time to scan the listener's tolerance of speech interruption

2. To torture the listener, to make him wriggle with impatience, to make him reject. This occurs especially in hostile, neurotic stutterers

3. Because he is caught midway in an approach-avoidance conflict. He wants to speak, but he fears the exposure of abnormality. These are usually silent postponements

4. To permit the fear or tension to ebb. To help him relax, to build up his courage. To combat time pressure

5. To take advantage of reactive inhibition in his rehearsal behavior

6. To revise the anticipatory behaviors, to modify the tremors and false postures which he feels will almost ensure stuttering

7. To regain some sense of self-contact and self-control. These are usually vocalized postponements or gestural rituals, coughs, yawns, etc. Feeling unable to utter the feared word, the stutterer does something else voluntarily to reassure himself

8. To bypass the moment of spasmodic breakdown if such moments exist

9. To plan a revised attempt to time the sound, syllable, or word and thus to reduce the probability of severe stuttering

10. As an equivalent of expected overt stuttering.

The automatization of postponement behaviors. Some very odd behaviors develop as postponement behaviors become automatic. One of our cases used a most peculiar vocalization of something like [l:m:si] prior to speech attempt on feared words. Often he would repeat this bit of jargon many times if he expected great difficulty. His parents said it was a contraction of "Let me see," a postponing phrase he had used very frequently and often inappropriately during his adolescence. Another stutterer showed no behavior other than the compulsive repetition of "Andodododoh . . . andoh . . . andoh . . . andodoh. . . ." His wife said that this behavior had begun only recently and that formerly he had used the phrase "And don't you know" in the "oddest places when he was talking." We have seen the decayed residue of the swallowing reflex similarly truncated and persisting in a stutterer who had formerly pursed his lips and swallowed to gain time. This behavior was socially acceptable, but he had overused it, and finally, like many anticipatory behaviors that become habitual and automatized, it had become compressed into a pursing of the lips and the elevation of the hyoid, though with no resulting completion of the swallow. We have watched the development of such postponement mechanisms in several cases, seen them originate in deliberate behavior, become stimulus-tied or bound, and finally observed them end in responses which were the bare skeletons, almost caricatures, of the former instrumental response. The key features of the original postponement are retained; the rest drop out. Many of the bizarre and strange behaviors of the stutterer are explained in such histories of habituated compression.

ABULIA

This term refers to the inability to make decisions or to act or perform certain voluntary movements. It is a sort of psychosomatic dyspraxia. It is the ultimate of procrastination and is well known in psychopathology. The stutterer, caught midway between two alternatives, both full of misery, just stays put. Abulia always represents a very advanced stage of the disorder and is a most difficult problem for the therapist to treat. The mand type of self-talk seems to be lacking. We have seen stutterers almost in a trance, almost cataleptic, their postures frozen and rigid. They tell us that in these states, their consciousness of self is very low and that often they do not even see or hear their listeners. Fortunately, most stutterers do not reach this stage. It is found more frequently in those who use silent postponements than in those who use vocalized ones.

TIMING DEVICES

Much has been written about the perseverating nature of the stuttering response. Repetitions and prolongations are by definition perseverations. Postponements also persist in time, but the time always comes when a stutterer must either give up communication altogether or finally make the speech attempt. The time pressure of the approach gradient increases with every instant and finally the stutterer dare not postpone any longer. What does he do then?

The answer is of course that he stops postponing and tries to say the word. It is at this point, however, that a new class of behaviors appears, instrumental responses designed to compel utterance at a specific moment in time. Otherwise, postponement would go on and on. It is difficult to stop postponing once you have started it, especially when its termination may be very unpleasant. Accordingly, certain timing devices or rituals are used to make the attempt mandatory. Anyone who has ever had to jump over a ditch or a stream that seemed wide can understand why the stutterer behaves this way. The variety of timing devices is endless. Some are quite socially acceptable. Many stutterers repeat words they have already spoken normally in order to get a running start so that the feared word is part of the total sequence. Others are very odd: head nods, foot twitches, sudden gestures, a facial grimace, a quick inhalation. Often the timing device used to end postponement is the same one that is used to interrupt a closure or postural fixation or a perseverative repetition. The stutterer may reason that if the interruptor trick occasionally works to get him out of the unpleasantness it may also aid him as a "starter," a term stutterers commonly use among themselves for this behavior. Sometimes starters may occur in organized sequences as ritualistic behavior, each component of which must be used before its successor is employed:

> In opposing his impediment, the stammerer has frequent recourse to starters and wedges. He may begin his sentences with such words as *Oh* or *listen*, or *well*, or *now;* he may use such phrases as *I say* or *let's see;* or he may use irrelevant sounds such as *ha-ha*—or *he-he*—or *uh-uh-uh-uh-uh.* One young man began his sentence with *it-tay-yer,* which he sing-songed, and repeated with rising pitch and increasing intensity (Bluemel, 1957, p. 48).

Many who stutter work out "starters" for themselves. Some pound with their foot, some make a certain grimace, some have trick sounds, or voice pitch. All of them deplore this and feel it to be unfortunate; but such things, which are considered voluntary, are often compulsive and are a part of the stutter (Blanton and Blanton, 1936, p. 77).

We know one stutterer who used an old nursery rhyme spoken in pantomime and accompanied by different gestures: "One for the money (head nod); two for the show (squeezing the lips); three to get ready (slow inhalation); and four to go! (suddenly hitting himself on the side)." The speech attempt was made always in unison with the last of these. Occasionally, after a long postponement in which he was usually completely silent and immobile, this stutterer would run through the sequence several times, and then the performance would be far more abnormal than if he had merely struggled through the utterance to begin with. No one who saw this behavior would ever think it was disorganized or breakdown behavior. It was highly integrated and stereotyped, although it was certainly difficult to believe it was useful. Nevertheless, this stutterer said, "it worked" (that is, he felt it prevented the most devastating experience of closure and tremor often enough so that he continued to use the routine.) Many stutterers continue to use starters that seldom "start," and much of their abnormality can be traced to these behaviors.

TRIGGER POSTURES

Langova (1967) and Moravek and Langova (1962) state that just prior to the stuttering block a greatly heightened tension (tonus) appears in the speech muscles and that it is this which comprises the essence of stuttering. According to these authors, the stutterer tries to overcome this pre-utterance tension by further tension (forcing) and of course cannot do so. If this initial tonus has been conditioned to certain situational and word cues, we can understand why the stutterer often uses what might be called *trigger postures*. Certainly they are frequently observed. The stutterer seems to pre-set his mouth and tongue for the first sound of the word to be spoken and then invests that preparatory posture with tension.

This presetting, of course, is quite normal. All of us put our muscles in readiness for any action before it occurs but the stutterer assumes the posture long before utterance, often sets it into tremor, and exaggerates its formation. Also, the preparatory postures that he assumes are often completely inappropriate to the sound he wishes to utter. It as though he cocks his speech gun to stutter. One of our clients consistently used a prolonged and tremorous /f/ posture just prior to attempting a word that he feared and it didn't matter whether that word began with that fricative or any other sound.

DISGUISE REACTIONS

We have been attempting to show that stuttering behaviors, despite their variability and inappropriateness, do make some sense if they are viewed as habituated attempts to cope with and escape from fixations and oscillations. There are certain reactions, however, that cannot be explained in this way. Why does one stutterer cover his mouth with his hand compulsively every time he stutters? Why does another laugh almost hysterically every time he stutters? Or a third turn his head far to the left? The answers are often in the histories of these behaviors. Initially they were adopted quite deliberately to hide or disguise the stuttering and then became automatized through the powerful force of intermittent reinforcement. One of our stutterers consistently cocked his head upward and to one side, wrinkled his brow, pursed his lips, and closed one eye whenever he had a severe blockage. The pattern was highly stereotyped and was very difficult to modify in therapy until we found that it had originally been a trick of pretending to think which he had often used in the past to disguise the fact that he was stuttering. Stutterers develop many ingenious ways of hiding their disorder. Some of these unfortunately become incorporated into it.

THE HISTORY OF ACCESSORY REACTIONS

In several cases we have been able to study the development of these instrumental responses. Most stutterers start off using behaviors that are socially acceptable and quite normal: the pauses, the use of "ah" or "um," the repetition of words previously spoken. Next appear the timing devices to terminate the postponement. Then these reactions change and become foreshortened, retaining only their dominant features in skeletal form, for example, the pursing of the lips and elevation of the larynx as the residue of a former swallowing reaction. As this compression of the response takes place, the reaction becomes more and more automatic and stereotyped. It becomes tied to word fear. It becomes habitual, even compulsive in response to the phonetic, durational, or semantic cues of a feared word, a part of the stuttering language he speaks. At this stage the stutterer feels unable to inhibit or even to vary the postponement behavior. The duration and form of the postponement reactions vary directly and automatically with the amount of the fear.

It is at this point that something new is added. The tremors, the closures, the postural fixations, and recoils that formerly had their locus in the actual speech attempt now move forward in time to invade the postponement behavior that was originally used to avoid them. When this happens, the stuttering, as may be imagined, increases greatly in severity. Now the postponement behaviors do not postpone but instead precipitate. The distraction devices no longer distract or prevent the occurrence of abnormality but rather contribute to it. The stutterer's starters do not start.

His timing tricks no longer facilitate utterance but only complicate it by their compulsivity. We have watched stutterers go up these steps, sometimes skipping one or two of them in the process, but the disorder always spirals in severity as the automaticity increases. In the most severe stutterers there is a final stage in which the stutterer either becomes interiorized and abulic or gives up all avoidance and resorts to intense struggle and interruptor devices. Some stutterers just stop talking. Of course not all stutterers run the entire gamut. Most in fact stop short of these final behaviors, but every therapist should be highly aware of the dangers involved in any therapeutic method that may enhance the natural tendency of stutterers to avoid or postpone their speech attempts

BIBLIOGRAPHY

ADAMS, M. R. 1974. A physiologic and aerodynamic interpretation of fluent and stuttered speech. *Journal of Fluency Disorders* 1: 35–47.

———. 1975. Clinical interpretations and applications. In *Vocal Tract Dynamics and Disfluency*, eds. L. M. Webster and L. C. Furst. New York: New York Speech and Hearing Institute.

———. 1978. Further analysis of stuttering as a phonetic transition defect. *Journal of Fluency Disorders* 3: 265–71.

———. 1975. Vocal tract dynamics in fluency and stuttering. In *Vocal Tract Dynamics and Dysfluency*, eds. L. M. Webster and L. C. Furst. New York: New York Speech and Hearing Institute.

———, S. RIEMENSCHNEIDER, D. METZ, AND E. CONTURE. 1974. Voice onset and articulatory constriction requirements in a speech segment and their relation to the amount of stuttering adaptation. *Journal of Fluency Disorders* 1: 23–9.

———, C. RUNYAN, AND A. R. MALLARD. 1975. Air flow characteristics of the speech of stutterers and nonstutterers. *Journal of Fluency Disorders* 1: 3–12.

AGNELLO, J. G. 1975. Laryngeal and articulatory dynamics of disfluency interpreted within a vocal tract model. In *Vocal Tract Dynamics and Dysfluency*, eds. L. M. Webster and L. C. Furst. New York: New York Speech and Hearing Institute.

AGNELLO, J. G. AND M. E. WINGATE. 1971. Air pressure and formants of stutterers and nonstutterers. Convention paper, ASHA, Chicago.

———. 1972. Some acoustical and physiological aspects of stuttered speech. Convention paper, ASHA, San Francisco.

——— AND L. MOULIN. 1970. Coarticulation patterns of stutterers and nonstutterers. *ASHA* 13: Abstract.

——— AND M. WENDELL. 1974. Voice onset and voice termination times of children and adult stutterers. *Journal of the Acoustical Society of America* 56: 362.

ALLEN, E. L. AND H. HOLLEIN. 1972. Vocal fold thickness in the pulse (vocal fry) register. *Folia Phoniatrica* 24.

ALLEN, G., R. PETERS AND C. WILLIAMS. 1975. Spectrographic study of fluent and stuttered speech. Convention paper, ASHA, Washington, D.C.

ANDREWS, G. AND M. HARRIS. 1964. *The syndrome of stuttering*. London: Heinemann.

BARR, H. 1940. A quantitative study of specific phenomena observed in stuttering. *Journal of Speech Disorders* 5: 277–80.

BLACK, P. C. 1957. A study of the consistency of sequences of stuttering behavior. Masters thesis, University of Pittsburgh.

BLANTON, S. AND M. G. BLANTON. 1936. *For stutterers.* New York: Appleton.

BLOODSTEIN, O. 1960–61. Development of stuttering. *Journal of Speech and Hearing Disorders* 25: 219–37; 366–76; 26: 67–82.

BLUEMEL, C. S. 1957. *The riddle of stuttering.* Danville, Ill.: Interstate.

BOOME, E. J. AND M. A. RICHARDSON. 1932. *The nature and treatment of stammering.* London: Methuen.

BRANKEL, O. 1961. Pneumotachographic studies in stutterers. *Folia Phoniatrica* 13: 136–43.

CHEVRIE-MULLER, C. 1963. A study of laryngeal function in stutterers by the glotto-graphic method. *Proceedings VIIe Congrès de la Société Française de Médecine de la Voix et de la Parole,* Paris.

CONTURE, E. G., G. M. MCCALL AND D. W. BREWSTER. 1977. Laryngeal behavior during stuttering. *Journal of Speech and Hearing Research* 20: 661–8.

DOUGLASS, E. AND B. QUARRINGTON. 1952. Differentiation of interiorized and exteriorized secondary stuttering. *Journal of Speech Disorders* 17: 372–88.

———. 1954. Development of stuttering and its diagnosis. *Canadian Medical Association Journal* 71: 366–71.

DRASEKE, J. 1921. Über Mitbewegungen bei Gesunden. *Deutsche Zeitschrift für Nervenheilkunde* 64: 340–46.

EDGREN, B., R. LEANDERSON, AND L. LEVI. 1970. A research program on stuttering and stress. *Acta Otolaryngologica* 263: 113–18.

FIBIGER, S. 1971. Stuttering explained as a physiological tremor. *Speech Translations Laboratory: Quarterly Progress and Status Report.* Royal Institute of Technology: Stockholm.

———. 1972. Further discussion on stuttering explained as a physiological tremor. *Speech Translations Laboratory: Quarterly Progress and Status Report.* Royal Institute of Technology, Stockholm.

FOLEY, T. H., C. D. MARSDEN, AND D. A. L. OWEN. 1967. Evidence for a direct peripheral effect of adrenaline on physiological tremor in man. *Journal of Physiology* (London) 179: 65–6.

FREEMAN, F. J. 1975. Fluency and phonation. In *Vocal Tract Dynamics and Dysfluency,* eds. M. Webster and L. C. Furst. New York: New York Speech and Hearing Institute.

———. 1979. Phonation in stuttering: a review of current research. *Journal of Fluency Disorders* 4: 79–89.

FREEMAN, F. J., G. BORDEN, AND M. DORMAN. 1976. Laryngeal stuttering: combined physiological and acoustic studies. Convention paper, ASHA, Houston.

FREEMAN, F. J. AND T. USHIJIMA. 1975. Laryngeal activity accompanying the moment of stuttering: a preliminary report of E.M.G. investigations. *Journal of Fluency Disorders* 1: 36–9.

———. 1978. Laryngeal muscle activity during stuttering. *Journal of Speech and Hearing Research* 21: 538–62.

FREUND, H. 1966. *Psychopathology and the problem of stuttering* Springfield, Ill.: Thomas.

FRICK, J. V. 1965. *Evaluation of motor planning techniques for the treatment of stuttering.* Final Report. Grant No. 82-48-0720-5003. U.S. Department of Health, Education, and Welfare.

————. 1970. *Motor planning techniques for the treatment of stuttering.* University Park, Pennsylvania: Pennsylvania State University Speech and Hearing Clinic.

FUJITA, K. Pathophysiology of the larynx from the viewpoint of phonation. *Journal of the Japanese Society of Otorhinolaryngology.*

————. 1966. Tremor control as a factor in stuttering. *Japanese Journal of Otology* 57: 287–91.

GAUTHERON, B., A. LIORZON, AND B. VALLANCIEN. 1973. The role of the larynx in stuttering. In *Neurolinguistic Approaches to Stuttering,* eds. Y. LeBrun and R. Hoops. The Hague: Mouton.

GERTNER, L. L. AND H. L. LUPER. 1967. A cinefluorographic study of the duration and number of lingual-alveolar articulatory contacts and reading time of stutterers and nonstutterers. Convention address, ASHA.

GREWEL, F. 1960. Balbuties (Stotteren). *Logopaedie et Foniatrie* 32: 109–15; 125–28; 145–52; 165–68.

GOTTLOBER, A. B. 1953. *Understanding stuttering.* New York: Grune and Stratton.

HENRICKSON, E. H. 1936. Simultaneously recorded breathing and vocal disturbances of stutterers. *Archives of Speech* 1: 133–49.

HILL, H. 1954. An experimental study of disorganization of speech and manual responses in normal subjects. *Journal of Speech and Hearing Disorders* 19: 295–305.

————. 1942. *Perseveration in normal speakers and stutterers.* Masters thesis, University of Indiana.

————. 1945. An interbehavioral analysis of several aspects of stuttering. *Journal of General Psychology* 32: 289–315.

HOOD, S. B. 1974. Clinical assessment of the moment of stuttering. *Journal of Fluency Disorders* 1: 22–34.

HUTCHINSON, J. M. 1975. Aerodynamic patterns of stuttered speech. In *Vocal Tract Dynamics and Dysfluency,* eds. L. M. Webster and L. C. Furst. New York: New York Speech and Hearing Institute.

JANSSEN, P. AND F. KRAAIMANT. 1977. The relation between stuttering and state anxiety. *Proceedings XVII International Congress of Logopedics and Phoniatrics,* Copenhagen.

JOHNSON, W. 1930. *Because I stutter.* New York: Appleton.

KANNER, L. 1942. *Child psychiatry.* Springfield, Ill.: Thomas.

KENYON, E. L. 1943. The etiology of stammering: the psychophysiologic facts which concern the production of speech sounds and of stammering. *Journal of Speech Disorders* 8: 337–48.

KIMMELL, W. 1938. The nature of effect of stutterers' avoidance reactions. *Journal of Speech Disorders* 3: 95–100.

KUSSMAUL, A. 1877. Die Störungen der Sprache. In *Cyclopaedia Medica,* ed. H. V. Ziemssen.

LANGOVA, J. 1967. Pathopsychological mechanisms in the initial tonus of stuttering. *HNO,* 15: 189–90.

———— AND M. MORAVEK. 1966. *An experimental study of stuttering and cluttering.* Prague: Academia.

————. 1964. Some results of experimental examinations among stutterers and clutterers. *Folia Phoniatrica* SVI: 290–96.

LENNON, E. J. 1962. *Le bégaiement: thérapeutiques modernes.* Paris: G. Doin.

LOHR, F. 1969. Visible manifestations of stuttered speech. Convention address, ASHA.

LUCHSINGER, R. AND G. E. ARNOLD. 1965. *Voice—speech—language.* Belmont, Cal.: Wadsworth.

MAKUEN, G. H. 1914. A study of 1,000 cases of stammering with special reference to the etiology and treatment of the affection. *Therapeutical Gazette* 38: 385–90.

McGLONE, R. AND T. SHIPP. 1971. Some physiological correlates of vocal fry phonation. *Journal of Speech and Hearing Research* 14: 769–75.

MONTGOMERY, A. A., AND P. A. COOKE. 1976. Perceptual and acoustic analysis of repetitions in stuttered speech. *Journal of Communication Disorders* 9: 317–30.

MORAVEK, M. AND J. LANGOVA. 1962. Some electrophysiological findings among stutterers and clutterers. *Folia Phoniatrica* 14: 305–16.

MOSER, H. M. 1942. Symposium of unique cases of speech disorders: presentation of a case. *Journal of Speech Disorders* 7: 173–74.

PLATT, L. J. AND A. BASILI. 1973. Jaw tremor during stuttering block. *Journal of Communication Disorders* 6: 102–9.

PRINS, T. D. AND F. E. LOHR. 1968. A study of the behavioral components of stuttered speech. Final Report Project No. 62302. Grant No. OEG 36062382-1882. U.S. Department of Health, Education and Welfare.

————. 1967. Behavioral dimensions of stuttered speech. *Journal of Speech and Hearing Research* 15: 61–71.

QUARRINGTON, B. AND E. DOUGLASS. 1960. Audibility avoidance in nonvocalized stutterers. *Journal of Speech and Hearing Disorders* 25: 358–65.

ROBINSON, F. B. 1964. *Introduction to stuttering.* Englewood Cliffs, N.J.: Prentice-Hall.

ROTTER, J. B. 1942. A working hypothesis as to the nature and treatment of stuttering. *Journal of Speech Disorders* 7: 263–88.

SCHILLING, A. 1960. Diaphragmatic radiokymograms in stuttering. *Folia Phoniatrica* 12: 145–53.

SCHRUM, W. F. 1967. A study of the speaking behavior of stutterers and non-stutterers by means of multichannel electromyography. Convention address, ASHA.

SCHWARTZ, M. F. 1974. The core of the stuttering block. *Journal of Speech and Hearing Disorders* 39: 169–77.

————. 1975. The core of the stuttering block. In *Vocal Tract Dynamics and Dysfluency,* eds. L. M. Webster and L. C. Furst. New York: New York Institute for Speech and Hearing.

SCRIPTURE, E. W. 1923. *Stuttering and lisping.* (2nd Edition). New York: Macmillan.

SHEEHAN, J. 1946. A study of the phenomena of stuttering. Masters thesis, University of Michigan.

————. 1951. Modification of stuttering through non-reinforcement. *Journal of Abnormal and Social Psychology* 46: 51–63.

————. 1958. Projective studies of stuttering. *Journal of Speech and Hearing Disorders* 23: 18–25.

————. 1958. Conflict theory of stuttering. In *Stuttering: A Symposium,* ed. J. Eisenson. New York: Harper.

————. 1974. Stuttering behavior: a phonetic analysis. *Journal of Communication Disorders* 7: 193–212.

SHEEHAN, J. G. AND R. B. VOAS. 1954. Tension patterns during stuttering in relation to conflict, anxiety binding and reinforcement. *Speech Monographs* 21: 272–79.

SKINNER, B. F. 1957. *Verbal behavior.* Englewood Cliffs, N.J.: Prentice-Hall.

SNIDECOR, J. C. 1955. Tension and facial appearance in stuttering. In *Stuttering in Children and Adults,* ed. W. Johnson. Minneapolis: University of Minnesota Press: 377–80.

STEIN. L. 1942. *Speech and voice.* London: Methuen.

STETSON, R. H. 1951. *Motor phonetics.* Amsterdam: North-Holland.

STUTENROTH, R. I. 1937. Specific reactions by which stutterers attempt to avoid stuttering. Masters thesis, State University of Iowa.

USHIJIMA, T., G. KAMIYANA, H. HIROSE, AND S. NIIMI. 1965. *Articulatory movements of the larynx during stuttering.* (Film) Tokyo: Research Institute of Logopedics and Phoniatrics.

VAN RIPER, C. 1936. A study of the stutterer's ability to interrupt stuttering spasms. *Journal of Speech Disorders* 1: 61–72.

————. 1937. Effect of devices for minimizing stuttering on the creation of symptoms. *Journal of Abnormal and Social Psychology* 32: 63–65.

————. 1937. The growth of the stuttering spasm. *Quarterly Journal of Speech* 23: 70–73.

————. 1937. The preparatory set in stuttering. *Journal of Speech Disorders* 2: 149–54.

————. 1936. Study of the thoracic breathing of stutterers during expectancy and occurrence of stuttering. *Journal of Speech Disorders* 1: 61–72.

————. 1974. The ablauf problem in stuttering. *Journal of Fluency Disorders* 1: 2–9.

———— AND R. MILISEN. 1939. A study of the predicted duration of the stutterer's blocks as related to their actual duration. *Journal of Speech Disorders* 4: 339–45.

VILLAREAL, J. J. 1962. The role of the speech pathologist in psychotherapy. In *The Psychotherapy of Stuttering,* ed. D. A. Barbara. Springfield, Ill.: Thomas.

WEBSTER, L. M. AND L. C. FURST (eds.) 1975. *Vocal tract dynamics and dysfluency.* New York: New York Institute for Speech and Hearing.

WEDBERG, C. F. 1937. *The stutterer speaks.* Magnolia, Mass.: Expression Co.

WINGATE, M. E. 1964. A standard definition of stuttering. *Journal of Speech and Hearing Disorders* 29: 484–89.

————. 1969. Stuttering as a phonetic transition defect. *Journal of Speech and Hearing Disorders* 34: 107–8.

————. 1976. *Stuttering theory and treatment:* New York: Irvington-Wiley.

WISCHNER, G. J. 1950. Stuttering behavior and learning. *Journal of Speech Disorders* 15: 324–35.

WYLLIE. J. 1894. *The disorders of speech.* Edinburgh: Oliver and Boyd.

YOUNG, E. H. 1928. *Help for you who stutter.* Minneapolis: Hill-Young School.

ZIMMERMANN, G. N. 1980. Articulatory behaviors associated with stuttering: a cine-radiographic analysis. *Journal of Speech and Hearing Research* 33: 108–21.

————. 1980. Articulatory dynamics of "fluent" utterances of stutterers and nonstutterers. *Journal of Speech and Hearing Research* 33: 95–107.

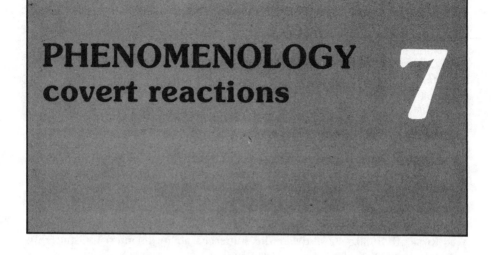

PHENOMENOLOGY
covert reactions
7

This chapter describes the feelings, reactions, and attitudes of those who stutter. It is a difficult task, almost an impossible one. There is an immense array of these responses to the fear and experience of stuttering. Moreover, their precise definition and measurement would require an objectivity that is impossible because they are covert and hidden. Research deals with them obliquely since the instruments for measuring emotional states are far from satisfactory. Much of our knowledge is based only on verbal testimony, on introspective accounts which themselves leave much to be desired. Those of us who have been stutterers may read our own experiences into these clinical accounts and distort them. It is very hard to find words that fit the squirting of our glands. Only poets have those words. Over a hundred years ago one of these poets wrote the following:

Come, I will show thee an affliction unnumbered among the world's sorrows,
Yet real and wearisome and constant, embittering the cup of life.
There be who can think within themselves, and the fires burneth at their heart,
And eloquence waiteth at their lips, yet they speak not with their tongue;
There be those whom zeal quickeneth, or slander stirreth to reply,
Or need constraineth to ask, or pity sendeth as her messengers,
But nervous dread and sensitive shame freeze the current of their speech:
The mouth is sealed as with lead, a cold weight presseth on the heart,
The mocking promise of power is once more broken in performance,
And they stand impotent of words, travailing with unborn thoughts,
Courage is cowed at the portal, wisdom is widowed of utterance:
He that went to comfort is pitied, he that should rebuke is silent,
And fools who might listen and learn, stand by to look and laugh:
While friends, with kinder eyes, wound deeper by compassion:
And thought, finding not a vent, smouldereth gnawing at the heart,
And the man sinketh in his sphere for lack of empty sounds.

There may be cares and sorrows thou hast not yet considered,
And well may thy soul rejoice in the fair privilege of speech:
For at every turn to want a word—thou canst not guess that want;
It is as lack of breath or bread; life hath no grief more galling (Tupper, 1861).

Nevertheless, enough students of the disorder have been able to record their impressions of the stutterer's covert behavior with enough similarity so that it can be described with some confidence. The aforementioned cautions, however, should be borne in mind.

FEARS

Perhaps the most common of the advanced stutterer's feelings is fear. Fear is the expectation of unpleasantness. This expectation ranges from vague doubt to complete certainty. The expected unpleasantness itself is also highly variable. The stutterer may be afraid of social penalty and stigma; he may dread listener loss or some other kind of rejection. Nonstuttering therapists often think these are the only things feared, but most of the stutterers with whom we have worked have told us that there is another more basic fear—the expectation of communicative inability and verbal impotence. What they fear most is the momentary loss of self-control. They dread the moment of muteness, of spasmodic contortion; they anticipate with foreboding the repetitions or fixations that seem both mysterious and involuntary. One stutterer called the moment of blockage the *petit mort*, the moment of the little death. The inability to move a muscle when you want to move it, a muscle that you can normally move with ease, is traumatic to the basic integrity of the self. Equally devastating is the experience of being unable to stop doing something that you don't want to do. As one of our stutterers said,

What really scares me is when I start to say a word and find myself saying the same syllable over and over again and I can't stop, or when I find myself making a yard of an *s* sound when I only want a quarter inch of it. I get petrified when I fear this sort of thing is going to happen. I feel as helpless as a ventriloquist's dummy. Something, somebody else is in charge of my mouth and I can't do anything about it.

This seems to be a very common and basic experience. We have seen little children stop suddenly after a perseverative repetition, cry uncontrollably, and run to their mothers for comfort. Their eyes, at least to us, seemed full of fear. In our opinion, this core experience is not simply frustration at stymied communication. That is present, of course, but something more traumatic is also occurring. It is the sudden loss of the ability to command oneself.

There are other unpleasant events to anticipate. Chief among these are the various punishing listener reactions. Few stutterers are able to run the verbal gauntlet of their days and years without receiving some hard blows from someone with whom they talk. Pity, rudeness, and rejection are commonly experienced. Most of our cases report having had listeners mock or humiliate them. Most have met at least a few vivid reactions of impatience and irritation. They remember the occasional cruel comment of a stranger, teacher, parent, or playmate. They have watched their friends be amused by some stuttering character on television and many came to think these reactions were universal, although perhaps kept hidden out of politeness. They have winced when, as children, they read about P-p-p-porky the p-pig in the comic strips. There are many jokes about stutterers, some of them very funny too—except to the stutterer. In short, most stutterers have been badly hurt by society's reaction to their disability. Most of them sense their deviance keenly. From India comes this account:

> The patients feel more unhappy by the treatment they meet at the hands of their fellow beings than by the ailment itself. Of course, the ailment itself is a great handicap to make them unhappy but the unsympathetic treatment adds to the misery of the patients. It is the sneering, zeering, and snubbing of the fellow beings . . . that make them feel the burden all the more heavy. And there is no dearth of persons who even take delight in copying a stammerer. The treatment . . . mentioned above creates an emotional mood in the patients. They become suspicious and quarrelsome or timid and shy (Mathur, 1960, p. 58).

But the stutterer often also finds rejection when it is not really there. Because he has difficulty communicating and is reluctant to reveal his sensitivity, he has few opportunities to test the reality of his suspicions. Most normal speakers find it frustrating to listen to a stutterer, but only a few ever show the marked rejection the stutterer attributes to them, simply because they are more concerned with other things. Nevertheless, imagined or real, social penalties are certainly important in the genesis and the maintenance of the stutterer's fears.

One of the more unpleasant aspects of stuttering is the ever present threat of exposure. Until he stutters, the stutterer looks and sounds quite normal. Since stuttering is intermittent and since there are many ways of hiding it, the mild stutterer always lives under the sword of Damocles, never knowing with certainty when the hair that holds it will break. Using his entire repertoire of avoidance and disguise reactions, he may be able to hide his impediment from many of his casual acquaintances or the strangers to whom he must talk briefly. But he always feels the threat of exposure. These stutterers live constantly in verbal jeopardy.

Although social penalties are unpleasant in themselves, the emotional reactions they generate in the stutterer are even more disagreeable. Feelings of unworthiness, embarrassment, shame, and guilt are common. Sometimes these feelings reverberate as the stutterer relives a traumatic experience over and over again, nursing his misery to keep it warm. Old wounds ache most when the wind blows cold. And when the stutterer feels moody or depressed for other reasons his stuttering curse seems intolerable. Some stutterers react to listener penalties with anger and hate. There are some very hostile stutterers, whose rage, bred of frustration and penalty, constantly seethes beneath the surface, occasionally breaking out in asocial attacks with a suddenness and vehemence incomprehensible to the listener. Other stutterers, less able to release their hostility outwardly, turn it upon themselves. Even little children sometimes slap their own faces or pinch themselves viciously after a volley of stuttering. Scripture gives a vivid picture:

> Few persons realize how terrible life becomes to a stutterer. One religious but stuttering lady finally demanded to be "cured or chloroformed." One boy often threw himself on the floor, begging his mother to tell him how to die. Many stutterers become so sensitive that they imagine everybody is constantly making fun of them. The stutterer prefers to be thought lazy or stupid rather than reveal the true nature of his trouble. A condition of mental flurry is usually present. When the patient starts to speak, he becomes partly dazed by his emotion and does not know exactly what he wants to say. This condition may be present even when he does not stutter; in trying to answer a question, for example, he cannot make up his mind just what he wishes to say. The embarrassment and sad experiences of the stutterer often lead to an abnormal mental condition. The patient is nervous, shy, easily embarrassed, retiring, odd in his ways, sad, etc. In some cases the change does not go beyond an increased sensitiveness. Many stutterers, especially young women and schoolboys, acquire a permanent facial expression that is typical of the profoundest sadness. The thought of suicide is frequent. It may be suggested that stuttering is a defect which tends to exclude the person from the society of his fellows, and that persons who already have this unconscious tendency instinctively seize upon such a means of encouraging it (1923, p. 3).

These emotional upheavals can be anticipated by the stutterer, and since they are not pleasant experiences, they are dreaded, whether the anticipation is one of hostility or shame or anxiety. Even fear can be feared.

THE PRECIPITANTS OF FEAR

Stuttering fears first begin as the consequences of these various unpleasant experiences. The context in which the unpleasant experience occurs determines the stimuli that will later precipitate fear. These stimuli fall into several categories: (1) characteristics of the listeners, (2) the content or implications of the message, (3) the words and their position in the utterance, and (4) the acoustic and motoric features of the sounds on which the stuttering occurs. Any of these, and any combination of them can serve as stimuli that will precipitate stuttering fears. It all depends on how the stutterer perceives them. Each stutterer develops his own particular pattern of fear-invested cues based on his perceptions, and these fears can generalize to other cues, following the laws of classical conditioning.

Much has been made of the role of the listener in stuttering since Wendell Johnson suggested that it began in the listener's ear rather than in the stutterer's mouth. Stuttering is apparently as much a disorder of communication as it is of speech; the receiver is at least as important as the sender in the interchange. There is a wealth of testimony from cases and research findings confirming the importance of the listener as a precipitator of stuttering fears. Stutterers scan their listeners with the intensity and care of a robber casing a bank. Again there are many individual differences. One stutterer's computer is programmed to read out FEAR if his prospective listener is of the opposite sex, is voluble, and is older; another's so that the facial expression of the listener, his size, and his probable vocation are inspected and responded to in that order. One of our stutterers found it impossible to speak to children without immediate fear. "I've had too many mothers who dragged their frightened children away from me," he said. One stutterer even found it easier to talk to listeners who interrupted him because, as he remarked, "I can sneak in what I have to say under the cover of their talking." Another told us that the one situation in which he *always* felt fear was when talking to school teachers. "Old or young, male or female, elementary, secondary, or college, whatever they are, teachers always petrify me."

It is difficult to generalize, considering the wide variety of conditionings, but it seems apparent that listeners whose rejection would have truly unpleasant consequences precipitate more fear than those whose opinion is less important. Accordingly, most stutterers are afraid of speaking to people in authority, prospective employers, parents, teachers, or prospective sexual mates. This generalization is also true for normal-speaking trainees in speech pathology who, as part of their practicum, are assigned to fake stuttering for a variety of listeners. One stutterer analyzed the content of 721 consecutive situation fears over a period of one month at the beginning of his therapy. These fears are given below, ranked in order of their frequency:

1. Fear of being ridiculed, smiled at, laughed at, viewed as being funny; 2. Fear of being exposed and classed as a stutterer, a deviant, an inferior, abnormal person, a speech defective; 3. Fear of being unable to communicate my message effectively in the allotted time, time pressure, frustration fear; 4. Fear of embarrassing my listener; 5. Fear of rebuke or impatience or rejection, either open or hidden, by my listener; 6. Fear that my listener will pity me; 7. Other (fear that I am not making progress; fear of relapse; fear that I will lose hope again, etc.)

The same stutterer rechecked his situation fears three months later, finding only 104 of them in the same period, and, although they were the same ones, the rank order had changed to 7, 3, 2, 5, 4, 6, 1. Much of the change resulted from reality-testing and the realization that most listeners are more curious than punitive. For example, his fear of mockery had been greatly exaggerated, and when a few listeners seemed to parrot him by opening their mouths when he gaped, or holding their breath when he did, it was more empathy than ridicule.

Many stutterers dread speaking to groups more than to individuals, probably because in a group there is a greater chance of at least one listener rejecting the stutterer. Even here, however, there are stutterers who react the opposite way, especially in situations where the stutterer is making a speech and possesses a captive audience. If he is especially vulnerable to listener loss, then he speaks better before a group. His listeners can't get away. To the beginning therapist in this field, who may feel overwhelmed by the diversity of stimuli that can precipitate the fear of stuttering, we can only say that each stutterer's phobic phenomena are unique because of his past conditioning and the particular patterns of generalization that have taken place. If we are to decondition and extinguish these fears, they must be identified for each individual. There are few rules and many exceptions. Yet these fears make sense. They have a history.

THE COMMUNICATIVE MILIEU: SITUATION FEARS

Stuttering does not occur in a vacuum but in an environment. This environment or milieu possesses distinctive features on which the stutterer may hang his dread. The telephone can become a frightening bugaboo if sufficient misery has been connected with its use. A doctor's office, a beauty parlor, a certain store can become dreaded places. The author of this text, long fluent, still feels fear when he sits in a certain chair of his old family home. For some children the schoolroom is colored with stuttering apprehension; others fear the playground. The bus station or airport, the employer's waiting room, even the church can be feared places. Again the patterns differ with different stutterers.

THE CONDITIONS OF COMMUNICATION

Stutterers also scan the conditions under which communication will occur for signs that mean approaching stuttering. Chief among these is temporal urgency, the time factor. When the stutterer knows in advance that he must finish his communication in a hurry, the red flare of fear arises. One of our stutterers, a soldier in combat, said that when going out on night patrol his major fear was not of the enemy but of being challenged to give the password on his return. Part of the fear of the telephone is due to the knowledge that the stutterer must begin to speak within a relatively short time or hear the click of a hung-up receiver at the other end of the line.

Since stuttering is a disorder of time, and the communication of messages is impeded by repetitions, prolongations, or any of the coping behaviors, most stutterers seem especially vulnerable to this time pressure. Under such stress, they usually stutter more, and longer, and with greater abnormality. The apochryphal story is told of the stuttering king of England who, while a young man and an officer on board ship, was marching his marines on the foredeck. When the front ranks had their forelegs about to step over the ship's side, and he was still completely blocked from all utterance, one of his fellow officers is reputed to have queried, "Gad, sir, aren't you even going to bid them goodbye?" Once again, however, some stutterers have surprised themselves and their listeners by being able to speak completely fluently under great urgency. One of our patients was a member of a submarine crew who discovered a malfunctioning of some of the controls and was able to give a series of directions and reports under great time pressure without a trace of his usual stuttering, though he claimed his hair began to turn grey as the result of the experience. We asked him how he could explain his fluency under such stress. "I'm not sure," he replied. "I guess I had no time even to think of stuttering, or what I was going to say. I just had to say it and did." Others in similar emergencies have testified that great fears or great necessities have wiped out the specific fears or rehearsal behaviors that trigger the stuttering response, and so for a moment they are able to be fluent.

Usually, the amount of stuttering varies with the meaningfulness of the message to be communicated. The greater the propositionality or meaningfulness, the more stuttering. Stutterers can often repeat what someone else has already said. "Small talk" in conversation provides little difficulty. Stutterers can often interject the little "asides," the bits of commentary on what they have said, with little stuttering.

For some stutterers the presence of certain types of masking noise arouses fear. One stutterer claimed that every time he rode in the back seat of a car he knew he would stutter and that he had the same apprehension in the hubbub of a cocktail party. "It's hard to make yourself understood in these situations," he said, "and if I stutter I know I'll have to say the whole thing over again which means more trouble. That's why I fear noise." Other stutterers, usually the milder ones with few silent closures, find that such situations are much easier than those in which silence must be broken.

Some stutterers fear oral reading or recitation of memorized material because there is little opportunity for avoidance or disguise. The words cannot be dodged; all pauses will be apparent. Other stutterers find the same activities much easier because no burden of responsibility for message formulation is required, and a certain amount of distraction from the stuttering is produced by the necessity for reading or remembering. Again, in all of these, we find the loci of the stutterer's fears determined by individual past experience.

The frequency, duration, and abnormality of stuttering varies with the listener's reaction as the stutterer perceives it, a perception which may not be realistic. In general, stutterers have more difficulty speaking to rejecting listeners, or to those who show impatience, irritation, pity, or embarrassment. The *threat* of possible punishment for stuttering seems to evoke more of it. Thus, speaking to a listener of higher status, or who has the power to facilitate or negate the stutterer's desires, ordinarily produces more stuttering. Nevertheless, some stutterers speak much better when confronted with a hostile, rejecting listener. As one of them said,

I won't let that bastard hear me stutter! Somehow, for a short time, I can rise to the occasion and summon up my energies and just refuse to stutter. I won't let him get the best of me. Of course, I couldn't keep it up very long, but I'd never put myself in a situation so I'd always have to be with a person like that.

A nice little old grey-haired lady once put her arm around the author when he had been stuttering badly to a store clerk, and said to him, "My son, oh you poor boy, do you always have to stutter like that, you poor thing." To his surprise, if not to his credit, he answered, and with complete fluency for once, "No, Madame, only when I talk!" Although many stutterers have more difficulty speaking to strangers, others have none in this situation. One of the latter said:

When I speak to a total stranger, one I have never seen before or expect to see again, I can talk perfectly, though I stutter badly to all the people who know me. I figure that the reason for this is that the stranger doesn't expect to hear me stutter—there's no reminder. For a short time I can pass as normal as I look.

Again, the variability seems due to different learning experiences.

THE COMMUNICATIVE CONTENT

There are also certain semantic variables that precipitate the fear of stuttering. We have much research which indicates that propositionality (the amount of meaning) in a word or utterance produces more stuttering. The stutterer knows this well, and so he scans his anticipated communication for signals of this sort. Nouns, verbs, and adjectives generate more fear than do articles or conjunctions. The key word or phrase of a joke is approached with more trepidation than other words. Vital utterances are more dreaded than casual ones. The words of a given sentence do not all carry the same load of meaningfulness, and the stutterer knows that more communicative disruption will occur when he stutters on an important word than on an unimportant one. A common trick used by some stutterers to defeat the expectancy of stuttering is to lead up to the main message with a few sentences of casual, meaningless conversation. Small talk is less to be feared than big talk. Indeed, many stutterers employ such meaningless gambit phrases or words ("Well," "You know," "What I mean is . . .") as devices to get started. Perhaps the reason most stutterers sing without trouble is that the content of the message sung is so low in information value, though there are other explanations too. The adaptation effect—the reduction in stuttering with repeated utterances of the same material—has been attributed variously to anxiety reduction, or to reactive inhibition, but also to the inevitable reduction in the meaningfulness of the material being spoken over and over again. Even the most frantic adolescent would find it difficult to maintain the same meaningfulness in the phrase "I love you" were he to say it sequentially one hundred times. Nevertheless, there are stutterers who find small talk very difficult, and most stutterers, when they are compelled to repeat what they have already said fluently, will show more stuttering. There are also stutterers who do not show the usual adaptation effect, and there are those who speak much better when they are especially concerned with the content of their communication. One of them told us, "When I can just quit thinking about stuttering and think about what I'm trying to tell the other person, I'm very fluent."

The emotional content of the message may also serve as a precipitant of stuttering fear. Bardrick and Sheehan (1956) and others have shown that emotionally loaded words produce more stuttering than either ordinary communication or nonsense material. Stutterers say they fear these emotional utterances. In part this fear may arise from anticipated listener rejection. One of our stutterers left the Catholic church because of his stuttering experiences during confession. "It was not, alas, that I had many sins to confess but the tremendous fear of having to suffer so much stuttering over and over again every time I went to confession." Almost all ordinary speech has some emotional content, but some utterances are filled with it, and on these the stutterer anticipates unpleasantness, not only because listeners may react unfavorably, but also because of the inevitable confrontation of his own miserable feelings. Unpleasant speech doesn't taste good. It is interesting and understandable that expressions of anxiety and guilt seem to be more feared than those of anger.

LINGUISTIC PRECIPITANTS

One of the most prominent features of the confirmed stutterer is his intense scanning of a prospective utterance for linguistic cues associated with stuttering. We should not be surprised to find this since, after all, stuttering does occur on sounds, syllables and words. Furthermore, no one stutters on every word or sound, so one would expect the stutterer to scrutinize his sounds and words and their placement for danger signals if only to avoid the consequences. We have said that this scanning is intense. It is very difficult for the normal speaker to comprehend the vigilance, the alertness, the complex pre-testing of stuttering probabilities that goes on in the mind of the stutterer. It is one of his greatest burdens. Kazin (1951) gives this autobiographical account:

> The word was my agony. The word that for others was so effortless and so neutral, so unburdened, so simple, so exact, I had first to mediate in advance, to see if I could make it like a plumber, fitting together odd lengths and shapes of pipe. I was always preparing words I could speak, storing them away, choosing between them. And often, when the word did come from my mouth in its great and terrible birth, quailing and bleeding as if forced through a thornbush, I would not be able to look the others in the face, and would walk out in silence, the infinitely echoing silence behind my back, to say it all cleanly back to myself as I walked in the streets . . . only then was it possible for me to

speak without the infinite premeditations and strangled silences I toiled through whenever I got up in school to respond with the expected, the exact answer (p. 67).

PHONEME FEARS

Of all the verbal stimuli that precipitate stuttering fears, phonemes and their distinctive features are probably the most vital. When stutterers remember their past experiences, the initial sounds of words stand out most clearly. "Words beginning with /b/, /p/, and /t/ consonants give me more trouble," one stutterer will tell you. Another may have a totally different set of feared phonemes. Again the past conditioning accounts for the variation. We even find stutterers claiming that 'h' words such as 'hour' are feared (although that word really begins with a vowel), thus indicating that the visual aspect of the spelling has come to be a stimulus. Stutterers may say that they fear the "s" sound when actually they produce that sound fluently far more often than they stutter on it. Some will inform you that vowel sounds are their "Jonah" or unlucky sounds but only when they occur in the initial position of a word. Others have generalized their feared stimuli to include all lip sounds or all tongue-tip sounds. The important thing to remember is that these stimuli are not distributed at random in any given stutterer; they have loci and foci; they have been conditioned.

Stutterers rarely fear the final sounds of words or syllables. Spencer Brown (1938) says:

> The beginning of a word has for the stutterer a far greater importance than the rest of the word. This is shown by the fact that of the spasms recorded in the data studied, 92 per cent were in relation to the initial sound of the words with only 8 per cent occurring at all other points. Other evidence showing this primacy for the stutterer of the initial part of the word is found in the introspections of stutterers. They report that they think of "*s* words" or "*k* words" and fear stuttering with relation to the initial sound of the word. Several stutterers who reported that they feared *s* words such as *see, seven, side*, etc., did not report such fears with relation to the *s* sound when it occurred at the beginning of the second or third syllable of a word, and questioned on the point said they did not fear the *s* in such words as *inside, consent, Robertson*, etc. Furthermore, many stutterers insist that they never stutter except at the beginning of a word (p. 113).

However they do have occasional fears of the sounds beginning accented syllables of longer words, especially on the sounds also feared in the initial position. Perceptually, each word presents to the stutterer a configuration of features any one of which may have been associated with unpleasant past experiences. The phoneme with which the word begins, the length of the word, the way it is spelled, its relative familiarity, its dominant syllable—any of these may signal danger quite apart from the word's propositionality or emotional loading. After a stutterer has fallen into the stuttering booby trap repeatedly and has been hurt, he scrutinizes his verbal terrain with great care lest unsuspectingly he fall into it again.

WORD FEARS

Stutterers develop fears of words as well as sounds. He fears the word as a whole because in the past his communication has been impaired by its utterance. For example, stutterers are often afraid to speak their own names or addresses, because on former occasions their inability to say these particular words provoked penalty and embarrassment. Some stutterers can recall very vividly the original experience that led to word fear. For most, however, the origin of the fear has been forgotten, and fear is magnified by mysteriousness.

Other word fears have their origin in the ambivalence of uncertain pronunciation as in foreign or unfamiliar words. Because of their need for synonyms, some stutterers have developed supervocabularies, many words of which they know only by sight but not sound. When they try to say them, mispronunciations add to the difficulty. Other words, such as the name of the disorder itself—*stuttering*—are feared because they are emotionally loaded. Some words seem to signal approaching stuttering merely because they are used so frequently in important communication. Child stutterers often show a word fear of "Mother" and adults of the pronoun "I" for this reason. These words have been used so often to initiate sentences concerned with emotional upheaval that the sand burrs of fear stick to them. Interrogatives such as *Where? Why? When? How?* are also often used under the same circumstances and become feared words. There are few valid generalizations about the type of words that stutterers fear but we can be sure that some words are feared as wholes and that stutterers scan them as such.

As though all this scanning were not burden enough, stutterers also search for and find danger signals in the *arrrangement* or positioning of the words within the prospective sentence. "It's the starting word that I fear," they tell us, and they mean not only the first word of a sentence but any word that follows a pause such as that used for verbal punctuation. The stutterer often responds to these perceptions of positional fear by rearranging the sequencing of his speech. He may attempt to bury the word that has evoked fear in the middle of the sentence instead of using it in the beginning as he originally intended, or he may preface it with some starting phrase such as, *"I believe that"* and thus reduces the positional cue on the feared first word. Words of high propositional value or emotional content are similarly shuffled about in the silent rehearsals that precede the speech attempt to lessen the certainty or expected severity of the anticipated stuttering. Sentences consist of configurations just as single words do. Certain features loom large: the starting word, the key word. The fear of stuttering lurks among these prominences.

RELATIONSHIP OF SITUATIONAL
TO WORD FEARS

Situational fears are fears that have become conditioned to features of interpersonal communicative relationship. Situational fears are energizers of word fears. They create the fund of fear that drains into and finds its focus in the word fears. Typically, the situation fears in the adult usually come first. The stutterer, confronted with an approaching speech situation, scans it for danger signals. "Oh, oh," he says to himself, "I'm going to have trouble. I'm going to stutter." At this point he anticipates his distress, the probable punitive audience reactions, and the communicative frustration. But these fears are often vague and without focus. It is only when the stutterer begins to formulate what he will say (and sometimes only as his speech unfolds) that the scanning for difficult words, sounds, and positional cues takes place. When these are identified, the fear gets suddenly stronger. It finds its focus. Tentative rehearsal behaviors then arise during which the stutterer rehearses his expected abnormality. He silently samples the approaching tremors and struggle reactions. He runs through his repertoire of possible avoidance strategies, selecting and discarding as time ticks on. Then finally he tries the first word of his utterance.

In Figure 9 we present a schematic drawing showing a hypothetical relationship between situational fears and the phonemic word fears of a stutterer as he says the same sentence in five different speech situations. The vertical lines represent the potential amount of phonemic word fear on each of the four words of the sentence. Thus, *Smith* is the most feared word; *stutterer* is less feared, and the amount of potential fear on the words *is* and *a* are minimal although present. The horizontal lines A through E represent the amount of situational fear. Thus baseline A (speaking alone) indicates a speaking situation in which little or no fear would be experienced; baseline B (speaking to a friend) might create some mild fearfulness; and baselines C, D, and E represent increasing fear gradients.

Figure 9. Schematic drawing showing interaction between phonemic-word fears and situational fears.

155

The length of the vertical above a given baseline may be viewed as representing the severity of stuttering upon that word. Since none of the verticals arise above baseline A, no stuttering would be evident when the stutterer says the sentence to himself. When speaking to a close friend, however, the short vertical above baseline B indicates that he would have a short, mild stuttering on *Smith* but not on the other words. When speaking to a therapist, he would have a longer more severe stuttering on *Smith* but still no stuttering on the other words. When speaking to a stranger, the vertical above baseline D is even longer, representing a further increase in stuttering severity on this word *Smith* but also another vertical, the one for the word *stutterer* has emerged above the baseline, and this indicates that he has stuttered mildly on this word too. Finally, when the situational fear is very intense as when speaking to a large audience, he would show some stuttering on every one of the four words of the utterance but again he would have his most severe blocking on *Smith* and the next most severe on *stutterer* while the words *is* and *a* would show only a little abnormality.

Figure 9 illustrates how situational and phonemic word fears may interact to account for the variance in frequency and severity of stuttering. It also may demonstrate the need to do more in therapy than merely reduce situational fears; we must also reduce those which have become conditioned to the phonemic, positional, and other features of the words.

CORRELATION OF FEAR WITH FREQUENCY AND SEVERITY OF STUTTERING

The correlation between expectancy and the actual occurrence of stuttering has been demonstrated many times. When the product of situational and word fears is large and much fear is experienced, stuttering occurs more frequently and more severely than when the fear is low. Stutterers seem to be able, in a given situation, to predict how much stuttering they will have and how severe it will be. The correlation may not be high but it is certainly positive, perhaps because the fears they sense determine the outcome of the speech attempt. Any therapy worthy of the name should try to reduce this correlation. It therefore seems unwise to ask the stutterer merely to "bounce" or "prolong" until he can say the word. If his fear is strong, he will have to repeat the same syllable many more times or to prolong the first sound much more than if his fear is weak. These differential experiences will not be lost on the stutterer, and further fear conditioning will take place. We must try to reduce the correlation between fear and severity, not to maintain or enhance it.

OTHER PRECIPITATING CONDITIONS

Many other factors seem to play a role in the precipitation of stuttering. Some stutterers report being able to speak better when thoroughly fatigued; others speak worse. Some stutterers speak better when they are ill than when they are well. Some stutterers speak better when they speak swiftly; others when they speak slowly. Usually the amount of stuttering is reduced under masking noise, but there are many instances where noise, especially at the lower intensities, creates more severe and frequent stuttering. Many stutterers speak more fluently when thoroughly relaxed or under the influence of alcohol; others speak better when highly tensed and mobilizing all their attentional resources and much worse when intoxicated. Even the weather has been shown to produce differences in the amount of stuttering. One of the first things any worker with stutterers finds out is that individual variability dominates this problem.

The only plausible explanation for such variability is different learning experiences. In its advanced stages, stuttering and the expectation of it have become conditioned to many different constellations of stimuli. The group trends toward more stuttering with multiple, authoritative, or rejecting listeners merely reflect the stutterer's general history of hurt; the effects of the time pressure and propositionality in creating more stuttering merely testify to conditions under which past stuttering became more frustrating. In short, the general consistencies can be explained in terms of the nature of the disorder as an interference to communication and the way society responds to it. The individual differences reflect the distinctive personal histories of the stutterers, the particular stimulus configurations with which his stuttering behaviors have been associated. The important point is that the symptomatology of advanced stuttering, despite its inconsistencies and variability, is no product of blind chance. Stuttering may be awful but also it is lawful, not chaotic, no matter how bizarre it looks or sounds. It has simply been differentially conditioned.

OTHER COVERT REACTIONS

So far we have dealt only with the stutterer's feelings before the moment of stuttering. This section deals with those that follow it. Different stutterers report different reactions to the experience of fluency breaks and abnormality. Chief among these are the feelings that may be placed somewhere on the continuum of embarrassment-shame-guilt. As the stutterer scans his listener for signs of rejection or distress, he projects his own feelings of stigma onto that listener. His sensors are hyperactive and often pick up and misinterpret the listener's responses. We worked with a hard-bitten gold miner from Alaska once who, when stuttering, watched his listener with an intensity which can hardly be imagined. At the slightest evidence of a smile, no matter how casual or sympathetic or humorous, he punched that listener in the nose. We got to know the city jail very well during his treatment. This man had plenty of hostility but very little embarrassment. Most stutterers, however, are just as super-sensitive to penalty but respond instead with feelings of shame and humiliation. All these reactions vary in intensity with the duration or the abnormality of the stuttering. The wilder and more spasmodic the struggle, the more the embarrassment. Some of the guilt feelings arise, they tell us, because the stutterers have sullied or tortured their listener with their grotesque display; others because they have "imposed upon the listener and taken up valuable time." Doubtless, there are often deeper reasons than these. Whatever their cause, the most common covert reactions that follow the moment of stuttering are embarrassment, shame, and guilt.

There are also brief feelings of relief. They are usually short in duration but they are there. A specific moment of stuttering has run its course and is finished. The obstacle has been overcome. There is a fragment of tension reduction, alas very transitory, a flicker of temporary peace. This may precede the shame or the generation of new fears. That particular feeling of frustration and abnormality has been overpassed and for a brief instant there is momentary relief. We do not feel however that this is a major part of the stutterer's experience.

FRUSTRATION

Our preceding discussion of the role of fear in the stutterer's problem may, by its length, overemphasize its importance. For there is another emotional response to stuttering that constitutes a major factor of the problem. This is frustration. Early in the development of the disorder it is frustration, rather than fear or shame, which dominates the child's reaction to his repetitions, prolongations, and stoppages.

It is very difficult for normal speakers to understand how powerful these feelings of frustration can be. Perhaps a faint inkling might be obtained by recalling the experience of trying to type swiftly when a few of the typewriter keys occasionally stick or will not work. Whenever an automatic sequence of movements is suddenly interrupted before completion, the experience is irritating and unpleasant. The cumulative effect of hundreds of these experiences of being balked and thwarted each day can profoundly affect a person who stutters. Indeed, many of the stutterer's fears are not so much fears of listener rejection as they are fears of being unable to say the word he wants to say when he wants to say it. It is hard to have to live with lips that stick, with a tongue that won't move when you want it to move, with a larynx that will not produce a sound upon command. When "gluency" rather than fluency dominates a person's communication, a life of frustration is his lot.

HOSTILITY

We have already mentioned another common covert reaction to the experience of stuttering—hostility. Hostility results partly from the aggressive feelings that accompany frustration and partly from the stutterer's natural resentment of the rejections and penalties shown by the listener. We hate our punishers. We get angry when we are blocked in carrying out a course of action. Many of our cases have revealed pronounced hostility once they felt it safe to do so. A few of them express their aggression overtly, but most seethe within. Vulnerable as they are to social penalty, they dare not add fuel to the flame of their distress by attacking their listeners—that would only bring on further penalty. Often the aggression is turned inward. Self-derogation, self-hatred often prevails and when it does the stuttering behavior is affected. We have seen stutterers bite themselves and hit their bodies in the throes of their struggle; we have seen them gag with symbolic revulsion. Even suicidal thoughts seem to appear more frequently than in the normal speaker. Profound dejection and depression are often the results of this self-attack.

It may seem that we have exaggerated the stutterer's feelings, that we have used only dark colors to draw the picture. Perhaps the stutterers we have known were the more severe ones. There may be many who consider the disorder only a minor nuisance. If so, they do not come to the speech clinic. Severe stuttering tends to make a person morbid. Once they trust you, most stutterers tell the same tale of fear, frustration, and shame. Here is one final account from one of our cases:

> In my thinking, and when I am alone, I can speak normally; but as soon as I am under threat or challenge, my world, my "facade" of normalcy collapses and leaves me to face the world of reality as a weak and too cowardly being behind a cellophane shell . . . it doesn't take much to trigger me off into my traditional reaction pattern.
>
> What's the matter with me. . . . I can't do anything right (at least to me). I've spent most of my life running away from everything, whether perceivable or not. I have little faith or trust in other people, much less in myself, and I don't feel that I am getting anywhere in the direction of planning and executing true goals and purposes of my life—rather, I survive from day to day, hour by hour, to be tyrannized by the real and imaginary dictates and reactions of others . . . instead of being the man that I want to be. I realize, to some extent, that I am sensitive, weak, and rather cowardly while still having big ambitions . . . , and yet I refuse in a thousand ways to lift myself from my life-sucking bog of self-imposed burden of resistance and resentment, yet my appetite for self-punishment seems to perpetuate itself in an unsatiable way.
>
> I have never—as far back as I can recall—been able, due to external pressures and my own inner conflicts, to really be myself . . . either I've been a "man of a thousand faces" or else an instrument of someone else, whether they have realized it or not. Now, when I want to find myself, I don't even know where or how to look or proceed.

RESEARCH ON COVERT FEATURES OF STUTTERING

Emotional arousal

The research on the emotional responses of stutterers has been mainly concerned with the relationship between fear and stuttering, although some of it focusses on general anxiety, shame, guilt, and hostility. Profound emotional reactions during stuttering were demonstrated long ago by

Robbins (1920) who placed a tambour over the hole in the head of a trephined stutterer and recorded a marked increase in the brain volume during stuttering. This evidence of vascular change also occurred when the subject was startled by a sudden gunshot and other such stimuli. A close correlation was shown between this increase and blood pressure and pulse rate during the period just prior to as well as during the moment of stuttering. Fletcher (1914) anticipated Robbins' study by showing a plethysmographic decrease in the finger blood volume during speaking by stutterers and correctly ascribed this to the fear and attendant emotion. He also found marked increases in pulse rate. Travis, Tuttle, and Cowan (1936) demonstrated that rapid changes in blood pressure occurred during stuttering. Changes in heart rate have been shown by other investigators to accompany stuttering, but, as Ritzman (1934) and Palmer and Gillette (1938) discovered, these do not characteristically appear when stutterers are silent.

Breathing disturbances commonly accompany stuttering and contribute to the distress. Many researchers have called attention to these disruptions. Nadoleczny (1927) pneumographically recorded the breathing of stutterers before and during stuttering and found breath-holding characteristic of the expectancy period. These fixations of the respiratory musculatures were also noted by Travis (1927), Murray (1932), Fossler (1930), Travis (1936), and Van Riper (1936). These authors and others have shown that prolongations of the inspiration and expiration phases of the breathing during both stuttering and its anticipation also occur. Trumper (1928) and Twitmeyer (1930) found shallow breathing in stutterers.

In the early thirties, considerable research focused on incoordinations of respiration. Normally contractions of the thoracic and abdominal musculature are parallel during speech. Fletcher (1914), Henrickson (1936), and Morley (1937), however, found them to be out of phase or in complete antagonism in stuttering. Some horizontal asynchrony in the muscles of the respiration during stuttered speech was found by Travis (1936) and Mosier (1944), but Mosier also found that the same behaviors occurred in normal speakers under communicative stress. Intermittent inhalatory gasps can be heard in most recordings of stuttered speech, and Hill (1944), in his excellent survey of the literature, stresses their importance in supporting his view of stuttering as a contraction pattern of shock, startle, or surprise. We have not found them to occur consistently, however, and much stuttering can occur without them. Furthermore, breathing irregularities take place not only during the moment of stuttering but during its expectancy too. Stutterers complain of being unable to "get the air out"; they speak of "butterflies in their stomachs," a subjective experience that may reflect tremors of the diaphragm. In 1928 Trumper observed such tremors fluoroscopically, and Schilling (1960), using roentgenkymography, found that 16 of 35 stutterers showed clonic fluttering of the diaphragm even during silent breathing.

The subjective experience of breathing irregularities coupled with pronounced vascular changes can be very disturbing to the stutterer. Most of them are doubtless the results of emotionality and struggle. They do not seem to be marked in the very young stutterer. Bloodstein (1961) has shown that they increase with age, and Starbuck and Steer (1953) found that the respiratory irregularities of stutterers decrease with adaptation in repeated readings of the same material. Van Riper (1936) discovered that many of the abnormal respiratory patterns shown during overt stuttering were actually rehearsed during the silent period just before the speech attempt, and he attributed them to stereotyped learned behaviors. Moore (1938) was able to produce in normal speakers many of the same types of breathing anomalies shown in his stutterers by associating a severe electric shock with the utterance of certain words. Hill (1954), using a red light which had been previously conditioned to shock, also found such disintegrations.

Further evidence of the emotions experienced by stutterers comes from research using the galvanic skin response (GSR), electroencephalography (EEG), and electromyography (EMG). Umeda (1960) found significant differences in GSR changes from silent to oral reading in his stutterers but not in his normal speaking controls. Lingwall (1967) found that his adult stutterers had a higher frequency of GSR's just before the signal to speak isolated words than did his normal speakers but was unable to find any significant GSR differences during the actual speech attempts. Kline (1959) found that GSR and reaction times to stimulus words correlated significantly with frequency of stuttering. Taylor (1966) compared stutterers with themselves before and after moments of stuttering, using GSR and pulse rate, but found no significant differences. An interesting study indicating that the anxiety shown by stutterers is associated primarily with speaking was performed by Valyo (1964). He had his subjects alternate speech and silence for one minute periods. In silence, GSR recordings showed no differences between stutterers and normal speakers, but during speech the stutterers' GSR's doubled while the controls showed no change.

Brutten (1963) used the Palmar Sweat Index (PSI), a measure of anxiety, to investigate the covert behavior of stutterers, finding a marked decrease in PSI during repeated readings of the same material (adaptation) and that this decrease was parallel to the decrease in expectancies of disfluency and to the number of disfluencies. He suggested that this was due either to anxiety reduction or to reactive inhibition. The normal speaking controls showed a similar decrease in nonfluencies but not the progressive decrease in palmar sweating. However, Gray and Brutten (1965), in a study of spontaneous recovery after adaptation found no direct relationship between changes in anxiety level as demonstrated by the PSI and changes in the frequency of stuttering. Hollander (1957) had stutterers reread a passage silently until adaptation occurred, then read it aloud. His argument was that if overt stuttering were related to expectancy, and if stutterers adapt in expectancy (and they did), then there should be a decrement in the subsequent overt stuttering. However, this did not occur. Karmen (1964) also used PSI in adaptation reading for 33 stutterers and their controls. There were no differences found either in initial PSI records, in adaptation rates, or in spontaneous recovery. If PSI is an index of general anxiety, not speech anxiety, stutterers seem to have no more of it than normal speakers.

Baron (1949) used an interesting, if oblique, approach to the problem of general anxiety, and found that when stutterers had to speak a given word one-half second after an eyelid conditioning trial, they conditioned much faster than the normal speaking controls. He attributed this facilitation to the speech anxiety felt by the stutterers. Karpf and Wischner (1960), in a similar experiment but using conditioned finger withdrawal, showed that stutterers conditioned faster than normals when speaking was done concurrently. Maxwell (1965) showed that the PSI was greater in an audience situation than when stutterers read to a single listener and that the PSI paralleled rather closely the amount of stuttering exhibited.

Emotion is often reflected in increased muscular tension, and there are many accounts of such tension in stuttering. The widespread use of relaxation methods in stuttering therapy suggests the importance of the stutterer's tension (or the therapists' belief in it). Jacobson (1938) showed long ago that anxiety is reflected in muscle tension, but the research is still sparse concerning tension and stuttering. Shackson (1936) using EMG found evidence of a latent tetany and muscle tremors of 50–60 per second in muscle-thickening records during stuttering. Brown and Shulman (1940) investigated the basal tension of stutterers in silence and found them no more tense than normal speakers under that condition, thus indicating that it could be speech anxiety rather than anxiety *per se* that was reflected in their usual tense struggling during speech. Although they were more concerned with the timing of the paired muscles than with the amount of tension, the EMG studies of both Travis (1934) and Williams (1955) showed evidence of increased tension during stuttering. Sheehan and Voas (1954) compared the masseter tension patterns during stuttering with those during normal speech and found that the tension built up to a peak just prior to the release. Shrum (1967) failed to corroborate the peaking of tension at this point in the stuttering block but he did show that tension was greater and lasted longer during stuttering than in normal fluency. This finding may reflect merely the struggling behavior of the stutterer rather than the tension produced by fear.

Evidence of strong emotion is also evident in the dilation of the pupils. Gardner (1937) and Luchsinger and Arnold (1965) both showed that this dilation occurred during most of the moments of stuttering and was not shown by nonstutterers when speaking. However, Gray and Williams (1969) did not find that widening of the pupils occurred just before the stuttered words were spoken.

Emotional arousal can also be demonstrated by urinary analysis. Edgren, Leanderson, and Levi (1970) had a group of stutterers speak in public and found evidence of extreme stress reactions as reflected by the urinary excretion of adrenaline and catecholamine. Chmelova, Kujalova, Sedlackova, and Zeleny (1975) checked the levels of adrenaline, noradrenaline, and dopamine in the urine of stutterers after rest and after stuttering.

These indications of emotional arousal were normal ai increased after stuttering.

Toomey and Sidman (1970) deliberately tried to creat stutterers by using a buzzer that was terminated by an electi the warning buzzer was set off during oral reading, one stu an increase in stuttering, two showed a decrease and the fou ...ed little change. This, along with other studies, seems to indica ...iat it is speech anxiety rather than general anxiety which is characteristic of the stutterer. There seems to be no doubt, not only from these researches, but also from our clinical impressions and the stutterers' testimony, that strong emotional responses often accompany the stuttering experience.

Situation Fears

Confirmed stutterers not only become anxious and aroused when they know they must begin speaking. They also dread certain speaking situations, usually those similar to ones in which they have experienced frustration or audience penalty in the past. While each individual stutterer shows his own pattern of situation fears based upon his past experience, there are some general commonalities: Speaking while alone is less feared than speaking to an audience; speaking to possibly punitive listeners is more dreaded than to those judged as being more accepting; having to speak in situations demanding specific responses (having to say one's name or address or making introductions) are felt to be more threatening than those which do not; situations requiring swift responses (time pressure) are more feared than those where the urgency is less; and situations involving interpersonal stress (arguing, apologizing, responding to criticism) are feared by many stutterers. We now cite some of the research that deals with these situation fears.

Travis (1928) found only a few individuals who stuttered when speaking to themselves. Other investigators have reported isolated instances of the same kind, but the most comprehensive investigation was done by Radol'skii (1965), who studied 125 stutterers of various ages and found that most preschool stutterers had as much stuttering difficulty talking to themselves as to others, and that only 11 of the older ones showed absolutely no stuttering when alone and speaking with normal tempo. The author of the present text, in his youth, stuttered severely when speaking to himself aloud and alone in the forest, and also recently, to his surprise, when reading a foreign language aloud to himself alone in his study. It was stuttering, not ambivalence or normal nonfluency. It is likely but not certain that in this solo stuttering, an imaginary critical audience exists.

Quinn (1971) found clear evidence that stuttering may occur when no listener is present. Langova and Svab (1973) found a reduction of stuttering when the stutterer was placed in an isolation booth but some stuttering did occur. On the other hand, more stuttering does seem to occur, and therefore more fear may be felt, in situations involving speaking to an audience.

Van Riper and Hull (1955) in a study performed in 1934, found an immediate increase in the frequency of stuttering after adaptation when the situation was changed by reading into a microphone or reading to an audience. Steer and Johnson (1936) replicated the study and reported as follows:

> ... the least stuttering occurred in situations in which there was either a familiar audience (of one person) or no audience at all. The most stuttering occurred in situations in which the audience was unfamiliar, or indefinite (phonograph recording), or relatively large (two to at least eight persons) (p. 36).

Hahn (1940) required his subjects to read a prose selection in different social situations and found that they had more trouble speaking to a seen rather than to an unseen audience, but there were many individual differences. Porter (1939) had stutterers read while alone, with two, four, and eight listeners, and also to listeners evaluated as being hard or easy to talk to. She also found that individual stutterers differed one from another but that in general they stuttered less alone and more with one, two, and four or more listeners. No differences between four and eight listeners were significant. Those listeners evaluated as "hard to speak to" evoked more stuttering. She also mentions that the stutterers expected to stutter more than they really did. Eisenson and Wells (1942) had their stutterers read in unison with the experimenter into "live" and "dead" microphones and found a decreased frequency in the latter situation. Shulman (1945) showed that adaptation to the speaking situation was retarded when the size of the audience was increased. Lerman and Shames (1965) used the Discomfort-Relief Quotients, a presumed measure of anxiety, to evaluate stutterer's responses before entering situations of various difficulty but could find no relationships. Siegel and Haugen (1964) measured the adaptation rates of stuttering in situations of increasing and decreasing complexity. They found that adaptation slowed as the audience increased but that no clear cut reversal occurred when the size of the audience decreased. In this connection, Maddox (1938) found that when stutterers read while observing themselves in a mirror, they had more difficulty than when reading just to the experimenter. The degree of self-confrontation that exists when speaking alone may determine the degree of stuttering in this condition.

Some listeners are more punitive or potentially punitive than others. Berwick (1955) found that when stutterers read to photographs of listeners they had previously judged as punitive, an immediate increase in stuttering resulted after a series of adaptation readings to the experimenter. Less stuttering occurred than when reading to photographs of nonpunitive listeners. It is probable that some stutterers may be highly punitive listeners to their own stuttering. Sheehan, Hadley, and Gould (1967) had stutterers repeatedly read matched passages to their peers and to authority figures. The authority listeners produced more stuttering and a slower adaptation than the peers.

Since communication always involves the dimension of time, it seems evident that those speaking situations in which time pressure is strong will be more feared than those in which it is not, Sheehan (1958) says:

> It is suggested that time pressure is a basic variable in stuttering, that it is through time pressure that the effect of interpersonal relations in stuttering is mediated. It is also through time pressure that anxiety and guilt and conflicts of all kinds come to play a part. When a stutterer feels in a subordinate or inferior role, or when speaking to an authority figure, he is likely to feel that he isn't really worthy of taking the other person's time (p. 143).

Stunden (1965) has demonstrated that stutterers were more vulnerable to time pressure than their controls. Forte and Schlesinger (1972) found that when time pressure was decreased by introducing a delay before being called upon to read, stuttering also decreased as the result of the postponement.

Scales of situational difficulty. Several attempts have been made to devise a standard rating scale of situational difficulty. One of the first of these was the *Speech Situation Rating Sheet for Stutterers* (Johnson, Darley, and Spriesterbach, 1963) wherein stutterers were to indicate which of 40 speaking situations they tended to avoid most or enjoy speaking in them the least. Shumak (1955) tried to validate and determine the reliability of this instrument but was unsuccessful. Trotter and Bergman (1957) used this Speech Situation Rating Sheet with 50 stutterers and 100 normal speaking controls finding that the two groups generally agreed on which situations were more difficult. One exception was telephoning. Renfrew (1952), using a similar list of speaking situations found great variability in situation fears from one stutterer to another but there was considerable consistency for each individual stutterer. Woolf (1967) devised the *PSI* (*Perceptions of Stuttering Inventory*), a questionnaire listing sixty items, many of which dealt with avoidance or postponement, thus indicating situation fears. The stutterer was to check the items "characteristic of me." More recently, Brutten (1973, 1975) reports the use of a *Speech Situation Check List* which contains a list of 54 speech situations and requires the stutterer to rank them in terms of emotional responses and history of fluency failures. Brutten and Janssen (1980) administered this checklist to separate groups of American and Dutch stutterers and found that the responses of two groups clustered in very similar ways. The stutterers showed agreement in their self reports of situational difficulty and fear. Again we find that speaking before an audience, making introductions, having to give specific information, and situations involving interpersonal conflict seemed to provoke more arousal of negative emotion, while talking with a friend or a young child, or speaking under the influence of alcohol did not.

Word Fears

Most of the research deals with word fears rather than phonemic fears although the stutterer has both types. (The latter will be summarized in our chapter on Loci.) The studies we report here seek to answer two questions: Is there evidence of emotional arousal just prior to the utterance of a stuttered word? Does it always occur?

In a respiratory study of stutterers' attempts on single words, Van Riper (1936) found evidences of rehearsal behavior during the period between word exposure and signal to speak. He also found a high inspiration-expiration ratio, a measure which is related to fear. He found further that although there is generally a high correspondence between the expectancy and the occurrence of stuttering, either can occur without the other. Johnson and Sinn (1937) had their stutterers do some adaptation reading, but after the first reading, they omitted all the words on which stuttering was expected. This procedure eliminated 98 per cent of the stutterings. Expectation occurred most generally on words previously stuttered. Milisen (1938), using both contextual and single words, found that in the sequential material (contextual) only 75 per cent of the stutterings were anticipated, as compared with 85 per cent for the single words. Of the words on which the stutterers signalled their prediction of stuttering, 61 per cent were stuttered in the contextual material as compared with 51 per cent for the single words. He concluded that stutterers were not able to anticipate all moments of stuttering.

Knott, Johnson, and Webster (1937) had their stutterers signal differently for certainty of stuttering, doubtful possibility, and certainty of fluency. They found a definite relationship between the degree of expectancy and stuttering. Eighty-eight per cent of anticipated (certain plus doubtful) words were stuttered and only 0.4 per cent of words for which fluency was expected showed stuttering. Sophisticated stutterers predicted less accurately than naive ones.

Johnson and Ainsworth (1938) had stutterers read silently, signalling expectancy or nonexpectancy on each word of a reading passage, and then do the same task again after two weeks. They found that the loci of expectancy on the second reading were generally the same and could not be accounted for by chance. Johnson and Solomon (1937) had stutterers mark copies of a reading passage to indicate words on which stuttering might occur. They found that stuttering occurred on 53 per cent of the words on which it had been anticipated and on only 10 per cent of those on which it had not. In an effort to account for the discrepancies between expectancy and occurrence of stuttering, Johnson and Solomon in the same study had 13 stutterers underline expected stutterings on different reading passages which were read immediately, then again after 15 minutes, after 15 more minutes, and after a one day interval. The percentage of anticipated and unanticipated stutterings remained much the same for all readings. Their conclusion that expectancy may operate at a low degree of consciousness seems forced from these data, but the article has been widely quoted. So also has the investigation by Johnson and Sinn (1937), who had their subjects reread a passage, speaking only the words on which no anticipation was present. They found that most of the unexpected stutterings occurred on words which had been stuttered in the previous reading. Milisen (1938) found that only three per cent of his stutterers were able to predict *all* of their stutterings and that the median stutterer could only predict 61 per cent, even when they were strongly shocked for failure to predict with accuracy.

Van Riper and Milisen (1939) showed that stutterers could predict with some accuracy the *duration* of their anticipated stutterings. Wischner (1952) showed that when stutterers *silently* read the same passage repeatedly and signalled expectancies of stuttering, a progressive decrease in the frequency of expectations occurred which appeared parallel to the adaptation effect usually shown by stutterers while speaking. Peins (1961) failed to corroborate the adaptation of expectancy, which had been reported by several other investigators. Martin and Haroldson (1967) had stutterers read a passage five times, rating each word on a five step expectancy scale. They found that words assigned a high expectancy value tended to be stuttered more consistently than those assigned a low expectancy. They state, however, that their data did not entirely support the frequently expressed view that in most instances stutterers can predict the occurrence of their blockings. In more than half of the instances where a word was assigned the highest expectancy value, no stuttering occurred. Lingwall (1967) reported that his GSR recordings, which are viewed by many as an indication of momentary fear or anxiety, showed no apparent relationship to given words or the ensuing stuttering on those words.

Silverman and Williams (1972) studied the ability of child stutterers to predict stutterings and found that only one child could accurately predict all stuttered words. Most of their subjects were able to predict only about half of them. McClean and Cooper (1978), exposing single words on a screen and requiring a yes-no judgment of expectancy prior to speaking found that when their subjects expected to stutter, they did so in 76 per cent of their utterances, and when they signalled they did not expect to stutter, they did not on 88 per cent of those words. Wingate (1975) found the concurrence of expectancy and stuttering to be very low as well as very variable from stutterer to stutterer. His critique of expectancy studies makes clear that there is no one-to-one relationship between word fear and stuttering.

We have some research which attempted to determine whether or not physiological evidence of emotional arousal occurs just prior to stuttering. Gautheron, Liorzou, Even, and Vallencien (1973) and Bar, Singer, and Feldman (1969) found increased subvocal laryngeal activity at this time but Shrum (1967) and McClean and Cooper (1978) did not. Peters, Love, Otto, Wood, and Bengnus (1976) showed altered EEG's on feared words. Ickes and Pierce (1973) found a decreased peripheral blood volume as stutterers approached words on which they stuttered.

Finally, there have been attempts to show that stutterers scan approaching speech for words that may cause them difficulty. Most researchers have studied the eye movements of stutterers during reading. Murray (1932) and Moser (1938) found stutterers had more fixations and regressive movements during silent reading than did their nonstutterers. Roland (1972) did not corroborate their findings but the subjects of Brutten and Janssen (1979) demonstrated longer average durations of eye fixations on those words which they had underlined as expecting to stutter. They concluded that stutterers search among the words to be spoken and sort out those on which they anticipate and do have difficulty. Certainly stutterers tell us that they scan approaching utterances for feared sounds and words.

This review makes clear that the correlation between word fear or stuttering expectancy and the actual occurrence of stuttering is far from being perfect. Other factors besides word fear must play a part in its precipitation, although word fear may still have some significant effects. Any theory of stuttering which holds that anticipatory struggle comprises its essence must contend with these findings. The proponents of this view (Johnson, 1955; Bloodstein, 1960) have placed strong emphasis on marginal consciousness of approaching stuttering and upon a subliminal awareness of difficulty, to explain the exceptions. The evidence for this view is not too convincing.

Frustration, Hostility, and Guilt

Although there are many clinical descriptions of the stutterer's emotions other than fear and anxiety, the research is meager. Some of it deals with frustration. Burstscher (1952) surveyed the information available at that time and concluded that a low tolerance for frustration accounted for much of the secondary characteristics of stuttering. Murphy (1952) also found that stutterers were significantly less resistant to frustration than their controls in a listening task involving competing messages. He also found differences between stutterers and nonstutterers on the Rosenzweig Picture Frustration Test. Quarrington (1953), however, replicated Murphy's investigation and found no differences. Madison and Norman (1952) found significant differences between their subjects and controls on the Rosenzweig, the stutterers being more "intropunitive" and less "extropunitive" and having lower "obstacle dominance" scores. However, no significant differences, using the same test, were found by four other investigators: Hirsch (1950), Lowinger (1952), Seaman (1956), and Emerick (1966). Emerick makes the point that this test may be unsuitable for measuring the kind of frustration stutterers experience.

Closely related to frustration are aggression and hostility. Krugman (1946) found pronounced aggression in his Rorschachs on stutterers. Santostephano (1960) found that stutterers obtained significantly higher hostility scores than nonstutterers on the Rorschach Content Test. This investigator also created a laboratory stress situation designed to evoke hostility and found that the stutterers showed significantly more hostility than the controls. Feldstein and Jaffe (1962) used anger-producing interviews with normal speakers and found no significant increase in "ah" and "non-ah" speech disruptions when this emotion was produced. Perkins and Haugen (1965) permitted open aggressive responses for half of a group of stutterers and prevented them for the other half. They found that open aggression produced less stuttering and less anger. Adams and Dietze (1965) found significant difference in stutterers' and nonstutterers' reaction times to words connoting aggression, depression, and guilt, the stutterers responding more slowly. Sheehan, Cortese, and Had using projective drawings, concluded that guilt feelings occurred during, and subsequent to the moment of stuttering, and were prevalent during the subsequent period.

BIBLIOGRAPHY

ADAMS, M. R. AND D. A. DIETZE. 1965. A comparison of the reaction times of stutterers and nonstutterers to items on a word association test. *Journal of Speech and Hearing Research* 8: 195–202.

AINSWORTH, S. E. 1939. Studies in the psychology of stuttering: empathic breathing of auditors while listening to stuttered speech. *Journal of Speech Disorders* 4: 149–156.

BAR, A., J. SINGER, AND R. G. FELDMAN. 1969. Subvocal muscle activity during stuttering and fluent speech. *Journal of South African Logopedic Society* 16: 9–14.

BARDRICK, R. A. AND J. G. SHEEHAN. 1956. Emotional loadings as a source of conflict in stuttering. *American Psychologist* 11: 391'(abstract).

BARON, M. 1949. The effect on eyelid conditioning of a speech variable in stutterers and nonstutterers. Doctoral dissertation, State University of Iowa.

BERLINSKY, S. L. 1954. A comparison of stutterers and nonstutterers in four conditions of experimentally induced anxiety. *Dissertation Abstracts* 14: 719 (abstract).

BERWICK, N. H. 1955. Stuttering in response to photographs of certain selected listeners. In *Stuttering in Children and Adults,* ed. W. Johnson. Minneapolis: University of Minnesota Press.

BLOODSTEIN, O. 1961. Development of stuttering. *Journal of Speech and Hearing Disorders* 26: 67–82.

BLUEMEL, C. S. 1957. *The riddle of stuttering*. Danville, Ill.: Interstate.

BOOME, E. J. AND M. A. RICHARDSON. 1932. *The nature and treatment of stuttering.* New York: Dutton.

BROWN, S. F. 1938. Stuttering with relation to word accent and word position. *Journal of Abnormal and Social Psychology* 33: 112–20.

BRUTTEN, E. J. 1963. Palmar sweat investigation of disfluency and expectancy adaptation. *Journal of Speech and Hearing Research* 6: 40–48.

——. 1973. Behavior assessment and the strategy of therapy. In *Neurolinguistic Approaches to Stuttering*, eds. Y. Le Brun and R. Hoops. The Hague: Mouton.

——. 1975. Stuttering topography, assessment and behavior change strategies. In *Stuttering: A Second Symposium*, ed. J. Eisenson. New York: Harper and Row.

—— AND P. JANSSEN. 1979. An eye marking investigation of anticipated and observed stuttering. *Journal of Speech and Hearing Research* 22: 20–28.

——. 1980. A normative and factor analysis study of the responses of Dutch and American stutterers to the speech situations check list. *Proceedings XVIII[e] International Congress Logopedics and Phoniatrics*, Washington.

BURTSCHER, H. T. 1952. The operation of frustration in the transition to and the development of secondary stuttering. *Speech Monograph* 19: 191.

CHMELOVA, A., V. KUJALOVA, E. SEDLACKOVA, AND A. ZELANY. 1975. Neurohumoral reaction in stutterers and stammerers. *Folia Phoniatrica* 27: 183–86.

ert Reactions

Stottern: *Eine Psychose* Leipsig.

me adjustment of stutterers versus nonstutterers. *Journal isorders* 14: 155–59.

N, AND L. LEVI. 1970. A research program on stuttering ngologie Supplement No. 263: 113–18.

LS. 1942. A study of the influences of communicative al speech situation for stutterers. *Journal of Speech Disorders*

EMERICK, L. 1963. A clinical observation on the "final" stuttering. *Journal of Speech and Hearing Disorders* 28: 194–95.

——. 1960. Social distance scale for stutterers. *Journal of Speech and Hearing Disorders* 25: 408–9.

ENDICOTT, J. 1957. An exploratory study of the relationship between recognition time of stuttered and nonstuttered words. Masters thesis, Ohio University.

FELDSTEIN, S. AND J. JAFFE. 1962. The relationship of speech disruption to the experience of anger. *Journal of Consulting Psychology* 26: 505–9.

FLETCHER, J. M. 1914. An experimental study of stuttering. *American Journal of Psychology* 25: 201–55.

FORTE, M. AND I. M. SCHLESINGER. 1972. Stuttering as a function of time of expectation. *Journal of Communication Disorders* 5: 347–58.

FOSSLER, H. R. 1930. Disturbances in breathing during stuttering. *Psychological Monographs* 40: 1–32.

FROESCHELS, E. 1961. New viewpoints on stuttering. *Folia Phoniatrica* 13: 187–201.

GARDNER, W. H. 1937. The study of the pupillary reflex with special reference to stuttering. *Psychological Monographs* 49: 1–31.

GAUTHERON, G., A. LIORZAN, AND B. VALLANCIEN. 1973. The role of the larynx in stuttering. In *Neurolinguistic Approaches to Stuttering*, eds. Y. Le Brun and R. Hoops. The Hague: Mouton.

GRAY, B. B. 1964. The relationship between anxiety level, fatigue, and stuttering adaptation. *ASHA* 6: 416 (abstract).

—— AND E. J. BRUTTEN, 1965. The relationship between anxiety, fatigue, and spontaneous recovery in stuttering. *Behavior Research and Therapy* 2: 251–59.

GRAY, K. C. AND D. E. WILLIAMS. 1969. Anticipation and stuttering: a pupilographic study. *Journal of Speech and Hearing Research* 12: 833–39.

HENRICKSON, E. H. 1936. Simultaneously recorded breathing and vocal disturbances of stutterers. *Archives of Speech* 1: 133–49.

HERREN, R. Y. 1931. The effect of stuttering on voluntary movement. *Journal of Experimental Psychology* 14: 289–98.

HILL, H. 1954. An experimental study of disorganization of speech and manual responses in normal subjects. *Journal of Speech and Hearing Disorders* 19: 295–305.

——. 1945. An interbehavioral analysis of several aspects of stuttering. *Journal of General Psychology* 32: 289–316.

——. 1954. An experimental study of disorganization of speech and manual responses in normal subjects. *Journal of Speech and Hearing Disorders* 19: 295–305.

——. 1944. Stuttering: II. A review and integration of physiological data. *Journal of Speech Disorders* 9: 289–324.

HIRSCH, B. 1950. A study of the responses of stutterers and nonstutterers to two kinds of personality tests. Masters thesis, Fordham University.

HOLLANDER, H. 1957. An investigation of the effects of silent adaptation to expectancy of stuttering on stuttering behavior. Masters thesis, University of Pittsburgh.

ICKES, W. K. AND S. PIERCE. 1973. The stuttering moment: a plethysmographic study. *Journal of Communication Disorders* 6: 155–64.

JACOBSON, E. 1938. *Progressive relaxation.* Chicago: University of Chicago Press.

JANSSEN, P. AND F. KRAAIMANT. 1977. The relation between stuttering and state anxiety. *Proceedings XVII International Congress of Logopedics and Phoniatrics,* Copenhagen.

JOHNSON, W. (ed.). 1955. *Stuttering in children and adults.* Minneapolis: University of Minnesota Press.

———, F. L. DARLEY, AND D. C. SPRIESTERSBACH. 1963. *Diagnostic methods in speech pathology.* New York: Harper and Row.

——— AND S. AINSWORTH. 1938. Studies in the psychology of stuttering: X, Constancy of loci of expectancy of stuttering. *Journal of Speech Disorders* 3: 101–4.

——— AND S. F. BROWN. 1935. Stuttering in relation to various speech sounds. *Quarterly Journal of Speech* 21: 481–96.

——— AND J. R. KNOTT. 1937. Certain objective cues related to the precipitation of the moment of stuttering. *Journal of Speech Disorders* 2: 17–19.

———, R. P. LARSON, AND J. R. KNOTT. 1937. Studies in the psychology of stuttering: III, Certain objective cues related to the precipitation of the moment of stuttering. *Journal of Speech Disorders* 2: 105–9.

——— AND L. S. MILLSAPPS. 1937. Studies in the psychology of stuttering: VI, The role of cues representative of past moments during oral reading. *Journal of Speech Disorders* 2: 101–4.

——— AND A. SINN. 1937. Studies in the psychology of stuttering: 5, Frequency of stuttering with expectation of stuttering controlled. *Journal of Speech Disorders* 2: 98–100.

——— AND A. SOLOMON. 1937. Studies in the psychology of stuttering: 4, A quantitative study of expectation of stuttering as a process involving a low degree of consciousness. *Journal of Speech Disorders* 2: 95–97.

KARMEN, J. L. 1964. A comparison between generalized anxiety adjustment and adaptation of stuttering behavior. Doctoral dissertation, University of Arizona.

KARPF, B. V. AND G. J. WISCHNER. 1960. An investigation of the effect of speech anxiety (drive) upon the conditioning of a finger withdrawal response. *ASHA,* 2: 367 (abstract).

KAZIN, A. 1951. *A walker in the street.* New York: Harcourt.

KLINE. D. F. 1959. An experimental study of the frequency of stuttering in relation to certain goal-activity drives in basic human behavior. *Speech Monographs* 26: 137 (abstract).

KNOTT, J. R., R. E. CORRELL AND J. N. SHEPHERD. 1959. Frequency analysis of electroencephalograms of stutterers and nonstutterers. *Journal of Speech and Hearing Research* 2: 74–80.

———, W. JOHNSON, AND M. WEBSTER. 1937. Studies in the psychology of stuttering: I, A quantitative evaluation of expectation of stuttering in relation to the occurrence of stuttering. *Journal of Speech Disorders* 2: 20–22.

KRUGMAN, M. 1946. Psychosomatic study of fifty stuttering children. *Journal of Orthopsychiatry* 16: 127–33.

LANGOVA, J. AND L. SVAB. 1973. Reduction of stuttering under experimental social isolation. *Folia Phoniatrica* 25: 17–22.

LERMAN, J. W. AND G. H. SHAMES. 1965. The effect of situational difficulty on stuttering. *Journal of Speech and Hearing Research* 8: 271–80.

LEUTENEGGER, R. R. 1957. Adaptation and recovery in the oral reading of stutterers. *Journal of Speech Disorders* 22: 276–87.

LINGWALL, J. B. 1967. Galvanic skin responses of stutterers and nonstutterers to isolated word stimuli. Convention address, ASHA.

LOWINGER, L. 1952. The psychodynamics of stuttering: an evaluation of the factors of aggression and guilt feelings in a group of institutionalized children. *Dissertation Abstracts* 12: 725 (abstract).

LUCHSINGER, R. AND G. E. ARNOLD. 1965. *Voice—speech—language.* Belmont, Cal.: Wadsworth.

MADDOX, J. S. 1938. Studies in the psychology of stuttering: VIII, The role of visual cues in the precipitation of moments of stuttering. *Journal of Speech Disorders* 3: 90–94.

MADISON, L. AND R. A. NORMAN. 1952. Comparison of the performance of stutterers and nonstutterers on the Rosenzweig picture frustration test. *Journal of Clinical Psychology* 8: 179–83.

MARTIN, R. R. AND S. K. HAROLDSON. 1967. The relationship between anticipation and consistency of stuttered words. *Journal of Speech and Hearing Research* 10: 323–27.

MATHUR, M. L. 1960. *Causes and cure of stammering.* Jodhpur, India: Navyng.

MAXWELL, D. L. 1965. A Palmar-sweat investigation of stuttering adaptation under two levels of audience complexity. Masters thesis, Southern Illinois University.

—— AND E. J. BRUTTEN. 1964. A Palmar-sweat investigation of stuttering adaptation and spontaneous recovery under two levels of audience complexity. *ASHA* 6: 416–17 (abstract).

McCLEAN, A. E. AND E. B. COOPER. 1978. Electromyographic indications of laryngeal area activity during stuttering expectancy. *Journal of Fluency Disorders* 3: 205–19.

McDONALD, E. AND J. FRICK. 1954. Store clerks' reactions to stuttering. *Journal of Speech and Hearing Disorders* 29: 306–11.

MILISEN, R. 1938. Frequency of stuttering with anticipation of stuttering controlled. *Journal of Speech Disorders* 3: 207–14.

MINUTE PHILOSOPHER. 1859. The irrationale of speech. *Fraser's Magazine,* July, 1859, pp. 1–14.

MOORE, W. E. 1938. A conditioned reflex study of stuttering. *Journal of Speech Disorders* 3: 163–83.

MORLEY, A. 1937. An analysis of associative and predisposing factors in the symptomatology of stuttering. *Psychological Monographs* 49: 50–107.

MOSER, H. M. 1938. A qualitative analysis of eye-movements during stuttering. *Journal of Speech Disorders* 3: 131–39.

MOSIER, K. V. 1944. A study of the horizontal disintegration of breathing during normal and abnormal speech for normal speakers and stutterers. Masters thesis, University of Indiana.

MURPHY, A. T. 1952. An electroencephalographic study of frustration in stutterers. Doctoral dissertation, University of Southern California.

MURRAY, E. 1932. Disintegration of breathing and eye movements in stutterers during silent reading and reasoning. *Psychological Monographs* 43: 218–275.

NADOLECZNY, M. 1927. Stuttering as a manifestation of a spastic coordination neurosis. *Archives of Psychiatry* 82: 235–46.

NEELLEY, J. N. AND R. J. TIMMONS. 1967. Adaptation and consistency in the disfluent speech behavior of young stutterers and nonstutterers. *Journal of Speech and Hearing Research* 10: 250–56.

NEWMAN, P. W. 1963. Adaptation performances of individual stutterers: implications for research. *Journal of Speech and Hearing Research* 6: 393–94.

————. 1954. A study of adaptation and recovery of the stuttering response in self formulated speech. *Journal of Speech and Hearing Disorders* 19: 312–21.

OXTOBY, E. T. 1946. A quantitative study of certain phenomena related to expectancy of stuttering. Doctoral dissertation, University of Iowa.

PALMER, M. AND A. M. GILLETTE. 1938. Sex differences in the cardiac rhythms of stutterers. *Journal of Speech Disorders* 3: 3–12.

PATTIE, F. A. AND B. B. KNIGHT. 1944. Why does the speech of stutterers improve in chorus reading. *Journal of Abnormal and Social Psychology* 39: 362–67.

PEINS, M. 1961. Consistency effect in stuttering expectancy. *Journal of Speech and Hearing Research* 4: 397–98.

PERKINS, W. H. AND C. HAUGEN. 1965. The relationship between frequency of stuttering and open expression of aggression. Convention address, ASHA., 1965.

PERRIN, E. H. 1954. Social position of the speech defective child. *Journal of Speech and Hearing Disorders* 19: 250–52.

PETERS, R. W., L. LOVE, D. OTTO, T. WOOD, AND V. BENINGUS. 1976. Cerebral processing of speech and non-speech signals by stutterers. *Proceedings International XVI Congress of Logopedics and Phoniatrics*. Basel: Karger.

PORTER, H. K. 1939. Studies in the psychology of stuttering: XIV, stuttering phenomena in relation to size and personnel of audience. *Journal of Speech Disorders* 4: 323–33.

PUROHIT, S. N. 1947. Why stammerers suffer. *Journal of Speech Disorders* 12: 419–20.

QUARRINGTON, B. 1953. The performance of stutterers on the Rosenzweig picture frustration test. *Journal of Clinical Psychology* 9: 189–92.

QUINN, P. T. 1971. Stuttering: some observations on speaking when alone. *Journal Australian College of Speech Therapists* 21: 92–94.

RAZDOL'SKII, V. A. 1965. On the speech of stutterers when alone. *Zhurnal Nevropatologii i Psikhiatrii* 65: 1717–20.

RENFREW, C. B. 1952. A questionnaire for stutterers. *Speech* (London) 16: 21–24.

RITZMAN, C. E. 1943. A comparative cardiovascular and metabolic study of stutterers and nonstutterers. *Journal of Speech Disorders* 8: 161–82.

ROBBINS, S. D. 1920. Comparative shock and stammering. *American Journal of Physiology* 52: 168–81.

————. 1936. Relative attention paid to vowels and consonants by stammerers and normal speakers. *Proceedings of the American Association for the Study of Disorders of Speech* 6: 7–23.

ROLAND, B. C. 1972. Eye movements of stutterers and nonstutterers during silent, oral and choral reading. *Perceptual and Motor Skills* 35: 297–98.

ROSENBERG, S. AND J. CURTIS. 1954. The effect of stuttering on the behavior of the listener. *Journal of Abnormal and Social Psychology* 49: 355–61.

SANTOSTEFANO, S. 1960. Anxiety and hostility in stuttering. *Journal of Speech and Hearing Research* 3: 337–47.

SCHILLING, A. 1960. Roentgen-Zwerchfell-Kymogramme bei Stottern. *Folia Phoniatrica* 12: 145–53.

SCHLESINGER, I. M., M. FORTE, B. FRIED, AND R. MELKMAN. 1965. Stuttering, information load, and response strength. *Journal of Speech and Hearing Disorders* 30: 32–36.

SCHLESINGER, I. M., R. MELKMAN, AND R. LEVY. 1966. Word length and frequency as determinants of stuttering. *Psychonomic Science* 6: 255–56.

SCRIPTURE, E. W. 1923. *Stuttering, lisping, and correction of the speech of the deaf.* New York: Macmillan.

SEAMAN, R. 1956. A study of the responses of stutterers to the items of the Rosenzweig picture frustration study. Masters thesis, Brooklyn College.

SHACKSON, R. 1936. An action current study of muscle contraction latency with special reference to latent tetany in stutterers. *Archives of Speech* 1: 87–111.

SHEEHAN, J. G. 1958. Conflict theory of stuttering. In *Stuttering: A Symposium*, ed. J. Eisenson. New York: Harper.

———. 1951. The modification of stuttering through nonreinforcement. *Journal of Abnormal and Social Psychology* 46: 51–63.

———, R. CORTESE, AND R. HADLEY. 1962. Guilt, shame, and tension in graphic projections of stuttering. *Journal of Speech and Hearing Disorders* 37: 129–39.

———, R. G. HADLEY AND E. GOULD. 1967. Impact of authority on stuttering. *Journal of Abnormal Psychology* 62: 290–93.

——— AND R. B. VOAS. 1954. Tension patterns during stuttering in relation to conflict, anxiety, and reinforcement. *Speech Monographs* 21: 272–79.

SHRUM, W. A. 1967. A study of speaking behavior of stutterers and nonstutterers by means of multichannel electromyography. Doctoral dissertation, University of Iowa.

SHULMAN, E. A. 1945. A study of certain factors influencing variability of stuttering. Doctoral dissertation, State University of Iowa.

SHUMAK, I. C. 1955. A speech situation rating sheet for stutterers. In *Stuttering in Children and Adults*, eds., W. Johnson and R. R. Leutenneger. Minneapolis: University of Minnesota Press.

SIEGEL, G. M. AND D. HAUGEN. 1964. Audience size and variations in stuttering behavior. *Journal of Speech and Hearing Research* 7: 383–88.

SILVERMAN, F. H. AND D. E. WILLIAMS. 1972. Prediction of stuttering by school-age children. *Journal of Speech and Hearing Research* 15: 189–93.

STARBUCK, H. AND M. D. STEER. 1953. The adaptation effect in stuttering speech behavior and normal speech. *Journal of Speech and Hearing Disorders* 18: 252–55.

STEER, M. D. AND W. JOHNSON. 1936. An objective study of the relationship between psychological factors and the severity of stuttering. *Journal of Abnormal and Social Psychology* 31: 36–46.

STUNDEN, A. A. 1965. The effects of stuttering as a time variable in the verbal behavior of stutterers. *Dissertation Abstracts* 26: 1784–85.

SVAB, L., J. GROSS AND J. LANGOVA. 1972. Stuttering and social isolation. *Journal of Nervous and Mental Diseases* 155: 1–5.

TAYLOR, J. A. 1951. The relationship of anxiety to the conditioned eyelid response. *Journal of Experimental Psychology* 41: 81–92.

TOOMEY, T. W. AND M. SIDMAN. 1970. An experimental analogue of the anxiety-stuttering relationship. *Journal of Speech and Hearing Research* 13: 122–29.

TRAVIS, L. E. 1934. Dissociation of the homologous muscle function in stuttering. *Archives of Neurology and Psychiatry* 30: 127–33.

———. 1928. The influence of the group upon the stutterer's speech in free association. *Journal of Abnormal and Social Psychology* 23: 45–51.

———. 1927. Disintegration of breathing movements during stuttering. *Archives of Neurology and Psychiatry* 18: 673–90.

———. 1957. The unspeakable feelings of people with special reference to stuttering. In *Handbook of Speech Pathology*, ed. L. E. Travis. Englewood Cliffs, N.J.: Prentice-Hall.

TRAVIS, L. E., W. W. TUTTLE, AND D. W. COWAN. 1936. A study of heart rate during stuttering. *Journal of Speech Disorders* 1: 21–26.

TRAVIS, V. 1936. A study of the horizontal disintegration of breathing during stuttering. *Archives of Speech* 1: 157–70.

TROTTER, W. D. AND M. F. BERGMANN. 1957. Stutterers' and nonstutterers' reactions to speech situations. *Journal of Speech and Hearing Disorders* 22: 40–45.

TRUMPER, M. 1928. A hematorespiratory study of 101 consecutive cases of stammering. Doctoral dissertation, University of Pennsylvania.

TUPPER, M. 1861. The stammerer's complaint. In J. Hunt, *Stammering and stuttering*. 1861. Reprinted, New York: Hafner, 1967, p. 3.

TWITMEYER, E. B. 1930. Stammering in relation to hemorespiratory factors. *Quarterly Journal of Speech* 16: 278–83.

UMEDA, K. 1960. The psychophysiological study upon stutterers. *Otology Fukuoka* 6: 377–91.

VALYO, R. A. 1971. Skin potential responses of stutterers and nonstutterers during speech and silence. *Dissertation Abstracts* 32: 1904–B.

VAN RIPER, C. 1963. *Speech correction: principles and methods*, 4th ed. Englewood Cliffs, N.J.: Prentice-Hall.

———. 1937. The influence of empathic response on frequency of stuttering. *Psychologic Monographs* 49: 244–46.

———. 1936. Study of the thoracic breathing of stutterers during expectancy and occurrence of stuttering spasms. *Journal of Speech Disorders* 1: 61–72.

——— AND C. J. HULL. 1955. The quantitative measurement of the effect of certain situations on stuttering. In *Stuttering in Children and Adults*, ed. W. Johnson. Minneapolis: University of Minnesota Press.

VAN RIPER, C. AND R. L. MILISEN. 1939. A study of the predicted duration of the stutterer's blocks as related to their actual duration. *Journal of Speech Disorders* 4: 339–45.

WELLS, P. B. AND M. T. MALCOLM. 1971. Controlled trial of treatment of 36 stutterers. *British Journal of Psychiatry* 119: 603–4.

WILLIAMS, D. E. 1955. Masseter muscle action current potentials in stuttered and nonstuttered speech. *Journal of Speech and Hearing Disorders* 20: 242–61.

WINGATE, M. E. 1975. Expectancy: basically a short term process. *Journal of Speech and Hearing Research* 18: 31–42.

———. 1976. *Stuttering: theory and therapy*. New York: Irvington.

WISCHNER, G. J. 1952. Anxiety reduction as reinforcement in maladaptive behavior: evidence in stutterers' representations of the moment of difficulty. *Journal Abnormal and Social Psychology* 47: 566–71.

WOOLF, G. 1967. The assessment of stuttering as struggle, avoidance and expectancy. *British Journal Disorders of Communication* 2: 158–71.

YOUNG, M. 1955. Audience size, perceived situational difficulty, and stuttering frequency. *Journal of Speech and Hearing Research* 8: 401–7.

THE LOCI OF STUTTERING AND THE ADAPTATION EFFECT

8

One of tne pieces of the jigsaw puzzle of stuttering that must be fitted into our overall understanding of the problem might be found in its loci—in the particular sounds or words on which stuttering behaviors occur. From the viewpoints of the listener, and the stutterer himself, stuttering occurs intermittently. No one seems to stutter on every word.* By locating the loci of the overt stutterings that do appear in the stream of speech we might be able to understand the disorder a bit better.

Most of the huge amount of research on loci has attempted to determine the special features and placement of stuttered words, syllables, and sounds. Usually, a fairly large sample or corpus of speech is procured, and then the molar moments of stuttering have been identified, and their locations analyzed. Many of the studies have used the oral reading of standard passages contrived to include all speech sounds but in some instances the corpus is composed of spontaneous or propositional speech but the speaking situation is not varied.

In the interest of clarity of exposition we shall postpone a detailed account of the many researches on the loci of stuttering and include it at the end of this section. Here we present two contrasting studies which seek to give us the answer to the question: How consistently do stutterers stutter on the same words?

The first of these researches is by Hendel and Bloodstein (1973) who had stutterers read the same passage twice, finding that, on the average, 48 per cent of a stutterer's stuttered words on one reading were also stuttered upon in the other reading. This was said to represent the *consistency* of the stutterings.

* We must be careful here because some research has shown that the apparent fluency which the stutterers show may not be like that of the fluency of nonstutterers. See Chapter 16.

In contrast, only 18 per cent of the same words were stuttered upon *by any one* of the sixteen other stutterers who read the passage. The *congruity* therefore was much lower than the consistency. This seems to indicate that the loci of stuttering must depend on something other than the features of the stuttered words themselves. Apparently, it is only for the individual stutterer that certain words are harder to say, and this may be because he has learned to fear them, a position held by Wendell Johnson and Oliver Bloodstein.

The basic position of these two authors (and many others) is that certain individuals develop fears of saying certain words because they have learned to associate disfluency with certain features of those words. Having stuttered on a word, that word is remembered and feared, and the fear provokes the struggling characteristics that identify the speaker as a stutterer. However, we must be cautious in accepting this position, first because, as we saw in our last chapter, the stutterer's ability to predict the words on which he stutters is not very great, nor is the consistency of stuttered words very high even in the individual stutterer when rereading the same passage in the same situation. Learned fears may explain a portion of the loci but not all.

Repeated *readings* of the same material in the same situation may inflate any measure of consistency. Our second research by Hamre and Wingate (1973) used instead a sentence construction task that approximated self-formulated, spontaneous speech and they found much lower consistency scores than did Hendel and Bloodstein or other authors who have used reading passages. Only 36 per cent of the stuttered words were consistently stuttered and most of these were uttered by the more severe stutterers. Moreover, many of the words on which stuttering repeatedly occurred were those that began sentences thus indicating that positional effects were important. Most of the words originally stuttered were spoken fluently later and many of the words that had previously shown no stuttering were stuttered upon later. In short, the consistency effect is not very strong either in reading or spontaneous speech; not strong enough, in our opinion, to provide a strong foundation for the anticipatory struggle hypothesis concerning the nature of stuttering. Learned fears may account for some of the loci but not for all. Let us now try to discover what other factors seem to determine what words are those on which the stutterer stutters.

POSITION OF THE WORD

Stutterers often ask their clinicians, "Why is it that I sometimes have trouble on a word and at other times can say it without any stuttering at all?" Unfortunately, at the present time we have no simple answer. The best one is that several factors contribute to the precipitation of stuttering on any given word. One of these is the position of the word within the sentence. First words, or words that come early in the sentence seem to be stuttered upon more often than those that follow. For once, the research is almost unanimous in this regard. It clearly shows that stutterers have more trouble "getting started" in their utterances.

Various explanations have been offered. One of the most prevalent holds that the stutterers' situation fears are focused at this moment of possible disclosure of his impediment, that this is when he fears he will be unmasked and revealed as a deviant. While this may be true in part, the same locus of stuttering on the early words of a sentence occurs even when the stutterer has already stuttered. It can also occur on the last sentences of a reading passage as well as on the first. Moreover, more stuttering tends to occur at the beginning of a clause within the sentence, as Quarrington, Conway, and Siegel (1962) and Soderberg (1967) have demonstrated, than on words within that clause.

Another explanation (Brown, 1938) claims that stutterers have more trouble on the first words of an utterance because these are more prominent and conspicuous. Trotter (1959) showed that word-conspicuousness was related to the severity of stuttering, presumably because conspicuous words would be remembered as being associated with difficulty more than nonconspicuous ones.

But we do not have to attribute consistency to fear alone. It is quite possible that the more often a word is stuttered, the more unstable its motor pattern will become, and therefore it will be more likely that stress of any kind might disrupt it. The fracture history of any given word may therefore determine the chances of its being stuttered upon again. This concept does not require the consistency effect to be attributed to learned fears alone. It can explain why stuttering may occur on an unfeared word and it helps us understand why children may stutter on some of the same words even though they show no signs of anticipating difficulty.

And there are other explanations. One of them attributes the word position effect to *uncertainty*. Various studies of normal speech show that hesitation pauses (including filled pauses such as the use of *uh, er,* and repetitions as well as silent gaps) tend to occur before the points of highest information uncertainty in the flow of speech. This has been shown by MacClay and Osgood (1959) and Goldman-Eisler (1958). These hesitations also are found at the junctures of the larger syntactical units such as sentences or clauses. They reflect decisions and indecisions about how the sentences or clauses are to be formulated and just which words are to be used. Quarrington (1965) found that the more unpredictable the word, the more likely it would be stuttered. As Taylor (1966) writes:

> In all their experience with language, speakers learn that earlier words of sentences tend to have high uncertainty. Stutterers will therefore approach the beginnings of sentences with a predisposition to stuttering based on their expectation that the early words will be hard to predict (p. 240).

There are several difficulties with this explanation. One is that when the first three words of a sentence are deliberately chosen to be function words, the characteristic increase of stuttering on the first three words of a sentence still occurs (Wingate, 1979). Since these function words have less uncertainty than the content words usually found early in the sentence, it is difficult to conclude that uncertainty can be the sole reason for the position effect.

Another explanation for the tendency of stuttering to occur early in the sentence is that this position is where most of the linguistic stress tends to be located—at least in the English language. By linguistic stress we refer to the emphasis on certain syllables and words. Stutterers often have difficulty in asking questions and the words *what, where, how, why,* and *when* always receive more linguistic stress. Also, the same concentration of sentence stress in the first words seems to be characteristic of declarative sentences, too, as Lieberman (1970) has demonstrated. Certainly we find it in imperative sentences.

But why should linguistic stress create more stuttering? We know that stuttering tends to occur on the accented syllables of words more than on the unaccented ones. When this finding is paired with the similar effect of sentence stress, it would seem to indicate that some information very important to our understanding of stuttering may be involved. All we have to offer are guesses. It might be possible that the coordinations of simultaneous and successive muscular contractions are integrated about the nucleus of the accented syllable (or word), and that when this integration is faulty, stuttering results. There is substantial evidence that stuttering may be a disorder of timing and of motor coordination. If so, we could expect that these loci for the integration of the sequential synergies of voice, articulation, and respiration would probably have their impact at the loci of stressed or accented syllables and words. Since these tend to occur early in the sentence, we have another possible explanation for the preponderance of stuttering early in the utterance.

How plausible are these explanations of the sentence position effect? To this reviewer, they are probably all mildly plausible but we also feel that all of them are only partial explanations. Perhaps each plays some part in determining why stutterers tend to have more stuttering on the first words of their utterances. All we really know is that stutterers do have more trouble getting started than in continuing to speak once they have begun.

LOCI WITHIN THE WORD: POSITIONAL EFFECTS

Similar to the unanimity of the research that showed stutterings to be clustered at the beginnings of sentences, we also find common agreement that the majority of instances of stuttering occur at the beginnings of words, rather than in their middles or ends. Because we know of no research to the contrary, we will list only a few of the many that support this finding. Johnson and Brown (1935) found that 92 per cent of stutterings occurred at the beginnings of words; Hahn (1942) 93 per cent; Taylor (1966) 97 per cent; Sheehan (1974) 96 per cent. When stuttering is shown later in the word, it seems to be located within the accented syllables, not those that are unstressed. Froeschels (1961), on the basis of "many thousand cases," insisted that stuttering never occurs "at the end of a word." Emerick (1963), however, describes a case showing "final stuttering" though he admits it is very rare, and Adams (1978) provides a wide band spectrogram showing an abrupt termination of phonation on a final sound prior to the appearance of a part-word repetition on the next word. Such abrupt terminations of phonation have been said (Stromsta, 1965) to be characteristics of the core behavior of stuttering.

PHONEMIC CHARACTERISTICS

Does the stutterer tend to have more difficulty on certain sounds than on others? Most confirmed stutterers would answer affirmatively, and when the phonemic characteristics of the first sounds of the stuttered syllables or words are examined for any individual stutterer, it is apparent that they are not randomly or evenly distributed. However, when the data from a large number of stutterers are pooled, these individual differences are obscured and therefore most of the research has shown no significant concentration on specific phonemes.*

Much of this information about the phonemic characteristics of loci must be considered with caution. For example, if a stutterer says, "Kuh-Kuh-Key," is he stuttering on the /k/ or is he having difficulty in initiating the vowel? He will tell you, and so would his naive listeners, that he is stuttering on the /k/. Again there is the stutterer who complains, "I can nnnnnnnnnnnnever say my *n* sounds" when he has actually held one far too long. Once more we meet the problem of definition and the need for a molecular or even a sub-molecular approach. A case could be made for locating stuttering on specific sounds if these sounds are suddenly interrupted or if they lack the coarticulatory features they need for making the transition into the next sound of the word but few of our studies of loci have included such information.

To those who consider stuttering a "phonetic transition" disability, the only sensible way to identify loci would be to examine the characteristics of the syllables on which stuttering occurs. Not much work has focused on this but some investigation has concerned the loci of stuttering on syllables requiring phonatory shifts in order to determine if stuttering may involve a coordinative difficulty in initiating phonation. Adams and Reis (1971) found that there was much less stuttering when subjects had to read a passage containing "all voiced" material than on a passage having a normal

---

* Vaane (1977), however, reported the results of her loci study showed that her Dutch stutterers as a group had more difficulty on words beginning with a vowel or semivowel than those beginning with consonants. She also found differences in loci according to the place and manner of articulation. Unfortunately her reading passages were neither phonetically nor linguistically balanced.

scatter of phonatory transitions. In analyzing their data, the authors found that the loci of stuttering tended to occur when the stutterer had to shift from silence to phonation or when uttering syllables containing shifts from unvoiced to voiced sounds. In a replication of their study, Adams and Reis (1974) again found similar results. About 35 per cent of the stutterings occurred on the first word of a sentence, on the first sound after a juncture, or on transitions from unvoiced to voiced sounds. Manning and Koufal (1976), however, found that syllables involving voiceless-voiceless shifts and voiced-voiceless shifts produced even more stuttering than occurred in the unvoiced to voiced transitions. Hutchinson and Brown (1978) and Vaane and Janssen (1978) also attempted a replication of the Adams and Reis experiment but could not corroborate their findings.

OTHER FACTORS DETERMINING LOCI

In general, the research supports the belief that longer words are more often the loci of stuttering than shorter words. This also holds for the disfluencies of nonstuttering children and adults as Silverman and Williams (1967) discovered. Suggested reasons for the length-of-word effect on loci are that longer words are more conspicuous loci for fear, or that their motor patterns are more complex and hence demand more precise timing, or that longer words are usually content words with high information value and so have greater uncertainty in encoding (Quarrington, Conway, and Siegel, 1962).

Another factor that may play a part, though perhaps a minor one, in the loci of stuttering is the *familiarity* of the word being spoken. Strange or unfamiliar words, or foreign words, tend to produce more stuttering. Perhaps this is due to the fact that the specific sequences of motor coordinations involved in speaking a completely unfamiliar word have never been practiced before and thus are more vulnerable to disruption. Perhaps, semantic uncertainty or the uncertainty as to how the word should be pronounced may help create the hesitancy. In any event, most of the research seems to show that stuttering varies inversely with frequency of word usage. Unfamiliar words tend to evoke more stuttering.

The meaningfulness of a word also contributes to the loci of stuttering. As Eisenson and Horowitz (1945) showed, propositional speech always yields more stuttering than nonsense material. In general, content words such as nouns, verbs, and adjectives tend to be stuttered upon more frequently than such function words as articles, conjunctions, and prepositions but word length may be involved here, too, since content words tend to be longer than function words. Our own impression, after reviewing all the research, is that grammatical class has only a minor effect in determining most of the loci of stuttering. Too many other factors such as position, linguistic stress, word length, familiarity, and information value all coalesce and combine to becloud specific relationships of any one of these to their loci.

COMBINATION OF FACTORS
DETERMINING LOCI

As we have suggested, it seems as though the loci of stuttering are determined by the influence of not one but several factors working simultaneously. This was the position held by Brown (1938), one of the first workers to investigate the problem of which words are stuttered. He proposed that by weighting any given word by combining word length, word position, grammatical structure, and the phonetic characteristics of its first sound, he could almost predict its probability of being stuttered. He showed, too, that severe stutterers showed more stuttering than milder stutterers when fewer of these characteristics were combined. Oxtoby (1946) and Trotter (1956) corroborated Brown's belief that the higher the word-weight, the more frequently stuttering occurred.

SUMMARY

So we come to the end of another trail in the forest of information where we have sought that elusive quarry: the nature of stuttering. Our study of the loci of stuttering has shown that they tend to occur at the beginnings of utterance and on the first or accented syllables of words. No single phoneme or class of phonemes or syllables seems more difficult than any other for all stutterers, a finding that apparently is in opposition to the belief that stuttering is a disorder of motor coordination. The consistency with which a given word or sound is stuttered is not very great (though it is present) and there is little congruity among different stutterers as to which words are repeatedly stuttered. Some learned fears of certain sounds and words probably account for some of the loci of stuttering but such other factors as position, accentuation, unfamiliarity, and uncertainty also contribute their share to the precipitation of stuttering on any given word. Perhaps the best explanation for all this information is that the words that are disrupted are those which are the loci of multiple stresses. The more stress that impinges on a word, the more likely it is that it will be stuttered upon.

RESEARCH ON LOCI

Consistency. Johnson and Knott (1937) were the first to study the tendency of stuttering to occur on the same words when the same reading material was read again. They found that 72 per cent of the words stuttered on the second reading had been stuttered on the first time, and they named this the consistency effect. A subsequent series of studies by Johnson and his students reported similar findings. This research was done with adult stutterers. To see if the consistency effect occurred also in young stutterers, Bloodstein (1960) had them repeat sentences and found that they too showed an average consistency of 77 per cent, and one of the children stuttered on the same words 100 per cent of the instances. However, Neelly and Timmons (1967), also using repeated sentences, found a lower consistency effect of 40 to 50 per cent and Williams, Silverman, and Kools (1969a) reported 45 per cent for their child stutterers. Hendel and Bloodstein (1973) indicate a 48 per cent level of consistency in rereadings by adults. Hamre and Wingate (1973) in the study we have previously reported, using a sentence construction task mainly with adults, found what might be called a consistency of 36 per cent but they sharply criticize the whole concept of consistency.

The consistency effect has also been evidenced by nonstutterers, both adults and children, in terms of the loci of their disfluencies. The researches of Neelly and Timmons (1967) and Williams, Silverman, and Kools (1969 found that these "normal disfluencies" had consistent loci on certain words in repeated sentences produced by children. As compared to the consistency of young stutterers however, the consistency is much lower in nonstutterers.

Position of the word in the sentence. Brown (1938) found more stuttering on the first word of a sentence, less on the second word, and even less on the third. This positional effect seems very well supported. Hejna (1955) found a gradual decrease in stutterings on consecutive words of a sentence in spontaneous speech but failed to find the most stuttering on the first word. He explained that in spontaneous speech, this first word was often a starter word such as *Well* or *And*, and not really a part of the sentence. Quarrington, Conway, and Siegel (1962) contrasted the amount of stuttering on first and final words of sentences, finding a significant difference in frequency with more stuttering on the initial words. Conway and Quarrington (1963) tried to control for other variables such as initial phonetic sound, grammatical class, and number of syllables by designing the sentences read by stutterers and also found that initial position had more stuttering than medial, and medial more than final position of words in the sentences. Quarrington (1965) found a correlation of .49 between position of the word within the sentence and decreasing frequency of stuttering. Taylor (1966b) showed that word position was a more important determiner of the loci of stuttering than either the length of the word or the phonetic characteristics of the syllables. Soderberg (1967) found more stuttering on the initial words of clauses than on subsequent words even though initial words were more typically function words and pronouns while final words were more often of the lexical class. Silverman and Williams (1967) found little differences between the loci of disfluencies in stutterers as compared with those of normal speakers except that the stutterers had more difficulties in the initial position, in getting started. Bloodstein and Gantwerk (1967) also found that very young stutterers had more trouble on the first words of their utterances.

Griggs and Still (1979) also discovered a tendency for stuttering to cluster about the beginnings of utterances, but marked individual differences existed. Wingate (1979) showed that although more stuttering occurred on the first three words of sentences, the position effect could be explained by the preponderance of words having linguistic stress which also has its loci in these first words.

Phonetic characteristics. Whether or not stuttering will occur seems to depend also on the characteristics of the first sound of the word, or the first sound of the syllable having primary accent. Johnson and Brown (1935) had stutterers read a long passage and then ranked the various speech sounds according to frequency of stuttering. Brown (1938) repeated the experiment using long lists of words out of context. He found that words beginning with consonants produced more stuttering than those beginning with vowels, although there was much individual variability about which sounds were difficult. Hahn (1942a) found a marked difference between consonants and vowels; only 2.9 per cent of the stutterings occurred on words beginning with a vowel. Quarrington, Conway, and Siegel (1962), using a special set of sentences in order to control for other factors, compared the occurrence of stuttering on four consonants, said by Johnson and Brown to be the most difficult ones, with four other consonants said to be least difficult. They found no significant differences in the amount of stuttering on the different sounds. Soderberg (1962) used word lists and found no significant differences in the frequency or duration of stutterings either between consonants and vowels, or between voiced and unvoiced consonants. His design, however, has been criticized by Taylor (1966a) as tending to minimize any vowel-consonant differences. Taylor (1966a), in her well-controlled study, found that consonants were stuttered much more frequently than vowels, but the particular consonantal contexts in which stuttering occurred were not those found by Brown or Hahn, no doubt because of individual variability.

Vaane and Janssen (1978), in an intensive investigation of the phonemic characteristic loci of stuttering in 48 Dutch stutterers, found that more stuttering occurred on words beginning with vowels than those beginning with consonants, and that the bilabial plosives seemed to provoke more stuttering than the other consonants.

Word length. Most of the research has indicated that longer words are stuttered upon more frequently than shorter words (Brown and Moren, 1942; Hejna, 1955; Soderberg, 1966). Schlesinger, Melkman, and Levy (1966) found that when words of one, two, or three syllables were spoken, stutterers had more difficulty as the word length increased. Similar findings were demonstrated by Soderberg (1971), Silverman (1972), and Griggs and Still (1979). To account for this rather consistent agreement, explanations have been couched in terms of conspicuousness, coordinative loading, and familiarity.

OTHER CHARACTERISTICS OF LOCI

Testing nonstuttering children, Cecconi, Hood, and Tucker (1977) found that as the difficulty of their reading passages increased, they showed more disfluencies. Following this lead, Blood and Hood (1978) tested young stutterers and reported that more difficult reading passages produced more stuttering. This implies that word familiarity plays a role in determining loci. Several studies including Hejna (1963); Soderberg (1966); and Schlesinger, Melkman, and Levy (1965) have shown that the frequency of word usage is related to stuttering frequency. Wingate (1967) found that the word frequency level was significantly related to stutterings on lists of short words but not on lists of longer words. Ronson (1976) concluded that only in severe stutterers was there a significant relationship between stutterings and word frequency level.

The linguistic characteristics of stuttered words have also been investigated. Propositional speech always seems to yield more stuttering than nonsense material, as Eisenson and Horowitz (1945) made clear. Bardrick and Sheehan (1956) had stutterers read one passage composed of numbers, another of ordinary meaningful prose, and a third of emotionally loaded words. The number of stutterings increased in that same order. In general, content (lexical) words such as nouns, verbs, adjectives, and adverbs are more frequently stuttered than function words such as conjunctions, prepositions, articles, possessive pronouns, etc. (Johnson and Brown, 1935; Brown, 1938; Hahn, 1942b; Hejna, 1955). However, as Quarrington, Conway, and Siegel (1962) have demonstrated, there is little agreement about the frequency of stuttering on the grammatical subclasses. Word length may account for the differences between lexical and function words, since lexical or content words are usually longer than function words. Taylor's (1966a) data supports this explanation. Lexical words also carry more information than function words and have greater statistical uncertainty in the speech sequence. Goldman-Eisler (1958) has shown that more hesitation pauses occur in normal speech before words of high information value and greater uncertainty than before words of low meaningful content and more certainty. Similar results were found by McClay and Osgood (1959). Soderberg (1967) found that prolongations occurred on lexical words while repetitions occurred with almost equal frequency on both lexical and function words. A study by Bloodstein and Gantwerk (1967) seems to corroborate Soderberg's results. Their 3–6 year old stutterers did not show the concentration of stuttering on nouns, verbs, and other content words but instead showed more difficulty on pronouns and conjunctions, function words. Williams, Silverman, and Kools (1969), however, with stutterers having a median age of nine years, found that the loci of their stutterings, like those of adults, clustered about content rather than function words. Griggs and Still (1979) found a minor group of their stutterers who had more trouble on the function words and they suggest that such minorities would not have been known in the usual studies which did not seek to determine individual differences.

ADAPTATION

Most of the research on loci involves the reading of the same material many times. When this is done, most stutterers show a progressive decline in the number of their stutterings. This has been called the *adaptation effect*, and formerly it was viewed as one of the unique features of the disorder. We now know that it is not, and that normal speakers also show a reduction in their disfluencies when saying the same thing over and over. Nevertheless, since it has been studied extensively, and because it demonstrates that stutterers can adapt to the stress of speaking, we include a short section on adaptation.

A representative adaptation curve is shown in Figure 10. It shows a very steep decrease in the number of stutterings from the first reading trial to the second, and then a slower decrease thereafter until a plateau is reached, usually on the fifth reading of the passage. Further trials yield no further decrement and often some small increase in the frequency of stuttering ensues.

The adaptation effect is usually transitory and unstable according to Cullinan (1963) and Bloom and Silverman (1979). It does not last very long. After a substantial interval of time such as a day or two, the frequency of stuttering returns to the level it showed when the stutterer first read the passage (Peins, 1961; Gray and Brutten, 1965). Also, the adaptation curves may be different on different days even for the same stutterer.

Moreover, not all stutterers show the adaptation effect, as Newman (1954) showed long ago. Prins and Lohr (1968), Bloom (1973), and Preus (1981) also discovered stutterers who did not adapt.

It is not only in the rereading of passages or lists of words that most stutterers show the adaptation effect. Neely and Timmons (1967) and others have used the repetition of sentences from memory. When the stutterer repeats his description of certain pictures or sketches or describes the same room in repeated telephone calls some adaptation has been demonstrated (Kroll and Hood, 1974). Spontaneous speech shows little

Figure 10. Typical adaptation curve showing frequencies of stuttering in rereadings of the same passage.

adaptation because what is said varies substantially (Kroll and Hood, 1974). Rousey (1958) had his stutterers talk continuously for five days and found only a little adaptation effect.

When single words are repeatedly uttered by a stutterer, some adaptation also occurs. Silverman and Williams (1972) showed that when consecutive oral repetitions of a single word which was stuttered were analyzed, the majority of the stutterers did not remain fluent even after complete fluency had been achieved. Instead they exhibited alternating fluent and stuttered productions of that word as they said it over and over again.

All of the early and most of the recent research on adaptation has been based on the counting of molar "moments" of stuttering. However, it is quite possible that specific behaviors included within the molar moments may adapt in different ways or not adapt at the same rate. Zenner (1971) discovered that while some of the stuttering behaviors did adapt, others did not or actually showed an increase on later trials. Silverman and Williams (1971) found that the course of adaptation was similar for part-word repetition, word repetition, phrase repetition, interjections, revision, and disrhythmic phonation. In contrast, Sakata and Adams (1972) showed that there were considerable differences in the way these specific types of disfluency adapted. Kroll and Hood (1974) concluded that specific stuttering behaviors did show adaptation but at different rates.

It might seem reasonable to suspect that those stutterers who adapt quickly and thoroughly to the repeated reading task would tend to have a better therapeutic prognosis than those who adapt more slowly or do not adapt at all. According to Lanyon (1965) who used a rating scale of severity rather than counting stuttered words, those stutterers who adapted the most showed more improvement. However, Prins (1968), Kroll and Hood (1974) and Bloom and Silverman (1979) found little predictive value in adaptation rates.

EXPLANATIONS OF THE ADAPTATION EFFECT

Many different explanations have been offered for the adaptation effect. It has been attributed to a decrease in fear or anxiety (Sheehan, 1951; Wischner, 1952), or explained as experimental extinction of learned behaviors (Leutenneger, 1957). Eisenson (1975) holds that much of the adaptation effect is due to the fact that in repeated readings, the meaningfulness of the material is decreased (there is usually more stuttering when the material being read is meaningful.) Peins (1961) and others have accounted for it in terms of reactive inhibition. Plausible as they may seem, these explanations do not appear to be particularly valid; certainly they all imply that the stutterer has learned his stuttering behaviors as a response to fear.

However, the adaptation effect is also shown by nonstutterers. Their disfluencies also decrease when they have to say the same thing over and over again. This is true not only of adults but also of children (Neely and Timmons, 1964; Williams, Silverman, and Kools, 1968; and Miller and Miller, 1977). Presumably, nonstutterers' fears of the situation or of the words are either non-existent or at most are very low. Moreover, even in stutterers, adaptation seems to vary independently of various measures of emotional arousal (Maxwell and Brutten, 1964).

An alternative explanation is that the adaptation situation provides an opportunity for practicing the coordinations involved in uttering the sounds and syllables and words when speaking the same material successively. If stuttering is a disorder of coordination, then such practice may help integrate the motor sequences involved. Whispered or silent rehearsals of a reading passage do not seem to enhance adaptation but repeated oral rereading does, as shown by Bruce and Adams (1978) and Besozzi and Adams (1969). As the stutterer or normal speaker practices the prosodic features of the material, the material becomes easier to speak. Well-memorized material promotes fluency, as most of us would agree, but it may not be just the increased familiarity with the material but rather the motor practice involved in the rehearsals which accounts for the improvement in fluency.

In our view, the most reasonable explanation has been offered by Wingate (1972). He attributes the adaptation effect to two factors: (1) an initial adaptation to the task or situation which takes place during the first reading and (2) a motoric practice effect which is shown on subsequent trials. We also feel that the first factor could include both situation and word fears if present in the stutterer, or merely the stress of unfamiliarity for the normal speakers, and that both improve because of practice. Most of the comparative studies have shown that the amount of first trial adaptation in stutterers is greater than in nonstutterers—which may support this speculation.

All in all, we feel that the tremendous effort and time spent in exploring the features of the adaptation effect have contributed very little to any *basic* understanding of the nature of stuttering. All it has shown is that stutterers stutter less under conditions of decreased stress or improve with practice. "If apprehension is what separates the abnormal disfluencies of stuttering from those which are normal, then one has trouble explaining how the consistency effect is an indicator of the stutterer's anxiety when this effect is also present in the relaxed disfluencies of the nonstutterer" (Perkins, 1980, p. 462).

BIBLIOGRAPHY

ADAMS, M. R. 1978.   Further analysis of stuttering as a phonetic transition defect. *Journal of Fluency Disorders* 3: 265–71.

———— AND R. REIS. 1971.   The influence of the onset of phonation on the frequency of stuttering. *Journal of Speech and Hearing Research* 14: 639–44.

————. 1974.   The influence of the onset of phonation on the frequency of stuttering: a replication and reevaluation. *Journal of Speech and Hearing Research* 17: 639–44.

BARDRICK, R. A. AND J. G. SHEEHAN. 1956. Emotional loading as a source of conflict in stuttering. *American Psychologist* 11: 391.

BESOZZI, T. E. AND M. R. ADAMS. 1969. The influence of prosody on stuttering adaptation. *Journal of Speech and Hearing Research* 12: 818–24.

———. 1978. Effects of two types of motor practice on stuttering. *Journal of Speech and Hearing Research* 21: 421–28.

BLOOD, G. W. AND S. B. HOOD. 1978. Elementary school-age stutterers' disfluencies during oral reading and spontaneous speech. *Journal of Fluency Disorders* 3: 155–65.

BLOODSTEIN, O. 1969. *A handbook on stuttering.* Chicago: National Easter Seal Society for Crippled Children and Adults.

———. 1960. The development of stuttering: changes in nine basic features. *Journal of Speech and Hearing Disorders* 25: 219–37.

——— AND B. F. GANTWERK. 1967. Grammatical function in relation to stuttering in young children. *Journal of Speech and Hearing Research* 10: 786–89.

BLOOM, C. M. 1973. Do all stutterers adapt? *Journal of Speech and Hearing Research* 16: 518–21.

——— AND F. SILVERMAN. 1979. Stability of performance of individual stutterers on oral reading adaptation tasks. *Journal of Fluency Disorders* 4: 39–44.

———. 1960–61. Development of stuttering. *Journal of Speech and Hearing Disorders* 25 (1960), 219–37, 366–76; 26: 67–82.

BROWN, S. F. 1938. A further study of stuttering in relation to various speech sounds. *Quarterly Journal of Speech* 24: 390–97.

———. 1937. The influence of grammatical function on the incidence of stuttering. *Journal of Speech Disorders* 2: 201–15.

———. 1945. The loci of stuttering in the speech sequence. *Journal of Speech Disorders* 10: 181–92.

———. 1938. Stuttering with relation to word accent and word position. *Journal of Abnormal and Social Psychology* 33: 112–20.

——— AND A. MOREN. 1942. The frequency of stuttering in relation to word length during oral reading. *Journal of Speech Disorders* 7: 153–59.

BRUCE, M. C. AND M. R. ADAMS. 1978. Effects of two types of motor practice on stuttering adaptation. *Journal of Speech and Hearing Research* 21: 421–28.

BRUTTEN, E. J. 1963. Palmar sweat investigations of disfluency and expectancy adaptation. *Journal of Speech and Hearing Research* 6: 40–48.

BRUTTEN, E. J. AND B. B. GRAY. 1961. Effects of word cue removal on adaptation and adjacency: a clinical paradigm. *Journal of Speech and Hearing Disorders* 26: 385–89.

BRUTTEN, E. J. AND D. J. SHOEMAKER. 1967. *The modification of stuttering.* Englewood Cliffs, N.J.: Prentice-Hall.

CECCONI, C. P., S. B. HOOD, AND R. K. TUCKER. 1977. Influence of reading difficulty level on the disfluencies of children. *Journal of Speech and Hearing Research* 20: 475–84.

CONWAY, J. K. AND B. J. QUARRINGTON. 1963. Positional effects on the stuttering of contextually organized verbal material. *Journal of Abnormal and Social Psychology* 67: 299–303.

COOK, M. 1968. Speech disturbance and length of utterance. *Psychonomic Science* 10: 125–26.

COPPA, A. AND A. BARR. 1974. Use of questions to elicit adaptation in the speech of stutterers and nonstutterers. *Folia Phoniatrica* 26: 378–88.

CULLINAN, W. L. 1963. Stability of adaptation in the oral performance of stutterers. *Journal of Speech and Hearing Research* 6: 70–83.

EISENSON, J. 1975. Stuttering as a perseverative disorder. In *Stuttering: A Second Symposium*, ed. J. Eisenson. New York, Harper and Row.

——— AND E. HOROWITZ. 1945. The influence of propositionality on stuttering. *Journal of Speech Disorders* 10: 255–59.

EMERICK, L. 1963. A clinical observation on the "final" stuttering. *Journal of Speech and Hearing Disorders* 28: 194–95.

FAIRBANKS, G. 1937. Some correlates of sound difficulty in stuttering. *Quarterly Journal of Speech* 23: 67–69.

FORTE, M. AND I. M. SCHLESINGER. 1972. Stuttering as a function of time of expectation. *Journal of Communication Disorders* 5: 347–55.

FROESCHELS, E. 1961. New viewpoints on stuttering. *Folia Phoniatrica* 13: 187–201.

GOLDMAN-EISLER, F. 1966. Discussion and further comments. In E. R. Lenneberg, *New directions in the study of language*. Cambridge, Mass.: M.I.T. Press.

———. 1958. The predictability of words in context and the length of pauses in speech. *Language and Speech* 1: 266–31.

GOLUB, A. 1955. The cumulative effect of constant and varying reading material on stuttering adaptation. In *Stuttering in children and adults*, eds. W. Johnson and R. Leutenneger. Minneapolis: University of Minnesota Press.

GRAY, B. B. AND E. J. BRUTTEN. 1965. The relationship between anxiety, fatigue and spontaneous recovery in stuttering. *Behavior Research and Therapy* 2: 251–59.

GRIGGS, S. AND A. W. STILL. 1979. An analysis of individual differences in words stuttered. *Journal of Speech and Hearing Research* 22: 572–80.

HAHN, E. 1942a. A study of the relationship between stuttering occurrence and phonetic factors in oral reading. *Journal of Speech Disorders* 7: 143–51.

———. 1942b. A study of the relationship between stuttering occurrence and grammatical factors in oral reading. *Journal of Speech Disorders* 7: 329–55.

———. 1940. A study of the relationship between the social complexity of the oral reading situation and the severity of stuttering. *Journal of Speech Disorders* 5: 5–14.

HAMRE, C. E. AND M. E. WINGATE. 1973. Stuttering consistency in varied contexts. *Journal of Speech and Hearing Research* 16: 238–47.

———. 1963. Stuttering frequency in relation to word frequency usage. *ASHA*, 5: 5 (abstract).

HEJNA, R. F. 1955. A study of the loci of stuttering in spontaneous speech. *Dissertation Abstracts* 15: 1674–75 (abstract).

HELMRICH, H. G. AND O. BLOODSTEIN. 1973. The grammatical factor in childhood disfluency in relation to the continuity hypothesis. *Journal of Speech and Hearing Research* 16: 731–38.

HENDEL, D. AND O. BLOODSTEIN. 1973. Consistency in relation to inter-subject congruity in the loci of stuttering. *Journal of Communication Disorders* 6: 37–43.

HOOD, S. B. 1974. Effect of communicative stress on the frequency and form types of disfluent behavior in adult stutterers. *Journal of Fluency Disorders* 1: 36–47.

HUTCHINSON, J. M. AND D. BROWN. 1978. The Adams and Reis observations revisited. *Journal of Fluency Disorders* 3: 148–59.

JOHNSON, W. AND S. F. BROWN. 1935. Stuttering in relation to various speech sounds. *Quarterly Journal of Speech* 21: 481–96.

JOHNSON, W. AND M. INNESS. 1939. Studies in the psychology of stuttering: 12. A statistical analysis of the adaptation and consistency of moments of stuttering in successive readings of the same material. *Journal of Speech Disorders* 4: 79–86.

JOHNSON, W. AND J. R. KNOTT. 1937. Certain objective cues related to precipitation of the moment of stuttering. *Journal of Speech Disorders* 2: 17–19.

JOHNSON, W. AND R. LEUTENNEGER, (eds.). 1955. *Stuttering in children and adults.* Minneapolis: University of Minnesota Press.

KROLL, R. M. AND S. B. HOOD. 1974. Differences in stuttering adaptation between oral reading and spontaneous speech. *Journal of Communication Disorders* 7: 227–38.

LANYON, R. L. 1969. Speech: relation of nonfluency to information value. *Science* 164: 451–52.

————. 1965. The relationship of adaptation and consistency to improvement in stuttering therapy. *Journal of Speech and Hearing Research* 8: 293–94.

LEUTENEGGER, R. R. 1957. Adaptation and recovery in the oral reading of stutterers. *Journal of Speech and Hearing Research* 1: 293–94.

LIEBERMAN, P. 1970. *Intonation, perception and language.* Cambridge: MIT Press.

MACCLAY, H. AND E. I. OSGOOD. 1959. Hesitation phenomena in spontaneous English speech. *Word* 15: 19–44.

MANNING, W. H. AND K. J. KOUFAL. 1976. The frequency of disfluencies during phonatory transitions in stuttered and nonstuttered speech. *Journal of Communication Disorders* 9: 75–81.

MAXWELL, D. L. AND E. J. BRUTTEN. 1964. A Palmar sweat investigation of stuttering adaptation and spontaneous recovery under two conditions of audience complexity. *ASHA* 6: 416–17.

MILLER, J. A. AND T. W. MILLER. 1977. Adaptation effect in nonfluent speech, behavior of controlled stutterers and normal speakers. *Journal of Fluency Disorders* 2: 305–310.

NEELLEY, J. N. AND R. J. TIMMONS. 1967. Adaptation and consistency in the disfluent speech behavior of young stutterers and nonstutterers. *Journal of Speech and Hearing Research* 10: 250–57.

NEWMAN, P. W. 1963. Adaptation performances of individual stutterers: implications for research. *Journal of Speech and Hearing Research* 6: 393–94.

————. 1954. A study of adaptation and recovery of the stuttering response in self formulated speech. *Journal of Speech and Hearing Disorders* 19: 312–21.

OXTOBY, E. T. 1946. A quantitative study of certain phenomena related to expectancy of stuttering. Doctoral dissertation, University of Iowa.

PEINS, M. 1961. Adaptation effect and spontaneous recovery in stuttering expectancy. *Journal of Speech and Hearing Research* 4: 91–99.

————. 1961. Consistency effect in stuttering expectancy. *Journal of Speech and Hearing Research* 4: 397–98.

PERKINS, W. H. 1980. Disturbances of speech flow. In *Introduction to Communication Disorders,* eds. T. J. Hixon, L. D. Shriberg, and J. H. Saxon. Englewood Cliffs, N.J.: Prentice-Hall.

PREUS, A. 1981. *Attempts at identifying subgroups of stutterers.* Oslo: University of Oslo Press.

PRINS, D. 1968. Pre-therapy adaption of stuttering and its relation to speech measures of therapy progress. *Journal of Speech and Hearing Research* 11: 740–46.

———— AND F. LOHR. 1972. Behavioral dimensions of stuttered speech. *Journal of Speech and Hearing Research* 15: 61–71.

————. 1968. A study of the behavioral components of stuttered speech. Final Report, Project No. 6-2382. Grant No. OEG-3-6-062382-1882. U.S. Department of Health, Education and Welfare.

QUARRINGTON, B. 1965. Stuttering as a function of the information value and sentence position of words. *Journal of Abnormal Psychology* 70: 221–24.

————. 1953. The performance of stutterers on the Rosenzweig picture frustration test. *Journal of Clinical Psychology* 9: 189–92.

————, J. CONWAY, AND N. SIEGEL. 1962. An experimental study of some properties of stuttered words. *Journal of Speech and Hearing Research* 5: 387–94.

REIS, R. AND M. R. ADAMS. 1978. Comments on the Adams and Reis observations revisited. *Journal of Fluency Disorders* 3: 299–302.

RONSON, I. 1976. Word frequency and stuttering: the relationship to sentence structure. *Journal of Speech and Hearing Research* 19: 813–19.

ROSSO, L. AND M. R. ADAMS. 1969. A study of the relationship between the latency and consistency of stuttering. *Journal of Speech and Hearing Research* 12: 389–93.

ROUSEY, C. L. 1958. Stuttering severity during prolonged spontaneous speech. *Journal of Speech and Hearing Research* 1: 40–47.

SAKATA, R. AND M. R. ADAMS. 1972. Comparison among various forms of individual stutterers' disfluency. *Journal of Communication Disorders* 5: 232–39.

SCHLESINGER, I. M., M. FORTE, B. FRIED, AND R. MELKMAN. 1965. Stuttering, information load and response strength. *Journal of Speech and Hearing Disorders* 30: 32–36.

SCHLESINGER, I. M., R. MELKMAN, AND R. LEVY. 1966. Word length and frequency as determinants of stuttering. *Psychonomic Science* 6: 255–56.

SHEEHAN, J. G. 1974. Stuttering behavior: a phonetic analysis. *Journal of Communication Disorders* 7: 193–212.

————. 1951. Modification of stuttering through nonreinforcement. *Journal of Abnormal and Social Psychology* 46: 51–63.

SHULMAN, E. 1955. Factors influencing the variability of stuttering. In *Stuttering in Children and Adults,* eds. W. Johnson and R. Leutennegger. Minneapolis: University of Minnesota Press.

SILVERMAN, F. H. 1972. Disfluency and word length. *Journal of Speech and Hearing Research* 15: 788–91.

———— AND D. E. WILLIAMS. 1972. Performance of stutterers on a single-word adaptation task. *Perceptual and Motor Skills* 34: 565–66.

————. 1971. The adaptation effect for six types of speech disfluency. *Journal of Speech and Hearing Research* 14: 525–30.

————. 1967. Loci of disfluencies in the speech of nonstutterers during oral reading. *Journal of Speech and Hearing Research* 10: 790–94.

SODERBERG, G. A. 1967. Linguistic factors in stuttering. *Journal of Speech and Hearing Research* 10: 801–10.

———. 1962. Phonetic influences on stuttering. *Journal of Speech and Hearing Research* 5: 315–20.

———. 1966. The relations of stuttering to word length and word frequency. *Journal of Speech and Hearing Research* 9: 584–89.

———. 1969. A comparison of adaptation trends in the oral reading of stutterers. *Journal of Communication Disorders* 2: 99–108.

———. 1971. Relations of word information and word length to stuttering disfluencies. *Journal of Communication Disorders* 4: 9–14.

TATE, M. W. AND W. L. CULLINAN. 1962. Measurement of consistency of stuttering. *Journal of Speech and Hearing Research* 5: 272–83.

——— AND A. AHLSTRAND. 1960. Measurement of adaptation in stuttering. *Journal of Speech and Hearing Research* 4: 321–40.

TAYLOR, I. K. 1966a. The properties of stuttered words. *Journal of Verbal Learning and Behavior* 5: 112–18.

TROTTER, W. D. 1959. Relationship between severity of stuttering and word conspicuousness. *Journal of Speech and Hearing Disorders* 21: 198–201.

VAANE, E. AND P. JANSSEN. 1978. Different types of disfluencies and some phonological features. *Logopedie en Foniatrie* 50: 14–20.

VAN RIPER, C. AND C. J. HULL. 1955. The quantitative measurement of the effect of certain situations on stuttering. In *Stuttering in Children and Adults*, eds. W. Johnson and R. Leutenegger. Minneapolis: University of Minnesota Press.

WELLS, G. B. 1979. Effect of sentence structure on stuttering. *Journal of Fluency Disorders* 4: 123–29.

WILLIAMS, D., F. SILVERMAN, AND J. KOOLS. 1968. Disfluency behavior of elementary school stutterers and nonstutterers: the adaptation effect. *Journal of Speech and Hearing Research* 11: 622–630.

———. 1969. Disfluency behavior of elementary school stutterers and nonstutterers: the consistency effect. *Journal of Speech and Hearing Research* 12: 301–07.

WINGATE, M. E. 1966. Stuttering adaptation and learning: I. The relevance of adaptation studies to stuttering as learned behavior. *Journal of Speech and Hearing Disorders* 31: 148–56.

———. 1966b. Stuttering adaptation and learning: II. The adequacy of learning principles in the interpretation of stuttering. *Journal of Speech and Hearing Disorders* 31: 211–18.

———. 1962. Evaluation and stuttering. *Journal of Speech and Hearing Disorders* 27: 106–15; 244–57; 368–77.

———. 1967. Slurvian skill of stutterers. *Journal of Speech and Hearing Research* 10: 44–48.

———. 1966. Prosody in stuttering adaptation. *Journal of Speech and Hearing Research* 9: 550–556.

———. 1979. The first three words. *Journal of Speech and Hearing Research* 22: 604–12.

———. 1979. The loci of stuttering: grammar or prosody? *Journal of Communication Disorders* 12: 283–90.

WISCHNER, G. J. 1952. Anxiety reduction as reinforcement in maladaptive behavior: evidence in stutterer's representations of the moment of difficulty. *Journal of Abnormal and Social Psychology* 157: 566–71.

ZENNER, A. A. 1971. A molecular analysis of stuttering and associated behaviors during massed oral readings of the same material: the adaptation and consistency of behaviors. Doctoral dissertation, Syracuse University.

THE SEVERITY OF STUTTERING

9

Once when we were video recording an adult stutterer reading a long passage for the first time, he only stuttered once and that one time was on the first word. Later we measured the duration of that moment of stuttering and it lasted only four tenths of a second. Anyone who listened only to the sound track would have been certain that the person was a normal speaker. And yet in that four-tenths of a second, his mouth gaped, his tongue protruded tremorously, his eyeballs bulged, and his whole face was contorted as he strained and struggled for utterance. Then he suddenly stopped the struggle and said the word. If we had measured the severity of his stuttering only in terms of frequency or duration, we would have concluded that he was a mild stutterer, even though the young man said it was one of the worst blocks he had ever experienced. We showed this segment of the videotape to a group of viewers and they unanimously agreed that it was the speech of a very severe stutterer.

This example illustrates some of the difficulties in devising adequate measures of severity. Another example may also be illuminating. A high school boy referred himself to our clinic saying that his stuttering was getting much worse. When we talked to his parents and teachers, they were surprised. All of them said he had improved greatly in previous weeks, that he now stuttered very rarely. One teacher did say that he was not reciting as much as he used to but that when he did, she seldom heard him stutter. What had occurred, of course, was that the youth had begun to hide his stuttering, to develop silent struggling, and to avoid speaking whenever he felt that he might have trouble. Before, he had been fairly unconcerned about his stuttering; now he was deeply ashamed of it, a reaction that stemmed from an unfortunate experience. He had asked a pretty girl for a date, and she had responded flippantly, "I'm not so hard up that I have to date a stutterer like you." We cannot always rely on listener judgments in evaluating the severity of stuttering.

We must also, in our judgments of how severely a person stutters, make sure that we get enough stuttering samples from varied situations, and not merely from that person's performance in the clinic. Silverman (1975) discovered that for half of his 115 stutterers their stuttering severity scores shown in a clinical or testing environment were underestimated. This has posed a real difficulty in evaluating the outcome or progress of treatment. Various strategies have been designed to reduce this tendency. Ingham and Andrews (1975), for example, found that covertly recorded speech samples showed significantly more severity than those that were overtly recorded. Boberg and Sawyer (1977), using a confederate to assess the speech of their stutterers, found more evidence of relapse after therapy than appeared in the clinic testing situation. Other methods such as requiring the stutterer to provide weekly reports by telephoning have also been used. There are many difficulties in obtaining a true measure of stuttering severity.

NEED FOR MEASURES OF SEVERITY

We urgently need good measures of stuttering severity. We need them in research, for some of the conflicting results of different investigations of the same problem probably result from different severity mixes. One investigator, with an unusually large proportion of very severe stutterers among his subjects, for example, may find that their coordination is inferior, while another, with a large proportion of very mild stutterers in his group, will get conflicting results. The adaptation curves of very severe stutterers differ markedly from those of mild stutterers, and there are many other reasons why we have to control for severity in research samples.

Similarly, in clinical practice, we constantly evaluate the stutterer's performance. How bad a stutterer is he? Is he getting better or worse? Are our methods effective? During the initial examination, severity must be evaluated so that appropriate therapy plans can be devised, clinicians assigned, and schedules of appointments set up in terms of need. Some stuttering problems are so severe that they exceed our competence level, and so we seek the help of others. When we do so, our referral letter should include some statement of stuttering severity. Descriptive terms such as "very severe," "severe," "moderately severe," "mild," or "very mild" may not be sufficient and further descriptive material such as that found in the following quotation from Gregory (1968b) should be added.

> Cora was a moderately severe stutterer. She manifested some severely tonic blocks, especially on bilabial sounds, that lasted as long as seven seconds. Articulation was slurred, and she rambled as she spoke—both characteristics were thought to be secondary manifestations of stuttering. She blocked on most of the consonant sounds and often on medial and final syllables. There were contortions of the face, squinting of the eyes, and very poor eye contact. Her eyes would water as she spoke. During speech she said her head "was hot." In summary, Cora was very anxious and tense as she spoke (p. 41).

In this account (which admittedly need not represent the reality) Gregory states that Cora was a "moderately severe stutterer." Unfortunately we do not know the markings on his scale of severity, nor do we know its upper and lower extremes. From this description of her other behaviors, we would say that Cora should be called "severe" or "very severe," but who are we to say that our estimates of severity or our terms representing severity are any better than those used by Gregory?

The need for measurements as well as impressions of severity is most evident in assessing the success of treatment. Measures of severity enable the clinician to determine if progress is being made. The comparison of different therapeutic regimes require them. Moreover, all studies of outcome should show a reduction of severity even if total fluency is not achieved. Boberg, Howie, and Woods (1979) in their review of operant programs, show that there are many deficiencies in the ways that severity before and after treatment have been assessed.

CLINICAL IMPRESSIONS OF SEVERITY

Although the phrases "very severe" and "very mild" might communicate the essence of a clinical impression, we are not so sure that this would be true for "moderate severity." Presumably, "moderate severity" describes the behavior of the average stutterer. But the average stutterer seen by a public school clinician would probably be less severe than one seen in a university clinic, and the latter less severe than one referred to a psychiatrist, so the population of each setting has to be taken into account too. Soderberg (1962) found that the majority of his 105 college stutterers were ranked as "mild" stutterers on the Iowa Scale of Severity and that the typical college stutterer actually has little overt speech difficulty in an oral reading situation. If, however, the samples had been taken from class recitation or job interviews, they would probably have shown more severity.

Our trouble in measuring severity lies first in this variability and second in the fact that we have no Bureau of Standards for stuttering. There is no standard stuttering kilo or centimeter. Each stutterer and each therapist has his own different internal yardstick, and what is worse, each one of them is more elastic than it is rigid. Moreover, some clinicians' subjective scales of severity have only three divisions—severe, average, mild—while others have five, or seven, or nine. In this connection, we might morosely contemplate the study in which Cullinan, Prather, and Williams (1963) used seven different rating methods to evaluate the severity of tape-recorded samples of stuttered speech. Their judges evaluated each sample twice, using five-point, seven-point, and nine-point equal-appearing interval scales. A seven-point scale with well defined judgment markings and a direct-magnitude-estimation ratio scale were also used. They found that even with only one judge, no one method was reliable enough to serve as an adequate predictor of severity for an individual stutterer, and none of the seven methods seemed to be any better than the others. Results such as these cast much doubt on the accuracy of the working clinician's judgments of severity. Actually, of course, few clinicians would ever be content to describe the severity of a client's stuttering as a scale value or with an adjective. Instead, they add descriptions of the behavior. Thus Robinson (1968) describes his case as follows:

> The overt stuttering he presented was of a relatively mild form consisting of two or three quick repetitions of word elements or, occasionally, brief fixations of articulatory postures accompanied by slight tremors. However, these signs of a stuttering problem were not evident frequently. He was admittedly clever at substitution and other verbal manipulations. Thus, he usually gave the impression of a person who stuttered only occasionally. He reported having many acquaintances and a few good friends who he was certain didn't know he was a stutterer. But he said his stuttering bothered him a great deal. It was very embarrassing, and he was always under a lot of tension and strain.
>
> When he read aloud, the "sticky" blocks were more frequent and somewhat more pronounced and his embarrassment was obvious. Yet the overt stuttering certainly wasn't severe, and as we talked with him we felt that treatment would be relatively easy, particularly after we explained our treatment approach and emphasized the importance of having him test the validity of his concern about the stuttering by stuttering openly and freely (p. 70).

In this descriptive account, we note that Robinson mentions such factors as the frequency of the stuttering, its duration ("two or three repetitions" and "brief fixations"), its characteristic form, its visibility, and finally the subject's reactions of avoidance and embarrassment, all of which contributed to his impression of a "mild" degree of severity. In the following passage, note that Sheehan (1968) concentrates primarily on form and frequency in describing the case of Leonard who was:

> . . . one of the severest stutterers I have ever encountered. Leonard's habitual pattern consisted of a violent tilting back of his head; rolling his eyes toward the ceiling; the muscles in his neck would stand out; he would become flushed; he would twist his face in a forced grimace; attempt various starters; some head jerks in an effort to release himself from the block; and also would accompany his stuttering with various bodily gestures. He had little fluency capacity and stuttered severely on almost every word. His name and words beginning with the same sound as his first and last names were especially difficult (p. 77).

In describing a "severe" stutterer, Gregory (1968a) mentions frequency, loci, form, and also the altered characteristics of the normal speech:

> The client was a severe stutterer (oftentimes he blocked on every other word in conversational speech). He stuttered mostly on initial sounds, but there was also blocking on medial and final syllables of words. He displayed considerable tension of the lips, tongue, jaw, and larynx as he spoke. Starters such as "uh," "wa wa wa," and "well uh" were used frequently. A gasping type inhalation was involved in approximately one of every three blocks. Breaking through a speech block was sometimes accompanied by a slight leg movement. Fluent words, or occasional fluent phrases, were spoken in a slow, labored rate (p. 47).

RATING SCALES OF SEVERITY

In the effort to impose some pattern on the chaos of clinical judgments of severity, Lewis and Sherman (1951) developed the first rating scale based on principles which had been used in designing handwriting scales. This scale unfortunately required multiple judges and much time and effort to be useful even in group comparisons, and so it was never widely used clinically. Starbuck (1954) developed a filmed audiovisual scale in which samples of stutterers in the act of stuttering were arranged sequentially to represent differing degrees of severity. Starbuck showed that five factors varied significantly with each successive step on his scale. They were: total words spoken in a given time, number of blockings, facial grimaces, accompanying limb movement, and eye shift or eye-blink. In actual clinical use, this scale, like the Lewis and Sherman scale, proved difficult primarily because it is difficult to match one stutterer against another. They stutter too differently. When matched with the criterion sample, whether filmed or tape recorded, the differences in behavior are more marked than the similarities. Handwriting samples can be matched against a series of model specimens much more easily than can stuttering samples. At any rate, neither of these scales has had any extensive clinical use.

An instrument, however, which has been used very widely is the *Scale for Rating the Severity of Stuttering* published in Johnson, Darley, and Spriestersbach's *Diagnostic Methods in Speech Pathology* (1963). Although the authors strongly emphasize the limitations of this scale and term it a "rough measure only" many speech therapists use it, not only in diagnosis but also for measuring therapeutic progress. We can understand why they do so for in many ways it assembles in one instrument most of the real indications of stuttering severity. Seven scale values are given with descriptive legends for each. To illustrate, we quote those for Scale values 2 and 5:

> #2 *Mild*—stuttering on 1 or 2 per cent of words; tension barely perceptible; very few, if any, disfluencies last as long as a full second; patterns of disfluency simple; no conspicuous associated movements of body, arms, legs, or head.
> #5 *Moderate to severe*—stuttering on about 8 to 12 per cent of words; consistently noticeable tension; disfluencies average about 2 seconds in duration; a few distracting sounds and facial grimaces; a few distracting associated movements (p. 231).

This Iowa scale is, in our opinion, deficient because of the way the variables are grouped. Unfortunately, neither the amount of tension, nor the duration, number, or kind of associated struggle movements increase equally or proportionately with increased severity. How would we rank a stutterer, for example, who stutters on only two per cent of his words and thus would fit scale value 2 of mildness, but who also shows consistently noticeable tension every time he does stutter, which would classify him as moderately severe with a scale value of 5? As the research, which we shall summarize later, has shown, these variables are not highly correlated with one another, although the scale indicates that they should be. Again we face the problem of fit. Our stutterers just do not seem to fit into these categories on all the alleged features for any one step of the scale.

However, we have revised this Iowa scale so that it can be used as a profile. As such, it is very useful, especially for measuring changes during therapy. Therapy progress is seldom even. The stutterer may make gains in reducing the duration of his blocks at the same time that the frequency of his stuttering increases. Or he may begin to show longer stutterings but have eliminated much of the tension or struggle. By charting the client's status at different times during therapy on these profiles, the therapist is often able to shape the treatment appropriately. We provide such profiles in the accompanying Figure 11.

Figure 11. Profile of stuttering severity showing changes as a result of therapy.

PROFILE OF STUTTERING SEVERITY

SCALE	FREQUENCY	TENSION- STRUGGLE	DURATION	POSTPONEMENT- AVOIDANCE
1.	Under 1%	None	Under $\frac{1}{2}$ sec.	None
2.	1-2%	Rare but present	Average $\frac{1}{2}$ sec.	Less than 5 %
3.	3-5%	Usual but mild	Average 1 sec.	5-10%
4.	6-8%	Severe	Average 2 sec.	11-20%
5.	9-12%	Very severe	Average 3 sec.	21-31%
6.	13-25%	Overflow to eyes and limbs	Average 4 sec.	31-70%
7.	More than 25%	Overflow to trunk	Longer than 5 sec.	More than 70%

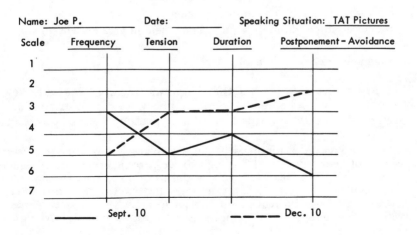

A SEVERITY EQUATION

These profiles are far from satisfactory and we hunger for some sort of unitary measure. Perhaps none is possible, but we have made two preliminary attempts to achieve a first approximation. In one attempt, we placed thermistors on various parts of the body to get summated readings of heat output which might reflect the contributions of duration, frequency, tension, and overt or covert struggle as well as emotion, but the technology involved defeated us. In the other, using recorded samples of severe, moderate, and mild stutterers as judged by a listener panel, we computed the numerical values of the following items: frequency of individual moments of stuttering expressed as a percentage; their average duration; the duration of the most severe moment of stuttering; the average amount of tension and struggle as judged on a five-step scale; the extreme amount of tension and struggle exhibited on the most severe moment of stuttering as judged on that scale and the number of avoidance reactions shown. Although all of these values could be ascertained with some objectivity and reliability, their combination to yield a single measure of severity poses many problems. The items need differential weighting but the weights were unknown. Should the items be combined algebraically or multiplicatively, or even exponentially? With these questions in mind, we offer the following equation as a conceptual model illustrating the factors that combine in some way to make up stuttering severity. It is not a quantification, but hopefully it will stimulate the research upon which quantification rests.

$$S = aF + bD_1 + cD_2 + dT_1 + eT_2 + fA + gE$$

where
F = frequency of stuttered words as a percentage of spoken words
D_1 = average duration of a stuttering moment
D_2 = duration of the longest stuttering moment
T_1 = average tension of a stuttering moment
T_2 = amount of tension in the stuttering moment of greatest tension
A = amount of avoidance
E = amount of emotional involvement

Van Riper (1968) describes the diagnostic picture of a very severe stutterer. A portion of the account is given to demonstrate that an assessment of severity in terms of such an equation might be possible:

> The symptomatic picture presented was as follows: Don stuttered on over 50 per cent of his words in oral reading and the percentage was much higher in propositional speech even in a relatively nonstressful situation. He showed very little adaptation on rereading or in repeating individual words, often an increase. There was no reduction in frequency under low frequency masking at 80 dB though there was some decrease in the duration of his blockings. The

average duration of his moments of stuttering in oral reading was 4 seconds; the longest one was 28. In propositional speech the durations were longer. Occasionally he would just have to quit speaking.

Except for the use of "um but" or "oh" or "um" or "ah" which he used to get started, there were few avoidances, "I see no point in substituting an easier word like the other guys often do. I don't have any. If I try one, I get hung up on that too." As with most of the severe stutterers, he had few specific phonemic or word fears, but his situation fears were very intense, often to the point of panic. Usually, Don plunged directly into the utterance, went into a prolonged tremor of the articulators, squeezed shut his eyes, jerked his jaw open very widely to interrupt the tremor, then did it again and again. Great tension accompanied this behavior and often it overflowed to the limbs and trunk. In his paroxysms, he would even stagger. Most of the grotesque behavior apparently seemed to serve as interruptor and escape devices. The tremors of the lips and jaws, which we were able to record electromyographically, ranged in frequency from 7 to 18 per second, with most of them oscillating at the first value. Often as a result of his longer blockings, he would become completely exhausted. Airflow was often interrupted at the laryngeal level as well as by the occluded tongue or lips. In some of his worst moments of stuttering, the tongue would protrude violently and show marked tremor (p. 101).

Several other authors have attempted to devise measures of stuttering severity that are based not only upon frequency, but on other factors as well. Janssen and Kraaimant (1978) did a factor analysis of stuttering behaviors and concluded that any measure of severity should take into account 1. total stutterings; 2. reading time (a measure of duration); 3. evidence of struggle; 4. tension and eyeblinks; 5. prolongations; and 6. tense silent blocks. Earlier, Prins and Lohr (1972) submitted their data from a frame by frame analysis of stuttering behaviors to a factor analysis and found one that they labeled the severity factor. The variables which loaded highly on this factor were moments of stuttering with long duration, high frequencies of stuttering moments, a slow labored rate of speech, lip tremors, and the number of different anatomical areas (face, arms, etc.) in which abnormalities occurred. Hood (1974) also devised an instrument for assessing the severity of stuttering. It was based upon a molecular analysis of stuttering behaviors and has been used to evaluate progress in therapy.

Perhaps the severity measure most often used—other than frequency counts—is the *SSI* Stuttering Severity Instrument by Riley (1972). Three measures of severity are used: the frequency of repetition and prolongation of sounds and syllables, the estimated duration of the three longest blocks, and a rating of the conspicuousness of the "physical concomitants" accompanying the stuttering. The latter refers to facial grimaces and other evidences of struggle. Numerical scores for each of these or a total score for all of them are obtained.

In the next sections of this chapter, we will try to describe how one might go about the diagnostic task of determining the weight of the components that contribute to the assessment of severity. We suspect that we will only be putting into words the kinds of processes that all therapists go through in arriving at their clinical impressions of the extent of a given stutterer's difficulty. We are fairly certain that we cannot cover all the diagnostic problems involved, and we are sure that no one will be entirely happy with the resulting evidence of our prescientific technology.

FREQUENCY OF STUTTERING

There is no doubt that one of the major contributors to a clinical impression of severity is the frequency of the moments of stuttering. The more often the stutterer stutters the more severe his problem seems to be. Although it is not the only factor, it is certainly one of the important ones. The stutterer reported by Bar (1967) who stuttered on 92.6 per cent of his words would be considered severe even if those stutterings were of short duration and contained little abnormality. All the research has shown positive correlations between frequency and rated severity, although they are not high enough to enable us to use frequency counts alone as the sole index of severity.

There are several difficulties in counting stutterings. In clinical practice, we can audiotape or videotape samples of the speech and then do our counting during several replays, a procedure which, as Aron (1967) and others have demonstrated, can yield highly reliable measures. As our summary of the research will show, combined audiovisual recordings yield higher frequency counts than either alone but audiotape recordings seem to be sufficient in most instances except when most of the stutterings are nonvocalized or are skillfully disguised.

VARIABILITY IN FREQUENCY

When estimating severity in the initial diagnosis or when ascertaining progress at different times during the course of therapy, it is important not to confine the speech samples to reading material. There are some very severe stutterers who can read with remarkable fluency. As we have seen, the amount of stuttering varies markedly in different speaking situations. The stutterer's performance in oral reading may not be representative of his real difficulty in communication. Sherman (1955) writes:

> Among a number of important considerations is the fact that stutterers typically vary from time to time in the severity of vocal characteristics of stuttering. They vary from day to day, from week to week, from month to month, regardless of whether they are undergoing therapy. . . An improvement in the reading situation, for example, does not necessarily indicate that there is also a comparable improvement in the spontaneous speech situation (p. 15).

To cope with some of this situational variability, Johnson, Darley, and Spriestersbach (1963) recommended using the Job Task (talking for three minutes about the person's actual or preferred vocation) or the TAT-Task in which Card 10 from the Thematic Apperception Test is presented to the stutterer, and he is asked to talk for three minutes about what is happening in the picture. We have used these successfully as well as other methods. Our customary diagnostic routine is to use a reading passage, a paraphrase of material read silently, a narration of some personal experience, and some telephone calls to procure information. Occasionally we use Rotter's Incomplete Sentences Test (1950), in which the stutterer reads aloud the first part of each unfinished sentence and then completes it, a procedure that gives an immediate comparison of reading and spontaneous speech, and also introduces some emotional stress. As Moore (1954) showed, topics such as parents, family, and speech experiences tend to elicit more stuttering than other subjects, and in getting our sample of spontaneous speech we often bring these into the interview.

Cyclic variations in severity of stuttering have also been found by Quarrington (1956) and by Quarrington as reported by Sheehan (1969) in this passage:

> Quarrington has recently gathered data on 39 young stuttering children, mean age 4 years, 4 months, observed over a 1-year period. In 32 of these, stuttering persisted over the 1-year period, during which their mothers supplied daily ratings of the frequency of stuttering . . . the resulting data curves revealed the presence of significant periodicities (p. 453).

Pittenger (1940), however, found no cyclic patterns in a given reading situation. These variations should not, then, markedly affect severity ratings based on frequency counts, since the cycles reported by Quarrington range in length from two to six months. There is also a fascinating article by the Hungarians Hirschberg, Kovacs, Palotas, and Szabo (1965) showing that certain "vago-tonic" stutterers stuttered more severely when a warm weather front passed over, while "sympathic-tonic" stutterers had more difficulty when a cold front came. Although we have not been able to assess the meteorology of stutterers, it is certain that more than a one-shot diagnosis of severity is needed. Stutterers are notoriously variable from situation to situation and from day to day, and repeated evaluations of severity are required no matter what methods are used to procure them.

SPEECH SAMPLING

It is also necessary to get a speech sample adequate in length for frequency counting. Obviously, too small a sample will not provide enough moments of stuttering to form any respectable basis for clinical judgment. Too large a sampling can be onerous. Our solution to the problem—probably not a very good one—is to use smaller samples for stutterers whose blockings are both frequent and full of struggle but larger ones for those with shorter and more repetitive behaviors. Generally speaking we seek a sampling of at least 400 words or ten moments of stuttering.

In order to survey the stutterer's difficulty, it is important to have reading materials that include words beginning with all of the different phonemes and also one contrived so that no one phoneme is loaded too heavily. Fairbanks' Rainbow Passage and that ancient composition entitled *Arthur the Young Rat* fulfill this criterion to some degree. The reason for using such material is that some stutterers have difficulty on only a few feared sounds, something to remember during initial interviews. An experienced therapist develops methods of eliciting spontaneous speech which also cover all the various phonemes, formulating his questions in such a way that the stutterer must use them all. Young and Prather (1962) found that 20-second samples of consecutive speech were sufficient for group analysis, but a much larger sample is necessary for diagnosing an individual case. Most clinical reading passages are 300–400 words long. If possible, the best technique is to talk long enough with the stutterer to evoke ten stuttering moments and then later, listen to a recording and count all the words he uttered to get a percentage. This procedure should be repeated in the telephone situation. Frequency counts are of course always expressed in percentages.

COUNTING STUTTERING BEHAVIORS

In procuring some estimate of severity by ascertaining the frequency of the stutterings, it is necessary to define what is being counted. Most workers in the past have used the molar "moments of stuttering" but there seems to be a growing trend to specify more precisely the molecular behaviors involved. A number of studies record the number of part word repetitions, prolongations or tense pauses; others merely report data on the percentages of words or syllables stuttered; still others report only the average number of stuttered words per minute of talking time. In our opinion, obtaining the percentage of *syllables* on which the basic behaviors of repetition or prolongation, or on which conspicuous avoidance and struggle have occurred, would seem to be the wisest course. The choice of syllables rather than words as the important data is, of course, due to the fact that multiple stuttering behaviors may be shown on a polysyllabic word such as *diadochokinesis*. The use of the number of stutterings per minute of talking time seems unwise because a single very severe instance of stuttering could take up that full minute and yet be recorded as having a very low severity. If all instances of stuttering were equal in severity, which they demonstrably are not, then counting stuttered words per minute might make sense.

With some training, the therapist can learn to count and estimate percentages fairly well, even without the aid of a tape recording, when conversing with the stutterer or listening to him as he telephones. Usually it is necessary to watch as well as listen while counting stutterings. Many of the inaudible abnormal postures, tremors, or facial twitches which are characteristic components of severe blockings may be found in fleeting miniature when the visual record is scanned. They should not be ignored in a frequency count.*

ORGANIZING FREQUENCY DATA

After the counting is completed there are several sets of figures that have to be turned into percentages. A certain stutterer may stutter on 18 per cent of his words in oral reading, on 32 per cent in talking about the TAT pictures, and on 60 per cent when talking over the telephone. Which percentage should be used in the profile or equation? Although all three should be recorded in the case files, it is best to use the highest percentage as the component figure in assessing the disorder's general severity. This ensures against underestimation, for stutterers can be very skillful at disguising the true extent of their problem, at least during the initial interview. During the course of therapy, however, as we reassess the severity using the same test situations, we often plot all three measures on a progress chart, finding perhaps that the frequency in oral reading had shown an early decrease which was not paralleled by a similar decrease in spontaneous speech. Other workers often average all three figures or consistently use only the highest one.

In concluding this section, it should be noted again that the frequency with which a person stutters is only one of several factors that contribute to severity. It is an important one but there are others too. Aron (1967) comes to the same conclusion:

> It can be generalized from the results here that we should differentiate more clearly between the terms "frequency" and "severity" of stuttering. There is no doubt that the amount of frequency of stuttering will contribute to an impression of its severity, but it would also appear that frequency as such should not be regarded as an independent and accurate measure of severity (p. 32).

DURATION AS A FACTOR IN SEVERITY

We suspect that clinicians, when judging severity, are much more influenced by the duration and struggle shown in the stutterer's blockings than by how often they occur. So, too, is the stutterer himself. He doesn't mind a lot of little stutterings half so much as he does a few long or grotesque ones full of tension. Subjectively, these hard blockings are the measure of his impediment. Some clinicians have been too concerned with simple countings when evaluating improvement. Severity involves much more

---

* One stutterer told this story when we called his attention to a tiny blocking which contained all the major features of his severe stuttering in miniature: "I guess you're right about that little block and I'm like the woman who upon marrying told her husband for the first time that she was already the mother of a baby. The man protested and became very angry. 'You should have told me that before we got married,' he shouted. Whereupon his wife answered, 'but it's only a little one.'"

than frequency counts. Personally, we have used the duration and abnormality of the three *worst* stutterings as our criteria for therapeutic improvement, and by "worst" we mean the longest and most struggled. When these become shorter and less abnormal, we feel that true progress is being made. The use of the three longest stutterings to serve as a measure of the duration factor in severity has also been demonstrated in studies by Myers (1978) and Preus (1981).

Stuttering has been called a speech impediment because the flow of speech is intermittently interrupted. Whatever the behaviors are that interrupt speech, we must know how long they last, or how much time they take away from communication in order to estimate the size of that impediment. If two stutterers both repeat the first syllable and prolong the /m/ in the word "psychometric" the one who repeats the syllable four times and prolongs the /m/ four seconds will show more severity than one who repeats the first syllable only two times and prolongs the /m/ only two seconds. The duration of the individual moments of stuttering is one of the basic components of any adequate index of severity. Like tapeworms, longer stutterings are worse than shorter ones.

Although Lewis and Sherman (1951) stated that severity would be best measured by evaluating moments of stuttering generally rather than by counting frequencies, only a few workers have measured the duration of the individual moments of stuttering. Doubtless this is because it is difficult to time short segments of audiotape with a stopwatch or measure spectrographic recordings with a ruler. Instead, indirect measures of stuttering duration, such as reading rate, are used more widely on the assumption that the longer the stutterer takes to say his words, the longer it will take him to read a passage. Generally, this is true although there are some stutterers who show a burst of speed after a moment of stuttering to compensate for the gap. These individuals flee hastily from the scene of their verbal crime and thus spoil the use of overall reading rate as a measure of severity.

We have found little difficulty in timing the durations of individual moments of stuttering. Indeed, it is easier than counting frequencies once the therapist has trained himself to count silently in seconds with some accuracy. The author is able to measure accurately the durations of individual moments of stuttering in terms of hippopotamuses or hippopotami. He has learned to say the word "hippopotamus" covertly in exactly one second. The longest stuttering block he ever measured lasted for 32 hippopotamuses all in a row and then the poor devil quit talking. Thus Sheehan's (1946) results showed that the average duration of repetitive blocks in his subjects could be stated as one "hippopotamus-hippopot" (1.6 seconds) in our counting-system, and the average duration of the prolongations was "hippopotam" or .87 seconds. A two- or three-hippopotami blocking is usually felt and sensed as a moment of severe stuttering.

Among the advantages of timing the durations of the individual stutterings is that it gives an impression of both the average and extreme fluency impediments. We can assess the variability in terms of standard deviations about the means. We can understand how badly the stutterer stutters at his worst. Total reading times or reading measures do not provide this important information. Furthermore, the extremes of duration may be highly significant in ¢valuating the stutterer's progress. A stutterer who is no longer having his old long, hard blocks will feel that he has made progress even if the average frequency and duration have remained much the same. As we shall see, subjective estimates of severity made by the stutterer himself do not correlate very highly with those made by the clinician. There are various reasons for this discrepancy, but one of them is that stutterers often measure their severity by their worst difficulties, not by their average ones. In the equation of severity, the extreme and the average duration of stutterings should probably be given equal weight. In clinical profiles we use either the average or extreme durations or the summation of both. How valid these procedures are will be determined by future research.

In timing durations, live or videotaped speech samples are best, since the beginning of the speech attempt, though highly visible, may not be audible. One caution should be mentioned. Filled time always seems shorter than empty time. Unless we actually count durations in stopwatch seconds or African beasts, the silent blockings will always seem longer than those that are vocalized. Repetitive stutterings normally seem longer than fixations. Though we have no research on the subject, our own unpublished data show that 90 per cent of normal speaking college students evaluate four-second stutterings as very severe; two-second stutterings as severe; one-second stutterings as moderate in severity; and one-half-second stutterings as mild.

Clinicians should evaluate the stutterer's reports of having very long blocks with some reservations. They usually overestimate their duration. Similarly, they also underestimate or completely fail to recognize the very short ones. This is reflected in the research of Ringel and Minifee (1966) who found that stutterers who were less able to make accurate judgments of time, either in silence or spontaneous speech, were the more severe.

TENSION AND STRUGGLE

As with measures of duration, we judge those moments of stuttering as more severe which are marked by tension or struggle. So does the stutterer. There is little research, but skilled clinicians can learn to make these judgments with some reliability as some of our own pilot studies with videotaped samples have shown. The presence of tremor, overflow movements, facial contortions, and even accompanying limb movements can be scanned, counted, and evaluated on improvised rating scales of severity. Again the clinician tries to estimate the amount of this tension and struggle shown on most of the moments of stuttering by a given stutterer, to compare this with that of other stutterers or with the picture remembered from earlier periods of therapy. Also, as with duration, we are interested in the most severe moments of tension and struggle, not just the average. Our research has shown a low but positive correlation between duration and tension judgments. That the correlation cannot be expected to be high is due to the fact that occasionally highly explosive and spasmodic blockings may be very short in duration. Electromyography can give objective measures of such tension for research purposes, but it is not very useful in routine clinical practice.

However, even though clinicians cannot be expected to use electrodes and amplifiers to procure accurate measurements of tension, they evidently can manage pretty well without them. In Denmark, Fibiger (1977) found that clinicians' severity ratings of individual stuttered words (on a ten point scale) closely reflected the amount of electromyographic activity (tension) even when they had to make their judgments sight unseen by listening to the stuttered words on tape recordings.

Severity can also be assessed in terms of visible abnormality though this is hard to quantify. Starbuck (1954) counted certain overt behaviors in devising his audiovisual scale of severity. In actual clinical practice this procedure is probably used very commonly in assessing severity. In his study of five days of continuous talking by stutterers, Rousey (1958) counted the number of visible symptoms (facial contortions, etc.) as one of his measures of severity and found the highest correlation (though it was only .62) between this item and the frequency of stuttering moments. The correlation was higher than that between frequency and either *rated* severity or the total output of words per eight hour day of talking. Clark and Murray (1962) suggest the use of a Behavior Analysis Chart in measuring therapeutic progress, that is, severity.

COVERT RESPONSES

Here we have real difficulty trying to be objective. How can we possibly provide figures for profiles or an equation which can represent the levels of anxiety, frustration, or shame? Once again we have outdistanced our research. Measures such as the psi (Palmar Sweat Index) and the gsr (Galvanic Skin Response) can give objective data, but they present many problems in interpretation and are not usually routinely available to the therapist. At present we are restricted largely to observation and inference. We can count how often the stutterer avoids words or postpones speech attempts. We can judge with some accuracy how reluctantly he enters a given speech situation. We can check his daily output of speech. We can see if he winces or blushes or averts his gaze or hangs his head when he stutters. We can listen to what he says about his problem as we carefully question him.

Sheehan (1970) has used the iceberg analogy to illustrate the fact that the visible and audible components of stuttering are only a small portion of the severity problem.

Nevertheless, we now have several instruments which purport to estimate the submerged portion of that iceberg, the covert responses. While no one of them is entirely adequate, they at least represent an attempt to measure the extent of this aspect of severity and they have been widely used.

The first of these, by Erickson (1969), consists of an *Adjective Check List* (ACL) and a *Severity Scale* (SS). Examples of these are given below. In the ACL, the items checked with an asterisk are those which significantly differentiated the more severe stutterers from those less severe.

ERICKSON ADJECTIVE CHECK LIST

Please check (√) the words in this list which best describe your characteristic feelings or behavior while you are talking with other persons in social conversation situations. Check as many or as few as seem appropriate.

*__Sensitive	__Spontaneous	__Modest	__Eager
__Aggressive	__Thoughtful	__Fearful	__Secure
__Boisterous	__Irritable	*__Awkward	__Comfortable
__Domineering	*__Short-spoken	__Lively	__Calm
__Extroverted	__Argumentative	__Indifferent	__Expressive
__Forward	*__Insecure	__Responsive	*__Nervous
__Cheerful	*__Introverted	*__Uneasy	__Restless
*__Tense	__Passive	__Jovial	__Hostile
__Boastful	__Poised	__Aloof	__Talkative

The Erickson instruments have been widely used and their reliability and validity were investigated by Andrews and Cutler (1974) who found that in general they were useful instruments for initial diagnosis but of less value in evaluating changes as the result of therapy. By deleting certain items, a shorter 24-item scale provided a more reliable and valid measurements of change in stutterers' attitudes toward communication.

Another instrument is the *Perceptions of Stuttering Inventory* devised by Rothenberg (1963) and Woolf (1967). Its abbreviation is PSI which should not be confused with the Palmar Sweat Index. This PSI consists of a 60-item battery of behavioral statements concerning struggle, avoidance, and expectancy, and the stutterer is asked to check those that are characteristic or not characteristic of his own stuttering problem. On the basis of the scores, profiles of tendencies are constructed which can be used to assess degrees of severity in the different dimensions and also therapeutic progress.

The PSI has also been widely used, not only in this country but abroad. Some questions as to its reliability and validity, at least in the Norwegian version, have been raised by Gimming (1979).

Lanyon (1967) also devised a severity of stuttering (SS) pencil and paper test, using groups of mild and severe stutterers and normal speaking controls to validate certain differentiating statements such as those provided in the following sample:

THE STUTTERING SEVERITY (SS) SCALE, WITH
DIRECTIONS FOR SCORING INDICATED IN PARENTHESIS

Read each of the following statements. Decide whether each is true or false as applied to you. If a statement is true, or mostly true, as applied to you, cross out the letter T for that statement. If a statement is false, or not usually true, as applied to you, cross out the letter F.
Make an answer to every statement, even though some of them seem not to apply to you. [These are samples from the test.]

1. When I talk I often become short of breath. (T)
2. When I have a hard time talking, I tend to look away from my listener. (T)
3. I am sensitive about my speech problem. (T)
4. I worry about the fact that I stutter. (T)
5. If I want to, I can be very fluent. (F)
6. There is something wrong with my speech. (T)
7. When I can't say a word, there are little tricks I can use to help me. (T)
8. People notice that I talk differently. (T)
9. I avoid meeting some people because I'm afraid I might stutter. (T)
10. If I did not stutter, I would probably speak much more than I do. (T)

These instruments are useful to the practicing clinician in many ways, but we would hate to have to rely on them alone without any personal observation of the stutterer in action. We once had someone else get the scores on all three of these scales for five stutterers whom we knew, and then we tried to identify them blindly but missed on every one. Someday we will have good measures of stuttering severity. These are the best we have today.

SUBJECTIVE SEVERITY

In the conclusions to her study of the severity of stuttering, Aron (1967) makes this remarkable statement: "The clinical impression that stutterers are poor judges of their own speech performance was borne out by the results of this study." She asked stutterers to rate the severity of their own stuttering immediately after they had read a passage, and again 30 minutes later when listening to the recordings. She found that the stutterers' self-ratings did not correlate very highly with those of the judges nor with reading rate or frequency counts. What is more significant, when the stutterers were asked to compare their performance during testing with the general severity of their stuttering for the same day prior to the experiment, the correlations were insignificant (.04–.32). From the experimenter's point of view, the stutterers were poor judges of their own severity, but it is also possible that, from the stutterers' point of view, the experimenter was the one making errors in judgment, no matter how objective her measures of frequency, word rate, or other data. Only the person with a bellyache knows how much it hurts. Aron recognized this point of view, stating that "the stutterer's feelings about his own performance should be viewed as a separate entity when comparing ratings and assessments of stuttering behavior." To cite just one of many similar observations in the literature, Naylor (1953) found no statistically significant relationship between his judges' evaluations of the severity of recorded samples of stuttering and the judgments of the stutterers who had recorded them. Indeed, they differed widely.

The clinician cannot afford to ignore the stutterer's subjective assessment of severity. For one thing it cannot be measured by the same yardstick at different times. In conditions where there is little time pressure for utterance, a moment of stuttering three or four seconds long would seem to the stutterer as being much less severe than a two-second blocking while trying to shout a warning to a child starting to cross a street in heavy traffic. Among familiar friends in casual conversation, ten moments of stuttering will seem less severe than three when answering a prospective employer's question, or than two while saying "I do" when getting married. Any clinician who thinks he can deny the validity of the stutterer's severity estimate is asking for resistance. Early in therapy, it is useful to ascertain the discrepancies between the stutterer's severity scale and our own. One way we do this is to sample enough of his moments of stuttering and ask him after each whether he would judge it to be more severe or less severe than his usual stuttering *in that particular speaking situation*. Later we ask him to demonstrate what he would consider a very severe, a severe, an average, or a mild "blocking," or we do the demonstrating. Through this exploration, we can get some crude idea of his internalized severity scale.

One should also recognize that during the course of therapy, the stutterer's severity yardsticks get shorter. One of our severe stutterers hardly recognized any three- or four-syllable repetition as a real moment of stuttering when he first came to us, for most of his difficulties consisted of very long (10–32 syllable) "runaways." Once he got in one of these reverberatory stutterings, he would yammer away almost endlessly before finally being able to continue. The little ones didn't count. However, four months later, he had improved so much that he would evaluate that same four-syllable repetition as being very severe. Clinicians often wonder why stutterers fail to recognize the very evident improvement they have made. They remain discouraged despite progress because their internal scales of severity have shrunk. It is for this reason that we always try to get audio- or videotapes at the beginning of therapy so that we can repeatedly show the stutterer his changes in severity.

Another observation should be of value to the beginning therapist. Stutterers do not base their subjective severity scales on oral reading but on live communication under pressure. Charting frequency counts or reading times at intervals during therapy will be considered by most stutterers a rather meaningless exercise. If they like you they will be polite, but their guts will cry nonsense. To them, oral reading in the laboratory or therapy room is only a remote and unreasonable facsimile of living speech.

REVIEW OF THE RESEARCH

Ratings of Severity

In this review, we will necessarily have to cover some studies already reported. Lewis and Sherman (1951) were the first to devise a scale based on listener judgment of recorded samples of stuttering. It had face validity and sufficient reliability for research purposes when applied with groups of judges. Sherman (1955) used a nine step scale of equal-appearing intervals composed of three-minute samples, each one rated at ten second intervals and concluded that a single judge could evaluate their severity with some reliability but that this reliability did not improve with training. Earlier, Sherman (1952) had discovered that five-minute samples could be rated with some reliability by a single judge. The reliability problem has been a difficult one, and it is even more troublesome when less objective scales are used. Also Sherman and McDermott (1958) found that different judges gave different ratings although a single judge could be consistent in his own ratings whether the sample included five, ten, fifteen, or twenty moments of stuttering.

Berry and Silverman (1972) reevaluated the Lewis and Sherman scale of severity and discovered that the intervals used were not equal as claimed, that the lower three intervals were much narrower than the upper three.

Cullinan, Prather, and Williams (1963) compared ratings of severity on four-, five-, eight- and ten-point scales, using different instructions. They found that the reliability of the rating scale was not good enough to use in individual prediction, even when a judge used his own standard sample as a yardstick (direct magnitude estimation). A group of judges, however, using several judgments of the same sample, can achieve reliable mean scale values. All these studies used tape-recorded samples. Young (1961) showed that the relationship between Iowa Scale ratings and the frequency of stuttering (or the total time taken to read a standard passage) is not high enough to justify the use of the scale values instead of frequency counts or speaking time measures. Martin (1965) found that direct magnitude estimation scaling judgments could yield fairly stable judgments of severity if a large group of judges were used but not otherwise. Trotter and Kools (1955) had a group of judges listen to the *same* samples of recorded stuttering three times and then rate them in severity. Their mean scale values of severity decreased with each new listening session. They caution that this tendency may affect a clinician's estimation of progress. The stutterer may not really be improving. Aron (1967) did a very careful study of various measures of severity. She found that it was possible to make reliable ratings with a nine-point scale and recorded samples. The experimenter's three separate severity ratings of the same reading passages were highly correlated with each other (.93 to .98). Since her ratings agreed well with those of five other judges she felt they had validity.

Hoops and Wilkinson (1973), using three groups of judges (teachers, speech pathology students, and other students), and a nine-point scale of severity found poor reliability in judgments of severity for half of the taped stuttering samples. An interesting attempt to correlate scale values of stuttering severity with eight physiological variables including heart rate, skin conductance, EMG activity and others was performed by Myers (1978). She found that "different subjects have different physiological variables that best correlate with the severity of their stuttering."

In rating the severity of individual moments of stuttering on single words, Spielberger (1956) procured a test-retest correlation of .85. Sherman and McDermott (1958) showed that a single judge could rate the severity of stuttering on single words with fair reliability, but that other observers would not give similar scale values on the same single words. Trotter (1953) found that the rated severity of a word was related to its phonemic, grammatical, and positional features.

Much research and clinical observation indicate that judgments of severity based on oral reading alone are far from representative. Harris (1942), Dixon (1947), Cohen (1952), and many others have shown that marked discrepancies in severity occur between oral reading and spontaneous speech. Most recently, Aron (1967) found a "marked disparity" between her ratings of the oral reading and the spontaneous conversation of her stutterers.

Since most of the studies have used judgments of audio-recorded samples, some distortion may have been introduced by the inclusion of the visible behaviors so prominent in severe stutterers. Tuthill (1946) and Moller (1957) found no differences in rated severity by judges who both saw and heard the subjects and those who only heard the tape-recordings of the stutterers. Luper (1959), however, found that his judges rated movies of stuttering samples as more severe when run silently than when the same samples were shown with sound. Williams, Wark, and Minifie (1963) found that audio samples and combined audiovisual samples were judged similarly either on rating scale values or frequency counts. Martin (1965) showed that groups of speech clinicians, stutterers, and naive students all rated audiovisual samples of stuttering as higher in severity than they did when listening to the same samples by audio-recordings alone. It is possible that some of the discrepancy here may be due to different kinds of stuttering behaviors. Generally, although audio-recordings are probably satisfactory, the combined audiovisual samples are more useful in clinical practice.

Frequency of Stuttering Moments

Frequency counts have been used for years as a gross measure of severity, and they serve as the basic measure of progress in operant conditioning methods of therapy. Certainly, if no moments of stuttering occurred, the severity would be nil. The relationship between frequency and listener judgments of severity, however, is not as high as might be expected. The following table presents the correlations between frequency counts and ratings of severity from six studies:

Study	Correlation
Shulman (1945)	.57
Sherman and Trotter (1956)	.61
Rousey (1958)	.51
Young (1961)	.76 (part word disfluencies)
Young (1961)*	.83 (prolonged sounds)
Aron (1967)	.46 to .71

Much variability in frequency counts occurs between reading and spontaneous speaking tasks. Sander (1961) discovered that, on the average, his stutterers stuttered on about 19 per cent of their words in spontaneous speaking but only on about 10 per cent in oral reading. The large standard deviations, however, demonstrated that a wide range of individual frequency counts was involved. Young (1961) found that his stutterers had a mean frequency count (also with wide variations) of 13 per cent for spontaneous speaking. Frequency norms expressed in deciles for oral reading and two Job Tasks are provided by Johnson, Darley, and Spriestersbach (1963). Frequency, however, is not the sole measure of severity as indicated by the findings of Berlin and Berlin (1964), who presented simulated samples of stuttering which were identical in frequency but differed in form. Listeners to these different kinds of stuttering judged them as differing in severity. Also, Cullinan (1963), found that frequency counts were not sufficiently stable from day to day to serve as adequate measures.

Rate of Utterance as a Measure of Duration

Since stuttering interrupts the forward flow of speech, it is not surprising to find that much research has focussed on the rate of speaking or oral reading as expressed usually in words per minute.** Pittelman (1942) and Roberts (1949) were among the first to try to verify this measure. Pittelman used passages that differed in emotionality. Stutterers read more slowly than inferior speakers or normal speakers on both types of materials, and all groups read the emotional passage more slowly than the nonemotional one. Roberts used adaptation reading of the same passage by both her stutterers and a control group and also measured total phonation times as well as reading times. She found, as did Pittelman, that stutterers read a passage slower than the normal speakers but more swiftly with each successive reading. What this indicates, of course, is that the frequency and/or duration of the stutterer's repetitions and voiced prolongations decreased as adaptation occurred. Meyer (1944) found that generally the

---

* In this connection, Prins and Lohr (1968) found that prolongations of sounds were the behaviors most highly correlated with other measures of severity.

** Minifee and Cooker (1964) concluded that counting syllables rather than words was a better measure since on polysyllabic words, stutterers could stutter more than once.

reading rate could be used as a crude index of severity. Bloodstein (1944) discovered that stutterers read more slowly than normal speakers not only for the whole passage but also for those segments of the passage on which they were fluent. Johnson and Colley (1945) found that frequency and duration were not highly related. Dixon (1947) revealed that, in adaptation readings, the reading times decreased proportionately with the decrease in numbers of stutterings. Liebman (1956) and Quarrington (1959) showed that test-retests of reading times correlated only about .69, thus indicating that such measures of severity were of small clinical use. Cullinan (1963) found the same thing, reporting that the overall reading rate was not stable enough to represent an individual stutterer's behavior.

Some of the more recent investigations have shown a positive relationship between reading and speaking times and other measures of severity. These may be summarized as follows:

Study		Correlation
Young (1961)	Speaking rate and frequency	.59
Sander (1961)	Speaking rate and frequency	.81
Bloodstein (1944)	Reading rate and frequency	.88
Young (1961)	Reading rate and frequency	.68
Sander (1961)	Reading rate and frequency	.86
Aron (1967)	Reading rate and frequency	.64 to .70
Young (1961)	Reading rate and scale judgments	.68
Aron (1967)	Reading rate and scale judgments	.72 to .88

Boehmler (1966) approached the matter differently in a pilot study. He measured the duration of silences and pause times for stutterers and normal speakers. The more severe stutterers showed more silent pauses and in different places than the less severe ones or the normal speakers. Mahl and Schultze (1964) summarize a series of studies related to silent pauses and other hesitation phenomena as a measure of anxiety in the speech of psychoneurotics and other individuals with emotional problems. In general they feel that such behaviors can be used to measure severity of emotional disorders.

Adaptation and Consistency as Measures of Severity

Johnson and Brown (1935) and Shulman (1945) report that the more severe stutterers had greater consistency in the loci of their stuttering. Leibman (1956), like Shulman, found a correlation of about .68 between consistency and severity, but he concluded that his consistency measures were too unreliable to yield accurate results. Tate, Cullinan, and Ahlstrand (1961) showed that of five different ways of measuring adaptation none was reliable or stable enough to use in measuring stuttering performance. Cullinan (1963) found that computing the weighted percentages of adaptation was the best method, but even this had a reliability of only .70. Lanyon (1965) found no significant relationship between this percentage measure of adaptation and the amount of improvement shown by stutterers at Iowa after a year of therapy. He also found that consistency (the tendency for stuttering to occur on the same words) was not related to improvement. Agnello (1966) found that if stuttering occurs on a certain kind of syllable consistently, it tends to be more severe. Leith (1954) points out various difficulties in identifying moments of stuttering in adaptation readings and questions the validity of adaptation measures.

Van Riper and Hull (1955) reported that the more severe stutterers had higher initial scores, higher plateaus, and more gradual rates of adaptation than those of milder stutterers. Luper (1950), however, found no relationship between adaptation rate and severity as judged by observers at the beginning and end of treatment. Brown (1945) suggested that we use word-weight measures of the loci of stuttering as indices of severity. Mild stutterers would require combined cues from position, length, grammatical class, and initial sound before stuttering on a given word; moderate stutterers would require only two or three of these, and severe stutterers only one to precipitate stuttering.

Other Measures of Severity

Froeschels and Rieber (1963) reported that stutterers who could not respond to visual and auditory signals to stop talking during a moment of stuttering were the more difficult cases. They showed greater "imperceptiveness." Ringel and Minifie (1966) found that those stutterers who were less able to make accurate judgments of time (protensity), either in silence or in spontaneous speech or oral reading, were more severe than those who could estimate time more accurately. Electromyography as a measure of the tension of individual moments of stuttering has been investigated by Shrum (1967). Brutten (1963) has suggested that a lack of decrement in palmar sweat measurements during adaptation readings may indicate greater severity. Attitude scales such as the Ammons-Johnson (1944) do not have enough reliability to use clinically except for exploration. The amount of time actually spent in talking each day has been suggested by Johnson, Darley, and Spriestersbach (1963) as a possible measure of severity, and Trotter and Brown (1958) showed that daily talking time increased as a result of therapy from an average of 26 minutes to 44 minutes per day. Naylor (1953) and others showed that the more severe stutterers spoke better under delayed auditory feedback than did the milder ones. Milisen (1938) found that severe stutterers were more able to predict the occurrence of stutterings than were the milder ones. The research of Leith (1954) suggests that the use of phonation time ratios and measures of pitch variability might be used to get some estimate of blockage and spontaneity.

Eventually we may have a battery of evaluative measures for severity which combine a few or many of these various factors. Young (1961) and Soderberg (1962) have suggested such a battery. Young even attempted to achieve a regression equation which would combine several factors but felt that it was not applicable to individual diagnosis.

BIBLIOGRAPHY

AGNELLO, J. G. 1966. Some acoustic and pause characteristics of nonfluencies in the speech of stutterers. Technical Report National Institute of Mental Health, Grant No. 11067–01.

AMMONS, R., AND W. JOHNSON. 1944. Studies in the psychology of stuttering: the construction and association of a test of attitude toward stuttering. *Journal of Speech Disorders* 9: 39–49.

ANDREWS, G. AND J. CUTLER. 1974. Stuttering therapy: the relationship between changes in symptom level and attitudes. *Journal of Speech and Hearing Disorders* 39: 312–19.

ARON, M. L. 1967. The relationships between measurements of stuttering behavior. *Journal of the South African Logopedic Society* 14: 15–34.

BAR, A. 1967. Effects of listening instructions on attention to manner and content of stutterers' speech. *Journal of Speech and Hearing Research* 10: 87–92.

BARR, W. 1940. A quantitative study of the specific phenomena observed in stuttering. *Journal of Speech Disorders* 5: 277–80.

BERLIN, S. AND C. BERLIN. 1964. Acceptability of stuttering control patterns. *Journal of Speech and Hearing Disorders* 29: 436–41.

BERRY, R. C. AND F. H. SILVERMAN. 1972. Equality of intervals on the Lewis-Sherman scale of stuttering severity. *Journal of Speech and Hearing Research* 15: 185–88.

BLOODSTEIN, O. 1944. The relationship between oral reading rate and severity of stuttering. *Journal of Speech Disorders* 9: 161–78.

BOBERG, E., P. HOWIE AND L. WOODS. 1979. Maintenance of fluency: a review. *Journal of Fluency Disorders* 4: 93–116.

———— AND L. SAWYER. 1977. The maintenance of fluency following intensive therapy. *Human Communication* 2: 21–28.

BOEHMLER, R. 1966. A normative study of durational distributions of speech and silence intervals during oral reading. Convention address, ASHA.

————. 1954. A quantitative study of the extensional definition of stuttering with special reference to the audible designata. *Speech Monographs* 21: 205 (abstract).

————. 1958. Listener responses to nonfluencies. *Journal of Speech and Hearing Research* 1: 132–41.

BROWN, S. F. 1945. The loci of stuttering in the speech sequence. *Journal of Speech Disorders* 10: 181–92.

BRUTTEN, E. J. 1963. Palmar sweat investigation of disfluency and expectancy adaptation. *Journal of Speech and Hearing Research* 6: 40–48.

————. 1973. Behavior assessment and the strategy of therapy. In *Neurolinguistic Approaches to Stuttering*, eds., Y. Le Brun and R. Hoops. The Hague: Mouton.

————. 1975. Stuttering: topography, assessment and behavior change strategies. In *Stuttering: A Second Symposium*, ed. J. Eisenson. New York: Harper and Row.

CLARK, R. M. AND F. P. MURRAY. 1962. The use of the self-concept as an adjunct to diagnosis and therapy. In *The Psychotherapy of Stuttering*, ed. D. A. Barbara. Springfield, Ill.: Thomas.

COHEN, E. 1952. A comparison of oral and spontaneous speech of stutterers with special reference to the adaptation and consistency effects. Doctoral dissertation, State University of Iowa.

CULLINAN, W. L. 1963. Stability of consistency measures in stuttering. *Journal of Speech and Hearing Research* 6: 134–38.

———, E. M. PRATHER AND D. E. WILLIAMS. 1963. Comparison of procedures for scaling severity of stuttering. *Journal of Speech and Hearing Research* 6: 187–94.

DIXON, C. 1947. The amount and rate of adaptation of stuttering in different oral reading situations. Masters thesis, State University of Iowa.

EMERICK, L. L. 1960. Extensional definition and attitude toward stuttering. *Journal of Speech and Hearing Research* 3: 181–86.

ERICKSON, R. L. 1969. Assessing communication attitudes among stutterers. *Journal of Speech and Hearing Research* 12: 711–24.

FIBIGER, S. 1977. Quantitative electromyographic evaluation of stuttering severity by means of description of the course of muscle activity in connection with labial stop consonants. *Proceedings XVII Congress of Logopedics and Phoniatrics.* Interlaken.

FROESCHELS, E. AND R. W. RIEBER. 1963. The problem of auditory and visual impercivity in stutterers. *Folia Phoniatrica* 15: 15–20.

GIMMING, O. 1979. A report on the test-retest reliability of the perceptions of stuttering inventory. *Nordisk Tidskrift for Logopedie og Foniatrie* 4: 33–40.

GREGORY, H. 1968a. A clinical failure: Fred. In *Stuttering: Successes and Failures in Therapy,* ed. H. Luper. Memphis: Speech Foundation of America.

———. 1968b. A clinical success: Cora. In *Stuttering: Successes and Failures in Therapy,* ed. H. Luper. Memphis: Speech Foundation of America.

———. 1972. An assessment of the results of stuttering therapy. *Journal of Communication Disorders* 5: 320–24.

———. 1970. *Stuttering: differential evaluation and therapy.* Indianapolis: Bobbs-Merrill.

HARRIS, W. E. 1942. A study of the transfer of the adaptation effect in stuttering. *Journal of Speech Disorders* 7: 209–21.

HEGDE, M. N. 1978. Fluency and fluency disorders: their definition, measurement and modification. *Journal of Fluency Disorders* 3: 51–71.

HIRSCHBERG, J., E. KOVAKS AND S. SVABO. 1965. Meteopathological observations of stuttering persons, *De Therapie Vocis et Loquellae* 2: 357–58.

HOOD, S. B. 1974. Clinical assessment of the moment of stuttering. *Journal of Fluency Disorders* 1: 11–34.

HOOPS, R. AND P. WILKINSON. 1973. Group ratings of stuttering severity. In *Neurolinguistic Approaches to Stuttering,* eds. Y. Le Brun and R. Hoops. The Hague: Mouton.

INGHAM, R. J. AND G. ANDREWS. 1973. Behavior therapy and stuttering: a review. *Journal of Speech and Hearing Disorders* 38: 405–41.

JANSSEN, P. AND F. KRAAIMANT. 1977. The relation between stuttering and state anxiety. *Proceedings XVII Congress of Logopedics and Phoniatrics.* Copenhagen: 189–97.

JOHNSON, W. 1961. Measurements of oral reading and speaking rate and disfluency of adult male and female stutterers. *Journal of Speech and Hearing Disorders,* Monograph Supplement 7: 1–20.

JOHNSON, E. AND S. F. BROWN. 1935. Stuttering in relation to various speech sounds. *Quarterly Journal of Speech* 21: 481–96.

JOHNSON, W. AND W. COLLEY. 1945. The relationship between frequency and duration of moments of stuttering. *Journal of Speech Disorders* 10: 35–38.

JOHNSON, W., F. L. DARLEY AND D. C. SPRIESTERSBACH. 1963. *Diagnostic Methods in Speech Pathology.* New York: Harper.

KIDD, K. K., R. C. HEIMBUCH, M. A. RECORDS, G. OEHLERT AND R. WEBSTER. 1980. Familial stuttering patterns are not related to one measure of severity. *Journal of Speech and Hearing Research* 23: 527–38.

LANYON, R. I. 1967. The measurement of stuttering severity. *Journal of Speech and Hearing Research* 10: 836–43.

———. 1965. The relationship of adaptation and consistency to improvement in stuttering therapy. *Journal of Speech and Hearing Research* 8: 263–69.

LANYON, R. I., R. J. GOLDSWORTHY AND B. P. LANYON. 1978. Dimensions of stuttering and relationship to psychopathology. *Journal of Fluency Disorders* 3: 108–13.

LEIBMAN, J. 1956. The test-retest reliability of adaptation and consistency scores. Masters thesis, Brooklyn College.

LEITH, W. R. 1954. An investigation of the adaptation phenomenon and certain concomitant voice alterations in stutterers and non-stutterers. *Dissertation Abstracts* 14: 2156–57.

LEWIS, D. AND D. SHERMAN. 1951. Measuring severity of stuttering. *Journal of Speech and Hearing Disorders* 16: 320–26.

LUPER, H. L. 1950. A study of the relationship between stuttering adaptation and improvement during speech therapy. Masters thesis, Ohio State University.

———. 1956. Consistency of stuttering in relation to the goal gradient hypothesis. *Journal of Speech Disorders* 21: 336–42.

———. 1959. Relative severity of stuttering ratings from visual and auditory presentations of the same speech sample. *Southern Speech Journal* 25: 107–14.

MAHL, G. F. AND G. SCHULTZE. 1964. Psychological research in the extra linguistic area. In *Approaches to Semiotics,* ed. T. A. Sebeok. The Hague: Mouton.

MARTIN, R. 1965. Direct magnitude-estimation judgments of stuttering severity using audible and audible-visible speech samples. *Speech Monographs* 32: 169–77.

MEYER, B. C. 1944. Psychology of stuttering: relationship between oral reading rate and severity of stuttering. *Journal of Speech Disorders* 9: 161–73.

MILISEN, R. 1938. Frequency of stuttering with anticipation of stuttering controlled. *Journal of Speech Disorders* 3: 207–14.

———. 1957. Methods of evaluation and diagnosis of speech disorders. In *A Handbook of Speech Pathology,* ed. L. E. Travis. Englewood Cliffs, N.J.: Prentice-Hall.

MINIFEE, F. D. AND H. S. COOKER. 1964. A disfluency index. *Journal of Speech and Hearing Disorders* 29: 189–93.

MOLLER, H. 1957. A preliminary investigation of the effects of secondary characteristics upon judged severity. Masters thesis, Queens College.

MOORE, W. E. 1954. Relations of stuttering in spontaneous speech to speech content and to adaptation. *Journal of Speech and Hearing Disorders* 19: 208–16.

MYERS, F. L. 1978. Relationship between eight physiological variables and severity of stuttering. *Journal of Fluency Disorders* 3: 181–91.

NAYLOR, R. V. 1953. A comparative study of methods of estimating the severity of stuttering. *Journal of Speech and Hearing Disorders* 18: 30–37.

PITTELMAN, R. K. 1942. A comparative study of oral reading rate of superior, normal, and stuttering speakers. Masters thesis, Purdue University.

PITTENGER, K. L. 1940. A study of the duration of temporal intervals between successive moments of stuttering. *Journal of Speech Disorders* 5: 333–41.

PREUS, A. 1981. Attempts at identifying subgroups of stutterers. Doctoral dissertation, University of Oslo Press.

PRINS, D. 1972. Personality, stuttering severity and age. *Journal of Speech and Hearing Research* 15: 148–54.

PRINS, T. D. AND F. E. LOHR. 1968. A study of the behavioral components of stuttered speech. Final Report Project No. 6-2382 Grant No. OEG-3-6-062382-1882. U.S. Department of Health, Education and Welfare.

———. 1972. Behavioral dimensions of stuttered speech. *Journal of Speech and Hearing Research* 15: 61–71.

QUARRINGTON, B. 1956. Cyclic variations in stuttering frequency and severity and some related forms of variation. *Canadian Journal of Psychology* 10: 178–83.

———. 1959. Measures of stuttering adaptation. *Journal of Speech and Hearing Research* 2: 105–12.

RILEY, G. D. 1972. A stuttering severity instrument for children and adults. *Journal of Speech and Hearing Disorders* 37: 314–22.

RILEY, G. D. AND J. RILEY. 1979. A component model for diagnosing and treating children who stutter. *Journal of Fluency Disorders* 4: 279–293.

RINGEL, R. AND F. MINIFIE. 1966. Protensity estimates of stutterers and nonstutterers. *Journal of Speech and Hearing Research* 9: 289–96.

ROBERTS, P. P. 1949. Speech sound time and oral reading time of college stutterers and nonstutterers. Masters thesis, Purdue University.

ROBINSON, F. B. 1968. A clinical failure: Harry. In *Stuttering: Successes and Failures in Therapy*, ed. H. Luper. Memphis: Speech Foundation of America.

ROTHENBERG, L. P. 1967. An exploratory study of adult stutterers' perceptions of their stuttering and their perceptions of the processes and outcomes of stuttering therapy. Quoted in G. Woolf, The assessment of stuttering as struggle, avoidance and expectancy. *British Journal of Disorders of Communication* 2: 158–71.

ROTTER, J. B. AND J. E. RAFFERTY. 1950. *Manual for the Rotter incomplete sentences blank, college form.* New York: Psychological Corporation.

ROUSEY, C. L. 1958. Stuttering severity during prolonged spontaneous speech. *Journal of Speech and Hearing Research* 1: 40–47.

SANDER, E. K. 1961. Reliability of the Iowa speech disfluency test. *Journal of Speech and Hearing Disorders*, Monograph Supplement 7: 21–30.

SHEEHAN, J. G. 1968. A clinical success: Leonard. In *Stuttering: Successes and Failures in Therapy*, ed. H. Luper. Memphis: Speech Foundation of America.

———. 1946. A study of the phenomena of stuttering. Masters thesis, University of Michigan.

———. 1969. Cyclic variation in stuttering. *Journal of Abnormal Psychology* 74: 452–53.

———. 1951. Modification of stuttering through nonreinforcement. *Journal of Abnormal and Social Psychology* 46: 51–63.

———. 1954. Rorschach prognosis in psychotherapy and speech therapy. *Journal of Speech and Hearing Disorders* 19: 217–19.

———. 1970. *Stuttering: research and therapy.* New York: Harper and Row.

SHEEHAN, J. G. AND R. B. VOAS. 1954. Tension patterns during stuttering in relation to conflict, anxiety binding, and reinforcement. *Speech Monographs* 21: 272–79.

SHERMAN, D. 1952. Clinical and experimental use of the iowa scale of severity of stuttering. *Journal of Speech and Hearing Disorders* 17: 316–20.

———. 1955. Reliability and utility of individual ratings of audible characteristics of stuttering. *Journal of Speech and Hearing Disorders* 9: 11–16.

——— AND R. McDERMOTT. 1958. Individual ratings of severity of moments of stuttering. *Journal of Speech and Hearing Research* 1: 61–67.

——— AND W. D. TROTTER. 1956. Correlation between two measures of the severity of stuttering. *Journal of Speech and Hearing Disorders* 21: 426–29.

SHRUM, W. F. 1967. A study of the speaking behavior of stutterers and nonstutterers by means of electromyography. Convention address, ASHA.

SHULMAN, E. A. 1945. A study of certain factors influencing variability of stuttering. Doctoral dissertation, State University of Iowa.

SHUMAK, D. 1955. A speech situation rating sheet for stutterers. In *Stuttering in Children and Adults*, ed. W. Johnson, Minneapolis: University of Minnesota Press.

SILVERMAN, F. H. 1975. How typical is a stutterer's stuttering in a clinical environment? *Perceptual and Motor Skills* 40: 458.

SNIDECOR, J. C. 1955. Tension and facial appearance in stuttering. In *Stuttering in Children and Adults*, ed. W. Johnson. Minneapolis: University of Minnesota Press.

SODERBERG, G. 1962. What is "average" stuttering? *Journal of Speech and Hearing Disorders* 27: 85–86.

SPIELBERGER, C. D. 1956. The effects of stuttering behavior and response set on recognition thresholds. *Journal of Personality* 25: 33–45.

STARBUCK, H. B. 1954. Determination of severity of stuttering and construction of an audio-visual scale. Doctoral dissertation, Purdue University.

TATE, M. W. AND W. L. CULLINAN. 1962. Measurement of consistency of stuttering. *Journal of Speech and Hearing Research* 5: 272–83.

TATE, M. W., W. L. CULLINAN AND A. AHLSTRAND. 1961. Measurement of adaptation in stuttering. *Journal of Speech and Hearing Research* 4: 321–29.

TROTTER, W. D. 1953. A study of the severity of the individual moments of stuttering under the conditions of successive readings of the same material. Doctoral dissertation, State University of Iowa.

TROTTER, W. AND L. BROWN. 1958. Speaking time behavior before and after speech therapy. *Journal of Speech and Hearing Research* 1: 48–51.

TROTTER, W. D. AND J. A. KOOLS. 1955. Listener adaptation to the severity of stuttering. *Journal of Speech and Hearing Disorders* 20: 385–87.

TUTHILL, C. E. 1946. A quantitative study of extensional meaning with special reference to stuttering. *Speech Monographs* 13: 81–98.

VAN RIPER, C. 1968. A clinical success: Don. In *Stuttering: Successes and Failures in Therapy*, ed. H. Luper. Memphis: Speech Foundation of America.

——— AND C. J. HULL. 1955. The quantitative measurement of the effect of certain situations on stuttering. In *Stuttering in Children and Adults*, ed. W. Johnson. Minneapolis: University of Minnesota Press.

——— AND R. MILISEN. 1939. A study of the predicted duration of the stutterer's blocks as related to their actual duration. *Journal of Speech Disorders* 4: 339–45.

WEST, R., M. ANSBERRY AND A. CARR. 1957.   *The rehabilitation of speech.* New York: Harper.

WILLIAMS, D. E., M. WARK AND F. D. MINIFIE. 1963.   Ratings of stuttering by audio, visual, and audiovisual cues. *Journal of Speech and Hearing Research* 6: 91–100.

WOOLF, G. 1967.   The assessment of stuttering as struggle, avoidance, and expectancy. *British Journal of Disorders in Communication* 2: 158–71.

YOUNG, M. A. 1961.   Predicting ratings of severity of stuttering. *Journal of Speech and Hearing Disorders,* Monograph Supplement 7: 31–54.

——— AND E. M. PRATHER. 1962.   Measuring severity of stuttering using short segments of speech. *Journal of Speech and Hearing Research* 5: 256–62.

———. 1970.   Anchoring and sequence effects for the category scaling of stuttering severity. *Journal of Speech and Hearing Research* 13: 360–68.

THE SELF-CONCEPTS OF STUTTERERS 10

We actively dislike the concept of self-concept. The abstraction is very difficult to make meaningful. Since the term *self-concept* has been used very loosely and in so many different ways it is hard to be sure we are really communicating when we use it. Psychological theories of the self have ranged from Moore's (1921) view of the self as the organized sum of all the individual's past experiences to Rogers' (1954) "the self the individual himself perceives, that is, his own attributes, feelings and behavior as observed subjectively and admitted to awareness (p. 85)." Tough old William James (1890) felt that the experience of the self was merely a complex of kinesthetic and organic sensations. Schilder (1950) stressed body image but did not omit the roles of emotion and evaluation in self-perception. With regard to the body image, he writes:

> The image of the human body means the picture of our own body which we form in our mind, that is to say, the way which the body appears to ourselves. These are sensations which are given to us. We see parts of the body surface. We have tactile, thermal, pain impressions. These are sensations which come from the muscles and their sheaths indicating the deformation of the muscle; sensations coming from the innervation of the muscles and sensations coming from the viscera. Beyond that there is the immediate experience that there is a unity of the body, a postural model of the body (p. 11).

Others have emphasized identity, continuity, evaluation, and social relationships as aspects of self-concept. Many writers protest the implication that the self-concept is unitary; they insist that we have as many selves as we have significant relationships. Others have said that we have "real-self" concepts and "ideal-self" concepts. Lowe (1961) reviewed the literature in an article called "Self-Concept: Fact or Artifact?" and came to no definite conclusions. Despite our distaste, however, we devote an entire chapter to the stutterer's self-concepts because there is no other hook on which to hang some very important information. Any therapist must deal with more than the stutterer's speech. Since stutterers have problems of identity, role, body image, and many other similar difficulties, we must try to understand them. We shall try to restrict our use of the term *self-concept* to self-awareness, self-identity, and self-evaluation, a restriction that probably won't restrict us much.

The literature on stuttering contains many statements to the effect that there is a unique "stuttering personality," although none of the various reviews of research have demonstrated that it exists. Nevertheless, although stutterers show a wide variety of personality patterns, perhaps as wide as that in the normal speaking population, there is no doubt that the person who says of himself, "I am a stutterer" formulates his self-concept in a way that implies compulsive deviancy. Such a self statement is almost as potent as a heroin user saying to himself for the first time: "I am an addict." This self-identification as a member of a minority and deviant group has been demonstrated by Zelen, Sheehan, and Bugenthal (1954) and others. As stuttering develops, there comes a time when, as a result of his own communicative frustration and the social rejection he gets from others, the stutterer comes to label himself as such. He finds the label pinned on him over and over again. He is classified and grouped with other people who have trouble talking. With that label, he is given an identity as a deviant. It is a bad moment, one that will be repeated often. Wendell Johnson (1946) puts it vividly:

> It is likely that if you have never been regarded as a stutterer, you can come nowhere near appreciating the uncanny, crushing power of the social disapproval of whatever is regarded as stuttering. It is probably one of the most frightening, perplexing, and demoralizing influences to be found in our culture (p. 458).

Many groups and associations of stutterers, both here and abroad, have been organized to provide opportunities for social interaction and to minimize the deviancy. Few of them have survived very long, however, perhaps because of the stigma that is felt when an overt identification is made that exceeds the relief. Many of the leaders of these groups, usually those with relatively more fluency but high degrees of situation fear, exploit their less fluent fellows by dominating the group meetings. In our experience they also tend to be highly punitive. Despite their loneliness, the severe stutterers soon find the situation intolerable, and unless new members appear the group breaks up. We know of two exceptions, one in Sweden, the Plus Club, and the National Council of Adult Stutterers based in Washington, D.C., which have existed for many years, and there may be others. In contrast to the prolific associations of other deviates, such as those for the blind, crippled, mentally retarded, or hard of hearing, where the deviancy is obvious and always present, stutterers' groups are based on a deviancy that is intermittent, easily disguised, and socially penalized, and the associations tend to be unstable. In this connection French (1966) writes:

> The fact is, and it is an important one, that stammerers cannot stand each other's company. For them there can be no equivalent of the invalid car rally [or] the homosexual bar. . . . Stammerers do not need each other—on the contrary, as I have mentioned before, they seek out and admire the fluent, as Moses was told by God to use Aaron and as Somerset Maugham needed his smooth, personable Gerald Huxton, his indispensable companion for twenty-five years (p. 74).

Indeed, the stutterer feels quite normal except when speaking—and even then provided he is not stuttering. The milder stutterer, as all clinicians soon discover, usually find it very difficult even to look at another stutterer, especially one who stutters severely. Although he classifies himself as a stutterer, he has little pride or comfort in the fact. And his fluent intervals make group identification with other stutterers difficult.

THE BODY IMAGE

At the core of the self-concept is the body image. Here too there is conflict and ambivalence. When silent, the stutterer has no marked difference to reveal his deviancy. When speaking, his facial contortions, abnormal postures, and struggling suddenly present a most abnormal picture, not only to others but to himself. One stutterer, a beautiful girl, said,

> I'd rather be blind or deaf, or have a huge birthmark on my face, or be bald than stutter. Then I would always have the trouble and I could get used to it. I'll never be able to accept a face that only sometimes suddenly jumps around and makes horrible sounds. How can you learn to bear something that comes and goes so erratically?

Another said, "It's like as though my body changes its color. Sometimes it's all right, then suddenly it's black or purple. That's how it feels to stutter."

As Shearer (1961) asserted, conflicting body images may be present in the advanced stutterer. When silent, or when fluent, he looks pretty much like anyone else. Unlike the crippled, the image he presents to others at these times shows no deviancy. It is only when he stutters that he becomes, as one of our cases said, "a monster." It is only then that his deviancy appears.

Body image develops through the evaluations of others, through the adjectives they use and the comments they make about us. One stutterer said that when he was nine years old, a friend of his had said that he looked like a pig when he stuttered. Lip protrusion still occurred on the bilabials, but his body image was more important. "When I stutter I have a snout, not a mouth. I'm repulsive." A Q-Sort investigation, with items culled from a universe pertaining to the body image, would be, in our opinion, very revealing.

We have collected the self-drawings of many stuttering children. Some are quite normal, but there are others with no mouth at all, or with black scribbling where the mouth should be, one with feces-like sausages emerging from the lips, and some with earless heads. Most of the deviations occurred around the mouth, the rest of the body being drawn in the usual fashion. Fitzpatrick (1959) had adult stutterers draw themselves while speaking and also draw a picture of the ideal speaker. Marked differences were found, many of which concerned facial expression. The self-drawings showed clear distortion. The projective drawings in the Wischner (1952) and the Sheehan, Cortese, and Hadley studies (1962), although used in testing other hypotheses, have similar distortions around the mouth regions. According to Schilder (1950), whose work on body image is still the classic, the perception of our own body is focused on the areas around the openings into that body. The tension and spasmodic movements of the mouth experienced by advanced stutterers doubtless play some part in centering an awareness of abnormality in this region.

One must also explain the common finding that many stutterers are unable to describe exactly what their mouths are doing when they stutter. They find it hard to tell you about, or to duplicate, their abnormal mouth behaviors, even immediately after the moment of stuttering. Much training is necessary before they can do so. The perception seems to be couched in terms of affect, of generalized distress. Many stutterers and observers of stuttering have noted the marked dissociation which occurs at the moment of stuttering. A sort of black-out, an imperception, a blotting out of awareness seems to take place at the moment of the stuttering struggle and contortion. One stutterer said, "When I get stuck and my mouth starts jumping around, I slip out of my skin and fly up and sit on a limb until the word finally comes out. Then I return." In very severe stutterers, the dissociation is so extreme as to resemble a psychotic episode. It seems probable that this denial of the body image, even when transitory, must have a profound effect on the integration of the self-concept.

The body is not static, and it is the body image that provides continuity for the body in motion. The stutterer's body image, the essence of his identity, does not provide this continuity. Instead it flip-flops between normality and abnormality, and much of his basic insecurity stems from this inconsistency. Stutterers use various strategies to minimize the distress caused by these shifts in body image. Some of them try to strengthen the normal image by extreme and incessant carefulness in grooming. We have come to dub them "Dr. Jekyll stutterers" for they deny the "Mr. Hyde." Clinicians should see if this strategy is being used before asking a stutterer to watch himself in the mirror or to maintain eye contact with his listeners while stuttering. Such stutterers will resist and sabotage these assignments unless careful desensitization procedures are used first. They find it very difficult to confront their stuttering as a problem. They tend to deny it, to disguise it. They shut their eyes or look away when blocking. They intellectualize about their disorder in abstract terms. They show pronounced avoidance behavior. The clinician must understand that self-confrontation of the stuttering behavior for these persons poses a real threat to the very foundation of their identities. This is not to say that such stutterers should be spared the inevitable confrontation that therapy requires, but the clinician must understand the deep nature of the resistance. As Shearer (1961) writes:

> When confronted by recordings of their own stuttering, they are amazed and horrified. When required to face themselves in front of the mirror and stutter, they show marked reluctance and resistance. One case said that he "felt like Dr. Jekyll suddenly seeing Mr. Hyde" (p. 115).

Other stutterers solve their body image dilemma in the opposite way. They magnify their stuttering moments. They suffer visibly, almost revel in their verbal misery. Written accounts of their discomfort portray a morbidity so extreme as to seem pathological. Old wounds are probed over and over again to renew the ache. When they do pseudostuttering, they overdo it. They exaggerate most unrealistically the negative reactions of their listeners. Indeed, they often watch listeners closely for any hint of rejection. Whenever we find stutterers with good eye contact, we probe for evidence of this suspiciousness. Most of their stuttering behaviors consist of struggle reactions, facial contortions, and interruptor devices. These "Mr. Hyde stutterers" avoid situations more than they do words. They often prefer to be unkempt, even dirty. They resist reassurance by the therapist; their aspiration levels are low. They find it difficult to recognize that the fluent fraction of their speech output may have importance. They minimize their successes and maximize their failures. Their relapses are sudden, severe, and frequent. Again, the clinician must understand this behavior in terms of the body image problem. These stutterers don't want to be torn apart by intermittent fluency.

We are of course describing the extreme cases. Most stutterers are somewhere in between. Also, a given individual may oscillate back and forth along a continuum of self-identifications, and, during therapy, shift from his original position to its opposite. Any stutterer who shifts this way has a more favorable prognosis than one who does not. The therapist's task is to help the stutterer reconcile his two self-images and create an integrated one. Our own solution to this conflict, at the beginning of therapy, has been to promote the image of a fluent stutterer with a tolerable minimum of abnormality when it does occur and an appropriate appreciation of the fluency that always exists and can be facilitated. During therapy, this provides at least a temporary solution to the identity problem.

THE SOCIAL ASPECT

Our self-concepts contain much more than body image. They also include our notion of the way others see us. We construct our personal identities by internalizing the reactions and evaluations of the people who play important parts in our lives—parents, siblings, mates, friends, employers, and fellow workers. What we think we see in the eyes of others often determines what and whom we think we are. We live in a spider web of human relationships and must find our identities therein. Our own part of the web is tugged and distorted by the forces which affect any other part and, alas, we must remember most spider webs contain some spiders.

Much of the stutterer's abnormal speech behavior is based on the evaluations of others and the way he perceives them. If his parents react to his disfluencies with anxiety or rejection, then the stutterer will develop behaviors of avoidance and struggle, indicating that he has accepted their value judgments. If others find him unspeakable, he will soon find it difficult to speak. Conceptions of self emerge from social interaction. Even one's body image is affected by the responses made to it by others as Wright's (1960) review of physical disability has made clear. However, in a larger sense, we also view our identities in terms of our social status as defined by others and in terms of the roles we play in the social groups to which we belong.

THE SOCIAL STATUS OF THE STUTTERER

Since the organization of social groups depends on communication, stuttering impairs a person's ability to find or maintain a satisfying place in a society such as ours. Social status in our culture is determined largely by occupation, education, and evidence of success as measured by wealth and possessions, and by the number of people upon whom the person has claims. Effective communication enhances the achievement of prestige in all of these, and stuttering, when severe, certainly interferes with it.

Many occupations require effective speech, and this fact screens out the stutterer or at least makes his participation very difficult. Any stutterer who wants to teach or be a salesman or a speech therapist must surmount formidable barriers. The vocational choices of stutterers have not been investigated thoroughly but, in general, the evidence indicates that stutterers usually choose vocations in which the lack of fluency will not jeopardize their success. This is not to say that stutterers prefer these occupations. Indeed, as Barbara (1954) maintains, they often see themselves as giants in chains. They dream of perfectionistic verbal achievements (the Demosthenes complex), and often they unrealistically prepare themselves for vocations they are obviously not fitted for. It is true also that a few gifted stutterers with special opportunity and great motivation have managed to attain success in all occupations. One of the most successful salesmen we ever knew was a severe stutterer. "I have an advantage over other salesmen," he said, "The people I contact never forget me. I've learned to put them at ease and sometimes when they get too frustrated by my stuttering they give me a sale just to get rid of me." These exceptions only prove the rule. Many, if not most, stutterers are denied the social status that accompanies the more prestigious occupations and professions.

Social status, of course, is not always determined by wealth or occupation. The Chinese distinguish between two kinds of status: *mien* and *lien*. When they save *mien* (*face*), they preserve the reputation of the family; when they save *lien* (also *face*) they protect their personal integrity and reputation. Both types of status are affected by stuttering. We have worked with both Chinese and Japanese stutterers and found that our major difficulties concerned *mien*. A Chinese stutterer who could not bear to watch his stuttering on videotape or even to listen to it on an audiotape recording said, "Every time I stutter, nineteen generations of ancestors cry out from their graves." A black stutterer said,

> Whenever I stutter, you become whiter and I blacker. Whenever I stutter to a white man, I shame my whole race. If I could only get my race off my back, I could handle my mouth.

The daughter of a millionaire said that she had avoided practically all contact with her "social inferiors" though at considerable cost of effort and ingenuity.

> In my own set, when I stutter, no one flickers an eyelash. We all pretend that nothing has happened. *Noblesse oblige*, you know, and *politesse*, and the old tale of the Emperor's clothes. But when I have talked to clerks while shopping, or even to our chauffeur or yardmen, they stare, or stop what they are doing, or look pityingly and I can't bear it. So I find ways of never talking to anyone out of my class.

A successful business man said,

> If I know I can fire them or buy them, I don't mind my stuttering so much and I don't stutter so hard. I'm on top and they're down under. Don't give a damn what they think. It's my equals that bother me.

The last excerpt illustrates an important point in the status dynamics of stuttering. As Sheehan, Hadley, and Gould (1967) have demonstrated, stutterers usually have more trouble speaking to authority figures or to their superiors than to the people upon whom they have claims. They do not expect as much rejection or penalty from the latter, and the rejection or penalty they do receive is not as meaningful. Many stutterers know this well. They do unwanted favors for others to put them in their debt; on the job, in the family, or in the clinic, they do the dirty work, so that obligations are contracted. We have watched some of them weave complicated webs of potlatch-like claims just so they could gain tolerance if not acceptance for their lack of fluency. Clinicians must always be aware of this tendency and beware of being entangled in the claim web.

SOCIAL IDENTITY AND SOCIAL CONTROL

Self-evaluation depends only partly on social status as determined by family position, occupation, wealth, or claims. It depends also on the attitudes and evaluations of the people who are important to us and with whom we interact daily. Their expectations are powerful forces in shaping our self-concepts, positively or negatively. Not all the people with whom we interact are equally important in this shaping process, but in each life there are always a few special persons and groups whose acceptances, approvals, or rejections are especially significant and potent in determining how we view ourselves.

One of the most important groups of course is the family. A large amount of research, some of it conflicting in its conclusions, has been focused on parental reactions to stuttering. In general, it supports the common belief that parents tend to interpret stuttering as noxious behavior and respond negatively to it. Kinstler (1961) has shown how important covert rejection can be, and the autobiographies of most of our stutterers attest to the traumatic effect of such parental reactions. Stutterers have been rejected, punished, mocked. They have been slapped and made to eat in the kitchen when company came. Their stuttering has provoked family conflicts. Their siblings have bedevilled them. Other stuttering children have been pampered and overprotected, indeed almost encapsulated, by their parents in the effort to spare them social penalty. This may cause other children in the family to feel jealous resentment, which they may show in many different ways. In some families, stuttering is never mentioned or overtly responded to, although the covert negative reactions of the family members are quite obvious. When the stutterer is aware that he stutters, a family conspiracy of silence makes him feel that stuttering is somehow so evil it cannot even be mentioned. These reactions have ill effects on the still plastic self-concepts of those children. They make the child feel abnormal and socially unclean. They make him feel deviant.

Other significant persons and groups are found on the playground and at school. Although the research here is sparse, plenty of anecdotal accounts indicate that teasing, mockery, and rejection are common experiences for the child who stutters. Brook (1957), a British therapist, writes:

> ... stammering is regarded as "socially taboo," "something nasty," or "something that just isn't acceptable." This attitude seems to be common to most countries and must have been handed down from ancient times. It is not merely to be explained away on the basis of sentiments passed on from parents to children. There seems to be something inherent in all of us (perhaps it springs from our racial unconscious) that causes us to view stammering, or the occasion of someone slipping on a banana skin, as something amusing (p. 105).

Stuttering has stimulus value. It is both visible and audible. Since it interferes with school recitations and the social play of children, it calls much unfavorable attention to itself, and few stutterers escape unscathed from the mockery and punishment of their peers. In the schoolroom or on the playground the child is on his own. There are no parents to protect him there; he feels the full force of the social controls against deviancy.

In adolescence, the stutterer's problems redouble. Try as he will to conform to the mores of his peer group in dress, hairdo, and rebellion, he finds it difficult to hold his own in the swift verbal interaction so important for this group. Adolescents are often the clinician's toughest cases. They cannot bear to confront their stuttering deviancy long enough to do anything about it. They resist being singled out. They want the security of peer group affiliation with an intensity which is almost overwhelming.

In adulthood, the important persons and groups are those of sexual partnership, marriage, and vocation. Here, too, the stutterer feels the force of negative evaluation. Often he selects a sexual partner who evaluates his speech with unusual tolerance, one who is impelled, by insecurity or value judgment to seek a spouse who is not a threat.

> I happened by chance to be working with three boys and a girl two years ago, all of whom were about to be married. I was struck by the fact that all four of them maintained that they never stuttered at all with their prospective spouses. Do you suppose they chose spouses with whom they were fluent? Was it that the positive emotion of young love obliterated fear? Or were they evaluating their speech through rose-colored earmolds?

There is little research on the wives or husbands of stutterers, and it would be most interesting to discover their bases for marital choice. A few stutterers, especially those who have been enrolled in a speech clinic, marry other stutterers, but in general, the stutterer seeks a partner who can both accept him and protect him against communicative trauma and stress. We have seen some very good marriages which satisfied these criteria.

THE STIGMA OF STUTTERING

The end result of all these negative reactions from the important people and groups in the life of a stutterer is that he usually comes to conceive of himself not only as an inefficient speaker but as an undesirable and reprehensible one. Society classifies people according to its normative standards of behavior. In communication, a function essential to group cohesiveness, the stutterer violates the norms. His stuttering is an attribute that makes him different from others in an undesirable way. Such a discrediting attribute is what sociologists mean by stigma. It is a negative behavioral valence applied to deviancy by members of a society.

Stuttering, however, is only one of many attributes in a given person. The stutterer may be tall and good-looking or very athletic. He may be a good dancer, a fine writer, a brilliant scientist. All of us have differences, some of which are assets and others liabilities. Others accept us or reject us first on the basis of their own needs in a particular relationship situation, and second on the basis of the algebraic summation of our assets and liabilities. Although stuttering is considered a stigma of sorts, the stutterer may have other attributes that are highly valued by the people he knows, and these attributes permit group acceptance despite the stigma. He might be unable to join the college debate team because of the emphasis this group places on verbal fluency, but he might be readily accepted on the basketball team if he can shoot well enough or is eight feet tall. It should be noted, however, that since most groups maintain their cohesion through communication, the stigma of stuttering requires an inordinate amount of compensatory assets to cancel its effect. The pervasiveness of this stigma often causes the stutterer to accentuate this one feature of his personality so that it colors his whole self-concept. Whatever else he may be, and surely he is many things, he often comes to consider himself first and foremost as a stutterer. He is the Ancient Mariner and stuttering is his albatross.

Once a stutterer defines himself as a stutterer, as belonging to a special category of persons, the new role changes his perceptions in many ways. He is not just a boy, or a son, or an athlete, or a student, or any other of his cluster of roles. The adjective "stuttering" becomes attached to each designation. The stutterer-role permeates and influences all other roles because speech is important in social relationships. It modifies his expectancies of others and of himself. The research on aspiration level indicates that, with certain exceptions, stutterers aspire to levels lower than those of normal speakers, not only in speech but in other goal-setting activities. This is easy to understand when one realizes that the stutterer tries and fails to speak without stuttering hundreds of times each day. The cumulative influence of this repeated failure, and the many avoidances of speaking opportunities has a profound effect on his self-esteem. Helplessness, hopelessness, and worthlessness dominate his life.

When the stutterer assumes the role of stutterer the consequences can

Figure 12.
Self-drawing by a six-year-old boy. "During the time I'm saying it, I feel like a monster. Feel all hot when I stutter. Sometimes feel like I'm going to tip over when I say it that way."

be devastating. Identity problems rear their ugly heads. Pretense, pseu-doidentities, and counterfeit roles are attempted and fail with exposure. Self-alienation, denial, and disavowal take their turn with self-hatred, depression, or fantasies of self-glorification. "If only I didn't stutter . . ." said the giant feeling his chains. "If only I could speak," sang the hermit thrush. Obsessed with the need to protect themselves from hurt, some stutterers withdraw from social interaction to lick their wounds and build the walls that will later imprison them. Or they fasten like leeches to the few of their companions who do not punish them. There are a hundred habitual patterns of behavior which result from assuming the role of stutterer. We cannot mention them all but any competent clinician soon learns to diagnose and assess them carefully.

STIGMA VISIBILITY

Students of physical disability and deformity have a concept we should consider here. It is "visibility." A stigma is assessed according to its degree of visibility or obtrusiveness. Stutterers vary markedly, one from another, in terms of this visibility-audibility concept. One single, long blocking accompanied by bizarre facial contortions, jaw jerks, and limb movements, even though it is followed by five hundred fluently spoken words, constitutes a more "visible" stigma than 50 short prolongations or repeti-tions of a sound spoken without struggle. Stutterers learn this fact very soon and many of them escape from the consequences of their stuttering stigma by complicated rituals of avoidance and by "interiorizing" their stuttering. These interiorized stutterers have been described very vividly by Freund (1935) and Douglass and Quarrington (1952). We asked one such stutterer a question and had to wait minutes before he answered. Not an expression crossed his face. No attempt at speech was visible although a slight straining of the neck muscles indicated that he had heard me. Finally and suddenly he blurted the answer and said, "Oh, that was a long hard one." These interiorized stutterers seem to suffer even more than those whose behavior is overt. They operate communicatively in an incredible state of tension and vigilance. Their long, silent gaps distress not only their listeners but themselves. But they do manage to keep their stuttering stigma fairly invisible and inaudible by using tricks. They are very difficult cases for the clinician to help. It is interesting that Douglass and Quarrington found that the majority of their interiorized stutterers came from families striving for upward mobility. In another interesting article Woods (1978) concluded that in many ways the stigma of the stutterer tended to shape his behavior. He found that clinicians and classroom teachers alike held stereotypes of the stutterer as being nonas-sertive, tense, and insecure. This corroborates similar studies by Woods and Williams (1971, 1976). Because teachers' expectations can become self-fulfilling prophecies, such a finding is worthy of attention.

SOCIAL EVALUATION
AND REACTIONS TO STUTTERING

Quite apart from the personal reactions of others to stuttering, which we have considered earlier, there are a number of stereotyped beliefs about the disorder, and most stutterers come to know them very well. One of these is that the stutterer is nervous, and needs calming. This belief probably comes from the nonfluency that most normal speakers exhibit under emotional stress. Perfect strangers will tell a stutterer to relax, to calm down, to take it easy. Another of these stereotypes is that stuttering is funny. Inevitably, the comic strips and television cartoons have exploited this, much to the suffering of stutterers who fail to see anything humorous about their disorder. Normally speaking children mock their stuttering playmates, call them "stutter-tongue" or sing the old song about K-K-K-Katy. There are many jokes about stuttering, a few of them even appropriate for polite company. There is another stereotype—that the stutterer is a bit insane or crazy. This one is usually reserved for those who show marked facial and bodily contortions. We have seen mothers snatch their children away from conversations with such stutterers. Another is that stuttering is a bad habit, like masturbation or thumb-sucking, which should be punished forthwith lest it continue. Another is that the stutterer is not very bright since he has not even learned to talk. Even babies learn to talk. Normally speaking persons who believe this speak very simply and carefully even to the adult stutterer and always a bit patronizingly. Many of our adult cases report that when they stutter upon asking directions to a bank or shop, the listeners will almost try to take them by the hand and take them there.

To dilute the demeaning impact which such listener reactions can have upon them, many stutterers develop intricate counterreactions. They restrict their social activity to groups that accept them, such as church organizations (or Boy Scouts), where they have the protection of an adult leader, or to clubs where they need take no active verbal part in the proceedings. When bidding for entrance into a new group, they contrive individual relationships with people who can later sponsor their membership without loss of group esteem. Stutterers often reconcile themselves to phantom membership, being present at the gatherings but never participating. Token belongingness is better than none, and they are careful not to run the risk of expulsion by opening their mouths. They become highly adept at scanning and evaluating the amount of group tolerance for their stuttering and do not exceed it.

A stutterer who feels like a marginal member of a social group may work hard at token identification. He may confine his utterance to the automatisms of small talk, or nonpropositional utterance. He often echoes what others have just said, begins to speak only under cover of the noises of their conversation, or uses many gestures and facial expressions to convey an impression of his interested participation. Or he may laugh a lot or even play the clown or fool to allay his hunger for social interaction. Some stutterers gain acceptance because they seem to be such good listeners. Other stutterers, in contrast, may pose as very taciturn individuals, speaking tersely, almost telegraphically, or starting to say something then pretending to think and hastily agreeing with the interlocutor who then finishes the sentence for them.

We have known stutterers who had become very adept in seeking entrance into new groups by mastering what might be called disclosure strategies. Even before they showed any actual stuttering they would, for example, casually or humorously comment upon the fact that they were stutterers. Or after the inadvertent disclosure of their impediment they would say something such as "Well, there I did it again. Thought I could keep from stuttering with you," or "Holy smoke, my tongue sure got tangled on that one, didn't it?" One of them, when asking a prospective employer for a job, would use this gambit: "Sir, could I have ten minutes of your valuable time to have a one minute conversation? I've got to say my name and introduce myself." Others have used a stuttering joke to break the ice and disarm a potential punisher. Others smile calmly after a moment of stuttering and repeat what they have previously said. They know an old truth, that the attitude of their listener is partly determined by the stutterer's own attitude. If the stutterer appears to accept his speaking disability without emotional stress, the odds are that the listener will, too. Stutterers become very skillful at computing odds, at estimating probabilities of listener responses.

LEVEL OF ASPIRATION IN STUTTERERS

One might expect that stutterers with a long history of communicative failure would show lower levels of aspiration if only to protect themselves from further failures. Sheehan and Zelen (1965) state:

> As part of its protective function, the disorder automatically keeps its possessor out of many kinds of dangerous competition. Through the stuttering, certain aspirations must be abandoned which would involve the threat of failure, or threat of success. The boy who feels impelled to follow his father's footsteps in becoming an eloquent lawyer, radio announcer, or community leader is spared the conflicts of successful or unsuccessful strivings in these areas (p. 83).

Using the Rotter Board Test of Aspiration Level, these authors did find that adult stutterers showed lower aspiration levels than the normal speaking controls, setting lower goals for themselves and thus avoiding risk of failure or success.

It has been suggested that these low aspiration levels might also be due to parental attitudes toward the stuttering child, that is that they would not expect or hope for as much achievement as they would if the child were less handicapped. But Goldman and Shames (1964) found instead that parents of older child stutterers made excessively high demands upon them for successful performance. Quarrington, Seligman, and Kosower (1969), however, in a similar study but with younger stutterers found no differences in goal setting by their fathers and actually lower goal setting demands by their mothers. The matter is, therefore, in doubt.

ROLE BEHAVIOR IN STUTTERING

The self-concept may be visually schematized as a mulberry shaped lump. Its core is the body image, but clustering about that center are the various roles assumed by the person. Some of these roles are the most prominent bumps on our mulberry of the self. The outward contours change with time as new roles are acquired and old ones discarded. Our ever-changing social relationships demand that we change our patterns of behavior to fit them. We walk through a series of different social worlds in the course of a life time, each of which makes certain demands, and we adjust our behavior accordingly. We often have to bid for entrance into new groups; our acceptance depends on how well we satisfy the groups' criteria for membership. Stutterers have trouble doing this.

The stutterer does not live, like Kipling's wolf, "by his wild lone." He too, despite his difficulty in communication, must live in a social matrix. We have known a few hermit stutterers but only a few. Most stutterers do what all of us must do, experiment with new roles and shape our behavior in terms of group expectations. The stutterer, however, because of his communicative impediment is subject to narrower limits in his choice of roles than most of us are. Some of the limitations are imposed by others; we hope, for example, that no stutterer serves as a traffic controller for any plane we might take. Some of the limits are self-imposed. We have known boys who refused to join the Boy Scouts because they knew they would stutter in saying the Scout oath or laws, youths who refused to be quarterbacks on football teams because they could not call signals fast enough, men who refused to get married for many reasons, all of which were based on their inability to communicate effectively. There are few social roles that do not require adequate speech. The stutterer soon learns and feels his limitations.

Nevertheless, most stutterers manage to acquire jobs and friends and mates and children, even though their choices (for all but the last of these) are more limited than for normal speakers. They have to work harder, tolerate more initial rejection, or accept a subordinate position in a new group. They must create compensatory assets in order to gain acceptance, and in general learn to live within their communicative limitations. A stutterer, once he has been able to master a new role and to know its satisfactions, often finds that role difficult to abandon, even when the social circumstances make it inappropriate. One stutterer, for example, reported his intense shame when he found himself clowning and laughing while telling a group of his friends that his brother had just been killed in an automobile accident. He had long used humor as a ploy to gain group acceptance. We know a stuttering scientist who spoiled one of our fly-fishing trips on the Gunnison River in Colorado by being unable to talk about anything except nuclear physics, even after he fell into a hole and wet his ears. It is our general impression that the more severe the stuttering, the fewer the roles undertaken. Perseveration in inappropriate social behavior may be largely due to the role rigidity created by stuttering.

At the same time, the stutterer also has a penchant for acting. Despite his difficulty in playing the new roles demanded by society, most stutterers speak more fluently when they escape from their real self-concepts by assuming phony roles. We have known stutterers to pass themselves off as policemen, ministers of the gospel, or visitors from foreign lands, and to be entirely fluent while playing these parts. Some very successful actors and actresses have been severe stutterers except on the stage or screen. Some stutterers are clergymen who are fluent only in the pulpit or in their ministerial robes. By playing roles, these stutterers free themselves temporarily from their histories of stuttering, from their stuttering selves. By altering their language and denying their identities they escape from the control of the self-centered stimuli to which much of their stuttering behavior has been conditioned. However, the jeopardy of possible exposure often creates its own anxiety and this, in turn, more stuttering. Few stutterers are able to play such roles long enough to incorporate them into their real self-concepts.

It is interesting to observe that when some stutterers in an unfamiliar situation, or as a result of therapy, are able to speak very fluently, they experience the same exposure-anxiety as when playing the false roles mentioned earlier. In them, the self-concept has become so colored by stuttering that prolonged and unexpected fluency is experienced as being almost traumatic. A role is a consistent pattern of behavior in a social context. Its use is governed primarily by group expectations. For years the adult stutterer has lived in groups which expected him to stutter and now suddenly he does not. Though relieved, he feels strange. Somehow, the integrity of the self feels threatened by that unexpected fluency. He does not feel like *him*. One stutterer said,

> Thank God! I'm glad that period of false fluency is over and I'm my old stuttering self again. The pressure was getting unbearable. Every new sentence, every new word I spoke, I thought would suddenly come out in the old horrible stuttering way and when they didn't, the pressure grew. I felt like a fake talking so easily and I knew it couldn't last. Odd as it may seem, now that I've relapsed, I feel calmer, more of a piece, even though I'm sorry it's gone.

Clinicians must deal with more than the *speech* of stutterers.

RESEARCH ON SELF-CONCEPT

The research dealing with the self-concepts of stutterers is scanty. An early investigation using questionnaires, interviews, and autobiographies by Johnson (1932) to study the stutterer's personality characteristics showed that wide varieties of personality patterns existed among his subjects. One of the first experiments on the problem, using the Q-Sort technique pioneered in England by Stephenson, was done by Fiedler and Wepman (1951) using ten stutterers (with only six nonstutterers as controls). They found no differences of statistical significance. A more thorough study using the Q-Sort was performed by Nelson (1955). It showed that the self-concepts of stutterers were more closely focused on stuttering than were those of a comparable group of student therapists. The stutterers tended to perceive themselves primarily in terms of their speech, that is, as stutterers. Rahman (1956) also used this technique but compared real and ideal self-concepts of stutterers and their controls, finding some few differences (primarily those dealing with social interaction) in the real self-concepts but very few in ideal self-concepts. Essentially both groups were similar. Clark and Murray (1965) present three case studies showing the use of the Q-Sort and other self-concept measures in diagnosis and prognosis. In another publication, Clark (1965) illustrates the clinical use of the Illinois Index of Self Derogation, a stuttering Behavior Analysis Chart, and the Draw-a-Person test.

Wallen (1973) used the Q-sort technique to ascertain the self concepts of a group of adolescent stutterers. They showed lower actual self-concepts as compared to their ideal self concepts. In Czechoslovakia, Pukacova and Comenius (1973) using the *Taylor Manifest Anxiety Scale* and the *Incomplete Sentences Test* with 74 child stutterers, found that 94 per cent had scores representing low self-esteem.

DO STUTTERERS DIFFER IN PERSONALITY?

As one surveys the many unpleasant social experiences a stutterer undergoes, it might seem that his personality might be shaped thereby and thus deviate from that of a normal speaker. Surprisingly, the research is almost unanimous in agreeing that this does not occur. Sheehan (1970) critically reviewed all the research prior to that time and concluded that "there were no demonstrable differences in personality between stutterers and nonstutterers, child or adult, or between their parents." Bloch and Goodstein (1971) in their review essentially agreed with this statement. Prins (1972) administered the California Test of Personality to 66 stutterers and found no significant personality maladjustment. The one possible exception to these findings is the review by Adams (1969) which found a few differences.

Another method of assessing the self-concepts of stutterers is the W-A-Y ("Who are you?") technique. Subjects are asked to answer this question repeatedly and differently each time. Zelen, Sheehan, and Bugenthal (1954) gave the test to 30 stutterers and 160 nonstutterers, finding some differences. One of the chief of these was in group membership. The stutterers conceived of themselves first as stutterers, and then in terms of other roles. The role-perception of adolescent stutterers was investigated by Buscaglia (1963) using a modified form of the Sarbin-Hardyck Test. He found that the stutterers were less able to perceive their own life roles, and the life roles of others, than were the nonstutterers. He suggested that the differences reflected the social inadequacy of the stutterers. Sheehan and Lyon (1974) criticized the Buscaglia study and, using the same test in its original form, found no differences between stutterers and normal speakers.

Other investigations of self-concept have used body image self-drawings (Clark, 1963; Fitzpatrick, 1959), the semantic differential (Hansen, 1964), and adjective checklists (Redwine, 1959) without yielding any firm conclusions about the self-concepts of stutterers as a group. Rieber (1963) presents a critical review of the general literature on stutterers' self-concepts. Silverman and Zimmer (1979), in addition to giving the California Test of Personality, also administered three semantic differential procedures to a group of adult female stutterers, a control group of male stutterers and another control group of nonstutterers. The female stutterers showed higher levels of self esteem than did the male stutterers or the nonstutterers.

Yairi and Williams (1970) studied the stuttering stereotypes of 127 speech clinicians, finding that 17 of the 26 most often mentioned personality traits of stutterers were undesirable. Similar stereotypes based on an adjective checklist were found by Woods and Williams (1976). Woods (1978), using the semantic differential procedure, demonstrated that both speech clinicians and classroom teachers held unfavorable stereotypes about stutterers in general; that is, stutterers were viewed as being nonassertive, tense, and insecure. Turnbaugh and Guitar (1979) had speech pathologists evaluate stutterers on a personality trait scale and found that they stereotypically ascribed negative personality traits to all stutterers no matter how mild or severe. Fransella (1970) describes the use of Kelley's Personal Construct Theory in the treatment of stutterers and designed a procedure intended to help the stutterer view himself in the role of a fluent speaker. As this view became accepted, the amount of stuttering declined. Many difficulties were reported. "The results of this study appear to put another nail in the coffin of the connection between an inferior personality and stuttering. Once again, persons who stutter do not seem substantially poorer in personality than persons who do not" (Prins, 1972, 132).

BIBLIOGRAPHY

ADAMS, M. R. 1969.   Psychological differences between stutterers and nonstutterers. *Journal of Communication Disorders* 2: 163–70.

BARBARA, D. A. 1954.   *Stuttering: a psychodynamic approach to its understanding and treatment*. New York: Julian.

BATTIN, R. R. 1977.   The M.M.P.I. as an adjunct to evaluation and treatment of the adult stutterer. *Proceedings XVII International Association of Logopedics and Phoniatrics*.

BLOCH, E. L. AND L. D. GOODSTEIN. 1971.   Functional speech disorders: a decade of research. *Journal of Speech and Hearing Disorders* 36: 295–314.

BROOK, F. 1957. *Stammering and its treatment.* London: Pitman.

BUSCAGLIA, L. F. 1963. An experimental study of the Sarbin-Hardyck test as indices of role perception for adolescent stutterers. *Speech Monographs* 30: 243 (abstract).

CLARK, R. M. 1965. Techniques for evaluating the self-concept of stutterers. *De Therapia Vocis et Loquellae* 1: 303–6.

———. 1960. The psychological implications for speech and hearing therapists of the characteristics of infantile thinking and body image. In *Psychological and Psychiatric Aspects of Speech and Hearing*, ed. D. A. Barbara. Springfield, Ill.: Thomas.

———. 1963. The self-concept of stutterers as shown by their drawings. *Journal of the Australian College of Speech Therapy* 13: 52–56.

——— AND F. M. MURRAY. 1965. Alterations in self-concept: a barometer of progress in individuals undergoing therapy for stuttering. In *New Directions in Stuttering*, ed. D. A. Barbara. Springfield, Ill.: Thomas.

DOUGLASS, E. AND B. QUARRINGTON. 1952. The differentiation of interiorized and exteriorized stuttering. *Journal of Speech and Hearing Disorders* 17: 377–85.

EMONDS, P. L. F. 1953–54. Stuttering. *Gawein* 2: 1–17; 43–47.

FIEDLER, F. E. AND J. M. WEPMAN. 1951. An exploratory investigation of the self-concept of stutterers. *Journal of Speech and Hearing Disorders* 16: 110–14.

FITZPATRICK, J. A. 1959. An investigation of the body image in secondary stutterers revealed by self-drawings. Doctoral dissertation, Denver University.

FRANSELLA, F. 1972. *Personal change and reconstruction.* London: Academic Press.

———. 1970. Stuttering: not a symptom but a way of life. *British Journal of Disorders of Communication* 5: 22–29.

FRENCH, P. 1966. The stammerer as hero. *The Encounter* 27: 67–75.

FREUND, H. 1935. Über Inneres Stottern. *Zeitschrift Ohrenheilkunde* 69: 146–48.

GOLDMAN, R. AND G. SHAMES. 1964. A study of goal setting behavior by parents of stutterers and parents of nonstutterers. *Journal of Speech and Hearing Disorders* 29: 192–94.

HANSEN, R. 1964. A study of the self-concepts of stutterers as evaluated by a semantic differential test. Masters thesis, Michigan State University.

HANSON, W. 1961. The self-related concept discrepancies of stutterers. Masters thesis, San Jose State College.

JAMES, W. 1890. *Principles of psychology,* Vol. I. New York: Holt.

JOHNSON, W. 1946. *People in quandaries.* New York: Harper.

———. 1961. *Stuttering and what you can do about it.* Minneapolis: University of Minnesota Press.

———. 1932. The influence of stuttering on the personality. *University of Iowa Studies in Child Welfare* 5: 1–140.

KINSTLER, D. B. 1961. Covert and overt maternal rejection in stuttering. *Journal of Speech and Hearing Disorders* 26: 145–55.

LEMERT, E. M. 1967. *Human deviance, social problems, and social control.* Englewood Cliffs, N.J.: Prentice-Hall.

———. 1951. *Social pathology.* New York: McGraw-Hill.

LOWE, C. M. 1961. The self-concept, fact or artifact? *Psychological Bulletin* 58: 525–36.

LUPER, H. L. 1968. An appraisal of learning theory concepts in understanding and treating stuttering. In *Learning Theory and Stuttering Therapy*, ed. H. H. Gregory. Evanston: Northwestern University Press.

MOORE, J. S. 1921. *The foundations of psychology*. Princeton: Princeton University Press.

MURPHY, A. T. AND R. M. FITZSIMONS. 1960. *Stuttering and personality dynamics*. New York: Ronald.

NELSON, L. 1955. An investigation of the changes in the self-concept of stutterers. Masters thesis, Western Michigan University.

PRINS, D. 1972. Personality, stuttering and age. *Journal of Speech and Hearing Research* 15: 148–54.

PUKACOVA, M. 1973. Psychological characteristics of stuttering children. *Psychologie a Patopsychologia Dietata* (Czecho-Slovakia) 8: 233–38.

QUARRINGTON, B., J. SELIGMAN, AND E. KOWSOWER. 1969. Goal setting behavior by parents of beginning stutterers and parents of nonstuttering children. *Journal of Speech and Hearing Research* 12: 435–442.

QUESAL, R. W. AND K. H. SHANK. 1978. Stutterers and others: a comparison of communication attitudes. *Journal of Fluency Disorders* 3: 247–52.

RAHMAN, P. 1956. The self-concept and ideal self-concept of stutterers as compared with nonstutterers. Masters thesis, Brooklyn College.

REDWINE, G. W. 1959. An experimental study of the relationship between self-concepts of fourth and eighth grade stuttering and nonstuttering boys. *Speech Monographs* 26: 140–41 (abstract).

RIEBER, R. W. 1963. Stuttering and self-concept. *Journal of Psychology* 55: 307–11.

ROGERS, C. B. AND R. F. DIAMOND (eds.). 1954. *Psychotherapy and personality change*. Chicago: University of Chicago Press.

SCHILDER, P. 1950. *The image and appearance of the human body*. New York: International Universities Press.

SHEARER, W. M. 1961. A theoretical consideration of the self-concept and body image in stuttering therapy. *ASHA* 3: 115 (abstract).

SHEEHAN, J. 1954. Self-perception in stuttering. Journal of Clinical Psychology 10: 70–72.

———. 1975. Conflict theory and avoidance reduction therapy. In *Stuttering: A Second Symposium*, ed. J. Eisenson. New York: Harper and Row.

———. 1979. Level of aspiration in female stutterers: changing times. *Journal of Speech and Hearing Disorders* 44: 479–86.

SHEEHAN, J. G., P. CORTESE, AND R. HADLEY. 1962. Guilt, shame, and tension in graphic projections of stuttering. *Journal of Speech and Hearing Disorders* 27: 129–39.

SHEEHAN, J., R. HADLEY, AND E. GOULD. 1967. Impact of authority on stuttering. *Journal of Abnormal Psychology* 72: 290–93.

SHEEHAN, J. G., S. L. ZELEN, AND J. F. T. BUGENTAL. 1954. Self-perception in stuttering. *Journal of Clinical Psychology* 10: 70–72.

SHEEHAN, J. G. AND M. LYON. 1974. Role perception in stuttering. *Journal of Communication Disorders* 7: 113–25.

SILVERMAN, E. M. AND C. H. ZIMMER. 1979. Women who stutter: personality and speech characteristics. *Journal of Speech and Hearing Research* 22: 553–64.

STARKWEATHER, C. W. 1970. Personal communication.

TRAVIS, L. E. 1957. The unspeakable feelings of people with special reference to stuttering. In *Handbook of Speech Pathology*, ed. L. E. Travis. Englewood Cliffs, N.J.: Prentice-Hall.

TURNBAUGH, K. R., B. E. GUITAR, AND P. R. HOFFMAN. 1979. Speech clinicians' attribution of personality traits as a function of stuttering severity. *Journal of Speech and Hearing Research* 22: 37–45.

WALLEN, V. 1973. A study of the self-concepts of adolescent stutterers. *Psychologia* 16: 191–200.

WEDBERG, C. F. 1937. *The stutterer speaks.* Magnolia, Mass.: Expression Company.

WILLIAMS, J. M. 1976. Strangers in our own land. *Hearing and Speech Action* 44: 8–10.

WISCHNER, G. J. 1952. An experimental approach to expectancy and anxiety in stuttering behavior. *Journal of Speech and Hearing Disorders* 17: 139–54.

WOODS, C. L. 1978. Does the stigma shape the stutterer? *Journal of Communication Disorders* 2: 483–88.

——— AND WILLIAMS. 1976. Traits attributed to stuttering and normally fluent males. *Journal of Speech and Hearing Research* 10: 267–78.

———. 1971. Reports of parental attitudes by stuttering and nonstuttering children. *Journal of Speech and Hearing Research* 16: 596–608.

WRIGHT, B. A. 1960. *Physical disability: a psychological approach.* New York: Harper and Row.

YAIRI, E. AND D. E. WILLIAMS. 1971. Reports of parental attitudes by stuttering and nonstuttering children. *Journal of Speech and Hearing Research* 14: 596–604.

———. 1970. Speech clinicians stereotypes of elementary school boys who stutter. *Journal of Communication Disorders* 3: 161–70.

ZELEN, S. L., J. G. SHEEHAN, AND J. F. T. BUGENTHAL. 1954. Self-perceptions in stuttering. *Journal of Clinical Psychology* 10: 70–72.

TYPES OF STUTTERERS 11

In seeking to understand the nature of stuttering, many workers have insisted that its wide variability from person to person can only be explained in terms of different types or subgroups of stutterers. They believe that stuttering is a syndrome, not a unitary disorder, and that the population of stutterers is not homogeneous but includes subgroups which can be differentiated one from another. This concept is not new. It has a very long history and its origins are lost in antiquity, yet we still find many contemporary authors and researchers accepting its explanatory power.

The Russian literature (Becker *et al.*, 1977) is full of references to types of stutterers and we find subgroups often described in European articles and books such as those by Dalton and Hardcastle (1977) in England, Preus (1981) in Norway, and Schmidt (1975) in Germany. In our own country, too, we find exponents of the concept that types of stutterers exist and many of these exponents are researchers who feel they have discovered clusters of subjects among their stutterers. Any idea so tenacious and widely held seems to merit a chapter of its own. Therefore, this chapter will seek to answer the question: Are there indeed subgroups of stutterers, each with its own well-defined and unique features which contrast and differentiate it from other subgroups? If so, many of our theoretical and clinical problems might be resolved.

Over 90 years ago Ssikorski (1889) made a statement which is still echoed today:

> The varieties of stuttering are so many and complex that the person interested in this neurosis must ask himself whether it is a single disorder or a number of disorders which have been grouped together because they have been insufficiently analyzed. The overt behaviors differ so much that it seems almost impossible to compare and classify the symptoms (p. 44).

245

Nevertheless, we must tackle typology with some caution. Kretschmer's (1925) effort to classify human beings into distinct physical types (asthenic, pyknic, etc.) created more problems than it solved, and Sheldon's later typology studies (1954), which correlated endomorphic, ectomorphic, and mesomorphic characteristics with personality traits has been shown by Tyler (1956) and others to be very vulnerable. There is some evidence to support the belief that some individuals tend toward more heightened sympathetic and others toward more parasympathetic arousal in terms of automatic balance and that these "constitutional" differences may be stable (Wenger and Wellington, 1943), but the differences exist on a continuum, and it is difficult to use them meaningfully to yield well-defined types. Typology has found much more support in the European than in the American literature on stuttering, and it is possible that our skepticism has prevented us from recognizing that subgroups of stutterers may actually exist.

Among many others, St. Onge and Calvert (1964) have strongly challenged the assumption that all stutterers are peas from the same pod. In their critical article they wax both vehement and eloquent:

> For example, it appears well within the realm of possibility that a population of dysrhythmic speakers could be found who possess no organic or psychological signs whatever, aside from markedly dysrhythmic speech. We usually do not know how many stutterers have or do not have serious organic or psychogenic signs, because investigators seldom trouble to perform the necessary diagnostic refinements. If some stutterers exist without other signs, perhaps the presence of an idiopathic group could be established. Alternatively, is there a group of stutterers whose pathology is primarily psychic, but in whom the dysrhythmia of speech looms large, and other and possibly more significant psychological signs are subordinated? Is there a psychogenic stutterer without organic signs? Also, is there a predominantly organic stutterer who on careful neurological examination would show many positive signs? The painful fact is that after over 2,000 studies we cannot answer these relatively simple questions with a substantial statement of how stutterers distribute themselves on either the psychological or organic side (p. 164).

But first let us review the literature. Most of it consists of arbitrary classifications based on clinical impressions. Stutterers have been grouped in terms of similar etiologies, similar stuttering behavior patterns, and similar therapeutic problems.

ETIOLOGICAL TYPES

One of the first efforts to distinguish different types of stutterers by their causes was that by Hieronymous Mercurialis (1530–1606). In his book on childhood diseases he describes two distinct stuttering types: *balbuties naturalis*, an organic disorder due to brain hyperexcitability, and *balbuties accidentalis* caused by fright and other emotions and made worse by them.

This dichotomy is still represented today. Very soon, however, the number of subclassifications grew as observers of stuttering found more and more apparent etiologies of stuttering. In his youth, this author translated an ancient and obscure German booklet, now lost, but which intrigued him greatly because it contained 99 different etiological and symptomatic varieties of stuttering, each with a Greek or Latin name. Why couldn't that author have found the hundreth variety if only for purposes of closure? Perhaps it was discovered later by Emerick (1968) who, with tongue in cheek, described a case of "spasmophemia porcus" in which the child began to stutter after his father's pigs got loose in the back seat of an automobile when he was taking them to market. Hunt (1861) lists 21 different etiological types of stuttering including "pneumognathoglosso-cheilomanis," a term that might cause anyone to hesitate. Klencke (1860), a contemporary of Hunt, was more conservative. He listed only five types: nervous, respiratory, constitutional, emotional, and habitual.

The incredible proliferation of types of stuttering finally led to a sensible counterreaction, so that Schulthess (1830) used only three classes: ideopathic (unknown etiology), symptomatic, and sympathetic, and Wyneken (1868) used ideopathic, deuteropathic (result of disease), and symptomatic (result of brain lesions). Throughout the literature we find this same magical triad of typology. (Why must we always classify things in threes?) In the twentieth century, Brill (1923), who defined stuttering as a psychoneurotic symptom, described three types: depressive, psychoneurotic, and psychopathic. Many authors with widely different ideas of the origin and nature of stuttering have found three categories.

MODERN ETIOLOGICAL TYPES

Our forerunners would not be particularly surprised to find typological classifications still popular today. They would feel quite comfortable in the six-fold typology given by Luchsinger and Arnold (1965): (1) The organic and inherited type with a strong cluttering component, (2) symptomatic stuttering in which the disorder reflects the disturbance caused by organic brain lesion, (3) developmental stuttering due to psychological shock or imitation during the speech learning period, (4) physiological stuttering arising from normal nonfluency, (5) traumatic stuttering resulting from great stress such as that produced by combat experience, and (6) hysterical stuttering. Luchsinger and Arnold present this classification without any research evidence, and it is presumably based on clinical impressions and case history material.

Another similar classification is given by Zaliouk and Zaliouk (1965). They examined 58 Israelic stutterers aged 6 to 15 years using a variety of tests and anamnesic inquiries. Though their data are not presented in a form which permits any real evaluation, they concluded that their stutterers fell into six groups, each having a unique and typical profile: tachylalic, spastic dysphonic, delayed language type, poor coordination type, dyslexicdysgraphic type, and psychogenic type. We provide, in the following quotations, sample descriptions of two of their types:

> *Tachylalic stutterers:* The speech pattern of this group was characterized by its excessive rate (5-7 words per second), while other motor patterns were equally very rapid, such as writing, walking, eating, etc. Most tachylalic children had other members of the family with either a similar type of stuttering or at least rapid speech and motor patterns. The speech was typical, mostly the clonic (cluttering) form of stuttering, or blurred speech with arhythmia and generally shallow breathing. Most of these children had extrovert personalities, and were hardly conscious of their speech defect, at least it did not interfere with their social and speaking activities. There were 11 (eleven) such cases. . . *Laterality-Motor Stuttering:* The common symptoms of this group were: lack of motor dominance, ambilaterality, reversed laterality, and poor motor coordination. The stuttering pattern was associated in many cases with other speech defects such as: dyslalias, blurred speech, rhinolalia. There were 7 (seven) such cases (p. 437).

In the Netherlands, Grewel (1960) has devised a most elaborate and detailed set of stuttering subgroups. He says,

> Stuttering is not a unitary disorder. There are different varieties of stuttering and different manifestations termed stuttering. These have different causes, different symptoms, and different courses of development.

Grewel describes a large number of subvarieties of broken speech which are often included in the stuttering category and cites cases representative of many of them. Among these are to be found the developmental form of stuttering (normal child disfluencies); the tachylalic; the cluttering type; a pseudocluttering variety in which auditory perception is impaired; a paraphrasic and paliphemic type in which the person finds difficulty in the encoding of speech; a neurotic variety in which fears of any kind precipitate stuttering behaviors; a type (school stuttering) marked by blockings confined to reading and spelling in the school situation; a pubertal form in which sexual conflicts are reflected in the speech; hysterical stuttering with predominantly oral symptoms; and others. Grewel also distinguishes between these conditions and the broken speech resembling stuttering shown in epilepsy and aphasia or dysarthria. He insists that careful diagnosis should lead to different forms of treatment for the different kinds of problems encountered. Thus for "literal" or "letter" stuttering which he describes as a "remarkable form of neurotic stuttering characterized by loci confined to the first letter of 'bad' or 'filthy' words or the person's own name and by a strong evidence of guilt and shame," Grewel maintains that any speaking exercises would be useless and that psychotherapy would be the treatment of choice.

The book by Becker, Vlassova, Asantiani, Beljakova, and Hey (1977) summarizes the newer typological studies in the Soviet Union, many of which stress pathological brain function as the main characteristic of one type. One of these studies, based on 37 stutterers, found three subgroups:

one with positive brain damage, one with possible brain damage, and a smaller group termed neurotic. The latter were more severe and more resistant to therapy. Another investigation on 152 stutterers found four subgroups: (1) 41 per cent who had suffered brain damage in childhood, (2) 37 per cent with neurotic symptoms, (3) 13 per cent with other psychopathology, and (4) 9 per cent with a slowly developing schizophrenia. The brain injured group had stuttered from the onset of speech; the disorder had progressed slowly and there were cluttering symptoms. The neurotic group was characterized mainly by logophobia with very strong situational and word fears.

A third study by one of the co-authors, Beljakova, using electromyography of the speech musculatures, found that the organic group could be distinguished from the neurotic group by the amount of abnormality in the myograms. The neurotic group had fewer recordings showing abnormalities than did the organic group. The treatment of stuttering advocated by this author differs according to the subgroup classification.

Also in Russia, Amirov (1960) describes only two types of stutterers: excitatory and inhibitory, both based upon Pavlovian conditioning theory. In Austria, Trojan and Weiss (1963) found four types: a neuropathic; a poorly coordinated type; a sensory variety with impaired auditory and kinesthetic perception such as that found in clutterers; and a psychopathological type.

We conclude this section on etiological stuttering types by returning to St. Onge (1963), who tentatively offers a triad of major alternatives to the view that stuttering is a unitary disorder, a position he finds unsupportable. Again the magical number three crops up, but it is perhaps of some interest that the three kinds of stutterers he describes seem to have their common items drawn from all the other collections. St. Onge's three types are as follows: "(a) the stutterer with no organic or psychogenic signs but who is simply phobic about speech; (b) the psychogenic stutterer for whom stuttering is a useful symptom of a larger disorder; and (c) the organic stutterer who is nonfluent because of organicity, or through organicity is unable to tolerate the normal fears associated with speaking." If we weren't all jaundiced by too many memories of the old mountain of nonsense written about stuttering, the fairly good consensus on these three types would be impressive, but we must remember that these typological statements were based on clinical impressions as remembered in arm chairs. They sound reasonable enough, but what real evidence do we have that these types exist or, for that matter, whether any subgroups of stutterers exist?

RESEARCH ON TYPES OF STUTTERING

In most of the research on types of stuttering, the subjects are analyzed to determine the presence or absence of certain phenomena. Usually these investigations consider only a single feature or at most two. For example, Fritzell, Peterson, and Sellden (1965) described two subgroups of children one of which showed paroxysmal EEG activity and the other of which did not. Similarly, Weiss (1967) found a subgroup of stutterers showing evidence of latent tetany and another group that did not. And Zerneri (1965) tested 102 stutterers under DAF and classified as organic all those who showed no disrupting effect of the delay. And Baldan (1965) distinguished subgroups of stutterers in terms of their reactions to motor-facial tests or induced nystagmus. Are these really subgroups? Such findings only show that differences exist among stutterers. One difference is hardly a sufficient criterion by which to distinguish a "type." These observations of differences do, of course, provide the material out of which distinctive clusters of features may yet be distilled to provide a basis for types or for a general syndrome.

In a few experiments the investigators deliberately selected subgroups of stutterers differing on certain designated features and then tested to see if these groups also differed on other related features. Graham and Brumlik (1961), for example, compared the stuttering behaviors of a small subgroup of stutterers known to have epileptiform spike discharges in their EEGs with two other groups, one of which had other abnormal EEGs and the other normal brainwave tracings. Those with the spikes had very mild and infrequent stutterings; those with the other kinds of abnormal EEGs had the most severe stutterings. Some showed no abnormality. The number of subjects was too small to permit any definitive conclusions, and we include the study here only to illustrate a possible methodology for future efforts to determine types. Gregory (1964) pioneered another possible method for defining subgroups. In his investigation of possible neural deficits in the auditory feedback system, he examined the performance of those subjects who scored lower than the lowest scoring normal speakers on his three basic filtered-speech tests to see if these same individuals also did poorly on tests of diadochokinesis, the Heath Rail-walking Test, the MMPI, etc. He failed to find any positive evidence for the existence of definite subgroups, but his method is interesting. Brankel (1961) suggests that it would also be important to test stutterers on several functions *simultaneously* (breathing, EEGs etc.) if we hope to get the data we need to determine types.

A careful investigation by Hinkle (1971) classified stutterers into three groups on the basis of their dichotic listening scores, which are said to reflect organicity, and then compared their group memberships on a set of twelve other variables including history, type of stuttering, and so on. Differences between three subgroups were shown to be present. Among the factors that distinguished the subgroups were tense versus mild stutterings, repetitive versus fixative behaviors, and severity during reading as compared with spontaneous speech. Hinkle concluded that the dichotic listening score based upon ear preference could be useful as a simple way for determining subgroups.* We have several other researches that seem to show that a subgroup of stutterers may exist whose members show

---

* A discussion of the dichotic research will be found on pp. 341–43.

reversed dominance in the dichotic listening task. The studies by Quinn (1972) and Sommers, Brady, and Moore, (1975) are representative.

Other researchers, too, have tentatively explained their findings as indicating that definite subgroups may exist. Tsunoda and Moriyama (1972) in their DAF test of auditory laterality, and Cohen and Hanson (1975) in their study of auditory-visual integration discovered some evidence of subgroups. In the latter research, for example, a subgroup of their stutterers performed much like nonstutterers who had suffered significant brain damage.

One truly comprehensive investigation of the typology of stutterers was performed by Berlin (1954). Although regrettably it was never published, it is probably the most definitive study that has been done, and it could well serve as a model for the future research which is so needed. At most we can only briefly present a glimpse of this work. Berlin selected three *mutually exclusive* groups of stutterers: those with pronounced family histories, those with definite evidence of brain damage, and those with psychogenic problems as defined by high scores on the MMPI. He then administered a questionnaire covering a large number of items about onset, speech symptoms, illnesses, and home environment, and he also gave the subjects certain tests of laterality and diadochokinesis. Berlin failed to find any hard evidence for the presence of different types, although a slight trend in the data indicated that a familial, perhaps organic, subgroup might be discerned. Berlin's study should be repeated with many other kinds of characteristics (adaptation types, EEG types, responses to masking and DAF, responses to certain drugs, speech characteristics, response to contingent punishment, arousal patterns and the like), and the sample of subjects should not be confined to adult stutterers. A better categorization of the groups and less reliance on questionnaire data would also be necessary.

Another respectable source of data bearing on typology is the study of Andrews and Harris (1964). By submitting their vast amount of data to factorial analysis, they were able to procure four possible factors that seemed to play an important part in the persistence of stuttering: a hereditary familial factor, a history of delayed speech, poor emotional home environment, and a "general lack of capacity to think, talk, and behave" appropriately (whatever that means). Andrews and Harris feel that there are definite subgroups in the population of stutterers and hope that future research will locate and define them.

The most ambitious and careful investigation of subgroups of stutterers was performed in Norway by Preus (1981). Using 100 stutterers and 29 possible predictors of subgroup differences, he subjected the data to sophisticated statistical procedures: the Automatic Interaction Detection (AID) and the Multiple Classification Analysis (MCA). Essentially Preus tentatively identified some eight subgroups of stutterers and made a strong case for designing different forms of therapy for each. One of these subgroups, for example, needed psychotherapy; another, cluttering therapy; another subgroup would be best treated by behavior modification;

another by non-avoidance therapy. Preus makes a plea for more research in this area and for varying the treatment approaches in terms of the stutterer's characteristics. He ends his paper with these words:

> A general conclusion of the study is that it has not been possible to prove the heterogeneity of stuttering in the sense that stuttering should be considered an aggregation of separate disorders that might be differentiated from one another. No *etiological* subgrouping has been substantiated (Preus, 1981, p. 288).

TYPES IN TERMS OF SYMPTOMS

Stuttering has been called a *syndrome*, meaning a set of symptoms that characterize a malady. This medical model may or may not be appropriate to stuttering. Certainly if stuttering is no more than a collection of learned behaviors, as some contend, the term *syndrome* must be stretched considerably. Nevertheless, there seem to be certain clusters of stuttering behaviors that lend themselves to categorization. Probably the most notable of these are found in two dichotomies, the first is divided into clonic and tonic stutterers, and the second into *interiorized* (masked unvocalized, or hidden) and *exteriorized* (vocalized) stutterers. Other symptomatological classes have also been described.

TONIC AND CLONIC STUTTERING

The terms *tonus* and *clonus* come from physiology, *clonus* referring to oscillatory and *tonus* to sustained contraction of muscle. Using these two terms to represent the wide variety of repetitive and fixatory behaviors of stutterers adds little precision to the description, but they have had wide usage, especially in Europe. One of the major difficulties lies in the overlap. Few pure clonic or pure tonic stutterers are to be found. According to Bloodstein (1960), even in young children, where repetitive stuttering behaviors apparently predominate, the presence of prolongations and "tonic blockings" are commonly discerned. In older stutterers, both clonic and tonic behaviors are usually seen in the same individual. Clonic repetitions predominate on stop consonants while tonic fixations occur more on continuants; in some stutterers, however, the reverse is true. Moreover, a moment of stuttering on a single word may include both tonic and clonic components. Finally, even the most tonic of all tonic fixations will show rhythmic alternations of tension in the accompanying tremors, if the latter are examined electromyographically. Is this clonus? Fletcher (1928), discussing tonic and clonic forms of stuttering says, "The fundamental difficulty in each of these cases is precisely the same . . . [any differences in symptoms are] purely incidental and superficial having nothing whatsoever to do with the basic character of this disorder."

Most modern investigators have accepted the impreciseness of the categories. Thus Froeschels (1943) (who did much to make the terms popular and who views tonus as the result of the child's struggle once he comes to believe that speech is difficult) has added the terms *tonoclonus* and *clonotonus* to take care of the varying predominance of the two features. Most of those who have conducted research with clonic and tonic stutterers have had to use the adverbial phrases "predominantly clonic" and "predominantly tonic" in defining their different groups of subjects since they were unable to isolate any pure types.

At any rate, there are four major studies which sought to relate the type of stuttering (tonic or clonic) to personality differences. They are by Matha (1938) in France, and Krugman (1946), Diamond (1953), and Emerick (1966) in the United States. The first three of these investigators failed to use matched controls and had other deficiencies in experimental design and in the interpretation of data, but they all found in general that the tonic stutterers tended to be more withdrawing and sensitive while the clonic ones were more extraverted and outgoing. Emerick's study was designed and controlled better, and he found no differences between his groups in responses to frustration or in goal setting. The sparseness of research, along with the imprecision of criteria, scarcely allows us to feel that clonic and tonic types of stutterers are useful categories. Certainly we should suspect the conclusions of Otsuki (1953) who found tonic stuttering to reflect masculinity and clonic stuttering femininity.

TYPES IN TERMS OF COVERT FEATURES

Several experiments have been designed to discover different types of stutterers with respect to anxiety, hostility, and other emotional aspects of the problem. Krantz (1954) explored 120 adult stutterers with a variety of tests to determine whether subgroups could be found with respect to manifest anxiety, hostility, and rigidity. She was unable to find any and concluded also that stutterers were far from constituting a homogeneous population. Gray and Karmen (1967) used the Palmar Sweat Index as a measure of anxiety during adaptation readings. They felt they had perhaps discovered subgroups of stutterers which differed in frequency of stuttering as related to nonverbal anxiety levels. Something of the same sort was found by Knott, Correll, and Shepherd (1959), who discovered two groups of stutterers whose EEGs differed from each other even more than either one differed from those of normal speakers. These authors attributed the variance to distinct differences in emotionality as reflected in the brainwaves. In England, Renfrew (1952) used Bloodstein's (1949) questionnaire to see if there were different types of stutterers in terms of the situations that evoked the most and least fluency. No discrete types of stutterers were found, and she concluded that "the situations which cause difficulty to each stammerer seem to be entirely individual and linked with his own special problems." This sad survey of the little we know about different patterns of covert features of stuttering certainly does not make us particularly optimistic that any real types of stutterers can be discerned by examining their emotional responses.

Another approach to a typology based on symptoms is found in Robinson's (1964, pp. 100–101) four common patterns of clinical problems shown by advanced stutterers. While he does not hold that these patterns represent all kinds of clinical problems, he feels that they are common ones, and he offers a somewhat different kind of therapy for each. No research has yet determined whether his four types are truly exclusive, but many clinicians feel they have some face validity. His schema is shown in Table 11.1.

Robinson advocates a different kind of treatment for each of the four subgroups of stutterers he classified in terms of overt and covert symptoms and this view is beginning to gain acceptance. Schmidt (1975) suggests using psychotherapy for the neurotic subgroup, a combined stuttering and cluttering therapy for those who show evidence of both disorders, and autosuggestion and direct speech training for the third—the "Hirnorganisches Glottis-Stottern" type. Kjeldsen (1972) describes diagnostic procedures for dividing children who stutter into two groups, one that would need non-avoidance therapy, and the other a different approach.

Eisenson (1975), who has long held that there were two types of stutterers, advocates using psychotherapy for his psychogenetic group but insists that the organic stutterer must learn to accept his stuttering and learn to cope with it. Kopf-Mehnert and Kellner (1974) provide diagnostic profiles of four subgroup classes based on rating scales of overt symptoms, speech fears, situational dependence, and other psychopathological symptoms. They maintain that these profiles permit the use of different forms of treatment according to need. Preus (1977) also advocated different

TABLE 11.1 Four Common Patterns of Clinical Problems

		COMMON AND PROMINENT	RELATIVELY RARE
Pattern I	Overt:	Devices to avoid, hide, disguise, deny, circumlocute. Ritualistic behavior; speech on residual air.	Long uninterrupted prolongations or repetitions or tremors. Facial contortions, "convulsive" movements.
	Covert:	Embarrassment, shame, specific word fears, some guilt.	Frustration, anger, hostility.
Pattern II	Overt:	Struggling, facial contortions, tremors, "convulsive" mannerisms, compulsive stuttering and talking.	Avoidance, postponement, disguise, giving up.
	Covert:	Frustration, anger, aggression, some guilt.	Embarrassment, word or situation fears, anxiety.
Pattern III	Overt:	Hesitancy, retrials, halfhearted attempts, abulia.	Struggle, severe contortions or tremors, disguise rituals.
	Covert:	Anxiety, frustration.	Hostility, guilt.
Pattern IV	Overt:	Weak speech attempts, extended prolongations or silent blocks, abulia.	Aggressive speech attempts, struggle, tremors, facial contortions.
	Covert:	Impotence, helplessness, frustration, low ego strength, guilt, anxiety, suggestibility.	Outwardly expressed hostility.

forms of therapy according to the subgroup to which the stutterer belongs. For example, he feels that behavior modification techniques would be most suitable for stutterers who have frequent overt stutterings but little avoidance or malattitudes; those with a cluttering component should have speech exercises and language training; those with psychopathology should have psychotherapy, and so on.

INTERIORIZED AND EXTERIORIZED STUTTERERS

Another attempt to distinguish types of stutterers in terms of characteristic behavior patterns is based on visibility and audibility. The most familiar of these attempts was that by Douglass and Quarrington (1952) in which, through observation, they differentiated two types of stutterers, the interiorized and exteriorized, in terms of the relative prominence of overt or covert features. According to these authors, the interiorized stutterer is the one who is able to conceal the overt manifestations of the disorder though at the price of constant vigilance, avoidance, and anxiety. This type is said to demonstrate a different course of development and different personality characteristics. The exteriorized stutterer is outgoing and extravertive, and his stuttering abnormality is readily apparent to the listener. No real research has since corroborated these findings of presumed types except for another study by Quarrington and Douglass (1960) and a negative finding by Doust (1956). Quarrington and Douglass compared vocalized and nonvocalized stutterers under one condition in which they were being heard and another in which they were not heard by listeners. They write, "The diagnosis of V (vocalized) or NV (nonvocalized) condition was made by an experienced speech pathologist after observing spontaneous and test-speech behavior of the subjects. Subjects who did not show a marked predominance of NV or V blocks were not included in this investigation." The NV (nonvocalized) stutterers showed a greater reduction of stuttering when they were not being listened to. Doust (1956) had a group of "nonvocalized-interiorized" and a group of "vocalized-exteriorized" stutterers undergo stress by using a breath-holding technique. He found no difference between the groups although they both differed from normals and neurotics. It is our general impression that interiorized-nonvocalized and exteriorized-vocalized forms of stuttering should be regarded not as different basic types but rather as different ways of responding to the same disorder, either because of different learning experiences or because of different personality patterns.

In Japan, Uenishi, Mori, Mizumachi, and Kubomura (1972) found three types of stutterers who responded differently to stress in terms of their maximum blood pressures. The "hesitating" type and the "spastic" type showed great changes in maximum blood pressure under stress; the "blocking" type did not. (We were unable to be sure of the characteristics of the types mentioned but the report indicates that the first two subgroups might be classified as exteriorized and the third subgroup as interiorized stutterers.)

Another attempt to differentiate interiorized from exteriorized stutterers was done by Kroll (1976). Kroll divided 53 adult stutterers into two *a priori* groups of exteriorized and interiorized stutterers, then collected data on eight variables including level of concern, level of awareness, and Rotter's test of locus of control. Using a hierarchial discrimination analysis technique he found three of the variables discriminated the exteriorized from the interiorized stutterers: communicative goals, group affiliation, and level of awareness. The exteriorized stutterer tends to speak freely, forms close relationships with his peer groups, and is highly aware of his stuttering. Interiorized stutterers avoid speaking, associate with persons of superior status, and are relatively unaware of their stuttering. This last finding seems surprising.

DEVELOPMENTAL TYPES

Stutterers have also been classified in groups according to the developmental stages or phases of the disorder. Thus Bluemel (1932) describes two types of stutterers, those having "primary stuttering" and those with "secondary stuttering." Primary stutterers showed only repetitions and prolongations; secondary stutterers were those who avoided certain sounds and words or showed evidences of struggle. Froeschels (1952) distinguished between "physiological stuttering" (normal childhood disfluency), imitative stuttering, and genuine stuttering. Van Riper (1954), unhappy with the classes of primary and secondary stuttering, inserted a third variety, transitional stuttering, to designate those who were aware of their disorder and struggled with it but showed little fear or avoidance. Still later, Bloodstein (1960) provided a fourfold list of phases based upon developmental characteristics. Unfortunately, none of these developmental types were discrete enough to merit their identification as specific subgroups, and the terms are rarely used today.

OTHER DIFFERENTIATING CHARACTERISTICS

Newman (1963) found a subgroup of stutterers who did not show the characteristic adaptation curve and suggested that these might comprise a different type of stutterer. Chevrie-Muller (1963), using glottography, found two groups—one which showed impaired laryngeal functioning and the other which did not. Murray (1966) similarly found two groups of stutterers, those who became fluent under masking and those who did not. Soderberg (1968) reviewed the research on delayed auditory feedback with stutterers and found possible evidence for types of stutterers in terms of their response to the delay. Other studies in this same vein have found marked differences among stutterers in motor coordination, in EEG abnormalities, in response to electronystography or photic stimulation, etc. All that these studies seem to show is that there is a lack of homogeneity in the population of stutterers. However, if different stuttering subtypes exist, it should be possible to tell one from another on more than a single trait or factor. There should at least be clusters of characteristic factors with minimal overlap between clusters. At present most of the research demonstrates only that stutterers differ one from another on one or two factors. There are many hints that subgroups of stutterers may yet be discovered, but at the present time we can only conclude that the typologies of stuttering based on etiology or symptomatology which have been proposed have only minimal supporting evidence.

BIBLIOGRAPHY

AMIROV, R. Z. 1960. Trigeminal, tricomponent method of studying higher nervous activity in man. *Zhurnal Vysshei Nervonoi Deiatel'nosti* 10: 468–72.

ANDREWS, G. AND M. HARRIS. 1964. *The syndrome of stuttering.* London: Heinemann.

BALDAN, G. 1965. Study of the vestibular function in a group of stutterers: electronystagmographic researches. *De Therapia Vocis et Loquellae* 1: 349–51.

BECKER, K. P., N. A. VLASSOVA, N. M. ASATIANI, L. J. BELJAKOVA, AND W. HEY. 1977. *Stottern.* Berlin: VEB Verlag Volk und Gesundheit.

BERLIN, A. J. 1954. An exploratory attempt to isolate types of stuttering. Doctoral dissertation, Northwestern University.

BLOODSTEIN, O. 1949. Conditions under which stuttering is reduced or absent. *Journal of Speech and Hearing Disorders* 14: 295–303.

————. 1960. Development of stuttering. *Journal of Speech and Hearing Disorders* 25: 219–37.

BLUEMEL, C. S. 1932. Primary and secondary stammering. *Quarterly Journal of Speech* 17: 187–200.

BRANKEL, O. 1961. Pneumotachographic studies in stutterers. *Folia Phoniatrica* 13: 136–43.

BRILL, A. A. 1923. Speech disturbances in nervous mental diseases. *Quarterly Journal of Speech* 9: 129–35.

CANTER, G. J. 1971. Observations on neurogenic stuttering. A contribution to differential diagnosis. *British Journal of Communication Disorders* 6: 139–43.

CHEVRIE-MULLER, C. 1963. A study of laryngeal function in stutterers by the glottographic Method. *Proceedings, VII Congrès de la Société Français de Médecine de la Voix et de la Parole,* Paris.

COHEN, M. S. AND M. L. HANSON. 1975. Intersensory processing efficiency of fluent speakers and stutterers. *British Journal of Disorders of Communication* 10: 111–22.

DALTON, P. AND W. J. HARDCASTLE. 1977. *Disorders of fluency.* London: Edward Arnold.

DASKALOV, D. 1962. Basic principles and methods of prevention and treatment of stuttering. *Nevropatologii e Psikhiatrii imeni S.S. Korsakova* 62: 1047–52.

DENHARDT, R. 1890. *Das stottern: eine Psychose.* Leipsig: Ernst Keil's Nachfolger.

DE PARREL, S. 1965. *Speech disorders.* Oxford: Pergamon Press.

DIAMOND, M. 1953. Personality differences between tonic and clonic stutterers. Doctoral dissertation, Syracuse University.

DOSTALOVA, N. AND T. DOSUZKOV. 1965. Über die drei Hauptformen des Neurotische Stotterns, *De Therapia Vocis et Loquellae* 1: 273–76.

DOUGLASS, E. AND B. QUARRINGTON. 1952. Differentiation of interiorized and exteriorized stuttering. *Journal of Speech and Hearing Disorders* 17: 372–88.

DOUST, J. W. L. 1956. Stress and psychopathology in stutterers. *Canadian Journal of Psychology* 10: 31–37.

DUNLOP, E. 1964. The choice of antidepressants in various types of depression. *Psychosomatic Medicine* 5: 107–110.

EISENSON, J. 1975. Stuttering as perseverative behavior. In *Stuttering: A Second Symposium*, ed. J. Eisenson. New York: Harper and Row.

EMERICK, L. L. 1966. A study of psychological traits in tonic and clonic stutterers. Doctoral dissertation, Michigan State University.

————. 1968. A clinical success: Mark. In *Stuttering:Successes and Failures in Therapy*, ed. H. Luper. Memphis: Speech Foundation of America.

FLETCHER, J. M. 1928. *The problem of stuttering*. New York: Longmans Green.

FREUND, H. 1932. Inneres stottern und einstalbewegungen, *Zeitschrift für Neurologie und Psychiatrie* 6: 1243–45.

————. 1966. *Psychopathology and the problems of stuttering*. Springfield, Ill.: Thomas.

FRITZELL, B., I. PETERSON, AND U. SELLDEN. 1965. An EEG study of stuttering and nonstuttering school children. *De Therapia Vocis et Loquellae* 1: 343–46.

FROESCHELS, E. 1943. Pathology and therapy of stuttering. *Nervous Child* 2: 148–61.

————. 1952. The significance of symptomatology for the understanding of the essence of stuttering. *Folia Phoniatrica* 4: 217–30.

GRAHAM, J. K. AND J. BRUMLIK. 1961. Neurologic and encephalographic abnormalities in stuttering and matched nonstuttering adults. *ASHA* 3: 342 (abstract).

GRAY, B. B. AND J. L. KARMEN. 1967. The relationship between nonverbal anxiety and stuttering adaptation. *Journal of Communication Disorders* 1: 141–51.

GREGORY, H. H. 1964. Stuttering and auditory central nervous system disorder. *Journal of Speech and Hearing Research* 7: 335–41.

GREWEL, F. 1960. Balbutiés (Stotteren) *Logopaedie et Foniatrie* 32: 109–15; 125–28; 145–52; 165–68.

HEESE, G. 1973. *Stammen: Behandlung og Forebyggelse*. Copenhagen: Borgens Verlag.

HINKLE, W. G. 1971. A study of subgroups within the stuttering population. Doctoral dissertation, Purdue University.

HUNT, J. 1967. *Stammering and stuttering*. (Original Edition, 1861) Reprinted. New York: Hafner.

KJELDSEN, P. 1972. Stammen–Diagnostik. *Nordische Titschrift for Tale og Stemme* 32: 21–34.

KLENCKE, H. 1860. *Die Heilung des Stotterns*. Leipsig.

KNOTT, J. R. R. E. CORRELL, AND J. N. SHEPHERD. 1959. Frequency analysis of electroencephalograms of stutterers and nonstutterers. *Journal of Speech and Hearing Research* 2: 74–80.

KOCHERGINA, V. S. 1965. Drug treatment of stammering in adults. *Zhurnal Nevropathologii i Psikhiatrii imeni S. S. Korakova* 65: 753–56.

KOPF-MEHNERT, C. AND H. J. KELLNER. 1974. Ein Vierdimensionales Deskriptives Modell fur die Diagnosie und Behandlung Jugendlicher und Erwachsener

Stotternder. In *Proceedings XVI Internation Congress of Logopedics and Phoniatrics.* Basel: Karger.

KRANTZ, J. 1954. A study of the interrelationships among manifest anxiety, manifest hostility, rigidity, duration of severity, and severity of stuttering within a group of stutterers. Masters thesis, Pennsylvania State University.

KRETSCHMER, E. 1925. *Physique and character.* New York: Harcourt.

KROLL, A. 1976. The differentiation of stutterers into interiorized and exteriorized groups. Doctoral dissertation, Purdue University.

———. 1978. The differentiation of stutterers into interiorized and exteriorized groups. In *Proceedings of XVIII International Congress of Logopedics and Phoniatrics,* Copenhagen.

KRUGMAN, M. 1946. Psychosomatic study of fifty stuttering children. *American Journal of Orthopsychiatry* 16: 127–33.

LANDOLT, H. AND R. LUCHSINGER. 1954. Language disorder, stuttering and chronic organic psychosyndrome; electroencephalographic results and studies of pathology of speech. *Deutsche Medizinische Wochenshrift* 79: 1012–15.

LUCHSINGER, R. AND G. E. ARNOLD. 1965. *Voice—speech—language.* Belmont, Cal.: Wadsworth.

MATHA, L. 1936. Demonstration de technique rééducation des troubles psychoneuro-moteurs du type bégaiement tonique. *Revue Française de Phoniatrie* 23: 99–126.

MURRAY, F. P. 1966. The effects of variably presented noise upon the speech of stutterers. Doctoral dissertation, Denver University.

NEWMAN, P. W. 1963. Adaptation performances of individual stutterers: implications for research. *Journal of Speech and Hearing Research* 6: 393–94.

ORTON, S. T. 1937. *Reading, writing, and speech problems of children.* New York: Norton and Co.

OTSUKI, K. 1953. A habit of stuttering. abstract no. 101 in G. Kamiyama, *A Handbook for the Study of Stuttering.* Tokyo: Kongo Shupan, 1967.

PREUS, A. 1981. *Attempts at identifying subgroups of stutterers.* Oslo: University of Oslo Press.

QUARRINGTON, B. AND E. DOUGLASS. 1960. Audibility avoidance in nonvocalized stutterers. *Journal of Speech and Hearing Disorders* 30: 358–65.

QUINN, P. T. 1972. Stuttering, cerebral dominance and the dichotic word test. *Medical Journal of Australia* 2: 639–43.

RENFREW, C. B. 1952. A questionnaire for stutterers. *Speech* (London) 16: 21–24.

ROBINSON, F. B. 1964. *Introduction to stuttering.* Englewood Cliffs, N.J.: Prentice-Hall.

SCHMIDT, H. 1975. Grundformen von Sprechablaufstorungen und Irhe Behandlungskriterien. In *Stottern-Poltern,* eds. K. H. Hahn and H. G. Muller. Hamburg: Wertenberg und Sohne.

SCHULTHESS, R. 1830. *Das Stammeln und Stottern.* Zurich: Hans Borg.

SHAPIRO, A. 1980. An electromyographic analysis of the fluent and dysfluent utterances of several types of stutterers. *Journal of Fluency Disorders* 5: 203–32.

SHELDON, W. H. 1954. *Atlas of men: a guide for somatotyping the adult male at all ages.* New York: Harper.

SODERBERG, G. A. 1968. Delayed auditory feedback and stuttering. *Journal of Speech and Hearing Disorders* 33: 260–67.

SOMMERS, R. K., W. A. BRADY, AND W. R. MOORE. 1975. Dichotic ear preference of stuttering children and adults. *Perceptual and motor skills* 41: 931–38.

SSIKORSKI, J. A. 1889. *Über das Stottern.* Berlin: Hirschwald.

ST. ONGE, K. 1963. The stuttering syndrome. *Journal of Speech and Hearing Research* 6: 195–97.

ST. ONGE, K. AND J. J. CALVERT. 1964. Stuttering research. *Quarterly Journal of Speech* 50: 159–65.

TROJAN, L. AND H. WEISS. 1963. Studien zur Stottertherapie. *Folia Phoniatrica* 15: 42–67.

TSUNODA, T. AND H. MORIYAMA. 1972. Specific pattern of cerebral dominance for various sounds in adult stutterers. *Journal of Auditory Research* 12: 216–227.

TYLER, L. E. 1956. *The psychology of human differences.* 2nd Ed. New York: Appleton-Century.

UENISHI, S., T. MORI, T. MIZUMACHI, AND M. KUBOMURA. 1972. Changes in maximum blood pressure in stutterers. *Psychosomatic Medicine* (Japan) 18: 418–23.

VAN RIPER, C. 1954. *Speech correction: principles and methods.* 3rd ed., Englewood Cliffs, N.J.: Prentice-Hall.

———. 1963. *Speech correction: principles and methods.* 4th ed. Englewood Cliffs, N.J.: Prentice-Hall.

WEISS, B. 1967. Neuromuscular excitability in stutterers. *Folia Phoniatrica* 19: 117–24.

WENGER, M. A. AND M. WELLINGTON. 1943. The measurement of autonomic balance in children: method and normative data. *Psychosomatic Medicine* 5: 241–53.

WOLF, A. A. AND E. G. WOLF. 1959. Feedback processes in the theory of certain speech disorders. *Speech Pathology and Therapy* 2: 48–55.

WYNEKEN, C. 1968. Über das Stottern und dessen Heilung. *Zeitschrift für Rationelle Medicin* 31: 1–29.

ZALIOUK, D. AND A. ZALIOUK. 1965. Stuttering: a differential approach in diagnosis and therapy. *De Therapia Vocis et Loquellae* 1: 437–41.

ZERNERI, L. 1965. Tentative d'applicazione delle voci retardata (DAF) della terapia della bulbuzie. *Bollettino Della Societa Italiana Di Fonetica Fonentria e Audiologia* 19: 125–30.

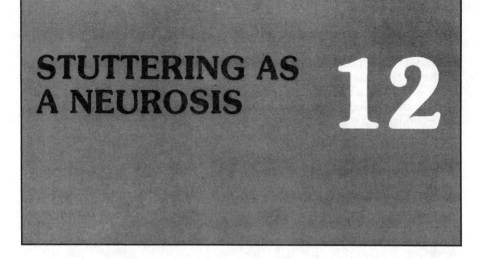

STUTTERING AS A NEUROSIS 12

In reviewing the world literature for the past decade we were surprised to find very few articles or books holding the view that stuttering is of neurotic origin. This contrasts sharply with the literature of previous decades though the number of authors espousing the neurotic origin of stuttering has been steadily declining since the early thirties when the concept had wide acceptance. To our knowledge there have been no new formulations as to the nature of the presumed stuttering neurosis and no experimental evidence to corroborate its existence. We find a few reports of individual stutterers with alleged neurotic etiology and occasional descriptions of the application of different kinds of psychotherapy to stutterers* but it is becoming very evident that most modern workers in the field of speech pathology no longer think of stuttering as a neurosis but instead they view it as either a set of learned behaviors or as an organic or a neuromuscular disorder.

Nevertheless, knowing how the thinking about stuttering has repeatedly changed over the years and often returns to earlier formulations, we feel it important to present the basic information on the neurotic aspects of stuttering. Indeed, to do otherwise would be to ignore some very prominent features of the problem.

A huge amount of the literature on stuttering is devoted to the neurotic aspects of the disorder. However, since many of the authors who consider stuttering a neurosis have divergent opinions about what kind of neurosis it is presumed to be, it is necessary first to clarify what is usually meant by the term. Neurotic behavior usually presents three major characteristics— unpleasant feelings, inability to understand or to accept the feelings, and

---

* Most of these have been reported in foreign journals from India, Japan, and the East European countries.

symptoms or patterns of behavior that symbolize and maintain them. Many adult stutterers fulfill these three criteria of neurosis. Do not forget, however, that most beginning stutterers, and some adult ones, show very marked and deviate speech behaviors without apparently manifesting any of these characteristics. The questions immediately presented are: If stuttering is neurotic in nature, is it a primary neurosis or a secondary one? Is the neurosis the source of the stutterer's difficulties or is it the consequence? Are all stutterers neurotic?

First let us explore the nature of neurotic behavior more closely. For many years, experimental neuroses have been produced in animals. Early in this century Pavlov trained dogs to make discriminations between such stimuli as circles and ellipses. When the differences between these stimuli were gradually reduced to the point where the discrimination was difficult or impossible, the dogs developed maladaptive and persistent behaviors which made them unfit for further conditioning. Since then, many other workers have created similar experimental neuroses. They have been produced in sheep by Liddell (1964) and in cats by Masserman (1943). They have also been deliberately produced in chickens by Watson and Rayner (1920) and by Krasnogorski (1925). The purpose in all these experiments is to set up a conflict between drives or cues so that an overt *adaptive* response could not be accomplished. When no appropriate responses can be made in such a conflict situation, strong autonomic responses occur as evidenced by cardiovascular changes, pupillary dilation, respiratory effects, and a variety of inappropriate motor behaviors. These autonomic responses and maladaptive motor patterns generalized rapidly to other stimuli and, once conditioned, were very difficult to extinguish.

Liddell describes a sheep made neurotic by conditioning:

> Here we see the diffused, agitated pattern of the classical experimental neurosis, continual head movement, bleating, left foreleg overreacting to the metronome. He had been taught to give no reaction to the metronome at 50 beats per minute, but here it shows that he cannot inhibit, and all differentiation between signals for shock and for no shock has been eliminated. The heart beat is irregular, with many premature beats. Moveover the heart of this animal is disturbed in the barn at night. The animal also loses its normal gregariousness and when alarmed by marauding dogs, will not run off with the flock but in another direction, and the neurotic sheep will often be mauled by the dogs (pp. 133–134).

Human neuroses generally have as their core an emotional upheaval of anxiety that seems unrelated to the stimuli which trigger it. All of us know fear and anxiety. When we are threatened by a dangerous situation, the autonomic response of anxiety is adaptive and useful. It is when apprehensiveness occurs in situations which should not normally produce it that we have neurotic anxiety. The symptoms of neuroses, so widely variable, are viewed by many writers as defenses against the distress of this unexplainable and inappropriate anxiety. In behavioral terms, they are nonadjustive habits which are continually reinforced by a temporary anxiety reduction. Mowrer (1950) has discussed neurosis in similar terms. Indeed, he speaks of the "neurotic paradox," wherein behavior which is obviously more punishing than satisfying seems to persist, and behavior which apparently ought to produce desirable consequences is abandoned. His main solution for the paradox is that neurotic behavior makes sense if we consider the timing of the rewards or punishments. If the rewards come later and are greater than the punishment, the maladaptive "neurotic" behavior will continue.

It is obvious that many of the behaviors of confirmed stuttering would fit these descriptions. It is not so clear that the original stuttering presents this picture or that it originates in such conflict situations in the majority of cases. We have studied very carefully the situations in which children began to stutter and have done so very soon after it appeared. A few of them demonstrated very clearly, so clearly that we cannot explain the origin in any other way, that the disorder had its roots in such situations and seemed to be the result of conflict-produced emotion. But this neurotic origin did *not* appear in most of the 44 children we were able to follow from onset to maturity (see Chapter V).

Neurotic anxieties and neurotic behaviors usually arise in conflict situations. Strong incompatible urges or responses compete, and when the conflict cannot be resolved, anxiety is generated. Dollard and Miller (1950) say that "an intense emotional conflict is the necessary basis for neurotic behavior." The suffering that comes from unresolved conflicts impels the person to react in various ways; those coinciding with a decrease in the suffering, however momentary, will tend to persist as neurotic symptoms.

It should also be pointed out that neuroses can also originate in trap situations, those in which the animal or person is repeatedly punished without being able to avoid or escape or react appropriately. For example, Liddell conditioned his sheep to flex its foreleg on the fifth or tenth or fifteenth beat of a metronome by administering the shock at these intervals. However, when he tried to condition them to an interval of 30 beats, the animal became "neurotic." The crucial factor in the production of neurosis may not always be unresolved conflict. It may also be centered in the inability of the animal to respond so as to minimize anticipated punishment. This has been shown by the experiments of Wolpe (1958) in which cats were confined in a cage and subjected to intermittent shocks that they could not escape. These cats demonstrated the same sort of persistent disturbed behaviors (crouching, random clawing, howling, and the autonomic responses of pupillary dilation, hair erection, etc.) which Masserman (1943) had previously termed neurotic and attributed to conflict. Thus, the feeling of helplessness due to communicative frustration may be as important as the ambivalence of conflict in the production of neurotic anxiety, and certainly the stutterer experiences great communicative frustration.

In his own words Coriat (1931) states a psychoanalytic view:

The anxiety in stammerers when they attempt or prepare to speak is not due to anticipation or to anxiety over a specific situation, but is caused by the fear of the ego being overwhelmed by the all-powerful auto-eroticism. This is particularly shown by the fact that stammerers frequently have literal dreams of nursing. Stammering becomes, therefore, a form of gratification of the original oral libido which continues as a post-natal gratification in talking. The confirmed stammerer tenaciously retains his earliest source of pleasure, that is, nursing; he reacts to the original oral binding of the mouth through a repetition compulsion localized in the speech mechanism, that is, in the tongue, lip, and jaw movements of the original physiological nursing mechanism (p. 155).

There are various views of the nature of the neurosis in stuttering. Even the psychoanalytic interpretations differ. Though Freud was unable to relieve the stuttering in one of his early cases, Frau Emmy, and felt that psychoanalysis was not an appropriate method for treating the disorder; many of his followers have not agreed. Stuttering has usually been regarded by the psychoanalysts as symptomatic of conflicts which have been resolved by fixations at anal or oral levels. To Coriat (1931), stuttering was the compromise symptom which partially solved the conflict between the instinctual need to remain an infantile suckling and the ego-need for more appropriate behavior. The anxiety, he felt, was due to the ego's fear of being "overwhelmed by the all-powerful oral eroticism." Stuttering behavior, according to Coriat, is related to the sucking and biting reactions of the infant at the nipple. Since speech also involves the lips and tongue, the compulsive repetition of movements performed by these organs allows even the adult stutterer to get his perverted oral pleasure as he talks.

Fenichel (1945), in contrast with Coriat, finds the essential conflict on anal rather than oral fixations. Stuttering is a pregenital conversion (hysterical) neurosis in that the early problems dealing with the retention and expulsion of the feces have been displaced upwards into the sphincters of the mouth. For the stutterer, according to Fenichel, speaking affords an opportunity to smear and soil his listener aggressively and with relative impunity. The attendant anxiety felt by the stutterer is due to his unconscious realization of the symbolic nature of his symptoms.

Heilpern (1941) presents a vivid picture:

> The patient's strong anal fixation is not surprising when one learns about his parent's personality. She made a habit of conversing with him when he was on the toilet. For a long time, even after he had begun to attend school, she examined his stools daily. In a rage, she once threw two quarters into the toilet, and then promised repentantly a piece of cake as a reward to him who would recover the money. The boy, almost grown up, did it. Humorous gifts, popular in this family, are toy chamber pots with little sausages in them. The mother can produce flatus voluntarily and does so jokingly to congratulate the father on the morning of his birthday. When she is in a rage, she pours out the chamber pot or even defecates on the floor (p. 97).

Glauber (1958) also rejected Coriat's restricted belief that the stutterer experiences perverted pleasure from his (stuttering) "act of nursing at an illusory nipple," as the complete explanation of the disorder. Instead, the basic conflict is between the id and the superego, the battleground lying in the ego-function of speech, for speech not only employs the oral pleasure-seeking (sucking) and aggression (biting), but it also serves as the basic mechanism for being able to live in a world of others. According to Glauber, it is the anxiety generated by all these conflicting drives that causes the stutterer to speak so haltingly. The result of this conflict is that the ego remains weak and arrested in its development and so does its most important function—speech. Stuttering as a symptom of the neurotic conflict shows features of regression as well as fixation and, at times, it reflects the person's need to defend himself against both of these solutions as well as the anxiety they create.

Barbara (1954), who has written much on stuttering, is one representative of the neoanalytic school, and much of his theory appears based on the position of Karen Horney. The basic conflict lies in the child's inadequate interpersonal relationships. Parental mishandling or perfectionistic demands or the lack of consistent tender loving care produces competing needs to comply, to avoid, or to react aggressively. Because these are incompatible with each other, ambivalence results and anxiety is generated. Since speech is the main vehicle for acquiring and maintaining interpersonal relationships, it reflects this ambivalence and anxiety in the form of hesitancy or stuttering. Barbara says:

> I feel that the symptom and the greater part of the ritual of stuttering itself is a major attempt toward an unconscious magical gesture with the purpose of symbolically demonstrating to others how the person who stutters suffers and is victimized (1954, p. 204).

Barbara also shows how a secondary stuttering neurosis can become overlaid on the primary one. Stutterers develop distinctive personality patterns (e.g., the Demosthenes complex) to prevent the anxiety from overwhelming them. In his fantasies:

> . . . as the individual who stutters soars to godlike heights, he is of necessity driven away from his real self. He becomes blinded by the compulsive need to have to prove himself—to become his Demosthenes image of himself (1954, p. 110).

Several other well-known American authors have used psychoanalytic principles in formulating their concepts of stuttering, although they have freed themselves somewhat from psychoanalytic terminology. Travis (1957), for example, as a result of his clinical experiences, considers the stutterer as one who is still caught in the conflict between the repressed urges to suck, eat, evacuate, and explore sexual pleasures and the parentally induced but reluctantly accepted inhibitions of these forbidden needs. Through stuttering the incompatabilities of love, hate, and fear can be resolved. It allows the stutterer to vent his forbidden impulses and to be punished for them without allowing them to be recognized for what they really are. Thereby the anxiety can be kept within bearable limits. The stutterer has difficulty in speaking because he has unspeakable feelings.

Murphy and Fitzsimons (1960) see stuttering as a "learned, noninte-grative, self-defensive reaction to anxiety or fear of threatening circum-stances with which the person feels incapable of coping." The child becomes hesitant in speech as well as in other functions because he has been belittled, dominated, rejected, and suppressed by the important persons (parents, etc.) in his environment and so fails to integrate his self-concept. The anxiety and guilt stemming from his feelings of inadequacy in interpersonal relationships make him hesitant in these interactions with others. Since this takes place at a critical stage in the child's development, this interpersonal hesitancy becomes reflected in his speaking, for speech always involves the display of the self. These authors seem to have applied to stuttering some of the concepts of the interpersonal theory of neurosis formulated by Harry Stack Sullivan. We present a brief quotation sum-marizing their position:

> We have maintained that the seeds of stuttering behavior are imbedded in the soil of early socialization experiences, and that stuttering's tap roots are intertwined most intimately with parent-child relationships. When nonverbal or verbal communicative or developmental task breakdowns germinate in these processes, the resulting disruptions to self-differentiation and integration are experienced by the child as feelings of apprehension or dread. . . . Stuttering can be defined as "what a person is." It tells us that self-defensive processes are in action, that anxieties or fears of diffused or specific character are operating, that the person is attempting not only to protect himself but to prove and improve himself also (Murphy and Fitzsimons, 1960, pp. 171–72).

Sheehan (1954, 1958) attempts to reconcile the psychoanalytic and learning theory points of view. He states that stuttering is one of the "neurotic reactions of a neurotic age." "It is a fault in the social presentation of the self, a self-role conflict." Applying the conflict theory of Dollard and Miller, Sheehan sees the disorder as a double approach-avoidance conflict with the stuttering repetitions and prolongations representing the precarious equilibrium between these two drives to speak and to keep silent. According to Sheehan, the approach-avoidance conflicts can occur on several levels: (1) the word level, (2) the situation level, (3) the expression of antagonistic emotions, (4) the level of interpersonal relationships (e.g., status), and (5) the ego-protective level. Anxiety can be generated by conflict at any of these levels, and stuttering is maintained by anxiety reduction since once the stuttering (which has become the symptomatic focus of all these fears) has occurred, the fear subsides. Guilt also plays a part in the generation of these conflicts. Sheehan feels that guilt serves as one of the original sources of the fear and the need to avoid speaking:

> Primary guilt would refer to the constellation of feelings which was behind the original appearance of stuttering, which the symptom formation has the function of handling. Secondary guilt refers to the feelings the stutterer develops as a result of his inevitable knowledge that his blocks are distressing to others, more so at times than to himself (1958, p. 135).

Sheehan also stresses the expressive nature of the symptom in advanced stuttering. The stutterer unconsciously chooses the type of stuttering which will best express his basic attitudes toward himself and toward his listeners.

STUTTERING AS A PHOBIA

Although the Russians generally hold the view that stuttering is of organic origin, they also recognize that a substantial number of stutterers show no neurological signs and these they class as being neurotic, as having developed learned phobias of speaking. Asamiani and Kazokov (1974) state that almost all of the adult stutterers they examined had developed logophobias whether their disorders were accompanied by brain damage or not. Becker *et al.* (1977) distinguished two subgroups of stutterers with psychopathology, one with neurotic speech phobias and the other with a slowly developing schizophrenia. The neurotic group was more resistant to therapy and developed powerful fears of situations and words very early. In Germany, Schmidt (1975) insisted that a neurotic subgroup of stutterers exists which must be treated by psychiatrists or psychologists. In India, Vishwanath (1970) describes stuttering as a learned maladaptive (neurotic) response having many symptoms common to other neurotic disorders.

Freund (1966) describes four major varieties of stuttering, two of which are neurotic in nature. The most common form of stuttering, according to Freund, belongs in the category of expectancy neuroses such as writer's cramp, stage fright, intermittent aphonia, certain forms of impotence, and other similar problems. The stutterer "experiences strange difficulties in the performance of an automatic skill (speaking) which previously he had been able to carry out with the greatest of ease." These difficulties may arise from many different stress factors (interpersonal conflicts, difficulties in verbal formulation and recall, physical and emotional traumatic experiences, social ambivalence, fear of listener reactions, and many others), but Freund stresses that the expectancy neurosis typically found in stutterers develops *after* the experience of communicative failure, not before. Freund writes:

> All of these forms of expectancy neurotic disturbances including stuttering have as a common characteristic that they are based upon actual "primary" traumatic experiences of failure in the performance of a learned skill or a simple motor or sensory act, often, though not necessarily, in socially embarrassing situations. The anticipation of their dreaded recurrence leads them, via inhibition, etc., to the establishment of a vicious spiral. In opposition to the phobias, the dread here is not of a symbolic nature but is based upon actual experience (1966, pp. 37–38).

The traumatic experiences of feeling blocked, of helplessness, of inability to cope, are sensed as a reflection of personal inadequacy, and the stutterer learns various defensive behaviors to protect his ego from being overwhelmed by the consequent anxiety. Freund points out clearly that the Freudian concepts of neurosis do not account for "the secondary 'neurotic' phase of actual stuttering—with the pathological defense system erected against the recurrence of communicative failure." Since the neurosis in "common stuttering" is born only after traumatic communicative failure has been experienced, it must be viewed as quite different from the "transference neuroses" of the psychoanalytic school. It is an expectancy neurosis.

We share with Freund the belief that the neurosis in confirmed stuttering most usually belongs in the category of expectancy neuroses. Unlike Freund, we do not feel that there is always a basic neurotic predisposition, and we cannot agree with this statement of his position:

> We feel that the behavior and inner experience of such stutterers is primarily determined by the nature of their personalities, not necessarily by a rigid and arbitrary progression of developmental stages. Some of these stutterers show this avoidance from the very beginning of the disorder. Most of them develop it very early. They tend to run away from other unpleasantnesses. Why should we expect them to do otherwise when confronted by stuttering? The fearful adult was a fearful child. This is not to say that this type (the most common type) of stuttering cannot appear as a terminal stage in the development of the disorder. We are certain that it can, but we feel that when it does, it represents the change in personality which stuttering itself can provoke. We would suspect, however, that even in such cases, there exists a basic personality structure which latently predisposes the person toward withdrawal and avoidance (1966, p. 138).

Our own position is that the neurosis in stuttering represents the end result of a learning process. We do not feel that most stutterers begin as neurotics. Certainly, the research has failed to show that stutterers have basically different personalities from normal speakers even after years of stuttering, and our clinical experience has convinced us that at onset and for some years later, most young stutterers do not show the features that are said to characterize neurosis. When they do appear, the "neurotic symptoms" stem from communicative frustration and social penalty. They are learned defenses designed to minimize the misery. They occur as responses to conflict and trap situations involving communication. They are secondary to the experience of unpleasant interruptions in uttering words. At first, they do lessen the unpleasantness, but as they become automatized, they contribute to it.

We do not, therefore, generally view stuttering as a symptom of some other neurosis—except in a few individuals. In most of our cases the fears have been learned; the behaviors which are so conspicuously maladaptive were once useful in minimizing the stutterer's difficulties. Through generalization, reinforcement, and automatization they have undergone a morbid growth and change. They persist despite their punishing

characteristics because they are continually reinforced by the consummation of communication. When we keep our eyes on what the stutterer
does, and understand what he is feeling, we find it very hard to hang the
label of primary neurosis around his neck. As Brutten and Shoemaker
(1967) put it, "Learning theory has shifted away from the idea that
individuals are neurotic or *have* neuroses and toward the idea that they
have learned maladaptive stimulus-response relationships." Most of our
stutterers have been pretty normal individuals—except when they had to
say something.

RESEARCH ON NEUROSIS

The research on stuttering generally, though voluminous, leaves much to
be desired when examined critically, but the research dealing with the
neurotic nature of the disorder is especially vulnerable to questioning.
One almost feels an urge to discard all the old studies and start all over.
Deficiencies in design, lack of control groups, an inadequate number of
assorted subjects, these and many other weaknesses make it difficult to
discern the grains of truth among all the chaff. Nevertheless it is worth
summarizing if only to help future researchers from making the same
mistakes. At the very least it demonstrates clearly that those who consider
stuttering a neurosis and only a neurosis have very little solid foundation
for their beliefs.

Are Stutterers Neurotics?

McDowell (1928) found no major differences between stuttering
children and their controls on three paper and pencil personality tests and
teachers' judgments. Johnson (1932), using the Woodworth-House Mental
Hygiene Inventory, found that stutterers as a group were not significantly
different in childhood maladjustment problems from normals, and they had
significantly less maladjustment than a comparison group of diagnosed
psychoneurotics. Bender (1939) administered the Bernreuter to 249 adult
stutterers and found them slightly poorer in social adjustment and speech
attitudes than normals. Bearss (1950) examined college stutterers with the
Rotter Incomplete Sentence Test and the Adam's Personal Audit but
found no differences between his subjects and their controls. Brutten
(1951) administered the Maslow Security Index to adult stutterers and
their controls and found no significant differences. Boland (1952) used
four scales and indices of anxiety and neuroticism and a test of speech
anxiety. No differences were found in general anxiety level or neuroticism,
but stutterers had more speech anxiety. Dahlstrom and Craven (1952)
administered MMPI to four groups of college subjects: stutterers, normal
speakers, normal speakers seeking counseling, and psychiatric patients.
They found that, although the stutterers were within the test norms, they

resembled the normal speaking students seeking counseling more than they did either of the other two groups. Several other similar MMPI studies by Pizzat (1949), Walnut (1954), and Thomas (1951) have shown the same tendency for stutterers to fall within the norms on most of the subscales of the test inventory. Certainly no marked tendency toward neuroticism has been shown by these MMPI investigations.

There are several studies in which the Bell Adjustment Inventory, the California Test of Personality, and other instruments whose validity is highly suspect were used, and we will list the authors here: Duncan (1949), Perkins (1946), Schultz (1947), Powers (1944), and Redwine (1959). Goodstein (1958) reviewed a number of the investigations of stutterers' personalities and concluded that they have not been shown to be severely maladjusted or to have unique personalities.

There have also been many investigations of stuttering using projective tests, especially the Rorschach and the TAT (Thematic Appreciation Test). Meltzer (1944) used the Rorschach with 50 child stutterers and their controls and discovered a number of differences between the groups, chiefly in negativism, fantasy, withdrawal, depression. Krugman (1946) also tested 50 child stutterers and a control group of children having other emotional problems. Using the Rorschach, he found that both groups showed strong evidence of neuroticism and instability. The stutterers were characterized as having rigid personalities, great anxiety, and obsessive-compulsive traits. It should be noted, as Sheehan (1958) pointed out, that the latter conclusion is not supported by Krugman's statistics. Both of these studies must be viewed with caution, especially since Wilson (1951), and Christensen (1952) using the child stutterer's sibling as his control, found no significant differences between siblings on the Rorschach or on the TAT insofar as neuroticism was concerned. Stroobant (1952) found no significant Rorschach signs of neuroticism in his New Zealand stutterers. Matsuoka (1964) in Japan administered the Rorschach to 20 fourth- to sixth-grade children and found that although they were "cautious, nervous, and anxious, their emotional control was not bad."

Adult stutterers, who according to Freund have already developed an expectancy neurosis, have also been subjected to projective testing. In 1944 Greene and Small found that "from 30 to 40 per cent of their stutterers showed Rorschach indications of marked emotional instability," but no data are provided. There are two studies by Pitrelli (1948) and Haney (1951) [which used no control group for their Rorschach investigations] that found indications of neurosis among stutterers, and one by Richardson (1944), which did use matched controls, but found no major significant differences between the groups. Sheehan (1970) critically reviewed most of the projective studies of stuttering and concluded that there was no firm evidence for the hypothesis that stutterers were neurotic.

In one of the most careful studies yet performed, Andrews and Harris (1964) explored in various ways the characteristics of children who stuttered as compared with their controls. Among the many items which failed to distinguish significantly between the groups were the following:

dependency, sensitivity, shyness, fears, enuresis, disturbing dreams, ability to form relationships with peers, mother-child relationships, and father-child relationships. If stuttering were indeed *only* a neurosis, surely some of these characteristics should have been shown to occur more frequently in the stutterers.

Do Stutterers Show Evidence of Oral or Anal Fixation?

We have been able to find only two studies which bear on the question of excessive orality. Meltzer (1933) found no Rorschach evidence to support Coriat's thesis, and Lowinger (1952), using the TAT, also found none in his study of institutionalized children who stuttered. Coriat cited the fact that stutterers generally had much more stuttering on the bilabial than on other sounds as evidence for his theory, but, as our review of the loci research has demonstrated, this is simply not true.

More work has concerned itself with excessive anality. Dickson (1954) used the Blacky Pictures Test (which shows dogs doing dirty deeds), a projective instrument of questionable validity, and found that more stutterers than nonstutterers had scores indicating anal-sadistic fixations. Carp (1962) also used the Blacky Test but failed to find excessive anal eroticism in the stutterers. The most extensive study was done by Keisman (1958). He used an Anal Trait Check List and an Anal Interest Picture Test (in which the time spent in looking at pictures of anal and non-anal activities was measured). The "findings were largely negative." This then seems to be the only experimental evidence for and against oral and anal fixation theory, and it hardly seems impressive, especially considering the work of Barnes (1951) and Sewell and Mussen (1952) who found little experimental evidence to support the Freudian view of oral and anal fixation.

Fisher (1970) presents a modern view of stuttering as an anal fixation as shown by stutterers' reactions to anal scenes and anal word stimuli. Dickson (1974) using the Blacky Test found no differences between stutterers and nonstutterers on oral fixation scores though they did show differences on other fixation scores.

Do Stutterers Show More Compulsivity Hostility, Anxiety, and Guilt than Normal Speakers?

Using the Rosenzweig Picture Frustration Test, Madison and Norman (1952) found that their stutterers, as compared against the test norms but not against a matched control group, showed more intropunitiveness and need persistence and less extrapunitiveness. Quarrington, a year later (1953), repeated the study on 30 stutterers and their controls but failed to find any significant differences between the groups. Santostefano (1960) found more hostility and anxiety in his 11 stutterers, using the Rorschach, and free associations to neutral and emotion-toned words. Brutten (1957) discovered no differences between stutterers and nonstutterers using the Palmar Sweat Index of anxiety when they were silent, but the data showed a trend that stutterers had more anxiety over speech. Riley and White (1967) gave the Objective Analytic Anxiety Battery to 17 stutterers and controls and found that the stutterers had more anxiety than the controls but that it was well below the neurotic level.*

Bharath and Ras (1970) applied the Eyesenck Personality Inventory to 100 stutterers in India and found significant indications of neuroticism and introversion. Hegde (1972), however, using the same test on 106 stutterers found that they scored within the normal limits on the neuroticism scale.

One final topic should probably be included in this summary of the research. Both Barbara (1946) and Pitrelli (1948) found a remarkably low incidence of stuttering among institutionalized psychotics and some evidence that a previously observed stutter had disappeared when the individual developed the psychosis. Since neuroses have been known occasionally to mask or to serve as a defense against psychosis, the implication was that these findings corroborated the neurotic nature of stuttering. However, Freund (1955), in a very scholarly review of the literature, showed clearly that the incidence of stuttering was three times as great (3.2 per cent) in 149 veterans who were schizophrenic than "among the general population."

If stuttering is a neurosis, then psychotherapy would seem to be the most appropriate treatment. A host of different psychotherapies have been used with stutterers over the years and we have described them elsewhere.* None of them seem to have been very effective. Perhaps the most devastating report of the outcome of psychotherapy with stutterers has been provided by Webster (1977). Of 648 stutterers treated only by psychotherapy, none were corrected, and 597 showed either no improvement or slight improvement. For other psychoneurotic disorders, psychotherapy seems to help about thirty per cent which is about the same figure obtained when no treatment of any kind is given and the patients recover spontaneously. Were stuttering solely a neurosis we would not expect such a miserable result.

Despite the fact that we have scrutinized all of these investigations with some care, it is difficult to fit them all together into a coherent judgment. So many of them fail to fulfill basic criteria of good research. So many of them contradict each other. The case for stuttering as a neurosis and only a neurosis has not been made.

* There are, of course, many case studies and reports which describe the hostile, anxious, and guilty feelings of stutterers or attempt to trace them back to early conflicts. Since it is impossible to present an adequate picture of such material in summary, we merely list some but not all of these references: Aikins (1925), Fogerty (1930), Fuchs (1934), Spring (1935), Wedberg (1937), Latif (1938), Heilpern (1941), Rotter (1942), Despert (1942), Usher (1944), Gustavson (1944), Harle (1946), Maas (1946), Naidu (1946), Bakes (1947), Renen (1950), Wallen (1961), and Massengill (1965). We have reread all these studies and conclude that, although some stutterers could certainly be called neurotic, we cannot accept the statement that all of them are.

* See Van Riper, *The Treatment of Stuttering* (1973), 140–176.

BIBLIOGRAPHY

ABBOTT, J. A. 1947. Repressed hostility as a factor in adult stuttering. *Journal of Speech Disorders* 12: 28–30.

ABBOTT, T. B. 1957. A study of observable mother-child relationships in stuttering and non-stuttering groups. *Dissertation Abstracts* 17: 1148–49.

AIKINS, A. 1925. Casting out the stuttering devil. *Journal of Abnormal Social Psychology* 18: 137–52.

ANDREWS, G. AND M. HARRIS. 1964. *The syndrome of stuttering*. London: Heinemann.

ASAMIANI, N. M. AND V. G. KAZOKOV. 1974. The clinical characteristics of adult patients with protracted forms of stuttering. *Zhurnal Nevropatologii i Psikhiatrii imeni S. S. Korsakova* 74: 574–79.

BAKES, F. 1947. Case of a stutterer. In *Case Histories in Clinical and Abnormal Psychology*, eds. A. Burton and R. Harris. New York: Harper and Row.

BARBARA, D. A. 1946. A psychosomatic approach to the problem of stuttering in psychotics. *American Journal of Psychiatry* 103: 188–95.

———. (ed.). 1965. *New directions in stuttering: theory and practice*. Springfield, Ill.: Thomas.

———. 1954. *Stuttering: a psychodynamic approach to its understanding and treatment*. New York: Julian.

BARNES, M. L. 1956. A study of the attitudes of parents and teachers toward children who stutter. Masters thesis, Ohio State University.

BEARSS, L. M. 1950. An investigation of conflict in stutterers and nonstutterers. Masters thesis, Purdue University.

BECKER, K. P., N. A. VLASSOVA, N. M. ASATIANI, AND W. HEV. 1977. *Stottern* Berlin: VEB Verlag Volk und Gesundheit.

BENDER, J. M. 1939. *The personality structure of stuttering*. New York: Pitman.

BERLIN, C. I. 1960. Parents' diagnoses of stuttering. *Journal of Speech and Hearing Research* 3: 372–79.

BERLINSKY, S. L. 1954. A comparison of stutterers and nonstutterers in four conditions of experimentally induced anxiety. *Dissertation Abstracts* 14: 719.

BHARATH, R. AND B. PRANESHA RAS. 1970. Some personality characteristics of stutterers. *Journal of the All India Institute of Speech and Hearing* 1: 7–13.

BLOODSTEIN, O., W. JAEGER, AND O. TUREEN. 1952. A study of the diagnosis of stuttering by parents of stutterers and nonstutterers. *Journal of Speech and Hearing Disorders* 17: 308–15.

BLOOM, J. 1958. Child training and stuttering. Doctoral dissertation, University of Michigan.

BOLAND, J. L. 1952. A comparison of stutterers and nonstutterers on several measures of anxiety. *Speech Monographs* 20: 144.

BRUNNER, M. 1936. Beeinflussung des Stotterns. *Zeitschrift für Psychoanalyse Padag.* 10: 360–65.

BRUTTEN, E. J. 1957. A colorimetric anxiety measure of stuttering and expectancy adaptation. *Dissertation Abstracts* 17: 2707–8.

———. 1951. Anxiety as a personality trait among stutterers. Master's thesis, Brooklyn College.

——— AND D. J. SHOEMAKER. 1967. *The modification of stuttering*. Englewood Cliffs, N.J.: Prentice-Hall.

273

BURTSCHER, H. T., JR. 1952.   The operation of frustration in the transition to and the development of secondary stuttering. *Speech Monographs* 19: 191 (abstract).

CARP, F. M. 1962.   Psychosexual development of stutterers. *Journal of Projective Techniques and Personality Assessment* 26: 388–91.

CHRISTENSEN, A. H. 1952.   A quantitative study of personality dynamics of stuttering and nonstuttering siblings. *Speech Monographs* 19: 144–45.

CORIAT, I. H. 1927.   The oral-erotic components of stammering. *International Journal of Psychoanalysis* 8: 56–69.

———. 1931.   The nature and analytical treatment of stuttering. *Proceedings of the American Speech Correction Association* 1: 151–56.

———. 1943.   The psychoanalytic concept of stammering. *Nervous Child* 2: 167–71.

DAHLSTROM, W. G. AND CRAVEN, D. D. 1952.   The Minnesota multiphasic personality inventory and stuttering phenomena in young adults. *American Psychologist* 7: 341 (abstract).

DARLEY, F. L. 1955.   The relationship of parental attitudes and adjustments to the development of stuttering. In *Stuttering in Children and Adults*, ed. W. Johnson. Minneapolis: University of Minnesota Press.

DESPERT, J. L. 1942.   A therapeutic approach to the problem of stuttering in children. *Nervous Child* 2: 134–47.

———. 1946.   Psychosomatic study of fifty stuttering children. *American Journal of Orthopsychiatry* 16: 100–113.

DICKSON, S. 1954.   An application of the Blacky test to a study of the psychosexual development of stutterers. Masters thesis, Brooklyn College.

DOLLARD, J. AND N. E. MILLER. 1950.   *Personality and psychotherapy.* New York: McGraw-Hill.

DOUGLASS, E. AND B. QUARRINGTON. 1952.   Differentiation of interiorized and exteriorized secondary stuttering. *Journal of Speech and Hearing Disorders* 17: 377–85.

DUNCAN, M. H. 1949.   Home adjustment of stutterers versus nonstutterers. *Journal of Speech and Hearing Disorders* 14: 255–59.

EYSENCK, H. J. AND S. RACHMAN. 1965.   *The causes and cure of neuroses.* London: Routledge and Kegan Paul.

FENICHEL, O. 1945.   *The psychoanalytic theory of neurosis.* New York: Norton.

FISHER, M. H. 1970.   Stuttering: a psychoanalytic view. *Journal of Contemporary Psychotherapy* 2: 124–27.

FOGERTY, E. 1930.   *Stammering.* New York: Dutton.

FREUND, H. 1966.   *Psychopathology and the problems of stuttering.* Springfield, Ill.: Thomas.

———. 1955.   Psychosis and stuttering. *Journal of Nervous and Mental Diseases* 122: 161–72.

———. 1934.   Über Inneres Stottern. *Zeitschrift Ohrenheilkunde* 69: 146–48.

FUCHS, E. 1934.   Zur Psychoanalyse des Stotterns. *International Journal of Psychoanalysis* 20: 375–89.

GLAUBER, I. P. 1943.   Psychoanalytic concepts of the stutterer. *Nervous Child* 2: 172–80.

———. 1954.   The nature of stuttering. *Social Casework* 34: 95–103.

———. 1958.   The psychoanalysis of stuttering. In *Stuttering: A Symposium*, ed. J. Eisenson. New York: Harper.

GOLDMAN, R. AND G. SHAMES. 1964. A study of goal-setting behavior of parents of stutterers and parents of nonstutterers. *Journal of Speech and Hearing Disorders* 29: 192–94.

GOODSTEIN, L. D. 1958. Functional speech disorders and personality: a survey of the research. *Journal of Speech and Hearing Research* 1: 359–76.

———. 1956. MMPI profiles of stutterers' parents: a follow-up study. *Journal of Speech and Hearing Disorders* 21: 430–35.

——— AND W. DAHLSTROM. 1956. MMPI difference between parents of stuttering and nonstuttering children. *Journal of Consulting Psychology* 20: 365–70.

GREENE, J. S. AND S. M. SMALL. 1944. Psychosomatic factors in stuttering. *Medical Clinics of North America* 28: 615–28.

GUSTAFSON, C. G. 1944. A talisman and a convalescence. Quarterly Journal of Speech 30: 1165–1471.

HANEY, H. R. 1951. Motives implied by the act of stuttering as revealed by prolonged experimental projection. *Speech Monographs* 18: 129.

HARLE, M. 1946. Dynamic interpretation and treatment of acute stuttering in a young child. *American Journal of Orthopsychiatry* 15: 156–62.

HEGDE, M. N. 1972. Stuttering, neuroticism, and extraversion. *Behavior Research and Therapy* 10: 395–397.

HEILPERN, E. 1941. A case of stuttering. *Psychoanalytic Quarterly* 1: 95–115.

JOHNSON, W. 1932. The influence of stuttering on the personality. *University of Iowa Studies in Child Welfare* 5: 1–140.

———. 1959. *The onset of stuttering.* Minneapolis: University of Minnesota Press.

KEISMAN, I. B. 1958. Stuttering and anal fixation. Doctoral dissertation, New York University.

KINSTLER, D. B. 1961. Covert and overt maternal rejection in stuttering. *Journal of Speech and Hearing Disorders* 26: 145–55.

KRASNOGORSKI, N. I. 1925. The conditioned reflexes and childrens' neuroses. *American Journal of Diseases of Children* 30: 756–68.

KRUGMAN, M. 1946. Psychosomatic study of fifty stuttering children. *American Journal of Orthopsychiatry* 16: 127–33.

LAFOLLETTE, A. C. 1956. Parental environment of stuttering children. *Journal of Speech and Hearing Disorders* 21: 202–7.

LATIF, I. 1938. Some aetiological factors in the pathology of stammering. *British Journal of Medical Psychology* 17: 307–18.

LIDDELL, H. S. 1964. The challenge of Pavlovian conditioning and experimental neuroses in animals. In *The Conditioning Therapies*, eds. J. Wolpe, A. Salter, and L. J. Reyna. New York: Holt.

LOWINGER, L. 1952. The psychodynamics of stuttering: an evaluation of the factors of aggression and guilt feelings in a group of institutionalized children. Doctoral dissertation, New York University.

MAAS, O. 1946. On the etiology of stuttering. *Journal of Mental Science* 92: 357–63.

MADISON, L. AND R. A. NORMAN. 1952. Comparison of the performance of stutterers and nonstutterers on the Rosenzweig picture frustration test. *Journal of Clinical Psychology* 8: 179–83.

MASSENGILL, R. 1965. Phobias present in three stuttering cases. *Perceptual and Motor Skills* 20: 579–80.

MASSERMAN, J. H. 1943. *Behavior and neurosis.* Chicago: University of Chicago Press.

MATSUOKA, T. 1964. Psychological study of young stutterers. Convention address, Japanese Psychology Association. Abstracted in G. Kamiyama, A handbook for the study of stuttering. 1967.

McDOWELL, E. 1928. *Educational and emotional adjustment of stuttering children.* Columbia University Teachers College Contributions to Education, No. 314.

MELTZER, H. 1943. Personality differences between stuttering and nonstuttering children as indicated by the Rorschach test. *Journal of Psychology* 17: 39–59.

MILLER, N. E. AND J. DOLLARD. 1941. *Social learning and imitation.* New Haven: Yale University Press.

MOLLER, H. 1960. Stuttering, predelinquent, and adjusted boys: a comparative analysis of personality characteristics as measured by the Wisc and the Rorschach test. Doctoral dissertation. Boston University.

MONCUR, J. P. 1952. Parental domination in stuttering. *Journal of Speech Disorders* 17: 155–65.

MOWRER, O. H. 1950. *Learning theory and personality dynamics.* New York: Ronald Press.

———. 1967. Stuttering as simultaneous admission and denial. *Journal of Communication Disorders* 1: 46–50.

MURPHY, A. T. 1952. An electroencephalographic study of frustration in stutterers. Doctoral dissertation, University of Southern California.

——— AND R. M. FITZSIMONS. 1960. *Stuttering and personality dynamics.* New York: Ronald.

NADOLECZNY, M. 1927. Stuttering as a manifestation of a spastic coordination neurosis. *Archives of Psychiatry* 82: 235–46.

NAIDU, P. S. AND S. K. AHMAD. 1946. Some excerpts from a clinical record of a case of stammering. *Indian Journal of Psychology* 21: 69–72.

PERKINS, D. 1946. An item by item compilation and comparison of the scores of 75 young adult stutterers on the California test of personality. Master's thesis, University of Illinois.

PITRELLI, F. R. 1948. Psychosomatic and Rorschach aspects of stuttering. *Psychiatry Quarterly* 22: 175–94.

PIZZAT, F. L. 1949. A personality study of college stutterers. Master's thesis, University of Pittsburgh.

POWERS, M. R. 1944. Personality traits of junior high school stutterers as revealed by the California test of personality. Masters thesis, University of Illinois.

QUARRINGTON, B. 1953. The performance of stutterers on the Rosenzweig picture frustration test. *Journal of Clinical Psychology* 9: 189–92.

REDWINE, G. W. 1959. An experimental study of the relationship between self-concepts of fourth and eighth grade stuttering and nonstuttering boys. *Speech Monographs* 26: 140–41 (abstract).

RENEN, S. B. V. 1950. Tongue troubles. *Journal of Logopaedics* (South Africa) 1: 16–19.

RICHARDSON, L. H. 1944. A personality study of stutterers and nonstutterers. *Journal of Speech Disorders* 9: 152–60.

RILEY, G. D. AND H. WHITE. 1967. "Anxiety among adults who stutter," convention address, ASHA, 1967.

ROTTER, J. B. 1942. A working hypothesis as to the nature and treatment of stuttering. *Journal of Speech Disorders* 7: 263–88.

———. 1944. The nature and treatment of stuttering: a clinical approach. *Journal of Abnormal and Social Psychology* 39: 150–73.

SANTOSTEFANO, S. 1960. Anxiety and hostility in stuttering. *Journal of Speech and Hearing Research* 3: 337–47.

SCHMIDT, H. 1975. Grundformen von Sprachablaufstorungen und Ihre Behandlungskriterien. In *Stottern-Poltern*, eds. K. H. Hahn and H. G. Muller. Hamburg: Wartenberg and Sohne.

SCHULTZ, D. A. 1947. A study of nondirective counseling as applied to adult stutterers. *Journal of Speech Disorders* 12: 421–27.

SEAMAN, R. 1956. A study of the responses of stutterers to the items of the Rosenzweig picture frustration study. Masters thesis, Brooklyn College.

SELIGMAN, J. 1966. The personality, attitudes and behavior of parents of children who stutter: an annotated bibliography. *Journal of Ontario Speech and Hearing Association* 2: 35–106.

SEWELL, W. AND P. MUSSEN. 1952. The effects of feeding, weaning, and scheduling procedures on childhood adjustment and the formation of oral symptoms. *Child Development* 33: 185–91.

SHEEHAN, J. G. 1954. An integration of psychotherapy and speech therapy through a conflict theory of stuttering. *Journal of Speech and Hearing Disorders* 19: 474–82.

———. 1958. Conflict theory of stuttering. In *Stuttering: A Symposium*, ed. J. Eisenson. New York: Harper.

———. 1968. Stuttering as self-role conflict. In *Learning Theory and Stuttering Therapy*, ed. H. H. Gregory. Evanston: Northwestern University Press.

———. 1970. *Stuttering: research and therapy*. New York: Harper and Row.

———. 1958. Projective studies of stuttering. *Journal of Speech and Hearing Disorders* 23: 18–25.

———. 1953. Theory and treatment of stuttering as an approach-avoidance conflict. *Journal of Psychology* 36: 27–49.

SHEEHAN, J. G., P. CORTESE, AND R. HADLEY. 1962. Guilt, shame, and tension in graphic projections of stuttering. *Journal of Speech and Hearing Disorders* 27: 129–39.

SNYDER, M. A., D. HENDERSON, M. MURPHY, AND, R. O'BRIEN. 1958. The personality structure of stuttering as compared to that of parents of stutterers. *Logos* 2: 97–105.

SPRING, W. J. 1935. Words and masses: a pictorial contribution to the psychology of stammering. *Psychoanalysis Quarterly* 4: 244–58.

STEIN, L. 1949. *The infancy of speech and the speech of infancy*. London: Methuen.

———. 1942. *Speech and voice*. London: Methuen.

STROOBANT, R. E. 1952. A psychological study of some stammering children. *New Zealand Speech Therapists Journal* 7: 8–13.

THOMAS, L. 1951. A personality study of a group of stutterers based on the Minnesota Multiphasic Personality Inventory. Masters thesis, University of Oregon.

TRAVIS, L. E. 1940. The need for stuttering. *Journal of Speech Disorders* 5: 193–202.

———. 1957. The unspeakable feelings of people with special reference to stuttering. In *Handbook of Speech Pathology*, ed. L. E. Travis. Englewood Cliffs, N.J.: Prentice-Hall.

——— AND L. D. SUTHERLAND. 1957. Psychotherapy in speech correction. In *Handbook of Speech Pathology*, ed. L. E. Travis. New York: Prentice-Hall.

USHER, R. D. 1944. A case of stuttering. *International Journal of Psychoanalysis* 25: 61–70.

VAN RIPER, C. 1973. *The Treatment of Stuttering*. Englewood Cliffs, N.J.: Prentice-Hall.

VISHWANATH, N. S. 1970. Learning, neurosis and stuttering. *Journal of the All India Institute of Speech and Hearing* 1: 92–103.

WALLEN, V. 1961. Primary stuttering in a 28 year old adult. *Journal of Speech and Hearing Disorders* 26: 394–95.

WALNUT, F. 1954. A personality inventory item analysis of individuals who stutter and individuals who have other handicaps. *Journal of Speech and Hearing Disorders* 19: 220–27.

WATSON, J. B. AND P. RAYNER. 1920. Conditioned emotional reactions. *Journal of Experimental Psychology:* 3: 1–14.

WEBSTER, L. M. 1977. A clinical note on psychotherapy for stuttering. *Journal of Fluency Disorders* 2: 253–55.

WEDBERG, C. F. 1937. *The stutterer speaks*. Redlands, Cal.: Valley of Fine Arts Press.

WILSON, D. M. 1951. A study of the personalities of stuttering children and their parents as revealed through projection tests. *Speech Monographs* 18: 133.

WOLPE, J. 1952. Objective psychotherapy of the neuroses. *South African Medical Journal* 26: 825–29.

———. 1958. *Psychotherapy by reciprocal inhibition*. Stanford: Stanford University Press.

WOLPE, J. A., A. SALTER, AND L. J. REYNA. 1964. *The conditioning therapies*. New York: Holt.

WRIGHT, B. A. 1960. *Physical disability: a psychological approach*. New York: Harper.

STUTTERING AS LEARNED BEHAVIOR

13

Almost all the current theories of stuttering have an ancient history. By knowing something about how these theories developed, one gets a perspective which can be acquired in no other way. We see concepts born, revised, and reborn. Our predecessors were eloquent in convincing themselves and their contemporaries of explanations which are at best only partial truths and at worst biased absurdities. We see also that many of our present beliefs, at least in germinal form, were formulated and even discarded long ago. We find concepts concerning stuttering as a learned response recurring again and again. It is a humbling experience to search through those old dusty books. Few who have done so can ever be very sure of the validity of their own beliefs. Some scholar two centuries hence, if by chance he comes across a tattered copy of this present book, will assuredly smile at our quaint benightedness—though not (we hope) at our hunger to understand.

At present we seem to be at the crest of a new wave of explanations of stuttering based on learning theory. Two earlier major waves, those of organicity and neurosis, have swept in and spent their energies on our theoretical shores, and far out on the horizon we discern the gathering force of servotheory. There will be other waves and these will repeat themselves too. Fortunately each one brings us some treasure as well as junk. So let us look back at the precursors of the present flood of learning theory.

Perhaps it was Amman (1700) who first stated flatly that stuttering was a bad habit. Indeed he called "haesitantia" a vicious one, claiming that there was nothing organically wrong with the tongue but that it had fallen into evil ways. In his therapy Amman sought to break the bad habit by training his stutterers to speak loudly and slowly, memorizing set passages and reciting them to friends. It was almost another hundred years before

Erasmus Darwin (1800), the grandfather of the stuttering Charles Darwin of evolution fame, attributed the disorder to emotionally conditioned interruptions of motoric speech, and suggested continual practice on the difficult sounds and learning to begin the plosives with loose contacts. In 1818 a Dr. Joseph Frank recommended that stutterers receive a good flogging for their exhibitions of abnormality. In the early decades of the nineteenth century, there were many workers interested in solving the puzzle of stuttering, and although the writers of that period usually attributed the cause of the abnormality to some debility of one or another of the "speech organs," they all felt that their stutterers required training to break the bad habits thereby engendered. One of the practitioners of that time was Madame Leigh (1825), who believed that the disorder was due to an abnormal tongue thrust habit and trained her patients to speak with the tonguetip up against the palate and used a pad of cotton to help it do so. And there was Arnott (1828) who sought to prevent the "spasm of the glottis" by teaching his stutterers to prefix each word with an "*e* vowel." And we find McCormac in 1828 saying that since stutterers habitually spoke with empty lungs, they should be trained to inhale deeply and exhale forcibly on each word. According to an old book by Potter (1882), Palmer in 1829

> divided speech defects into two classes, organic and functional; the latter (including stuttering) being chiefly due to irregular muscle action, which being established from habit, becomes independent of the original cause and closely resembles chorea in its nature and phenomena. His treatment was one of moral discipline, with varied details for each case (p. 48).

In this brief sampling of the literature, we find the basic rationale for the retraining of improper breathing, incorrect articulation, or inadequate voice, according to the bias of the particular author.

By the middle of the century, at about the time of our Civil War, the belief that stuttering was a bad habit had attained widespread acceptance especially in Britain and the United States. Alexander Melville Bell (1853), the inventor of Visible Speech and the father of Alexander Graham Bell of telephone fame, wrote several books dealing with stuttering. At first, Bell found it very difficult to get others to believe in his view that stuttering was a learned response. He writes, "The popular impression is that the impediment is 'organic,' or altogether 'in the nerves,' and its eradication beyond the reach of art." Bell was outraged by the surgical mutilations of his time and spoke his mind. He insisted that since speech is learned, so must be its defects:

> Speaking is an artificial process—an acquirement, not a natural instinct—and its defects can only be amended by the same means through which its exercise is first obtained—by imitative education. . . . The impediment has been shown to be a habit; it is therefore beyond the province either of medical or surgical treatment, and within that, exclusively, of the educator (p. 47).

As Bell's belief that stuttering was only a bad habit took hold, others besides physicians began to treat it. A large number of laymen, usually former stutterers, set up treatment centers in their own homes and conducted a private practice. Among the best of these were the Hunts, father and son, who were evidently highly successful practitioners. A fascinating article in Fraser's Magazine by "A Minute Philosopher" (who was probably Charles Kingsley, the famous orator and preacher, who himself had stuttered severely) describes the Hunt method as one in which the stutterer was trained "naturally and without dodge or trick to speak consciously as other men spoke unconsciously." The abnormal behaviors of the lips, tongue, jaw, and breath were compared with the normal behaviors and the latter were then strongly reinforced in a kindly environment.

Among these practitioners, however, were many ruthless charlatans who used all sorts of tricks and speech-exercise rituals based on distraction and suggestion to prey on their victims. Their secret methods of cure were jealously guarded, with the stutterers being sworn to "eternal secrecy" before being accepted into one of their "stammering institutes." For our purposes here, it is enough to say that these persons all felt that stuttering was a bad habit which could be extinguished by penalizing it and replacing it with strongly reinforced normal speech. Ignoring the fact that every stutterer can speak normally under certain conditions, they believed that by getting completely fluent speech and practicing it often enough and strongly enough, the old bad habit of stuttering would be weakened and finally broken. To achieve this fluency, they used rhythmic speech, breath control, a lalling form of utterance, syllable tapping, a cork between the teeth, abnormal inflections, and a host of other devices and routines. Some of these techniques are still being advocated today (Andrews and Harris, 1964; Beech, 1967; Goldiamond, 1965) and essentially for the same reasons—to create a nucleus of stutter-free speech which can then be strengthened.

There were also some early beginnings to the modern learning-theory concept that stuttering is due to approach-avoidance conflicts. Mendelssohn in 1729 attributed the disorder to a conflict between ideas and emotions. Wyneken (1868) writes: "Stammering consists of a temporary clumsiness in the managing of the voice, a clumsiness which can be conditioned by various influences." He also has this to say about the conflicts in speaking:

Should I attempt to give an explanation, then I would say that, with reference to the muscles which are active in speech, the will is more or less bound, and that by doubt. The stutterer is thus a doubter of speech. If he dares the word which seems difficult to him, then however his will is partially paralyzed by doubt, in a manner, can also be called a will, and one which is directly opposed to the will proper. The muscles which underlie respiration, phonation, and articulation often are not sure, if I may express myself thus, whom they should obey, and as a consequence thereof do not fulfill their functions with the necessary synergy, and stuttering occurs. The relation is similar as when somebody, for example, wants to venture a jump, but in the very moment in which he leaps doubts that he will succeed. Often he can no longer stop the leap, but also does not jump with sufficient assurance (*l'aplomb nécessaire*), and so does not reach his goal. A striking analogue to the influence of doubt upon speech we find in the influence of doubt upon sexual potency. Many people, says Niemayer, are impotent only because they doubt their sexual potency; when the doubt is overcome: then there is nothing the matter with them (pp. 20–21).

A similar point of view is expressed by Denhardt (1890) in these words:

> If we examine the mental processes during stuttering, we see that the disturbance typifies the struggle between two opposing forces. The volition which tries to convert the thought into speech is pitted against the belief that we are unable to accomplish what we intended. One drives, the other restrains. The will to speak initiates the impulse toward movement; at the same time fear prevents it. From their conflict and the desire of the stutterer to gain a victory for his desire to speak, result the total characteristics of stuttering. Finally the will to speak wins out and produces the word which had been withheld by the stutterer's lack of faith in his own expressive ability (pp. 176–177).

An early example of the modern desensitization and counterconditioning sort of therapy advocated today by Wolpe (1958) and Eysenck and Rachman (1965) is found in the writing of Sandow (1898), Sandow believed that each spasmodic moment of stuttering was triggered by "psychic" stimuli, usually those invested with emotion. He insisted that through relaxation and calming procedures, these stimuli would become unable to produce the stuttering paroxysms and that this was the way stuttering should be extinguished. A quotation illustrating the importance of this use of relaxation as a counterconditioner may make his position clear:

> Every stutterer should treat himself—or if very young should be treated—as one afflicted with serious neurasthenia. . . . With every movement of the body he should keep this serious manner of treatment in mind. He should act with extreme slowness and self-comfort, and with as much nonchalance and indifference as possible. . . . Not any kind of slowness in the use of arms and legs is meant hereby for there is more than one meaning to "slowness." One person walks slowly because an ambling person in front of him is blocking the way. Another walks that way because he is too sleepy to want to, or be able to do otherwise. A comfortable slowness similar to this latter one of quiet inner satisfaction must become second nature to the patient (p. 35).

As we enter the present century, we find a growing emphasis on stuttering as learned behavior, although during its first three decades, due to the influence of Freud, the most commonly held theory of stuttering, at least in this country, was that it was a neurosis. As late as 1936, Blanton made a survey of all the important American authorities on stuttering and found only one (Bluemel) who believed that stuttering was learned. But other voices had also made themselves heard. Dunlap (1932) made no bones about his certainty that stuttering was a habit. He felt that it stemmed from parental corrections, interruptions, or verbal conflicts.

He had no patience with corrective speech exercises which merely tried to reinforce normal speech, saying:

> Since every stammerer has a habit of correct speech, along with his stammering habit, manifesting one habit in some circumstances and the other habit in other circumstances, we can understand why no cases can be remedied by the procedure so often advised by persons who had not worked with stammerers, who say, "All you need to do is to form the habit of correct speech. . . ." In order to extend the patient's habit of correct speech to the situations in which he now stammers, the stammer must be attacked directly (p. 273).

And Dunlap did attack it directly through the voluntary practice of stuttering—his *beta*-hypothesis. "The patient is instructed also that when the critic commands 'again' he is to say the word over (or to say the initial syllable again, if stopped on a syllable) in the same way as that in which he said it before, or in a way as near as possible to the erroneous way." After using this negative practice several times, the therapist then commands "right!" and the stutterer then attempts to say the word without stuttering. This use of the moment of reactive inhibition anticipates such present day practices as cancellation.

Bluemel (1935), who had previously discarded his earlier organic theory of stuttering as a transient auditory aphasia, outlined a learning theory of stuttering based on Pavlovian conditioned inhibition. He held that since speech had been learned, it could be considered a conditioned reflex. By applying to stuttering the principles of conditioned inhibition derived from Pavlov's experiments, he sketched how the disorder could be generated and maintained. Bluemel also distinguished between "pure or primary stammering," which was the result of conditioned inhibition, and "secondary stammering" which also included many habituated strategies for coping with the interruptions. With a little stretching, he may be considered to have been the person who first discovered the two-factor theory of stuttering. As McDearmon (1966) has pointed out in his review of Bluemel's contribution, his writings did much to lay the groundwork for the favorable reception that modern learning theory approaches to stuttering have had in this country.

Finally, we should certainly mention two European workers, Hoepfner (1912) and Froeschels (1943, 1955, 1964), who described how stuttering may develop out of normal childhood disfluency through a learning process and who opposed the organicists and the psychoanalysts who had dominated the field. It is probably difficult for any contemporary student of stuttering to appreciate the contributions of all these men. All of them met powerful opposition. The author remembers well how viciously he was criticized when he published a paper (Van Riper, 1937a) showing how many of the most abnormal behaviors of stuttering were learned instrumental responses used to avoid, minimize, or escape from expected or experienced speech interruptions. At that time everyone spoke of "stuttering spasms." All breathing abnormalities were viewed as neurological dysfunctions. If a stutterer said, "um-um-um-uh-er-no" the breakdown began with that first "um." If he jerked his head to time the moment of the speech attempt, that head jerk was part of the neurological spasm. The idea that these reactions were only the habituated residues of behaviors once deliberately used to cope with the fear or experience of speech interruptions was heresy. Other correspondents were less abusive but just as certain that only ignorance or stupidity could lead anyone to believe that these behaviors were something more than symbolic symptoms of a deep seated neurosis. Symptomatic therapy (the unlearning of these coping behaviors) was viewed as completely inadequate and probably dangerous since conversions to more abnormal reactions would assuredly result.

MODERN CONCEPTS OF STUTTERING AS LEARNED BEHAVIOR

Most of the current thinking about stuttering reflects the influence of learning theory. Few writers today deny that learning plays some part in determining the patterns of behavior shown by advanced stutterers. The different varieties of stuttering reactions, the changes that occur as the disorder develops, the role of situational and verbal cues in its precipitation, all these and many other features of the problem testify to the influence of learning.

There is much disagreement, however, about the exact role that learning plays. Is the original stuttering learned, and, if so, how is it learned? How is stuttering maintained? How is it shaped? How can it be unlearned? There are different answers to these questions, and consensus is far away. We find explanations of stuttering based on classical conditioning, operant conditioning, cognitive learning theory, and many combinations of these.

This situation with regard to stuttering merely reflects the confused state of current learning theory which has been in great flux. The drive reduction concepts of Hull (1951) have been under attack. The views of Tolman and Guthrie and the Gestaltists refuse to roll over and stay dead. Learning theorists such as Mowrer revise their thinking so often that it is difficult to discern their current concepts. Attempts to translate the Freudian concepts of conflict into behavior theory as illustrated by Dollard and Miller (1950) have added further complications. All theoretical positions are under severe challenge and most of them seem vulnerable. Controversy is rampant among psychologists as evidenced by the criticisms of Chomsky (1959) and Breger and McGaugh (1965) and the countering stout defense by Wiest (1967). No learning theory yet seems to account for all the facts of learning, so we should not be surprised to find different explanations for how stuttering is learned, shaped, and maintained. At the present time most of the learning theories of stuttering are based on classical conditioning, operant conditioning, or both despite evidence that neither has been shown to be entirely acceptable. Let us first consider the operant point of view.

STUTTERING AS OPERANT BEHAVIOR

Most of the operant explanations are based on the assumption that stuttering results from the reinforcement of normal disfluencies. Thus Flanagan, Goldiamond, and Azrin (1959) say:

> Stuttering has often been considered an emotional blocking; it can, however, be regarded as a unit of verbal behavior; that is, breaks, pauses, repetitions, and other nonfluencies can be considered operant responses, having in common with other operants the characteristic of being controllable by ensuing consequences. For the chronic stutterer, such nonfluencies may have immediately been followed by consequences which did not occur in connection with regular speech, thereby becoming isolated as response units. Some consequences, such as attention on the part of the listener, noninterruption, and the like, may increase the likelihood of occurrence—that is, may be reinforcing (p. 979).

It should be stated that this position is not held exclusively by operant theorists. Wendell Johnson, Froeschels, and many others have also felt that stuttering was the problem child of the family of normal disfluencies. And Bloodstein, Alper, and Zisk (1965) state that: ". . . stuttering as a clinical disorder is simply an exaggeration or extension of certain kinds of disfluency to be heard in the speech of normal children" (p. 63).

Even though stuttering disfluencies are largely confined to syllabic repetitions or phonemic prolongations, so that other forms of disfluency are less prominent, the crucial point made by those who hold the operant view is that all children and all adults occasionally emit these behaviors. The stutterer emits too many of them because somehow they have been rewarded and reinforced. Of all the possible types of disfluency, why must these particular ones somehow be singled out to receive special reinforcement that finally predominate in stuttering? No other explanation of the change in distribution of types of disfluencies is consistent with the operant view. But why should the syllabic repetitions and phonemic prolongations be reinforced so exclusively? This is a question which evidently has not been considered by operant conditioners although it is a vital one. Indeed no systematic theory of stuttering based specifically on operant conditioning has yet been formulated.* Laboratory demonstrations that the frequencies of stuttering behavior may be increased or decreased by operant strategies, and investigations in the application of operant conditioning principles to actual stuttering therapy, compose the major bulk of the literature.

Nevertheless, the basic assumption on which these advocates of operant explanations usually seem to base their reasoning is that the core behavior of stuttering originally consisted of the same kind of syllabic repetitions and phonemic prolongations which all children (and all adults) experience

---

* Theory construction has been deliberately eschewed by most adherents of operant conditioning. They seem to feel that their behavioral science is in its early stages and prefer to stick to observables. Theoretical constructs are not observable. The closest approach to an operant theory of behavior is in B. F. Skinner's book *Verbal Behavior* (1957).

occasionally. We must remember that this is an assumption. The only research we know which bears on the subject is that of Stromsta (1965), who showed that sonograms of the original syllabic repetitions of children who were still stuttering ten years later were markedly different from those of children who had "outgrown" the disorder. Admittedly this research is hardly crucial and we urgently need longitudinal studies in which the specific "stuttering" behaviors of children who do or do not become stutterers can be repeatedly compared.

Actually the operant framework does not require that the original reinforcement had to be a consequence of normal disfluency. All that it demands is that broken words occur, that they are emitted. If emitted, a behavior can be shaped into another form. Operant behaviorists are not particularly concerned about the causes of behaviors, although occasionally they may speculate a bit, as this quotation from Shames and Sherrick (1963) illustrates:

> The conditions surrounding the original emission and early development of nonfluencies in the speech of infants are still quite obscure and in need of detailed observation. It is possible that the repetitions observed in later speech may be related to the vocal behavior emitted by infants during their early speech development (babbling and chaining of syllables). . . . It is also possible that nonfluency in speech is a characteristic of the human organism because of its physiological limitations (p. 5).

Thus Shames and Sherrick (1963) apply operant conditioning principles to stuttering and suggest that when childhood disfluencies are emitted but have no important consequences, the child is and will remain a normal speaker no matter how many syllabic repetitions he exhibits or what kind they are. On the other hand, these authors state that if the normal disfluencies produce desired consequences (gaining parental attention, permitting the child to speak without interruption, etc.) they will increase in frequency until they become a major feature of his communication. Then, if they get punished through rejection or frustration, the child will start doing things to avoid or escape them, and whatever he does (if it leads to less unpleasantness) will also increase. It may be the use of a stalling trick or a sudden head-jerk or anything else. There are gaps in the reasoning here but some of them can be filled. On the one hand listener reactions (attention, concern, etc.) are so positively reinforcing that they create the stuttering problem by increasing the normal disfluencies. On the other hand, listener reactions are so punishing that successful efforts to escape them are negatively reinforced. This could be true if the child's listeners changed their behavior from attending to rejecting, or from concern to punishment as soon as the frequency of stutterings increased beyond a certain cut-off point. This may indeed take place, although we have no evidence that it does.

Adherents of the operant position are not particularly concerned about the antecedents of behavior. All they require is that a specified behavior be emitted and subjected to contingent reinforcement. If it increases or decreases as its consequences are reinforcing or punishing, respectively, the behavior is to be considered an operant. It operates, has effects upon, the environment. According to Shames and Sherrick, disfluency of any kind, normal or abnormal, can be considered an operant because it can be increased or decreased, or shaped into varied forms by differential reinforcement. These authors make a strong case for shaping when they point out that the adult stutterer shows a markedly different form of stuttering than he did when he was a child. What changed his stuttering? According to the operant conditioners, specific reinforcements which followed (were contingent upon) the deliberate or chance variations in the disfluent behavior were the agents which caused the modification.

Let us give some oversimplified illustrations. If a stutterer happens to shut his eyes in a block, he may thereby shut out the impatient or mocking looks on the listener's face that have been punishing him. Thus this negative reinforcement (the termination of punishment) is contingent on the eye-closing since it follows it, so that eye-closing is strengthened and maintained. Or, if a stuttering child hungers for a parent's attention and gets it whenever he repeats a syllable several times, then repeating syllables receives positive reinforcement. Even if these reinforcements occur only occasionally they can maintain the stuttering. This is an explanation for the shaping of stuttering that comes as the disorder passes through its developmental stages; it is also an explanation for its maintenance.

WHY DO PUNISHED BEHAVIORS PERSIST?

But the stuttering gets punished more and more as it grows in severity and frequency, and punishments (contingent aversive stimuli) usually weaken a response. Why doesn't the stuttering then diminish or get suppressed? The operant therapists explain that most of the so-called secondary symptoms are instrumental responses used to cope with the aversive stimuli given by the listener. The postponement tricks which eventually become habitual are intermittently reinforced because, occasionally by using them, the stutterer can escape the listener's punishment. An avoidance trick enables the stutterer to avoid listener rejection. A head-jerk that terminates a long prolongation would be strongly reinforced because it *ends* the listener's shocked expression, the punishment. So, through enough negative reinforcements, the head-jerk becomes stronger and stronger. It may occur not once but many times if the punishing listener's look continues. As Ayllon and Azrin (1965) state:

> It appears that human behavior can be maintained by punishment if the punisher has been given discriminative or conditioned reinforcing properties. These results provide an experimental basis for interpreting clinical phenomena such as "masochism" wherein an individual seeks out punishment and does nothing to avoid it (p. 418).

Thus, even though stuttering gets punished by the listener, the things (all his avoidance and struggle behaviors) that the stutterer does to try to escape that punishment—and they are by far the greatest part of the abnormality—get strengthened. Every time we do something that enables us to escape punishment, that behavior will be reinforced and maintained. No person likes aversive stimuli whether they be electric shocks or the shocked expressions on a listener's face.

The same sort of reasoning may apply to the punishing characteristics of the stuttering itself quite apart from any listener reaction. The presence of repetitions and prolongations and gaps in the forward flow of speech, when they continue long enough to produce communicative frustration, and when there are too many of them, can be viewed as punishing. They are unpleasant to the speaker as well as to the listener. If the stutterer in responding to this unpleasant experience, suddenly exhales and manages to emit the word on the end of his breath that sudden exhalation coincides with the escape from unpleasantness. It will therefore be strengthened by negative reinforcement. If a long tremor of the lips is terminated by a sudden lip protrusion, the lip protrusion will be similarly reinforced, and when tremors appear in the future, the stutterer will be likely to stick out his lips again . . . and again. When stutterers are asked why they do these bizarre things, they answer, "because sometimes they work." As all students of conditioning know, intermittent reinforcement produces responses that are more resistant to extinction than continuous reinforcement. It is not necessary therefore for the attempt on the end of the breath or the lip protrusion or any other such behavior to coincide each time with the final emission of a stuttered word. It is sufficient that they do so occasionally.

We must also point out, however, that conjoined with this escape from punishment is the ability to continue talking, a positive reinforcement added to the negative reinforcement we have been illustrating. We not only get relief but also reward for using these "secondary symptoms." After all, the purpose of talking is to communicate a message. Stutterers desire the consummation of communication with an intensity that normal speakers can hardly fathom. Deprivation creates drive. Only the desert wanderer knows the wonder of water. The stutterer wants badly to complete the message he is sending. Anything that seems to further that end will be positively reinforcing. Thus the head-jerk that coincided with the final utterance of the word not only ends his frustration, but it also enables him to continue. Reinforcement is both negative and positive. This double dose of relief and reward is sufficient to instate a host of inappropriate behaviors and to maintain them at high emission levels. This, and other learning theory explanations of stuttering, explains clearly why confirmed stutterers show such a wide variability of behaviors. The set of instrumental responses that happens to get reinforced differs from one stutterer to the next. We all cope with our troubles in different ways. Stutterers experiment with different strategies of avoidance and escape. Certain ones receive the double-barrelled reinforcement we have mentioned, and these become the major features of the stuttering he exhibits. It is in this way that different stuttering patterns are shaped. It is in this way that stuttering grows. Escape from punishment and communicative progress, in our opinion, are sufficiently reinforcing to account for most of what Wingate called the accessory features of stuttering, but we find it very difficult to explain the core behavior of stuttering in these terms. We can do so with a lot of stretching but we are not happy with the result. A temporally distorted word requires some other explanation.

It should be strongly stated that these applications of conditioning principles to stuttering do not rest on a very substantial foundation of research. As we shall see in the section on the research that has been done with stutterers, the results are far from substantiating these attractive explanations of how the disorder is created, developed, and maintained. Indeed the experimental foundation is most insecure, probably because it is fairly new, and hastily built. It has been clearly demonstrated that the frequency of stuttering behaviors can be manipulated in a controlled laboratory situation by arranging their consequences and perhaps their antecedents, but this is far from sufficient evidence that the same or similar consequences or antecedents are responsible for the acquisition of all the features of the disorder. A theory that explains only selected portions of an assembly of related phenomena is not an adequate theory, particularly when the evidence for it is so meager and has been gathered under conditions that differ so much from the conditions surrounding the phenomena the theory seeks to explain.

THE EXPERIMENTAL PRODUCTION OF "STUTTERING"

If stuttering is only learned behavior—nothing else—then we ought to be able to demonstrate not only how it is shaped or maintained but also how it can be originated (or "instated," to use the jargon.) The evidence here is insubstantial and unsatisfactory. It is difficult and even dangerous to do such experiments. We have enough stutterers without trying to produce them in the laboratory. Nevertheless, the attempt has been made. Moore (1938) administered severe electric shocks to 18 stutterers and their normal speaking controls as the subjects uttered nonsense syllables according to a predetermined set of intervals. He found that both groups of subjects showed similarly disintegrated breathing during speaking. Moore also demonstrated that these breathing disruptions could be conditioned, for they appeared later on when the subjects listened silently to a recording of the syllables.

In an unpublished study, Van Riper in 1954 administered a very severe shock for failure to choose the correct word from three possibilities in the utterance of consecutive sentences such as this: "The (1. boy; 2. girl; 3. child) was playing in the (1. yard; 2. grass; 3. snow.)" Without foreknowledge of which word was correct, and with a series of very strong shocks as a penalty for not completing the sentence within a set time, two subjects were run, a man and a woman, both highly fluent students and individuals who were fond of the author. To our surprise, despite the approach-avoidance conflicts, which were very evident, and the many severe shocks and profound emotional upheaval experienced by the subjects, no stuttering appeared. Then, appalled by what he was doing to his friends, this author said, "Here, let me share the shock. I can't stand to have you take it alone." And then suddenly real stuttering, uncontrollable repetitions and blockages, appeared as a consequence of the shocks. What is even more painful to recount, this behavior intermittently persisted for months in the man. Three years later, the woman reported she was having an occasional runaway repetition or complete blockage. We never ran another subject and could not account for the result until long afterward we read the research of Brady (1958) in which the executive monkeys got the ulcers rather than the monkeys who got the shocks.

During a complicated serial motor task performed by his normal speaking subjects, Hill (1954) paired a red light with a shock until the light became a conditioned stimulus, and it was then administered while the subjects were speaking. He reported the occurrence of repetitions and prolongations indistinguishable from stuttering.

These three reports can probably best be explained through the principles of classical conditioning, but we also have one in which strictly operant procedures were used. Flanagan, Goldiamond, and Azrin (1959) administered a persistent shock to three normal speaking subjects who had previously been trained to depress a key for each nonfluency while reading. During the experimental condition, the subjects could free themselves from the continuous shock by depressing the key, and it was found that their nonfluencies increased markedly and persisted for a short time even when the shock was removed. They disappeared, however, as soon as the subjects left the laboratory. According to the authors, "Stuttering was defined as any hesitation, stoppage, repetition, or prolongation in the rhythmic flow or vocal behavior" and, from their brief report, it is difficult to be certain that stuttering rather than normal disfluency was the behavior that was "instated." The study evidently showed that an increase in frequency of disfluencies of all types occurred when negative reinforcement was employed. It did not show, however, for example, that the number of syllable repetitions per word increased or that the prolongations became longer, or that coarticulation failure occurred within the syllables, or that airflow or voice was interrupted. It is even possible that the only behaviors which increased were deliberately faked disfluencies which the subjects used to stop the continuous shock. Bloodstein and Shogan (1972) reported that by increasing the tension of their articulators, stutterers could throw themselves into "real" blocks with a feeling of loss of control so perhaps this is what occurred.

These reports of the deliberate creation of stuttering-like behaviors do not seem sufficiently applicable to explain the usual onset of stuttering. Any hard evidence that stuttering *originates* through operant conditioning procedures is lacking. The view that *all* of the behaviors shown by the adult stutterer are maintained and shaped by their consequences has also not been satisfactorily established. As our review of the research will show, punishment of normal or abnormal disfluencies does not always decrease them, nor does the positive reinforcement of fluency always make a stutterer more fluent. Sometimes it makes him worse.

It is true that some, but not all, of our research shows that certain stuttering behaviors can be brought under stimulus and experimenter control to a certain degree in the laboratory, but even the most effective punishments used in the Minnesota experiments by Siegel, Martin, and others never seemed to have suppressed it or extinguished it completely. Carry-over to normal communicative situations outside the laboratory has also been very disappointing despite the use of tokens and wrist straps and the like. Similarly, the application of operant principles in treatment has been less than satisfactory as the reviews by Boberg, Howie, and Woods (1979) and Ingham and Andrews (1973) have demonstrated. Moreover we were not at all impressed with those operant studies which use rhythmic and rate controlled forms of speech as a replacement for the stuttering response. *If operant conditioning is truly effective, we should be able to reinstate normal speech and extinguish stuttering without having to use these hoary old methods which for hundreds of years failed our ancient predecessors.* In half an hour any therapist can get a stutterer to speak without stuttering temporarily by using rhythmic speech or relaxation or suggestion or any of a hundred other such procedures. Sometimes the fluency may last a half hour or even more if the suggestion is very effective or the stutterer very suggestible. To use the precarious fluency achieved by such procedures as a proof that stuttering is nothing more than an instrumental response controlled by discriminative stimuli seems at worst sophistry or at best naiveté.

This criticism may have been too vehement and may therefore have given the erroneous impression that we feel operant conditioning plays no part in the stuttering problem. Quite the contrary, we are convinced that most of the so-called "secondary" symptoms of stuttering, the most abnormal features of the disorder in the confirmed stutterer, are probably *maintained* by the positive reinforcement of communicative consummation and by the negative reinforcement of decreased frustration. We are not so sure that these behaviors were originally learned in this way, but once they occurred or were deliberately used in the search for relief, the chances are that they persist because of their consequences. Operant conditioning explains only a part of the problem but it does explain a very important part.

RESPONDENT LEARNING THEORY: CLASSICAL CONDITIONING

Some learning theorists attribute the core behavior of stuttering to the disruptive effects of negative emotion on the sequencing of speech. As they see it, strong emotions such as those accompanying the expectation of imminent unpleasantness, punishment, or frustration are disintegrative, and they produce breakdown not only in the formulation of messages but also in their motoric expression. For example, if one is consumed with fear or anxiety, it is difficult to organize the flow of thought sufficiently to produce fluent speech. Also, if the fear is great enough, it tends to disrupt the intricate coordination patterns required for fluency so that broken speech results. In the stutterer any stimulus previously associated with the emotions that originally produced such breakdown would tend to create fear and also to disrupt speech. In this view stuttering is learned in the same way that dogs learn to stop eating and to jump spasmodically when a tone is presented which was previously paired with an electric shock. If this is its origin, stuttering has been classically conditioned. Brutten and Shoemaker (1967) describe the learning process in this way:

> . . . disintegration created by negative emotion is fundamental to any discussion of that specific form of fluency failure termed stuttering. In this light, stuttering is not seen as an instrumental response that depends on reinforcement for acquisition or maintenance, but as a fluency failure caused by the cognitive and motoric disorganization associated with negative emotion. Whatever else may be involved in stuttering, the speaker is engaged in the performance of a motor act that requires fine coordination and this performance is disrupted. The disorganization is seen as part of the generalized autonomic response complex which in essence defines negative emotion. . . . This learning to respond with negative emotion to stimuli takes place through classical conditioning. In essence, then, it is hypothesized that when an individual stutters, he is experiencing learned negative emotion (autonomic activity) which is disrupting to his normally fluent speech behavior (p. 30).

This explanation—that the basic behaviors of stuttering are produced by emotion that has been conditioned to certain stimuli—differs from the operant point of view in several important ways. First of all, this account does not assume that the original stuttering behavior was normal disfluency,* so it does not have to explain *why* the syllabic repetitions and phonemic prolongations received so much more reinforcement than the other types of normal disfluency. Secondly, this theory of stuttering states that the original fluency breaks consist of disorganized forms of previously integrated behaviors, a concept which we will remember was held by Bluemel.† Thirdly, this classical conditioning theory of stuttering considers the antecedents of stuttering to be as important as its consequences. Certain stimuli produce emotional upheaval and that upheaval disrupts speech. When neutral stimuli are paired with those that originally produced the emotional upset, these become the antecedents of stuttering. The stuttering is the byproduct of this emotional learning. Thus Brutten and Shoemaker (1967) state: "We have taken the position that stuttering is that form of fluency failure which results from conditioned negative emotion." This is respondent rather than operant learning. It is based on the

---

* It assumes instead that the disfluent behaviors of nonstutterers are not "normal," which makes the distinction between stutterers and nonstutterers imprecise.

† Bluemel (1957) explained the early onset of "stammering" as being due to the fact that in childhood speech was not yet thoroughly integrated and was therefore more vulnerable to emotional stress.

association of stimuli with other stimuli. To cite some oversimplified examples: One of the children we studied shortly after the onset of stuttering was reported to have stuttered first at mealtime in a summer cabin. On the table was a lighted kerosene lamp. The boy had just begun to say "Mummy, I . . ." when he knocked over the lamp and set fire to the cabin.

The parental report seemed pretty clear that immediately afterward, when he tried to talk, especially to his mother, and most often at mealtimes, the first word of each utterance showed very frequent syllabic repetitions, and that complete blocking often occurred especially when he used the words "Mummy" and "I." (Let us say immediately that this report is hardly typical of the onset histories we have seen, and that we use it here only to illustrate the respondent learning explanation.) The occasions on which these words were appropriately uttered contained stimuli which were similar, or had been paired with those which originally resulted in broken speech because they triggered a discharge of negative emotion which had come to have the power to break it.

It is apparent that this view of the nature of stuttering has an ancient history and that there is a decided folklore flavor to it. "He began to stutter when he was scared by a horse." "He began to stutter when a tramp came to the door." Every speech therapist has heard such tales, but those of us who have investigated many of these accounts usually find that others had recognized stuttering in the child long before the alleged traumatizing incident occurred and so we have become a bit cynical and suspicious of such evidence. We have, however, found reason to believe that some few of these accounts were indeed true and that some stuttering problems did apparently arise in this way.

In general, this belief that stuttering is the by-product of conditioned negative emotion rests on the assumption that the original moments of stuttering were produced by unpleasant emotional upheaval, and that they represent disruptions and disorganizations of normal speech. Is this assumption true? Do the first stutterings always occur under conditions of emotional stress? Do the first stutterings always show the same sort of features characteristic of other stress-produced disorganization? Do these repetitions and prolongations of a syllable or sound really deserve the term "disintegrated behaviors?" In the beginning stutterer, they do not appear to be highly random or chaotic. An extensive review of the research and our own clinical experiences make us reject the adverb "always." As Johnson (1959) has shown in his monumental study of the onset of stuttering, most stuttering does not originate in situations involving emotional trauma, nor does it begin suddenly, nor does it involve marked disruptions in verbal behavior. Rather it seems, in most instances, to be discovered first in fairly normal communicative situations, to show a gradual course of developmental increase and initially to be characterized by rather stereotyped syllabic repetitions. Brutten and Shoemaker have pointed to breathing abnormalities, especially the sharp inhalation characteristic of startle, as evidence of emotionally produced disruption, but we have not found these to be characteristic of most beginning stutterers.

Most of the literature dealing with beginning stutterers indicates that the initial behaviors do not show the profound disorganizations that characterize stress responses. They are not accompanied by great emotional upheaval. Beginning stuttering most often is reverberatory and fixative. It does not show the picture of startle or panicky awareness, nor is it random struggle.

Because information about the beginning stutterer is sparse, those theorists who attribute the core behavior solely to emotional disruption have again assembled data from adult stutterers to support their hypothesis. Most of them have punished or threatened to punish stutterers on certain words or for each moment of stuttering, using electric shock, or noxious noise, or simple verbal responses such as "No" or "Wrong!"* Unfortunately, even these adult studies have failed to show conclusively that threatened punishment (which should produce emotional disruption) consistently increases stutterings or disfluencies. Some researchers find that it does; others that it has no effect; still others that punishment (or its expectation) decreases disfluencies. Some of the confusion may be due to differences in research design or to the difficulty in creating in the laboratory the appropriate kinds of punishment to which adult stutterers are especially vulnerable. When we think of how many children have been punished during the act of speaking and how many children have had to speak in the throes of profound emotion, we wonder why so few stutterers have been produced. If originally stuttering is created by trying to talk under the influence of negative emotion, all of us should be stutterers.

We feel that the real contribution of classical conditioning theory as it is applied to stuttering lies in its ability to explain the development of the disorder. The spread and generalization of situational and word fears is probably due to the linking of antecedent stimuli. The intricate avoidance strategies employed deliberately by the confirmed stutterer are triggered by conditioned stimuli which were previously associated with negative emotion. We are not so sure that the basic disruptions in the speech of stutterers are always necessarily the product of emotional upheaval. Stuttering can occur when no anxiety or other evidence of negative emotion seems to be present, not only in the beginning stutterer but also in the adult at times. To restrict the term stuttering to that class of fluency failure created by conditioned negative emotion may be convenient to the theorists but it fails to account for a large part of the problem.

TWO-FACTOR THEORIES OF HOW STUTTERING BEHAVIOR IS LEARNED

For purposes of clear exposition in describing the application of classical conditioning to stuttering, we have neglected to state that few theorists today believe that everything the stutterer does and feels can be explained with classical conditioning concepts. The stereotyped avoidance and strug-

---

* A summary of this research is provided in the last section of this chapter.

gle reactions, which Wingate (1964) called the accessory symptoms of stuttering, are not considered by any modern writer as breakdown phenomena. The stutterer who characteristically says, "ah . . . ah . . . ah . . . um" prior to making a speech attempt is not caught in the throes of panic-produced disintegration. He is deliberately postponing an expected unpleasantness. The typical stuttering patterns in the adult seem to be too individualized and too organized to fit such an hypothesis. Accordingly, Brutten and Shoemaker (1967), applied Mowrer's (1950) two-factor learning theory to stuttering. In their formulation, they combine both the operant and classical kinds of conditioning. They feel that the core behavior, the disruption of the motor sequences of speech into repetitions and prolongations, are precipitated by classically conditioned negative emotions as described in our last section. They also feel that the stutterer learns various methods for coping with the threat or experience of broken speech and that these reactions of avoidance and escape are instrumental responses which have been conditioned through their reinforcing consequences. Brutten and Shoemaker say, "We have proposed that the stutterer may evidence two classes of learned behavior. The first class includes the conditioned negative emotion that tends to disrupt fluent speech. This conditioned emotionality may lead to the second class, escape or avoidance behavior" (p. 62). In various other statements they make clear that in their view the onset and development of involuntary stuttering behaviors can be accounted for best by the classical conditioning of negative emotion, whereas the voluntary coping reactions with which the stutterer tries to solve his problem are instrumentally conditioned. About the latter, they write: "Although these learned instrumental responses are not found among all stutterers, in many they are more prevalent and more dramatic than the repetitions and prolongations that define stuttering. These instrumental responses are often nonverbal behaviors such as facial tics, body twitches, or leg movements" (p. 61). In their therapy, Brutten and Shoemaker use classical conditioning procedures, such as counter conditioning (reciprocal inhibition) or deconditioning to weaken the conditioned negative emotion, and massing or negative practice to weaken the instrumental behaviors through nonreinforcement. They feel, however, that the basic target should be the classically conditioned negative emotion, since if this is eliminated, much of the utility served by the instrumental responses would be lost. When the latter continue to be demonstrated, Brutten and Shoemaker conveniently attribute their persistence to the past history of intermittent reinforcement.

WISCHNER'S ANTICIPATORY THEORY OF STUTTERING

Not all the theories of stuttering which are based on learning theory fit exactly into the templates of classical or operant conditioning or even two-factor theory. One of these other theories is that tentatively formulated by Wischner (1947, 1950, 1952). Wischner applied the Hullian concepts of drive-reduction to account for the maintenance of stuttering behaviors, the main drive being that of anxiety. Wischner adopts Johnson's position that stuttering begins when the child, because of parental disapproval or other penalties, begins to react to his normal disfluencies with tension, anxiety, and avoidance. Wischner, however, in contradistinction to Johnson, states that the stutterer is not trying to avoid the now noxious normal disfluencies but instead to avoid "the original consequences which attended the original nonfluent behavior,"—the feelings of anxiety, hurt, and shame. Certain situational or verbal cues come to precipitate these learned anxieties, and the person takes steps to reduce them by various avoidance behaviors. "This anxiety possesses drive properties and motivates the child to activity designed to avoid the noxious stimulation." Since the avoidance behaviors do keep the original disfluencies out of the stutterer's mouth (even though they may appear to the listener to be much more abnormal) the learned anxiety-tension connected with these disfluencies does not arise. It is in this way that the stutterer's avoidance behaviors are actually able to lessen anxiety while speaking. Through anxiety reduction, these avoidance reactions are strongly reinforced and thereby developed and maintained.

Certainly, avoidance behaviors do occasionally avoid unpleasantness. They are successful often enough. The stutterer who substitutes the nonfeared word "youth" instead of "boy" terminates the specific fear that was connected with the latter word. Or, if the stutterer utters "um-um-um-er-um" before a word colored black by learned anxiety, sometimes, if he postpones long enough, that specific anxiety goes down, and he experiences no stuttering whatsoever. Any behavior that reduces the anxiety drive gets strongly reinforced. The performance of these stuttering rituals thus becomes a major feature of stuttering. Like whistling in the dark as you pass a graveyard, if nothing evil happens, you are more likely to whistle the next time you pass that place—and, if the fear is greater, to whistle louder and longer. Each successful avoidance strengthens the probability that it will be used again.

But these anticipatory struggle and avoidance behaviors are themselves punished by listeners. Why then do they persist? Wischner answers this question by saying that the punishment occurs after the anxiety reduction, since the listener's punishment is usually perceived after the utterance is completed. He also uses the concepts of anxiety confirmation and secondary gains to explain why stuttering behaviors persist. With regard to the latter, he writes:

> Clinical experience reveals a wide variety of material benefits that may accrue to the stutterer without his necessarily being aware of them. Thus there may be "considerate" teachers who excuse Jimmie from recitation. Or Bill may receive a medical discharge from the Army on the basis of his speech with a disability pension attached. All of these may well serve to reinforce stuttering behavior. It seems important from a therapeutic standpoint to investigate very carefully the possibility of secondary gain in each stuttering case. To accept the stutterer's

negative reply at face value to the question, "Does your stuttering bring any rewards?" is inadequate, since the stutterer very often is not directly aware of the benefits that he might be deriving from his speech behavior (1950, p. 332).

Wischner says that the punishment doesn't occur until after the anxiety reduction has occurred. We doubt this. This social punishments may come later, as Wischner says, but an equally strong punisher, frustration, comes immediately.

SHEEHAN'S APPROACH-AVOIDANCE CONFLICT THEORY

Like most of the other explanations of stuttering in terms of learning theory, Sheehan's theory (1958) is an application of an earlier formulation, in this instance the approach-avoidance conflict theory of Dollard and Miller (1950). Unresolved conflict is always unpleasant. Ambivalence, indecision, uncertainty are noxious emotional states. They are as unpleasant as pain, hunger, or other human miseries. There are various kinds of conflict. The child in a candy shop, torn between buying a lollipop or chocolate, has an *approach-approach* conflict. He wants both but must choose. A fisherman suddenly confronted by a mother bear with cubs wonders whether to lie down in the water, to run upstream, or downstream, or cross the river to the other side. He is in an *avoidance-avoidance* conflict— and he isn't particularly happy. Some of the most unpleasant conflicts in life are *approach-avoidance* conflicts—like going to the dentist. One is caught in a tug of war between opposing needs and drives. The conflict is only resolved by certain behaviors which permit one urge to become stronger than the other and these resolving behaviors are thereby strongly reinforced. Anything we do that reduces our unpleasantness is reinforced. One of the main unpleasant features of conflict is the tension and the oscillation or fixation which occur when the opposing forces are about equal. You find that the closer you come to the dentist's office, the stronger is the opposing urge to run the other way and so you find yourself in the uneasy and miserable balance of conflicting forces. In Sheehan's words:

> Caught as he is in a double approach-avoidance conflict, the stutterer is caught between two choices, each one of which threatens the bitter along with the sweet. He can speak, thus achieving his aim of communication, but at the cost of the shame and guilt he has learned to attach to his stuttering. Or he can remain silent, abandon communication, and suffer the frustration and guilt that such a retreat carries with it (1958, p. 126).

Thus Sheehan claims that in stuttering we have double approach-avoidance conflicts. No only is there the approach-avoidance conflict in which there is a desire to speak and at the same time a desire not to speak, but also another one going on at the same time: the desire to be silent and the fear of silence (silence being equated with death and impotence).

Considering the onset of stuttering, Sheehan (1958) maintains that when an individual experiences guilt, he also experiences the conflicting needs to express himself and to be silent. This Sheehan would also call an approach-avoidance conflict. It is created by opposing needs, and it leads to oscillations and fixations in behavior. In speech these become the repetitions and prolongations found in stuttering. In other words, since the verbal expression of guilt is the focus of the conflict, the turmoil of the inner self is revealed in the verbal nonfluencies of the child. Since the child feels rejected, he believes that he has done something wrong, and this reaction leads to an unhappy choice: either he must believe his parents are mean and unjust (which decreases his security) or else he must justify their rejection by doing something that deserves their rejection. Stuttering may be that thing.

This tug of war between opposing forces, according to Sheehan, shows up on various levels; (1) the word level (saying sounds or words which have been feared, or are hard to pronounce as "statistics," or carry unpleasant meanings); (2) the situation level, where communicative situations are such that you both desire to enter or avoid them; (3) the level of emotional expression in which opposing desires to express hate and love, etc., are involved; (4) the level of interpersonal relationships, e.g., wanting to impress the boss and fearing he may reject you; (5) the ego-protective conflicts that result in the oscillations and fixations of speech. The more of these conflicts that are involved in any moment of stuttering, the harder and longer one stutters. The more equal the approach-avoidance drives in a speaking task, the more likely one will fixate or oscillate, that is, stutter.

Sheehan's basic treatment is to bring the therapist's force to bear toward strengthening the approach gradient and weakening the avoidance one. His is basically a classical conditioning therapy since he holds that the stutterer should experience the stimuli (which originally produced the conflict or were associated with it) in a therapeutic situation where no conflict would occur. Speak even though you do stutter. Enter the feared situations even though you fear them. Accept the challenge even though you fear you'll fail. Say the dirty word or the feared word. And do all of these in group therapy with other stutterers or in the presence of an accepting therapist so you won't feel the miseries of conflict. Experience the buzzer without the shock. Test the reality; it isn't as bad as you think. Decrease all avoidance behaviors at all levels. Learn to live with a minimum of ambivalence.

Sheehan sets up two principal hypotheses: (1) the conflict hypothesis—that the stutterer blocks or stops or repeats whenever the conflicting approach and avoidance tendencies (on any level) reach a precarious equilibrium, and (2) the fear reduction hypothesis—that the stuttering itself reduces the fear of the occurrence of stuttering sufficiently to permit the release from the blocked word, thus resolving the conflict momentarily and so enabling the stutterer to continue.

SUMMARY

Although the theoretical positions of Sheehan and Wischner, based on familiar Hullian concepts, are very attractive, they have found limited acceptance. The research cited in their support, consisting mainly of projective drawings, is not impressive. They have not shown that stuttering can be produced in the fashion they claim it is produced. Also, if stuttering is reinforced every time it occurs, repeated readings of the same material should increase not decrease their frequency of occurrence. As Beech and Fransella (1968) point out, their position that the stuttering reduces the fear that triggers it is not convincing even when we take into consideration the possibility that the punishment may come later than the relief, a proposition that has not been substantiated. Approach-avoidance conflicts doubtless play some part in stuttering, but many fractured words occur without such conflicts being evident. Both of these writers fail to provide satisfactory accounts of the onset, development, sex ratio, loci, and many other basic features of the disorder. One feels that they have crammed the poor stutterer into the Procrustean beds of their theoretical models so very hard that, though a good portion of his trunk is encompassed therein, his head and limbs are missing.

COGNITIVE LEARNING THEORIES OF STUTTERING

Not all those who feel that stuttering behaviors are learned attribute all of that learning to the various associative relationships between stimuli and responses. The same is true of many psychologists concerned with learning. Although they do not deny that habits may be acquired through classical or operant conditioning, they feel that these models do not account adequately for all the intricate and complex kinds of learning found in human beings, or for that matter even in the lower animals. Tolman (1951) showed long ago, for example, that a rat running a maze seems to be learning a kind of map of the terrain rather than a set of serial turning habits. Latent learning, one-trial insightful learning, exploratory behavior, and a good many other problems in the acquisition of responses present considerable difficulty for the S-R conditioning theorists. Pavlov himself noted these and attempted to solve them by positing a second signal system—the use of overt or covert language—for the control of human behavior, and many behaviorists today are investigating the possibility of conditioning language themes as ways of reconciling their theory with more of the facts. Most cognitive learning theorists organize their positions on the concepts of perception and information theory and the organization of cognition consisting of models, maps, systems, strategies, or programs, and the like. This text cannot possibly explore these old and new developments in detail, but explanatory concepts such as Miller, Galanter, and Pribam's (1960) TOTE hypothesis, Festinger's (1957) cognitive dissonance theory, and Feigenbaum's (1959) EPAM all seem to indicate that sooner or later we will have a cognitive learning theory for stuttering.

At present there is no comprehensive cognitive theory of stuttering. The closest attempt is that by Smith (1966). He bases his preliminary theoretical formulation on Festinger's (1957) belief that behavior is always directed toward a reduction of cognitive dissonance. Cognitive dissonance is present when there is an incompatibility between opinons, beliefs, or attitudes; or between expected performance and actual performance, or between stored information (expectations) and incoming stimuli, or between goals and plans. The brain as a computer is inherently programmed to seek always a reduction in cognitive dissonance by varying the output of the system until the incongruity no longer exists. The relationship of this view to information theory is obvious, and Miller, Galanter, and Pribam (1960) even go so far as to describe a possible brain mechanism which could account for this reduction of error signalling in the form of two feedback loops which comprise a feedback comparator system. Smith, in applying this theoretical construct to stuttering, does not seem to us to be very successful. He employs the concept of the GIAL. (General Incongruity Adaptation Level) developed by Driver and Streufert (1965) who state: "Organisms with past experiences rich in general incongruity would develop high GIAL's and those with very predictable peaceful pasts would evolve very low GIAL's" (p. 50). A brief excerpt from Smith's work may communicate its disappointing flavor:

> Let it be assumed that the parents have begun calling attention to the child's speech through pressure to speak more fluently or to stop "stuttering." The incongruity created by the pressure may represent an overload which could produce one of the radical shifts in the GIAL. . . . However, if the child has responded to the pressure of his parents by trying to speak as they would prefer, the incongruity thereby induced by his parents may not be resolved through a new, higher GIAL because he may not be developmentally able to speak more fluently. Conscious efforts to control speech may only compound the difficulty. Therefore the incongruity from the environment persists or even intensifies, and, even though the GIAL may be rising, it does not resolve the conflict. For that reason, the child may find himself in a dilemma: he cannot adjust to the incongruity coming from his parents through a higher GIAL (General Incongruity Adaptation Level) because his efforts to control his speech fail, which can create even more incongruity which would require still more change in the GIAL (p. 21).

Two other cognitive learning theories of stuttering, although they have rarely been viewed as such, are those by Emil Froeschels and Wendell Johnson. When their writings are closely examined, it seems apparent that both of these men base their explanation of the disorder on misperception. Froeschels, for example, in several articles stresses the role of the misperception that speaking is difficult. He says that this wrong belief leads a child to respond to his physiological stuttering (normal disfluency) by struggle and avoidance, thereby creating the real disorder. Froeschels (1952) writes:

The child, believing in speech difficulty, and perhaps being asked not to iterate (repeat), will try to overcome the "difficulty" by using more muscular energy. In this way the iterations will be spoken with strongly contracted muscles, and the single iterations will therefore proceed more slowly than the iterations without pressure. . . . As time goes on, new signs and symptoms are developed. It is the author's opinion that every stage in the development of the clinical picture is caused by the patient's belief in his inability to speak normally (p. 113).

Froeschels also makes the point that all of the accessory struggling movements are those which can be made voluntarily, and he seems to say that initially at least they are deliberately used as strategies to cope with the illusory inability.

Although Johnson shifted his theoretical beliefs several times during his productive lifetime—indeed all the way from the cerebral dominance theory to an interactionist position—he is best known for his semantogenic theory, a representative account of which is found in his book *People in Quandaries* (1946). Johnson's basic thesis was that stuttering is the result of misperception and misevaluation, that it has its onset in the parent's misjudging the child's normal disfluencies as being abnormal and unacceptable. Again, once the stutterer has interiorized these misevaluations, has labeled them inappropriately, and has begun to think about them in a language which is full of semantic errors, he adopts various strategies of avoidance to lessen his distress. Even Johnson's therapy uses a cognitive approach.

IS STUTTERING LEARNED THROUGH OPERANT CONDITIONING?

A substantial number of studies seems to support the view that stuttering can be considered as belonging to the operant class of learned responses because it decreases when aversive stimuli are applied contingently. Among the contingent aversive stimuli that have been used are electric shocks, delayed auditory feedback, a burst of very intense light or sound, the interruption of communication (time-outs), verbal reprimands, and different response costs (the loss of money, etc.). Let us review some of this research.

Flanagan, Goldiamond, and Azrin (1958) had three stutterers read for about 30 minutes until adaptation had occurred and a base-rate seemed stabilized. Then a 105 dB tone was presented continuously through earphones except that each stuttering moment turned off the sound for five seconds (negative reinforcement). All three subjects showed an increase in stuttering. When the contingent tone was omitted, the frequency of stuttering decreased to the baseline rate. Then the noxious tone of one second-duration was administered contingent upon each stuttering moment, and the stuttering decreased, one subject becoming entirely free there in the laboratory. In a similar study, Goldiamond (1965), using delayed auditory feedback as a "punishment" instead of the loud tone, showed that when a short pulse of DAF was made contingent upon stuttering, stuttering decreased.

The DAF produced a slower rate and increased fluency—which is about what we would expect from our knowledge of the fluency-facilitating effects of DAF. In an attempt to replicate Flanagan, Goldiamond, and Azrin's research, Biggs and Sheehan (1969) used a 108 dB high frequency tone as an aversive stimulus in three conditions: presented contingently with a moment of stuttering, presented randomly, and stopping it when stuttering occurred. Since they found that stuttering decreased under all three conditions they attributed the decrease mainly to distraction.

Several studies from the University of Minnesota have also dealt with punishing stuttering. Using three stutterers, Martin and Siegel (1966b) studied the effects of administering contingent shock for different types of stuttering behavior (nose-wrinkling, tongue-protrusion, etc.) and found that these specific stuttering behaviors decreased but returned to baseline as soon as the contingent shock was removed. However, at the same time, an increase in prolongations occurred. In another experiment (Martin and Siegel, 1966a) with two male stutterers these authors simultaneously "punished" stuttering by the words *not good* and rewarded fluency by the word *good*. Both of these contingencies increased the fluency, and when they were no longer used, more stuttering occurred. A nylon strap used as a discriminative stimulus was shown to have some effectiveness. Brady (1967) shocked his subjects contingently for each moment of stuttering while reading a 1,000 word passage and found that there was less stuttering in this condition than when no shock was employed. Quist and Martin (1967) used the word *wrong* as a consequence for any repetition and prolongation in one stutterer and for "uh" or prolonged "n" sounds in two others after baselines had been established. They reported reductions in frequency of stuttering under these contingencies. The responses returned to base-rates when the contingencies were removed. Hegde

Figure 13. Number of tongue protrusions and S-prolongations emitted by subject O each two minutes during session B. (Reproduced by permission from Houghton-Mifflin Co., publishers of H. N. Sloane and B. D. Macaulay (eds) (Operant Procedures In Remedial Speech and Language Training. Chapter 16 by R. Martin "The Experimental Manipulation of Stuttering Behaviors.")

(1971) found that contingent shock reduced stuttering in oral reading. According to Gross and Holland (1965) contingent electric shock produced a decrease in stuttering but also shocking the listener had the same effect. Haroldson, Martin, and Starr (1968) used a contingent "time-out" or period of silence, as an interruption to communication, and found a decrease in stuttering in their four subjects.

Not all of the research has corroborated the usual findings that contingent punishment decreases stuttering. Timmons (1966), using an experimental and a control group of stutterers, gave the first group the word *wrong* as a punishment contingent upon stuttering in the middle series of repeated readings of the same material. The controls received no "punishing" word. No significant increases or decreases in stuttering were found. Daly and Cooper (1967) studied adaptation readings in which shock was administered first during, and then after each moment of stuttering, and then in a third condition no shock was given. Differences among conditions were not significant. Stevens (1963) gave a sample shock prior to the stutterers' readings and found no significant change as a result of making it contingent on the stuttering moment.

Several studies by Cady and Robbins (1968); Cooper, Cady, and Robbins (1970); and Daly and Kimbarrow (1978) have shown that the contingent use of such words as *right!*, *wrong!* or *tree!* all produce the same decrease in stutterings or in normal disfluencies. Why should a presumably neutral word such as *tree* decrease stuttering? According to the operant conditioners, all three words must be been punishing since they produced a response decrement. A more meaningful explanation is probably that they called attention to stuttering. As alerting devices they may simply have eliminated some of the minor stutterings. Or perhaps all these words, including *tree* interrupted the preparatory sets to stutter or served as distractors.

PUNISHMENT OF NORMAL DISFLUENCIES

Perhaps because it is difficult to get stutterers to be subjects in experiments requiring contingent punishment, several studies have used normal speakers. Bilger and Speaks (1959) paired a green light with a tone that had been associated with electric shock and then used the light to "punish" their disfluencies and found that more disfluencies occurred when the light was given.

Brookshire and Martain (1967) used *wrong, no* and *uh-uh* paired with normal speakers' disfluencies and found a temporary suppression of the latter which varied somewhat depending on which "punishing" word was used. Siegel and Martin (1965a) found no significant differences when shock was made contingent on disfluency in two experiments, but in a third study using oral reading they found that random shock slightly increased disfluencies although unexpected contingent shocks significantly reduced them. These investigators then used nonshock "punishments" (Siegel and Martin, 1965b and 1966)—the words *right* and *wrong*, and a buzzer. These contingencies including the buzzer, decreased the normal disfluencies. The word *right* did not increase them. Brookshire (1968) used bursts of randomly presented aversive noise as normal speakers read aloud one day and aversive noise contingent upon disfluencies the other day, the order of conditions being counterbalanced. The subjects who received the contingent noise after having experienced the random noise did not show the usual decrease in disfluencies. In a somewhat similar study, Brookshire and Eveslage (1969) used contingent random noise and contingent *no* whenever their normal speakers were disfluent. The random noise increased disfluency and the *no* decreased it. Siegel and Martin (1968) used verbal punishment of spontaneous speech and found a similar decrease in disfluency and also a slowing down in rate—the subjects probably became more careful in how they talked. There have been other experiments of this sort but their pertinence depends on the assumed equivalence of normal disfluencies to those of stuttering, an assumption which we do not feel has been validated.

These operant punishment studies had a profound effect upon workers in the field of stuttering and soon their impact was seen in the devising of operant methods for treating stutterers. Since our concern here is the nature of stuttering rather than its treatment, we will not review them but instead call attention to some representative reports. Those by Ryan (1971), Shames, Egolf and Rhodes (1969), and Andrews and Ingham (1971) are most noteworthy.

DOUBTS ABOUT THE OPERANT NATURE OF STUTTERING

During the decade of the seventies, studies began to appear which cast some doubt on the operant nature of stuttering. Many of these examined the effect of contingent punishment on the molecular components of the molar moments of stuttering, and they found that punishment had different effects on such behaviors. Contingent aversive stimuli did not reduce sound and syllable repetitions or prolongations as it usually does with such accessory responses as iterations, eye blinking, nose wrinkling, tongue thrusts, or sudden arm movements. Behaviors belonging to the latter class of behaviors usually show a decrease in frequency under punishment but the basic behaviors often increased or remained unchanged. Two studies by Brutten (1980) and by Bastijens, Brutten, and Stes (1978) are illustrative. In the former, Brutten found that a contingent verbal reprimand resulted in an increase, not a decrease, in prolongations; in the latter, Bastijens *et al.* showed that contingent verbal reprimand was able to suppress (though not completely) the stutterer's compulsive arm movements. These reports, of course, support Brutten's two factor theory which maintains that the basic behaviors are classically learned whereas the accessory behaviors are learned intrumentally or operantly.

The two researches just mentioned are not the only ones which indicate that the operant view of the effect of contingent punishment may not be entirely valid. Studies by Webster (1968), Starkweather (1970), Zenner and Webster (1975), and Janssen and Brutten (1973) also showed that certain specific component behaviors in the molar moments of stuttering do not always decrease under punishment. Some decrease, some increase, and some remain unchanged.

Moreover, when the performances of individual subjects under contingent punishment is examined, we find that some of them do not show the expected decrease in frequency. For example, Martin, St. Louis, Haroldson, and Hasbrouck (1975) found that, of their five stutterers, the percentage of words stuttered increased for two subjects, decreased for two others, and remained the same for the fifth one under contingent punishment. Such individual differences in responding to punishment have also been reported by other researchers.

The nature of the aversive stimuli used in some of the operant punishment research may account for some of the contradictory results. Starkweather (1970) found that mild contingent shocks decreased stuttering but very severe ones increased its frequency. Short term experimental sessions may show suppression, but long term application of aversive stimuli may instead show an increase (Hegde, 1979).

There are other difficulties for the operant view of the nature of stuttering which concern the scheduling of consequences. Williams and Martin (1974) reported no significant differences in the decrease of stuttering between immediate delivery of the aversive stimulus and delayed delivery. In terms of operant learning theory, immediate delivery should have produced more decrease (Azrin and Holz, 1966). Williams and Martin (1974), however, did show that contingent electric shock had some effect in reducing the frequency of stuttering.

The nature of the aversive stimuli used in the operant studies has also raised questions. For example, how aversive are time-outs? Adams and Popelka (1971) found that six of their eight subjects who showed a decrease under contingent time-out "attributed their decreased stuttering to a more relaxed confortable state." The time-outs gave them a chance to calm themselves.

Finally, some of the operant studies have been criticized because of their use of unstable base-rates or base-rates founded on too small samples. Thus Adams (1970) claimed that the reported base-rates in the Haroldson, Martin, and Starr (1968) study were so unstable that their findings should be considered doubtful. Starkweather (1971) in his article, "The Case Against Base-Rate Comparisons in Stuttering Experimentation," showed that a real problem existed.

The operant model also requires that positive reinforcement (reward) should *increase* the frequency of stuttering behaviors. Here the evidence is not substantial. Ryan (1967) found an initial decrease then later an increase in stuttering when his single subject was paid a penny every time he stuttered. Starkweather (1978), using tokens redeemable for other rewards, administered them contingent upon stuttering and found that three of his four subjects showed a *decrease* in stutterings while only one of them showed an increase, the latter probably because he "faked" stuttering to get the reward.

Escape from punishment (negative reinforcement) may also be viewed as rewarding. In the study by Goldiamond (1965), when the continuous "punishing" DAF was turned off whenever the person stuttered, the expected increase in stuttering did not take place. Biggs and Sheehan (1969) found that stuttering decreased when a continuous and very loud tone was turned off contingent upon stuttering. According to the operant paradigm, it should have increased.

The studies by Cady and Robbins (1968); Cooper, Cady, and Robbins (1970); and Daly and Kimbarrow (1978) that we have mentioned earlier showed that the contingent administration of *right!* when stuttering occurred resulted in less stuttering just as the verbal reprimand *wrong!* or the neutral word *tree!* had done. As Bloodstein (1979) remarked, "To observe it (the word *right*) acting as a punisher is anomalous and contradictory" (p. 666). Van Riper (1957) reported that when a male stutterer was rewarded for quotas of stuttering by being kissed by a pretty girl, an immediate and dramatic decrease, rather than an increase, in stuttering occurred. He also reported that when a very hostile boy stutterer was rewarded for stuttering moments by being contingently allowed to give Van Riper a very severe electric shock, the stuttering again did not increase but was almost eliminated. Stevens (1963) found no significant increase in stuttering when verbal approval was made contingent upon stuttering. Lanyon and Barocas (1975) showed that contingent monetary gain for moments of stuttering decreased stuttering rather than increased it. All in all, it seems evident that most of this positive and negative reinforcement research does not support the view that stuttering consistently behaves according to the operant model.

OTHER EXPLANATIONS
FOR THE PUNISHMENT EFFECT

There are other alternative explanations for the decrease in stuttering resulting from contingent punishment. The first of these is that the punishment calls the stutterer's attention to his moments of stuttering and he simply tries not to stutter as often. That this self instruction not to stutter or to speak as fluently as possible can be successful in decreasing (though not eliminating disfluencies completely) has been demonstrated by Wingate (1959), Goldiamond (1965), Martin and Siegel (1966), Siegel and Martin (1968), and Martin and Haroldson (1979). Oelschlaeger and Brutten (1974) found that instructions "to try not to interject" reduced the frequency of interjections but that instruction to "try not to repeat" did not. It is possible therefore that when molar "moments of stuttering" are used as the target behaviors for contingent punishment, some of the decrease may be due to the elimination of these more normal disfluencies.

Siegel (1970) in his review of punishment studies, recognized that all of the various forms of contingent punishment that reduced stuttering had one property in common—they made each moment of stuttering or disfluency more conspicuous to the speaker. Using the term "high-lighting" to refer to the focusing of attention on the disfluencies, he suggests that the reason high-lighting does decrease them is because they thereby become "carriers of their own punishment." This sounds plausible but if it is true, then stuttering should extinguish itself unless the stutterer is masochistic or unless the punishment becomes the signal for future reward.

Another way of accounting for the suppressing of stuttering behaviors through contingent punishment is that the introduction of a shock or reprimand or time-out simply serves as a distraction. Bloodstein (1975) pointed out that stuttering tends to be reduced when any kind of strong or novel stimulus is introduced into the speaking situation. Perhaps the stutterer becomes so afraid of the shock that he does not scan for approaching stuttering and so has fewer phonemic or word fears. Perhaps it is due to external inhibition which Pavlov claimed occurred when the strength of a conditioned response decreased because of a novel stimulus (for example, the slamming of the laboratory door) during the process of conditioning. Many stutterers tell us that they try to use distractions to counter their fears and that if they can just stop thinking about stuttering they stutter less. Biggs and Sheehan (1969) attributed the decrease in stuttering when a tone was presented randomly, contingently, or in escape conditions to distraction. Williams and Martin (1974) consider distraction to be one possible reason for their findings which showed that both contiguous and non-contiguous shock for stuttering produced about the same decrease, and that the shock did not have to be administered immediately after the stuttering to be effective. Operant principles would have predicted that this would not have happened. The whole concept of distraction is a slippery one, and its nature is so unclear that many workers fail to consider it seriously. Boers-van Duk (1973) provides a summary of treatment methods for stuttering whose effectiveness has been attributed to distraction and she rejects its validity as a reasonable explanation.

IS STUTTERING SELF-REINFORCING?

Theorists have always had difficulty in explaining why stuttering—presumably an unpleasant experience not only to the listener but to the stutterer himself—persists. Various explanations have been offered. Wischner (1952) suggests several possibilities beside the old one of secondary gains such as attention-getting: 1. the unpleasant tension built up during prior expectancy ceases once the feared word has been spoken. (If you are terribly afraid the bear will bite you, *that specific fear* disappears once the bear does bite.) 2. If stuttering is, as Johnson suggested, an avoidance of normal disfluency which has been colored by unpleasant parental concern, the successful avoidance (even though the behavior is abnormal) is more rewarding than were the normal disfluency to have occurred. Even though the stuttering behavior gets punished, the reward precedes it and so has more effect. Sheehan (1953) attributes the persistence of stuttering to negative reinforcement. Stutterers are caught in unpleasant double approach-avoidance conflicts on various levels; the stuttering behavior immediately precedes the resolution of the conflict and so it is reinforced. Since most of these conflicts are solved by reducing the avoidance by the actual stuttering, the fear reduction that occurs during the stuttering reinforces the behavior.

The pertinent research in support of these views is very scanty. Sheehan and Voas (1954) found that masseter action current records showed a buildup in tension that peaked just before the stuttering ended. Shrum (1967), however, failed to corroborate this peaking in his electromyographic study, finding instead that the tension often persisted even after the word was spoken. Wischner (1952) (unconvincingly to us at least) interpreted a series of projective drawings done by his stutterers just before, during, and after a moment of stuttering to indicate that tension, anxiety, and stress built up before and during the block but subsided when it was completed. Sheehan, Cortese, and Hadley (1962) in a similar study also had their stutterers "draw" their own behavior before, during, and after a moment of stuttering. They found self-pictures which they "interpreted" as indicating that tension-reduction did occur following the blockage in some but not all stutterers, and that often the release was followed by the increased unpleasantness of guilt and shame. These few conflicting and rather dubious studies are hardly enough to allow us to feel confident in the adequacy of such explanations. If stuttering is self-reinforcing, we will probably have to look elsewhere for the reinforcement.

Perhaps the self-reinforcement for stuttering behaviors may lie in the fact that when the moment of stuttering is terminated and when the word is finally uttered, some progress in communicative consummation has been accomplished. Presumably when a stutterer begins to say a sentence he wants to complete it, since the basic drive in speaking is to communicate. Thus Silverman (1976) suggests that stuttering behaviors are reinforced because the stutterer does complete the transmission of his message. Moreover, when a moment of stuttering is followed by fluency, as often occurs, the latter may serve as its positive reinforcement. Halvorson (1971) found that when he additionally rewarded (with money points) each instance when a moment of stuttering was followed by a fluent word, the frequency of stuttering in *some* of his subjects decreased more than when the moments were just punished. This might be interpreted as weak evidence for consummation of communication as a positive reinforcer. The time-out studies of Haroldson, Martin, and Starr (1968) and others may be interpreted as showing that the stuttering-suppressing effect of time-outs may be due to their counteracting the communicative progress that would otherwise follow the stuttering. Sheehan (1951) interrupted communication by insisting that his stutterers repeat any stuttered word until it was spoken normally before they could continue speaking and found that stuttering decreased more rapidly in adaptation readings when this was done. It might also be mentioned that Van Riper (1957) devised his cancellation procedures in part to prevent the moment of stuttering from being immediately rewarded by the consummation of communication.

IS STUTTERING LEARNED AND MAINTAINED BY CLASSICAL CONDITIONING?

We now review the studies that deal with the classical conditioning of stuttering. Those who advocate this view feel that negative emotional states (fear, anxiety, frustration) lead to the breakdown of the motoric integrations of speech and that stimuli associated with this negative emotion become able to produce that breakdown.

Our own investigations of onset were reported in Chapter IV and indicated that only rarely did the first stutterings appear in emotionally loaded situations. The only other significant research is that done at Iowa. In a comprehensive interview investigation of the onset of stuttering in 246 children, Johnson (1959) found only a very few instances in which its onset was reported by the parents to have occurred in association with "illness or injury, shock or frights, as a consequence of imitation, or under any other unusual or memorable, or dramatic circumstances." Indeed most of the parents interviewed found it difficult to recall the circumstances under which the disorder first appeared. This is sparse evidence indeed.

One group of researches sought to determine whether or not the speech of nonstutterers is affected by negative emotion. Hill (1954) found that when a light was paired with shock and then administered to normal speakers, they became significantly more disfluent. Savoye (1954) had her nonstutterers read aloud, then repeatedly introduced a tone followed by a shock while they were speaking. They had more disfluencies during the ten seconds following the tone than during a ten second period midway between the shocks. Stassi (1961) found that when she continuously kept saying "Wrong!" while nonstutterers were speaking, they had more disfluencies than when she did not say it or when she said it only a few times. Brookshire (1968) found that when a sudden burst of white noise was introduced randomly, not contingently, his normal speakers showed more repetitions of all types. Brookshire and Eveslage (1969) found that stuttering increased under random shock but decreased when a contingent "No!" was given.

Turning now to stutterers, we find some evidence that the threat of punishment or even noncontingent punishment can increase stuttering. The first experimental approach was performed by Van Riper (1937). Finding it impossible, in a pilot experiment, to administer electric shock so that it would be truly contingent upon stuttering, he instead gave a sample shock then threatened to give another shock for each moment of stuttering which occurred during an adaptation reading. The subject was told that the shocks would be given at the end of the reading, but actually were not administered. A reversal of the adaptation effect and an increase in stuttering was found during the reading in which shock was threatened.

Frick (1952) had stutterers read single words, comparing the frequency of stutterings under four conditions: 1. no shock or threat; 2. contingent shock; 3. threatened shock per stuttering moment which was actually administered at the conclusion of the reading; and 4. shock administered after every word whether stuttered or not. Frick found no decrease in stutterings in any condition, but the combined shock conditions showed more stuttering than the control condition. Shock, contingent or threatened, did not suppress stuttering.

An experiment by Reed and Lingwall (1976) provided results that oppose Brutten and Shoemaker's (1967) contention that repetitions are resistant to contingent punishment. Not only did they decrease under this condition but the accompanying galvanic skin responses increased or remained stable. On the other hand, Janssen and Kraaimant (1978) present evidence showing a strong relationship between fast repetitions (but not prolongations) and measures of emotional arousal. Toomey and Sidman (1970), using a warning buzzer signalling severe shock, found only one of four stutterers showing more stuttering during the warning condition.

One of the requirements of a classical conditioned response is that it must be shown to be linked to antecedent stimuli. For example, stuttering should be closely associated with certain features of a speaking situation involving unpleasantness.

Johnson and Sinn (1937) eliminated 98 per cent of the subjects' stutterings by having them omit those words on which they had stuttered on a previous reading. Johnson and Knott (1937) had their stutterers read the same passage after an interval of time and found that 72 per cent of the moments of stuttering occurred on the same words previously stuttered in the first reading. Berwick (1955) showed that the frequency of stuttering was greater when the subjects spoke to photographs of preselected listeners evaluated as "difficult" than when they spoke to those evaluated as "easy listeners." Connett (1955) attempted, through suggestion, to increase the perception of the consonant /t/ as a difficult sound and found a slight but not significant increase in the frequency of stuttering on words beginning with this sound in adaptation readings.

The research on the relationship between expectancy and subsequent stuttering has already been reviewed. To summarize it briefly in this context: the studies of Knott, Johnson, and Webster (1937); Johnson and Inness (1939); Johnson and Ainsworth (1938); Milisen (1938); Van Riper (1936); Van Riper and Milisen (1939); Dixon (1947); and such recent ones as those by Brutten and Gray (1961), Brutten (1963), and Martin and Haroldson (1967), and others show very clearly that a substantial positive relationship between expectancy and subsequent stuttering has been demonstrated at least for adults. The research also shows, however, that *expectancy is not always followed by stuttering* and that stuttering can occur even when no expectancy is subjectively experienced. After all, all expectancy *proves* is that the stutterer knows the conditions under which stuttering has occurred in the past. Nevertheless, in general, the loci, the frequency, and the severity of stuttering seem to be somewhat predictable on the basis of the conditions preceding utterance, thus providing some evidence that those conditions are related to the occurrence of stuttering.

Stimulus generalization of the antecedent cues also seems to point in the direction of respondent learning. Fierman (1955) and Johnson, Larson, and Knott (1937) showed that a colored border associated with an adaptation reading passage in which stuttering occurred seemed to precipitate more stutterings than an equivalent sheet without the distinctive border. Johnson and Millsapps (1937) showed some tendency for stuttering to be linked to inkblots representing previously stuttered but deleted words. Brutten and Gray (1961) demonstrated that, by inserting words (which had previously been stuttered upon several times) into lists of words that had been fluently spoken, less stuttering occurred on the previously stuttered words. These authors attributed the decrease to the generalization of positive emotion to adjacent words and seem to feel that their view of stuttering as a stimulus contingent response had been supported by the results, an interpretation which seems less than secure.

Better evidence for stimulus generalization is found in a study by Peters and Simonson (1960). Using a memory drum to expose word-pairs to be memorized by their stutterers, these investigators selected words of high and low "stuttering potential" as rated by the individual subjects, then arranged them so that the first member of the pair of words to be exposed was always a word of low stuttering potential while the second member of the pair was, in half the instances, another word of low stuttering potential and in the other half, a word of high potential. The results of this verbal memory task showed that stuttering occurred more frequently on words learned in association with words of high stuttering potential than those with low potential. Associative learning through stimulus contiguity seemed to have taken place. This would also support the respondent learning hypothesis.

We have already reviewed the studies which seem to show that all the behaviors in stuttering do not seem to be operant responses. The basic behaviors of part word repetitions and prolongations do not appear to respond consistently to contingent punishment or reward as do the accessory ones. But this does not mean at all that they therefore must be classically conditioned responses. They may not be learned; they may merely reflect the stutterer's difficulty in coordinating the basic synergies of respiration, phonation, and articulation under stress. The research supporting the belief that stuttering is learned through classical conditioning is just too thin to be convincing.

CONCLUSIONS

When each of these studies is subjected to the critical analysis they require, many more questions are raised than are answered. Why do these investigations of punishment and stuttering yield such disparate results?

How important is the problem of the definition of stuttering? What was punished, the core behavior, or the associated struggle and avoidance reactions? Perhaps both normal and abnormal disfluencies were punished? Was the punishment truly contingent or contiguous? Were the punishments truly punishing? Are there other explanations for the reduction of stuttering under punishment? Subjects differ in vulnerability and attitude toward shock; electrode contacts shift; the utterance of the word *wrong!* can be spoken in many ways, and in the laboratory situation it may possess little real unpleasantness. Are these punishments anything like the ones usually encountered by the stutterer in the outside world? Was he merely playing the experimenter's game? Can we be sure that these stimuli were not merely alerting devices, or, on the other hand, distractors? How truly stable were the base-rates? Why did punishment produce only limited decreases in stuttering and have such temporary and restricted effects? Was the noxious noise effective because of its lingering masking effects? Did not DAF or its residual effects facilitate fluency quite apart from its presumed punishing characteristics? How representative of the general stuttering population were the subjects? What controls were made for possible experimenter bias? How important was the role of awareness? Did the fear of punishment wipe out the fear of stuttering?

This author has asked these and many other similar questions about each experiment, and his conclusion is to him a disappointing one. It is this: The research has not yet established that stuttering behavior can be entirely explained by present learning theory, neither its origin nor its maintenance. Neither classical nor operant conditioning nor their combination (as in Brutten and Shoemaker's two-factor theory) are completely explanatory. Each of these accounts for some of the phenomena of stuttering but not for all. No one today would deny that stutterers learn to use various behaviors in coping with their stigmatized and frustrating speech difficulties. Fifty years ago all stuttering behaviors were thought to be unlearned spasmodic disintegration (an era this author remembers well), but that era has long passed and rightly so. Stuttering behavior is not simply convulsive seizure activity. Let us say again that much of it is learned. We are convinced that much of the behavior which goes under the name of stuttering is learned behavior. We can account for its variability of symptoms and its consistency of patterning in no other way. We have watched it being learned. We have taught different kinds of stuttering. We have extinguished stuttering behaviors of many varieties. Our own experiments in therapy have been based on learning theory, and we know that stuttering behavior can be modified by applying its principles. We are convinced that proper scheduling of appropriate reinforcements and punishments can alter the frequency with which certain avoidance and struggle behaviors are emitted. However, let us make it very clear that we are also convinced that though both respondent and operant learning are involved in stuttering, the core behavior (especially in its form at onset) requires some other explanation. Our questions still remain: does learning theory account for the genesis or the complete phenomenology of stuttering? Does it adequately explain how children begin to stutter? Does it account for all the behaviors? We really regret that we cannot give these questions affirmative answers on the basis of the explanations presently offered, or the research that is available. We wish we could.

BIBLIOGRAPHY

ADAMS, M. R. 1970. Some comments on 'time-out' as punishment for stuttering. *Journal of Speech and Hearing Research* 13: 218–20.

——— AND G. POPELKA. 1971. The influency on 'time-out' on stutterers and their disfluency. *Behavior and Therapy* 2: 334–39.

AMMAN, J. O. C. 1965. *A dissertation on speech* (1700). Reprinted 1965, New York: Stechert-Hafner.

ANDREWS, G. AND M. HARRIS. 1964. *The syndrome of stuttering.* London: Heinemann.

ANDREWS, G. AND R. J. INGHAM. 1972. Stuttering: an approach to the evaluation of stuttering therapy. *Journal of Speech and Hearing Research* 15: 296–302.

APPELT, A. 1912. *The real cause of stammering and its permanent cure.* London: Methuen.

ARNOTT, N. 1828. *Elements of physics.* Edinburgh: Adams.

AYLLON, T. AND N. H. AZRIN. 1965. The measurement and reinforcement of behavior of psychotics. *Journal of Experimental Analysis of Behavior* 8: 357–83.

AZRIN, N. H. AND W. C. HOLZ. 1966. Punishment. In *Operant Behavior, ed.* W. K. Konig. New York: Appleton-Century-Crofts.

BASTIJENS, P., G. J. BRUTTEN, AND R. STES. 1978. The effect of punishment and reinforcement procedures on a stutterer's factor II avoidance response. *Journal of Fluency Disorders* 3: 77–85.

BEARSS, M. 1951. An investigation of penalty on the expectancy and frequency of stuttering. Masters thesis, Purdue University.

BEASLEY. B. 1879. *Stammering: its treatment.* London: Hamilton.

BEECH, H. R. 1967. Stuttering and stammering. *Psychology Today* 1: 49–51; 61.

BEECH, H. R. AND F. FRANSELLA. 1968. *Research and experiment in stuttering.* New York: Pergamon.

BELL, A. M. 1853. *Observations on defects of speech, the cure of stammering, and the principles of elocution.* London: Hamilton-Adams.

BERWICK, N. H. 1955. Stuttering in response to photographs of certain selected listeners. In *Stuttering in children and adults,* ed. W. Johnson. Minneapolis: University of Minnesota Press.

BIGGS, B. AND J. SHEEHAN. 1969. Punishment or distraction? Operant conditioning revisited. *Journal of Abnormal Psychology* 74: 256–62.

BILGER, R. C. AND C. E. SPEAKS. 1959. Operant control of nonfluent speech in normal talking. *ASHA* 3: 97 (abstract).

BLANTON, S. 1936. The treatment of stuttering. *Proceedings of the American Speech Correction Association* Vol. 6, No. 1: 24–31.

BLOODSTEIN, O. 1960–61. The development of stuttering. *Journal of Speech and Hearing Disorders* 25: 219–37; 366–76; 26 (1961), 67–82.

———. 1975. *A handbook on stuttering.* rev. ed. Chicago: National Society for Crippled Children and Adults.

————. 1979. The operant model of stuttering. *Journal of Speech and Hearing Research* 22: 665–66.

BLOODSTEIN, O. AND R. L. SHOGAN. 1972. Some clinical notes on forced stuttering. *Journal of Speech and Hearing Disorders* 37: 177–86.

BLOODSTEIN, O., J. ALPER, AND P. ZISK. 1965. Stuttering as an outgrowth of normal disfluency. In *New Directions in Stuttering: Theory and Practice*, ed. D. E. Barbara. Springfield, Ill.: Thomas.

BLUEMEL, C. S. 1935. *Stammering and allied disorders*. New York: Macmillan.

————. 1940. Stammering and inhibition. *Journal of Speech Disorders* 5: 305–8.

————. 1957. *The riddle of stuttering*. Danville, Ill.: Interstate.

BOBERG, E., P. HOWIE, AND L. WOODS. 1979. Maintenance of stuttering: a review. *Journal of Fluency Disorders* 4: 93–116.

BOERS-VAN DUK, M. 1973. Distraction. In *Neurolinguistic Approaches to Stuttering*, eds. Y. Le Brun and R. Hoops. The Hague: Mouton.

BOLAND, J. L. 1953. A comparison of stutterers and nonstutterers on several measures of anxiety. *Speech Monographs* 20: 144 (abstract).

BOOMER, D. S. AND D. W. GOODRICH. 1961. Speech disturbance and judged anxiety. *Journal of Consulting Psychology* 25: 160–64.

BRADY, J. V. 1958. Ulcers in executive monkeys. *Scientific American* 199: 539–40.

BRADY, W. 1967. *The effect of electric shock on the frequency of stuttering*. Masters thesis, Pennsylvania State College.

BREGER, L. AND J. L. McGAUGH. 1965. Critique and reformulation of "learning theory" approaches to psychotherapy and neurosis. *Psychological Bulletin* 63: 338–58.

BROOKSHIRE, R. H. 1968. Simple and interactive effects on random and response contingent aversive stimuli upon disfluencies of normal speakers. Convention Address, ASHA.

BROOKSHIRE, R. H. AND R. A. EVESLAGE. 1969. Verbal punishment of disfluency following augmentation of disfluency by random delivery of aversive stimuli. *Journal of Speech and Hearing Research* 12: 383–88.

BROOKSHIRE, R. H. AND R. R. MARTIN. 1967. The differential effect of three verbal punishers on the disfluencies of normal speakers. *Journal of Speech and Hearing Research* 10: 496–505.

BRUTTEN, E. J. 1963. Fluency and disfluency. *ASHA* 3: 781 (abstract).

————. 1957. A colorimetric anxiety measure of stuttering and expectancy adaptation. *Dissertation Abstracts* 18: 2707–8.

————. 1963. Palmar sweat investigation of disfluency and expectancy adaptation. *Journal of Speech and Hearing Research* 6: 40–48.

————. 1975. Stuttering: topography, assessment and behavior change strategies. In *Stuttering: a second symposium*, ed. J. Eisenson. New York: Harper and Row.

————. 1980. The effect of punishment on a factor I stuttering behavior. *Journal of Fluency Disorders* 5: 77–85.

BRUTTEN, G. J. AND P. JANSSEN. 1979. An eye-marking investigation of anticipated and observed stuttering. *Journal of Speech and Hearing Research* 22: 20–28.

BRUTTEN, E. J. AND B. B. GRAY. 1961. Effects of word cue removal on adaptation and adjacency: a clinical paradigm. *Journal of Speech and Hearing Disorders* 26: 385–389.

BRUTTEN, E. J. AND D. J. SHOEMAKER. 1967. *The modification of stuttering.* Englewood Cliffs, N.J.: Prentice-Hall.

CADY, ·B. AND C. J. ROBBINS. 1968. The effect of the verbally presented words 'wrong,' 'right' and 'tree' on the disfluency rates of stutterers and nonstutterers. Convention Address, ASHA.

CHOMSKY, N. 1959. Review of B. F. Skinner, "Verbal Behavior." *Language* 35: 26–58.

CONNETT, M. H. 1955. Experimentally induced changes in the relative frequency of stuttering on a specified speech sound. In *Stuttering in Children and Adults,* ed. W. Johnson. Minneapolis: University of Minnesota Press.

COOPER, E. B., B. B. CADY, AND C. J. ROBBINS. 1970. The effect of the verbal stimulus words *wrong, right* and *tree* on the disfluency rates of stutterers and normal speakers. *Journal of Speech and Hearing Research* 13: 230–244.

CURLEE, R. F. AND W. H. PERKINS. 1968. The effect of punishment of expectancy to stutter on the frequencies of subsequent expectancies and stuttering. *Journal of Speech and Hearing Research* 11: 787–95.

DALY, D. A. AND E. B. COOPER. 1967. Rate of stuttering adaptation under two electroshock conditions. *Behaviour Research and Therapy* 5: 49–54.

———— AND J. V. FRICK. 1972. The effects of punishing stuttering expectations and stuttering utterances: a comparative study. *Behavior Therapy* 1: 228–39.

———— AND M. L. KIMBAROW. 1978. Stuttering as operant behavior: effects of *wrong, right* and *tree* on the disfluency rates of school-age stutterers and nonstutterers. *Journal of Speech and Hearing Research* 21: 581–97. '

DARWIN, E. 1800. *Zoonomia.* London.

DENHARDT, R. 1890. *Das Stottern: eine Psychose.* Leipsig.

DIXON, C. C. 1947. The amount and rate of adaptation of stuttering in different oral reading conditions. Masters thesis, State University of Iowa.

DOLLARD, J. AND N. E. MILLER. 1950. *Personality and psychotherapy.* New York: McGraw-Hill.

DONAHUE, I. 1941. Change in stuttering frequency under specified conditions. Masters thesis, State University of Iowa.

DRIVER, M. AND S. STEUFERT. 1965. *The "General Incongruity Adaptation Level" (GIAL) hypothesis: an analysis and integration of cognitive approaches to motivation.* Lafayette, Ind.: Purdue University Institute for Research in the Behavioral, Economic and Management Sciences.

DUNLAP, K. 1932. The technique of negative practice. *American Journal of Psychology* 55: 270–73.

EGOLF, D. B., G. H. SHAMES, AND H. SELTZER. 1971. The effects of time-out on the fluency of stutterers in group therapy. *Journal of Communication Disorders* 1971. 4: 111–18.

EVESLAGE, R. A. AND R. H. BROOKSHIRE. 1968. Verbal punishment of disfluency following augmentation of disfluency by random delivery of aversive stimuli. Convention Address, ASHA.

EYSENCK, H. J. AND S. RACHMAN. 1965. *The causes and cures of neuroses.* London: Routledge and Kegan Paul.

FEIGENBAUM, E. A. 1959. An information processing theory of verbal learning. RAND Report P-1817, Santa Monica, Cal.: RAND Corporation.

FESTINGER, L. 1957. *A theory of cognitive dissonance.* Evanston, Ill.: Row, Peterson Co.

—— AND D. BRAMEL. 1962. The reactions of humans to cognitive dissonance. In *Experimental Foundations of Clinical Psychology,* ed. A. J. Bachrach. New York: Basic Books.

FIERMAN, E. Y. 1955. The role of cues in stuttering adaptation. In *Stuttering in Children and Adults,* ed. W. Johnson. Minneapolis: University of Minnesota Press.

FLANAGAN, B., I. GOLDIAMOND, AND N. H. AZRIN. 1959. Instatement of stuttering in normally fluent individuals through operant procedures. *Science* 130: 979–81.

——. 1958. Operant stuttering: the control of stuttering behavior through response contingent consequences. *Journal of Experimental Analysis of Behavior* 1: 173–77.

FREDERICK, C. H. 1955. An investigation of learning theory and reinforcement as related to stuttering behavior. Doctoral dissertation. University of California, Los Angeles.

FRICK, J. V. 1952. An exploratory study of the effect of punishment (electric shock) upon stuttering behavior. *Speech Monographs* 19: 146–47.

FROESCHELS, E. 1955. Core of stuttering. *Acta-Oto-Laryngologica* 45: 115–19.

——. 1943. Pathology and therapy of stuttering. *Nervous Child* 2: 148–61.

——. 1964. *Selected papers (1940–1964).* Amsterdam: North-Holland.

——. 1952. The significance of symptomatology for the understanding of the essence of stuttering. *Folia Phoniatrica* 4: 217–30.

GOLDIAMOND, I. 1965. Stuttering and fluency as manipulatable operant response classes. In *Research in Behavior Modification,* eds. L. Krasner and L. P. Ullman. New York: Holt.

GOLUB, A. J. 1951. The influence of constant and varying word stimuli on stuttering adaptation. Masters thesis, State University of Iowa.

GOSS, A. E. 1956. Stuttering behavior and anxiety as a function of experimental training. *Journal of Speech and Hearing Disorders* 21: 343–51.

GRAY, B. B. 1965a. Theoretical approximations of stuttering adaptation. *Behavior Research and Therapy* 3: 171–85.

——. 1965b. Theoretical approximations of stuttering adaptation: statement of predictive accuracy. *Behaviour Research and Therapy* 3: 221–27.

—— AND E. J. BRUTTEN. 1965. The relationship between anxiety, fatigue, and spontaneous recovery in stuttering. *Behaviour Research and Therapy* 3: 251–59.

GRAY, B. B. AND J. L. KARMEN. 1967. The relationship between nonverbal anxiety and stuttering adaptation. *British Journal of Communication Disorders* 1: 141–51.

GREGORY, H. H. (ed.). 1968. *Learning theory and stuttering therapy.* Evanston: Northwestern University Press.

GROSS, M. S. 1968. The effects of punishment and reinforcement on the disfluencies of stutterers. Convention Address, ASHA.

—— AND H. L. HOLLAND. 1965. The effects of response contingent electroshock upon stuttering. *ASHA* 7: 376 (abstract).

GUTHRIE, E. R. 1935. *The psychology of learning.* New York: Harper.

HALL, J. 1966. *The psychology of learning.* New York: Lippincott.

HALVORSON, J. A. 1971. The effects on stuttering frequency of pairing punishment (response cost) with reinforcement. *Journal of Speech and Hearing Research* 14: 356–64.

HAROLDSON, S., R. MARTIN, AND C. D. STARR. 1968. Time-out as punishment for stuttering. *Journal of Speech and Hearing Research* 14: 356–64.

HEGDE, M. H. 1972. The effect of shock on stuttering. *Journal of the All India Institute of Speech* 2: 104–10.

————. 1977. Stuttering as operant behavior. *Journal of Speech and Hearing Research* 22: 667–69.

HILGARD, E. R. AND R. C. ATKINSON. 1967. *Introduction to Psychology.* New York: Harcourt.

HILL, H. 1954. An experimental study of disorganization of speech and manual responses in normal subjects. *Journal of Speech and Hearing Disorders* 19: 295–305.

HOEPFNER, T. 1912. Stottern als assoziative Aphasie. *Zeitschrift für Pathopsychologie* 1: 448–553.

HULL, C. L. 1951. *Essentials of behavior.* New Haven: Yale University Press.

HUNT, J. 1967. *Stammering and stuttering, their nature and treatment* (original ed., 1861). Reprinted, New York: Hafner.

INGHAM, R. J. AND G. ANDREWS. 1973. Behavior therapy and stuttering: a review. *Journal of Speech and Hearing Disorders* 38: 405–41.

JANSSEN, P. 1974. The effects of response-contingent shock on stuttering behaviors. Convention Paper, ASHA, Las Vegas.

———— AND G. J. BRUTTEN. 1973. The differential effects of punishment of oral prolongations. In *Neurolinguistic Approaches to Stuttering*, eds. Y. Le Brun and R. Hoops. The Hague: Mouton.

JANSSEN, P. AND F. KRAAIMANT. 1978. The relation between stuttering and state anxiety. *Proceedings XVII Congress of Logopedics and Phoniatrics.* Copenhagen.

JOHNSON, W. 1946. *People in quandaries.* New York: Harper and Row.

————. 1959. *The onset of stuttering.* Minneapolis: University of Minnesota Press.

———— AND S. AINSWORTH. 1938. Studies in the psychology of stuttering: X. constancy of loci of expectancy of stuttering. *Journal of Speech Disorders* 3: 101–4.

JOHNSON, W. AND M. INNESS. 1939. A statistical analysis of the adaptation and consistency effects in relation to stuttering. *Journal of Speech Disorders* 4: 79–86.

JOHNSON, W. AND J. R. KNOTT. 1937. Certain objective cues related to the precipitation of the moment of stuttering. *Journal of Speech Disorders* 2: 17–19.

JOHNSON, W., R. P. LARSON, AND J. R. KNOTT. 1937. Studies in the psychology of stuttering: III. Certain objective cues related to the precipitation of the moment of stuttering. *Journal of Speech Disorders* 2: 105–9.

JOHNSON, W. AND L. S. MILLSAPPS. 1937. Studies in the psychology of stuttering: VI. The role of cues representative of past stuttering in the distribution of stuttering moments during oral reading. *Journal of Speech Disorders* 2: 101–4.

JOHNSON, W. AND A. SINN. 1937. Studies in the psychology of stuttering: V. Frequency of stuttering with expectation of stuttering controlled. *Journal of Speech Disorders* 2: 98–100.

KINGSLEY, C. 1859. Irrationale of speech. *Frazer's Magazine* London.

KLINGBEIL, G. M. 1939. Stuttering and stammering. *Journal of Speech Disorders* 4: 115–32.

KNOTT, J. R., W. JOHNSON, AND M. J. WEBSTER. 1937. A quantitative evaluation of expectation of stuttering in relation to the occurrence of stuttering. *Journal of Speech Disorders* 3: 20–22.

LANYON, R. I. AND V. S. BAROCAS. 1975.   Effects of contingent events on stuttering and fluency. *Journal of Consulting and Clinical Psychology* 43: 486–93.

"LEIGH, MME.," IN J. HUNT. 1967.   *Stammering and stuttering* (Original Ed., 1861). Reprinted, New York: Hafner.

LINGWALL, J. B. 1967.   Galvanic skin responses of stutterers and nonstutterers to isolated word stimuli. Convention Address, ASHA.

LOHR, F. E. 1969.   Visible manifestation of stuttered speech. Convention Address, ASHA.

LUPER, H. L. 1950.   A study of the relationship between stuttering adaptation and improvement during speech therapy. Masters thesis, Ohio State University.

———. 1968.   An appraisal of learning theory concepts in understanding and treating stuttering. In *Learning Theory and Stuttering Therapy*, ed. H. H. Gregory. Evanston: Northwestern University Press.

———. 1954.   The consistency of selected aspects of behavior in the repetitions of stuttered words. Doctoral dissertation, Ohio State University.

MAHL, G. F. 1961.   Measures of two expressive aspects of a patient's speech in two psychotherapeutic interviews. In *Comparative Psycholinguistic Analysis of Two Psychotherapeutic Interviews*, ed. L. A. Gottschalk. New York: International Universities Press.

MARTIN, R. R., 1968.   The experimental manipulation of stuttering behaviors. In *Operant Procedures in Remedial Speech and Language Training*, eds. H. W. Sloane and B. D. Macaulay. Boston: Houghton-Mifflin.

——— AND S. K. HAROLDSON. 1967.   The relationship between anticipation and consistency of stuttered words. *Journal of Speech and Hearing Research* 10: 323–27.

———. 1977.   Effect of vicarious punishment on stuttering frequency. *Journal of Speech and Hearing Research* 20: 21–26.

———. 1979.   Effects of five experimental treatments on stuttering. *Journal of Speech and Hearing Research* 22: 132–46.

MARTIN, R. R. AND G. M. SIEGEL. 1966a.   The effects of simultaneously punishing stuttering and rewarding fluency. *Journal of Speech and Hearing Research* 9: 466–75.

———. 1966b.   The effects of response contingent shock on stuttering. *Journal of Speech and Hearing Research* 9: 340–53.

———. 1969.   The effects of a neutral stimulus (buzzer) on motor responses and disfluencies in normal speakers. *Journal of Speech and Hearing Research* 12: 73–82.

MARTIN, R. R., K. ST. LOUIS, S. HAROLDSON, AND J. HASBROUCK. 1975.   Punishment and negative reinforcement of stuttering using electric shock. *Journal of Speech and Hearing Research* 18: 478–90.

MARTIN, R. R. AND R. J. INGHAM. 1973.   Stuttering. In *Modification of Speech and Language*, ed. B. Lahey. Springfield, Ill.: Thomas.

McDEARMON, J. 1966.   C. S. Bluemel and the learning theory approach to stuttering. *Western Speech* 30: 106–11.

MILISEN, R. 1938.   Frequency of stuttering with anticipation of stuttering controlled. *Journal of Speech Disorders* 3: 207–14.

MILLER, G. A., E. GALANTER, AND K. H. PRIBAM. 1960.   *Plans and the structure of behavior*. New York: Holt.

MILLER, N. E. AND. J. DOLLARD. 1941.   *Social learning and imitation*. New Haven: Yale University Press.

MOORE, W. E. 1938. A conditioned reflex study of stuttering. *Journal of Speech Disorders* 3: 163–183.

MOWRER, O. H. 1950. *Learning theory and personality dynamics.* New York: Ronald Press.

NEELLEY, J. N. AND R. J. TIMMONS. 1967. Adaptation and consistency in the disfluent speech behavior of young stutterers and nonstutterers. *Journal of Speech and Hearing Research* 10: 250–56.

NEWMAN, P. W. 1963. Adaptation performances of individual stutterers: implications for research. *Journal of Speech and Hearing Research* 6: 293–94.

OELSCHLAEGER, M. L. AND G. J. BRUTTEN. 1978. The effects of response contingent stimulation on the frequency of part-word repetition of four stutterers. *Journal of Fluency Disorders* 3: 10–17.

OWEN, T. V. AND M. G. STEMMERMANN. 1947. Electric convulsive therapy in stammering. *American Journal of Psychiatry* 104: 410–13.

PETERS, R. W. AND W. E. SIMONSON. 1960. Generalization of stuttering behavior through associative learning. *Journal of Speech and Hearing Research* 3: 9–14.

POTTER, S. O. L. 1882. *Speech and its defects.* Philadelphia: Blakeston.

PRINS, D. AND F. E. LOHR. 1969. Behavioral dimensions of stuttered speech. Convention Address, ASHA.

QUIST, R. W. AND R. R. MARTIN. 1967. The effect of response contingent verbal punishment on stuttering. *Journal of Speech and Hearing Research* 10: 795–800.

REED, C. B. AND J. B. LINGWALL. 1976. Some relationships between punishment, stuttering and galvanic skin responses. *Journal of Speech and Hearing Research* 19: 197–205.

ROUSEY, C. 1958. Stuttering severity during prolonged spontaneous speech. *Journal of Speech and Hearing Research* 1: 40–47.

RUBIN, M. 1957. A study of the consistency and adaptation effects in ten to thirteen-year-old stutterers. Masters thesis, Brooklyn College.

RYAN, B. P. 1967. The effects of positive reinforcement on the frequency of stuttered behaviors. Convention paper, ASHA.

———. 1971. Operant principles applied to stuttering therapy for children. *Journal of Speech and Hearing Disorders* 36: 264–80.

SANDOW, L. 1898. *Mechanik des Stotterns.* Norhansen: Edler.

SAVOYE, A. L. 1954. The effect of the Skinner-Estes Operant Conditioning Paradigm upon the production of nonfluencies in normal speakers. Masters thesis, University of Pittsburgh.

SHAMES, G. H. 1975. A behavioral perspective of stuttering. In *Stuttering: a second symposium,* ed. J. Eisenson. New York: Harper and Row.

———, D. B. EGOLF, AND R. C. RHODES. 1969. Experimental programs in stuttering therapy. *Journal of Speech and Hearing Disorders* 34: 30–47.

——— AND C. E. SHERRICK. 1963. Discussion of nonfluency and stuttering as operant behavior. *Journal of Speech and Hearing Disorders* 28: 3–18.

SHEEHAN, J. G. 1958. Conflict theory of stuttering. In *Stuttering: A Symposium,* ed. J. Eisenson. New York: Harper and Row.

———. 1951. The modification of stuttering through non-reinforcement. *Journal of Abnormal and Social Psychology* 46: 51–63.

———. 1953. Theory and treatment of stuttering as an approach-avoidance conflict. *Journal of Psychology* 36: 27–49.

————, P. CORTESE, AND R. HADLEY. 1962. Guilt, shame, and tension in graphic projections of stuttering. *Journal of Speech and Hearing Disorders* 27: 129–39.

SHEEHAN, J. G. AND R. B. VOAS. 1954. Tension patterns during stuttering in relation to conflict, anxiety binding, and reinforcement. *Speech Monographs* 21: 272–79.

SHRUM, W. F. 1967. A study of the speaking behavior of stutterers and nonstutterers by means of multichannel electromyography. Convention Address, ASHA.

SHULMAN, E. 1955. Factors influencing the variability of stuttering. In *Stuttering in children and adults*, ed. W. Johnson. Minneapolis: University of Minnesota Press.

SHUMAK, I. C. 1955. A speech situation rating sheet for stuttering. In *Stuttering in children and adults*, ed. W. Johnson. Minneapolis: University of Minnesota Press.

SIEGEL, G. M. 1970. Punishment, stuttering and disfluency. *Journal of Speech and Hearing Research* 13: 677–714.

————. 1965b. Verbal punishment of disfluencies in normal speakers. *Journal of Speech and Hearing Research* 8: 245–51.

————. 1966. Punishment of disfluencies in normal speakers. *Journal of Speech and Hearing Research* 9: 208–18.

————. 1968. The effects of verbal stimuli on disfluencies during spontaneous speech. *Journal of Speech and Hearing Research* 11: 358–64.

————. 1967. Verbal punishment of disfluencies during normal speech. *Language and Speech* 10: 244–51.

———— AND R. R. MARTIN. 1965a. Experimental modification of disfluency in normal speakers. *Journal of Speech and Hearing Research* 8: 235–44.

SILVERMAN, F. H. 1976. Communicative success: a reinforcer for stuttering. *Perceptual and Motor Skills* 43: 398.

SKINNER, B. F. 1953. *Science and human behavior.* New York: Macmillan.

————. 1957. *Verbal behavior.* Englewood Cliffs, N.J.: Prentice-Hall.

SMITH, R. W. 1966. A cognitive motivation approach to stuttering: an initial formulation. Masters thesis, Purdue University.

SOLOMON, R. I. 1964. Punishment. *American Psychologist* 19: 239–53.

STARKWEATHER, C. W. 1970. The simple, main, and integrative effects of contingent and noncontingent shock of high and low intensities on stuttering repetitions. Doctoral dissertation, Southern Illinois University.

————. 1971. The case against base-rate comparisons in stuttering experimentation. *Journal of Communication Disorders* 4: 247–58.

———— AND J. LUCKER. 1978. Tokens for stuttering. *Journal of Fluency Disorders* 3: 167–80.

STASSI, E. J. 1961. Disfluency of normal speakers and reinforcement. *Journal of Speech and Hearing Research* 4: 358–61.

STEER, M. D. AND W. JOHNSON. 1936. An objective study of the relationship between psychological factors and the severity of stuttering. *Journal of Abnormal and Social Psychology* 31: 36–46.

STEVENS, M. M. 1963. The effect of positive and negative reinforcement on specific disfluency responses of normal speaking college males. Doctoral dissertation, State University of Iowa.

STROMSTA, C. 1965. A spectrographic study of dysfluencies labeled as stuttering by parents. *De Therapia Vocis et Loquellae* 1: 317–20.

TIMMÒNS, R. J. 1966. A study of adaptation and consistency in a response-contingent punishment situation. Doctoral dissertation, University of Kansas.

TOLMAN, E. C. 1951. *Collected papers in psychology.* Berkeley, Cal.: University of California Press.

TOOMEY, G. L. AND M. SIDMAN. 1970. An experimental analogue of the anxiety-stuttering relationship. *Journal of Speech and Hearing Research* 13: 122–129.

VAN RIPER, C. 1937a. Effect of devices for minimizing stuttering on the creation of symptoms. *Journal of Abnormal and Social Psychology* 32: 63–65.

―――. 1937b. The effect of penalty upon the frequency of stuttering. *Journal of Genetic Psychology* 50: 193–95.

―――. 1937c. The growth of the stuttering spasm. *Quarterly Journal of Speech* 23: 70–73.

―――. 1936. Study of the thoracic breathing of stutterers during expectancy of occurrence of stuttering. *Journal of Speech Disorders* 1: 61–72.

―――. 1957. Symptomatic therapy for stuttering. In *Handbook of Speech Pathology,* ed. L. E. Travis. Englewood Cliffs, N.J.: Prentice-Hall.

――― AND C. J. HULL. 1955. The quantitative measurement of the effect of certain situations on stuttering. In *Stuttering in Children and Adults,* ed. W. Johnson. Minneapolis: University of Minnesota Press.

――― AND R. L. MILISEN. 1939. A study of the predicted duration of the stutterers' blocks as related to their actual duration. *Journal of Speech Disorders* 4: 339–45.

WEBSTER, L. M. 1968. A methodological investigation of the contingent stimulation of stuttering moments. Convention Address, ASHA.

―――. 1968. A cinematic analysis of the effects of contingent stimulation on stuttering and associated behaviors. Doctoral dissertation, Southern Illinois University.

―――. 1966. An audio-visual exploration of the stuttering moment. Masters thesis, Southern Illinois University.

――― AND G. J. BRUTTEN. 1974. The modification of stuttering and associated behaviors. In *Communication Disorders: Remedial Principles and Practices,* ed. S. Dickinson. Glenview, Ill.: Scott Foresman.

WENDAHL, R. W. AND J. COLE. 1961. Identification of stuttering during relatively fluent speech. *Journal of Speech and Hearing Research* 4: 281–86.

WIEST, W. M. 1967. Some recent criticisms of behaviorism and learning theory. *Psychological Bulletin* 68: 214–25.

WILLIAMS, J. D. AND R. D. MARTIN. 1974. Immediate versus delayed consequences of stuttering responses. *Journal of Speech and Hearing Research* 17: 569–75.

WINGATE, M. E. 1964. A standard definition of stuttering. *Journal of Speech and Hearing Disorders* 29: 484–89.

―――. 1959. Calling attention to stuttering. *Journal of Speech and Hearing Research* 2: 326–35.

―――. 1966. Stuttering adaptation and learning: I. The relevance of adaptation studies to stuttering as "learned behavior." *Journal of Speech and Hearing Disorders* 31: 148–56.

WISCHNER, G. J. 1952. Experimental approach to expectancy and anxiety in stuttering behavior. *Journal of Speech and Hearing Disorders* 17: 139–54.

————. 1947.   Stuttering as learned behavior: a program of research. Doctoral dissertation, University of Iowa.

————. 1950.   Stuttɛ .ng behavior and learning. *Journal of Speech and Hearing Disorders* 15: 324–35.

WOLPE, J. 1952.   Experimental neuroses as learned behavior. *British Journal of Psychology* 43: 1–9.

————. 1953.   Learning theory and abnormal fixations. *Psychological Review,* 60: 111–16.

————. 1958.   *Psychotherapy by reciprocal inhibition.* Stanford: Stanford University Press.

WYNEKEN, C. 1868.   Über das Stottern und dessen Heilung. *Zeitschrift für rationelle Medizin* 31: 1–29.

YOUNG, M. A. 1964.   Identification of stutterers from recorded samples of theiɪ "fluent" speech. *Journal of Speech and Hearing Research* 7: 302–3.

ZENNER, A. A. 1971.   A molecular analysis of stuttering and associated behaviors during massed oral readings of the same material. Doctoral dissertation, Syracuse University.

———— AND L. M. WEBSTER. 1975.   The molar and molecular effects of contingently stimulating the stuttering moment. *Stuttering: A Second Symposium,* ed. J. Eisenson. New York: Harper and Row.

ORGANICITY IN STUTTERING   14

There are many who reject the possibility of an organic basis for stuttering. Among these are not only psychologists and psychiatrists (who perhaps should remember their former assumption that schizophrenics had no organic involvement), but there are many, possibly a majority, of speech pathologists, too, who refuse to accept any organic explanation of the disorder. Among these was Wendell Johnson (1967) who listed twelve features of stuttering which he felt were incompatible with organicity. Some of the items on his list were its intermittency, its momentary duration, its early onset, its spontaneous recovery, its variability, and its reduction under certain conditions such as singing, whispering, and talking to oneself. However, Hamre (1972) showed that there were other disorders of known organic etiology which had comparable features. Epileptics, to cite just one example, can appear quite normal between attacks; some petit mal episodes may be very brief; seizures often do not occur until after three years of age; and the symptoms are often precipitated by stress. Other known organic disorders show the other features. Sander (1975) points out that recovery from stuttering need not rule out organicity:

> Dyslexics can be taught to read but their success in transcending their problem does not argue against its organic basis. When stutterers enhance their fluency by monitoring themselves more carefully or altering their speaking style, the results may well bespeak a successful compensation (p. 261).

EARLY VIEWS OF ORGANICITY

There is something about the sight of an adult in the throes of a severe moment of stuttering which immediately suggests that there must be something organically wrong with him. As he gasps, forces, and jerks, his bizarre spasmodic behavior seems so utterly inappropriate to the task of saying one little word that it is very difficult to believe that he could possibly possess a normal speaking mechanism. This impression, of course, is not given so readily by most beginning young stutterers, but even they have so many broken words, under conditions which hardly seem stressful, that one wonders whether there may not be something basically defective about them, too. All of us stumble occasionally in our walking, especially if there is an unexpected doorsill to trip over, but if someone stumbles often and when striding over what appears to be a smooth surface we might infer some fundamental difficulty in coordination. Even though such a person demonstrates that he can at times walk normally, the more often he stumbles, the more sure we are that there is something organically wrong. Indeed, one of the first signs of myasthenia gravis or muscular dystrophy may be this intermittent difficulty in locomotion.

Throughout the centuries this belief in the organic nature of stuttering has persisted—probably because of these first intuitive impressions. For more than a thousand years of recorded history, the tongue was felt to be the villain. Aristotle (384 B.C.)* attributed the disorder to tonguetie or tongue weakness: "the tongue is too sluggish to keep pace with the imagination." Celsus, the most famous of Roman physicians, who lived at the same time as Christ, insisted on gargling and massaging the tongue to strengthen it. Galen (A.D. 200) felt that the tongue was too cold and wet and so lacked strength. In the sixth century, Aetius of Amica recommended cutting the lingual frenum. De Chauliac (1336) felt that a person stuttered because of transitory convulsions and paralysis of the tongue. Mercurialis (1584) described two types of stutterers, those with too wet and those with too dry a tongue, and treated them accordingly with blistering substances or gargles. Francis Bacon (1627) thawed the stiff tongues of stutterers with hot wine, thereby producing more fluency as one might expect.

These older beliefs concerning the tongue as the culprit began to fade with the beginning of the nineteenth century, although some treatments persisted for a time—Itard's ivory fork. Madame Leigh's secret pad of cotton placed under the tongue tip, and the infamous surgical operations of Dieffenbach (1841), which divided or excised chunks from the tongue. By midcentury, this ancient belief in a defective tongue had pretty well subsided, but the quest for organicity had not. Let us trace some of the other theories of organic causation.

Structures other than the tongue were also blamed for stuttering. Hahn (1736) and Morgagni (1761) felt that the hyoid bone was the culprit. Yearsley (1841) attributed the difficulty in speaking to a narrowed airway caused by enlarged tonsils and uvula, and he removed these structures, as many other surgeons have since, in seeking the cure for stuttering. Velpeau, a contemporary of Dieffenbach, and also a tongue slitter, insisted

---

* In preparing this historical account, we read as many of the original references as we were able to procure. For the remainder, we have relied primarily on the following sources: Haase (1846), Hunt (1870), Appelt (1911), Bluemel (1913), Klingbeil (1939), Froeschels (1943b), Larson (1949), and Freund (1966).

that stuttering was due to an overly small mouth cavity caused by a palate which was too low.

Since even casual observation reveals that the tongues and other oral structures are no different in stutterers than in normal speakers, we find in the early 1800s some of the old writers beginning to speak of malfunctioning rather than defective organs. Thus Bertrand (1828) views the disorder as a "spasmodic nervous affection" and Serre d'Alais (1829) and Arnott (1829) found its source in a chronic "spasm of the glottis." Serre d'Alais described two types of stutterers, those with choretic and those with tetanic spasms and thus laid the foundation for the concepts of clonic and tonic varieties of stuttering still current today. This view of stuttering as a form of chorea (St. Vitis Dance) became very popular during the first half of the nineteenth century, because it superficially explained the intermittent nature, the repetitive form, the spasmodic behaviors, and the tremors. It enabled the physicians of the day to throw away the outworn and patently false belief in defective organs but retain the concept of organicity. Moreover, the concept of localized spasm had ancient authority behind it. Avicenna (1037), the most famous of Arabian physicians, from whom many of the medieval European physicians procured their medical knowledge, attributed stuttering to brain lesions which in turn were the cause of the spasms of the epiglottis which produced the stuttering symptoms.

As one might expect from the common appearance of breathing abnormalities in stutterers, many of the older writers located the source of stuttering in the respiratory apparatus or its neurological governors. Thus Sir Charles Bell (1832) speaks of stuttering as a partial chorea resulting in respiratory incoordinations. Becquerel (1847) ascribed the disorder to deficiencies in the nervous centers governing thoracic breathing that caused a premature escape of air. Coen (1875) believed that stutterers were subbreathers and that the breath spasms were the result of pathological changes in the respiratory apparatus. His remedy was to have the stutterer bare his chest, stand against a wall, and do breathing exercises. Many other writers held similar views and even as recently as 1930 Twitmeyer held that an abnormal state of neurological imbalance, created originally by emotion, produced the breathing abnormalities which triggered stuttering.

Another group of writers attributed stuttering to biochemical differences. Hippocrates (370 B.C.), the father of medicine, believed that stuttering was caused by an accumulation of "black bile," and he applied varices (substances which scarred or blistered the skin) which, by creating skin ulcers, would allow the evil (pus) to drain away. During the Middle Ages, the use of leeches and bloodletting for the relief of stuttering was also based on the belief that there was something wrong with the composition of the blood or "humours." Since the science of biochemistry appeared relatively recently, most of the organic theories that focus on differences in body fluids do not belong in this history. The research bearing on biochemical differences between stutterers and nonstutterers will be reviewed in a later section of this chapter.

In the nineteenth century a few writers began to ascribe stuttering to a malfunctioning or damaged brain. According to Hunt (1870), Rullier (1821) felt that "the cerebral irradiation which follows thought and puts the vocal and articulating organs in action gushes forth so impetuously and rapidly, that it outruns the degree of motility possessed by the muscles concerned, which are thus, as it were, left behind." Hence the latter are thrown into that convulsive and spasmodic state which characterizes stuttering. This quaint description may apply more to cluttering than to stuttering, but it shows the sort of medical thinking current only 150 years ago. Voisin (1821) and Astrie (1824) also believed that stuttering was due to disordered brain function, but their treatment of the disorder consisted of pressing the thumb against the cheek while talking and the use of Itard's fork under the tongue. Lichtinger (1844) distinguished between cerebral and spinal stuttering, and in his work we find the beginnings of the view of defective cortical inhibition of the lower brain centers. Rosenthal (1861) located the cause of the breathing abnormalities shown by stutterers in the malfunctioning of the medulla oblongata caused by psychic shocks during childhood. Kussmaul (1877) defined stuttering as a syllabic dysarthria produced by a lack of coordination of voice, respiration, and articulation, due to neurological deficits. He viewed it as a form of aphasia. Of the three Gutzmanns who wrote extensively on stuttering, H. Gutzmann, Senior, in his book *Das Stottern* (1898), which became the classical work on stuttering of his age, promulgated the concept that there was a deficiency in the cerebral cortex which impaired syllabic coordination and thus produced the clonic and tonic spasms. Gutzmann also collected a series of cases of aphasic stuttering to support his position of cerebral etiology. In this country Swift (1932) attributed stuttering to lesions in the cuneus (a wedge-shaped convolution at the base of the occipital lobe of the cortex), which impaired the visual imagery of stutterers and so produced the blockages. Bluemel (1913), however, felt that it was the auditory imagery of stutterers which was deficient, and he defined the disorder as a transient auditory aphasia or amnesia. The stutterer had difficulty speaking because he had temporarily lost the auditory image of the word. Bluemel later dropped this explanation when it was pointed out how frequently stutterers could substitute synonyms, a fact that demolished his theory and led subsequently to his revised theory based on conditioned inhibition.

Most noteworthy of the later neurological explanations of stuttering was the cerebral dominance theory first espoused by Orton (1927) and developed by Travis (1931) and Bryngelson (1935).* Since all of the muscles used to produce speech are paired structures, and those on the right side receive motor impulses originating in the left hemisphere of the cortex while those on the left side from the right hemisphere, and both streams of impulses must be synchronized to produce smooth movements,

---

* According to Kistler (1930) both Sachs and Stier as early as 1911 hypothesized that the battle for predominant control of speech between the right and left hemispheres was the cause of stuttering.

it was hypothesized that this synchronization could only be achieved if one of the cortical hemispheres had a sufficient margin of dominance to enable it to impose its timing patterns over the other and thereby achieve the desired synchronization. These authors believed that stutterers had lower margins of cerebral dominance than normal speakers and that the thalamic static of accompanying emotion could further reduce that margin. When this occurred, dysynchronies ensued and neurological blockages and spasms resulted. It was an ingenious theory and stimulated much research, some of which seemed to support it, but it fell from grace primarily because homolateral motor tracts were discovered, because both right- and left-handed subjects seemed to have left-hemisphere dominance, because the basic research was challenged, and because the presumed shift of handedness which had been thought to account for the reduced margin of dominance was not corroborated. One of the basic problems of the theory was that it was untestable except in terms of peripheral laterality. Some recent research which we will review in a later section indicates that a revision of the theory may again find some acceptance.

At about the same time, other organic concepts of the nature of stuttering were presented. Seeking some explanation for the sex ratio, the strong hereditary factor, the apparently poor diadochokinesis of stutterers, and certain biochemical differences brought out in the research of Kopp (1934), Robert West (1943) introduced the concepts of spasmóphemia and dysphemia.

> Stuttering is a manifestation of a fundamental atypia, or divergence from human norms, that, though not often interfering with the performance of the basic animal functions of the organism, often, however, interferes with the peculiarly human function of speech. This atypia is not usually adequate to produce stuttering without the complicity of certain contributory factors.

West's view of the dysphemic atypia was that it was either a mild or latent epileptiform disorder called pyknolepsy which could be precipitated by various kinds of stress, or a mild "form of subclinical cerebral palsy."

In Europe, Szondi (1932) investigated 100 stutterers, using a variety of neurological and serological tests, and concluded that they were constitutionally different in that 20 per cent showed signs of brain pathology and a high proportion demonstrated other evidences of neurovascular difficulties. Seeman, in a series of publications (1934; 1947; 1959) developed the concept that stuttering was the result of disturbed functioning in the striopallidar system rather than in the cortical centers. He felt that in stutterers there was a basic imbalance in the functioning of the sympathetic and parasympathetic parts of the autonomic nervous system, the sympathetic being overactivated. He writes:

> An attack of stuttering develops as a result of dynamic functional deviations of the striopallidum, the normal activity of which is impaired by acute affective and emotional influences of the subcortical region and thus the coordination of speech movements is impaired. It may thus be said that a paroxysm of stuttering is objectively characterized by an orthosympathetic reaction (1966, p. 430).

As this quotation indicates, Seeman's theory should really not be included in the category or organic theories since the disturbed functioning of the autonomic nervous system is seen as the result of strong emotional experiences. We have seen fit to mention it here primarily because its emphasis on the striopallidum offers another site for organic etiology. Moreover, in his emphasis on hereditary factors, Seeman often seems to be implying some sort of organic predisposition.

Another organic theory was advocated by Weiss (1950), who held that stuttering always stemmed from cluttering and that the latter was an inherited stage of language imbalance based perhaps upon submicroscopic lesions in the striopallidum, as Seeman maintained, or upon delayed maturation of the nervous system. A related point of view is that of Karlin (1947) who theorized that stuttering was due to delayed myelinization of the nerve sheaths.

As we review this historical material, we are impressed by the ludicrousness of some of the beliefs that were stated so positively by the greatest authorities of the past, and we become highly aware of the limits of our own present information concerning the organicity of stuttering. We simply do not have the basic understanding of how motoric speech is organized and programmed in time. None of our predecessors' organic theories make much sense today, and those that are still current are more speculative than substantiated. Nevertheless, the continuing quest for an acceptable, organically based theory of stuttering is impressive.

Modern attempts to investigate the possibility of an organic component in stuttering have concerned themselves with studies of motor coordination, servo system feedback, malfunctioning of the cerebral processes responsible for motor speech, biochemical differences between stutterers and nonstutterers, and hereditary predisposition to stutter. In this chapter we shall concern ourselves with the last three and begin by presenting what we know about hereditary factors.

HEREDITARY PREDISPOSITION TO STUTTER

While it is possible to have an organic cause for a disorder which is not inherited (as in a traumatically produced aphasia), a hereditary predisposition is usually considered evidence of organicity. As we observed in our discussion of incidence, most of the research has shown a higher degree of familial incidence in stutterers than in nonstutterers. Let us now go into the matter more deeply.

The research on hereditary factors. Many of the early writings on the hereditary causes of stuttering reported the familial history in fairly general terms. Stutterers were interviewed to determine how many of their immediate ancestors or siblings stuttered. No control groups were used. Only the unanimity of their findings make them worth mentioning here. Mygind (1898) reported that 42 per cent of his stutterers had stutterers in their families. Makuen (1914) reported that 39 per cent of 1000 stutterers had relatives who stuttered. Scripture and Glogau (1916) found that 25 per cent of their stutterers had stuttering relatives. Bryant (1917) gives a figure of 50 per cent for an incredible 20,000 patients; Tromner in Germany (1929) raised the ante to 80 per cent. In England, Boome and Richardson (1932) found 34 per cent of 522 of their cases had stuttering "heredity." Bryngelson and Clark (1933) reported 75 per cent of the 127 stuttering Minnesota children they personally examined had stuttering in their immediate families. Abe (1934) lists 24 per cent of 225 stuttering Japanese soldiers as reporting familial incidence. Some 42 per cent of the stutterers examined by Ingebregtsen (1936) had stutterers in their immediate families. Meyer (1945) found ten times more stuttering ancestors in the families of stutterers. Freund (1952) reported that 88 immediate relatives of 121 stutterers also stuttered and that other neurotic signs were found among them. Otsuki (1958) claimed that 42 per cent of his stuttering subjects showed familial incidence. Streifler and Gumpertz (1955) discovered stuttering in the immediate relatives of 56 per cent of their stutterers. In France, de Ajuriaguerra, Diatkine, Gobineau, Narlian, and Stambak (1958) found that 31 of their 92 stutterers had family histories of stuttering. Luchsinger (1959) found a family history of stuttering in 33 per cent of his 272 Swiss stutterers. Hirschberg (1965) found 51 per cent of 151 Hungarian stutterers to have family histories of stuttering. Mussafia (1964) found 39 per cent of 241 Belgian⁄stutterers to have stuttering in their immediate families. Daskalov (1962) gives a figure of 32 per cent for the familial history of stuttering in 850 Russian stutterers.

One of the first hereditary studies using control groups of normal speakers was performed by Wepman (1939). He found that 71 per cent of 127 stutterers reported stuttering in the immediate family as compared to only 13 per cent of the controls. Bryngelson and Rutherford (1937) reported that 46 per cent of 74 stutterers had stuttering relatives as compared with only 18 per cent of the 74 controls. In a further compilation of data Bryngelson (1935) compared 152 stutterers with their controls and found that stuttering occurred in 51 per cent of the stutterer's families but in only 13 per cent of the normal speakers. Pierce and Lipcon (1959), in a careful study, compared the family histories of 36 naval stuttering recruits with 36 matched normal speakers and found that 20 of the stutterers had family members who stuttered but none of the normal speakers had family members who stuttered. Johnson (1959) in his onset of stuttering study found that over five times as many parents of stutterers reported stuttering in their immediate families as compared with that reported by parents of the normal speaking children, the difference being significant beyond the 1 per cent level of confidence. Stutterers had five times as many stuttering fathers, for example, as did their normal speaking controls.

There are two researches that should be considered as being especially well done, those by Andrews and Harris (1964) and by Kenneth K. Kidd and his associates (1977, 1978, 1979). The first of these by Andrews and

Harris reported that the risk of stuttering was 5.8 per cent for mothers also stuttering, 19.1 per cent for fathers, 8.4 per cent for sisters and 20 per cent for brothers. When the stutterers were compared with their controls, 39 per cent of the stutterers had family histories of stuttering as compared with only 1.4 per cent for the normal speakers.

The Yale University geneticist, Kenneth Kidd, has probably carried out the most extensive and careful study of the inheritance of stuttering. With his coworkers, the families of over 500 stutterers have been investigated and in a series of reports (Kidd 1977; Records, Kidd, and Kidd 1977; Kidd, Kidd, and Records 1978; Kidd and Records 1979) we have some of the best information to date. For male stutterers, over 21 per cent had fathers who stuttered but only 6 per cent had mothers who stuttered. Of the female stutterers, 22 per cent had fathers who stuttered and 12 per cent had mothers who did. When all of the first-degree relatives (2524) are considered, 14.8 per cent of them stuttered. This *incidence* is so much greater than that found generally in the population (about 5 per cent) that it is difficult to believe that environmental factors alone could account for the results.

Beyond this general finding, the data analysis by Kidd, Kidd, and Records (1978) shows that six criteria for a sex-modified mode of inheritance are fulfilled. The transmission cannot be explained by the simple Mendelian models of autosomal dominant, autosomal recessive, or X-linked traits but there are other models (multifactorial and single major locus) that seem to fit the data on stuttering. Essentially, what is inherited is a threshold tendency to stutter, the males having a lower threshold (thus being more susceptible to environmental precipitants) and the females having higher thresholds. The authors also examined the possibility that the transmission might be due to cultural roles or learned through imitation. Both were found to be unsatisfactory explanations. With regard to the latter, Kidd, Kidd, and Records write:

> There remains the possibility that stuttering may be a learned or imitative behavior based on sex-role models. We have examined our family data to determine how many of our index cases had a parental model to imitate. We found that 140 of the 511 index cases had one or both parents who stuttered. Of the 148 parents who stuttered, 87 no longer stuttered by the time the index case was born. Thus, only 61 of the 511 index cases (12%) had a stuttering parental model to imitate (1978, p. 18).

The role of imitation or morbid family attitudes has often been used to explain the tendency for stuttering to run in families. This does not seem to be supported by most of the researches. Nelson (1939) investigated the familial tendency (siblings, parents, grandparents) to stutter in two groups of 204 each, one composed of stutterers and the other of normal speakers. No significant difference in incidence was found between the percentages of those from either group who had had close association with other stutterers. There were 58 stutterers who had stutterers in their immediate families but who had never had personal contact with them. In another study, by Andrews and Harris (1964), 13 of 80 stutterers as compared with only 1 of 80 controls had a positive family history of stuttering. In addition, 17 of 80 other stutterers had a positive family history with prolonged contact with another stuttering member of the family, but there were no normal speakers in this category. In a much-quoted investigation, Gray (1940) compiled the family trees of two branches of a stuttering family for five generations. The Iowa branch had 8 stutterers, 3 former stutterers, and 16 nonstutterers; the Kansas branch had only 1 stutterer and 16 nonstutterers. The differences in frequency of stuttering (although even the Kansas branch with its 1 stutterer represents an incidence of 4 per cent which is greater than in the general population) was attributed to semantogenesis—as a family curse.

We have several other family tree studies showing a substantial number of stuttering relatives. Figure 14 from Kidd, Kidd, and Records (1978) provides the family trees of four of their stutterers.

Other family tree studies have also shown a preponderance of stutterers occurring for several generations. One by Gedda, Branconi, and Bruno (1960) revealed that a pair of male twins who stuttered had a maternal grandfather, a paternal uncle, and a paternal great uncle who stuttered. Weissova and Handzel (1962) report a fascinating study of a family characterized by both a parathyroid gland insufficiency and stuttering. The father and all three sons had both problems.

The hereditary factor in stuttering and cluttering. It is possible, of course, that only certain subgroups of stutterers show a hereditary strain. We have

Figure 14. Selected pedigrees of families with stuttering. Squares are males; circles are females; solid symbols represent individuals who ever stuttered. The arrow indicates the index case (proband); a number in a symbol indicates that there are that many siblings of that sex. (From Kidd, Kidd, and Records, 1978, by permission.)

previously (Chapter 11) mentioned several studies indicating that a cluttering type of stutterer may be identified. If so, these stutterers may be the ones who show more stutterers or clutterers in their families. Weiss (1964) provides the family tree in Figure 15 to show the relationship.

It has been suggested repeatedly by various authors that the family strain of stuttering is strongly associated with cluttering. Freund (1952) studied the families of 95 stutterers and the families of 26 "stutterer-clutterers." In the first group he found 36 stammerers (over a third) and 12 tachylalics (individuals with very hasty speech). Of the stutterer-clutterers, there were 12 stutterers (almost one-half) and ten others who had tachylalia. Berry (1937) found that there was a tendency for stuttering to occur more in families containing twins and also that in families containing both twins and siblings, it occurred more frequently among the twins. Luchsinger and Arnold (1965) gave family trees showing the high prevalence of both stuttering and cluttering in these families. Pfändler (1952) summarizes the genetic studies on stuttering and cluttering and concludes, as we do, that it is very difficult to disregard this evidence of some constitutional factors.

Twin studies. A genetic hypothesis concerning the nature of stuttering may also be supported by evidence that identical twins (monozygotic) have a greater incidence of stuttering than fraternal or dizygotic twins. As we have seen in our chapter on incidence, stuttering does seem to have a greater incidence in twins generally than in nontwins. In one of the first twin studies Seeman (1937) found that of 14 monozygotic (identical) twins, 9 of them were stutterers, whereas of 5 dizygotic (fraternal) twins only 1 child stuttered. Luchsinger (1944) found that if stuttering occurs in

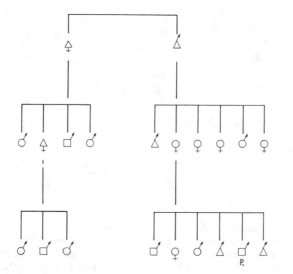

Figure 15. Mixed heredity of cluttering and stuttering. (From D. A. Weiss, 1964.)

monozygotics it occurs in both, whereas in dizygotics it occurs in only one. Nelson, Hunter, and Walter (1945) found that of 200 twin pairs, 20 per cent stuttered, a much higher incidence than in the normal population. They also found that of the identical twins, 14 per cent stuttered as compared with 22 per cent of the fraternal twins. However, Graf (1955), in a study conducted in Iowa found only 21 of 1104 twins who stuttered, an incidence of 1.9 per cent, only about twice as high as in the normal population.

Perhaps the most careful study we have of concordance in twins was done by Howie (1976) who found that it was higher in identical twins (58 to 63 per cent) as compared to fraternal twins of the same sex (13 to 19 per cent). Nevertheless, the matter is still in doubt for Howie also discovered that in about half of the identical twins, one was a nonstutterer.

In addition to these researchers we can add an unpublished study of our own. Over the course of years, we have been collecting data on the children of the stutterers with whom we have worked. In the course of their therapy, some of them met and later married other stutterers receiving treatment. We can report that in all but 1 of 14 married pairs of stutterers (in which both mates stuttered) at least 1 child stuttered. Of the total number of their children (29), 20 of them went through a period of stuttering sufficiently severe to have their parents bring them to us for examination and recommendations. This is a tremendously high incidence.

The sex ratio. One of the features of stuttering that has been used to support the belief that stuttering must have some sort of organic etiology is the sex ratio. As we have seen in our study of incidence, there are always more males than females who stutter. This holds true at all age levels. Attempts to account for this universally shown fact in terms of cultural roles or errors in sampling or diagnosis have not been persuasive. Kidd, Kidd, and Records (1978) examined these alternative explanations and, finding them inadequate, suggest instead that a sex-modified trait for susceptibility to stutter may be inherited. Their evidence in support of that view based on family pedigrees, seems to indicate not only that the sex ratio is real but also that it is probably biologically determined. Any theory of the nature of stuttering that refuses to accept the possible organicity of the disorder must account for this sex ratio.

It is very difficult to explain why three or four times as many males stutter as do females in terms of excessive parental demands or expectations of speech proficiency that might produce enough hesitation to become learned behaviors. It is hard to believe that so many more males than females have neurotic tendencies so early. On the other hand, an explanation couched in terms of differential motor coordination ability between the sexes in the early years may possibly seem more plausible. Girls do seem to acquire verbal skills and facility earlier than boys at the time stuttering usually begins. Perhaps the trait that is inherited is a disability in integrating the very complex coordinations needed for speech.

In concluding this section we would like to quote from Sheehan and Costley's (1977) review of the research on the hereditary factor in stuttering:

> Repeated studies over the years have established to a significant degree that stuttering runs in families. Taking different studies into account and allowing a rough correction for probable methodological error in a few of the studies, the proportion of stutterers who reveal a family history of stuttering is about one-fourth to one-third. . . . It should be noted that familial incidence may be interpreted as either a genetic or a cultural factor. However, the proportion of cases, at least one-fourth of all stutterers, is difficult to explain on a solely cultural learning, or sociopsychological basis. It does provide some support for a genetic factor, at least in some sub-typology of the disorder.

Sheehan and Costley also, suggest on the basis of studies by Sheehan and Martyn (1966) and Cooper (1972), that more spontaneous recovery occurs in those stutterers who do not have a family history of stuttering.

While no one has yet discovered a stuttering gene or allele and the exact mode of inheritance is still in doubt, it would seem unwise, in the light of this evidence, to summarily dismiss the possibility that organicity may exist, at least in some stutterers.

CEREBRAL DOMINANCE

An ancient concept which has recently been resurrected sought to explain the stutterer's difficulty in achieving smoothly coordinated speech in terms of a central asynchronization of the motor impulses due to a lack of, or a confusion in, cerebral dominance. Since all of the muscles used in speech are paired and both sets must be activated simultaneously as well as successively, it was proposed that a lack of such central dominance would lead to lags or blockings that would produce stuttering behaviors. The lack of a cerebral processing center on one side of the brain which was powerful enough to impose its timing patterns on the other hemisphere was viewed as the basic, organic factor in stuttering. Normal speakers were said to have a wide margin of lateral dominance; stutterers, a much narrower one. Moreover, emotional stress was seen as being able to reduce that margin, thus explaining the effect of fear and other negative emotion. In this early formulation, the cerebral dominance theory was completely untestable, and it soon became identified with peripheral handedness. Stutterers were said to be persons who lost their natural margin of dominance because they had changed their handedness from the natural hand to the other or that, by using the unnatural hand in writing, they created even more havoc with the integration of their speech movements.*

The original cerebral dominance theory was first published by Stier (1911) and Sachs (1924) in Germany but it received its early acceptance through the writings of Orton (1927) and Travis (1931). It generated a

---

* It is difficult now (even for the author who wore a plaster cast on his right arm and wrote thousands of pages of verbalized sentences with his left hand for many months) to recall the enthusiasm with which this organic view of stuttering was accepted.

substantial amount of research, much of it concerning whether stutterers generally were left-handed individuals who had been shifted.

PERIPHERAL SIDEDNESS IN STUTTERERS

The whole literature on handedness is full of hazards as well as hints, probably because preference can be influenced by many environmental factors. The downfall of the Orton-Travis theory came because it was tested in terms of handedness, a peripheral and motor function, and because some of its advocates blamed stuttering on a forced shift in handedness, a most irrelevant concept since hemispheric dominance does not always reflect itself in peripheral sidedness.

One hates to start digging again in the old boneyard of the laterality research on stuttering. Let us see what we can unearth. First of all, dominance is peripherally represented not only by hand preference but also by foot, ear, and eye preference, all of which have been included under the term *sidedness*. (In addition to these motor aspects of cerebral dominance, there is also some evidence of laterality differences in perception.) Hand preference has been the one motor aspect most commonly investigated. Our first question is whether stutterers tend to fall into the categories of left-handed and ambidextrous, since it is in these that central ambilaterality (two-hemispheric control center for speech) has been demonstrated. Unfortunately hand preference is not always easy to determine. As Van Riper (1935) and Subirana (1964) showed, few individuals are completely right-handed or left-handed. Using some overly demanding criteria, the latter author found only 8 per cent to be completely right-handed and only one single individual out of the 600 subjects he examined was completely left-handed. Most of the reports indicate an incidence of from 8 to 15 per cent of left-handedness in the general population. Some evidence of a hereditary factor exists in handedness (Bryngelson, 1935), and identical twins usually show opposite hand preference. This has been used to explain the occurrence of left-handed individuals, the right-handed individual being thought to be the surviving member of a pair of embryonic twins. Animals are also predominantly right-handed (Peterson, 1931) but left-handed and ambidextrous rats are to be found. (We had a left-handed rat once that starved to death rather than reach for food readily available to its right paw, and we achieved a strain of completely left-handed mice after seven generations of selective breeding.) Adequate measurement of handedness is difficult. Van Riper (1935) devised an angle board device which is one of the few tests that permit the quantitative measurement of *how* left-handed or *how* right-handed a person is. Although the distribution of hand preference is highly skewed in favor of the right hand by any of the methods used to determine it, most individuals show mixed laterality rather than complete unilaterality. Footedness and eyedness are even more mixed.

The early studies are difficult to evaluate since the data were obtained by questionnaire. Representative of these is one by Ballard (1912) who stated that four times as many stutterers were found among children whose only right-handed activity was in writing as the result of a questionnaire study of 13,000 school children. Another was performed by Quinan (1921; 1938), who reported three times as many stutterers in predominantly left-handed subjects. Bryngelson (1934), using a 20-item hand preference questionnaire with 700 stut·erers classified 61 per cent of them as being ambidextrous. Bryngelson and Rutherford (1937) compared 74 stutterers with 74 normal speaking controls. The percentages of right-handed, left-handed, and ambidextrous normal speakers were 75 per cent, 16 per cent, and 8 per cent respectively, and for the stutterers the figures were 61 per cent right-handed, 4 per cent left-handed, and 34 per cent ambidextrous. Bryngelson reported that a very high incidence of shift of handedness in both of these studies had occurred among those stutterers classed as being predominantly right-handed. Hirschberg (1965) stated that of 151 stutterers he found 66 per cent who were right-handed, 5 per cent left-handed, and 4 per cent who were ambidextrous. De Ajuriaguerra and others (1958) found only 30 per cent of their stutterers as compared with 68 per cent of their normal speakers to be thoroughly right-handed. Also, 51 per cent of the stutterers (ages 11 to 14 years) showed mixed handedness as compared to 21 per cent of the normal speakers.

In an effort to escape the contamination of possible shifts of handedness which may have occurred early in life, several investigators attempted to find other ways of testing handedness than hand preference for writing, shaving, fork handling, and the like. Orton and Travis (1929) recorded the precedence of the action currents to both forearms in simultaneous contraction; Travis and Herren (1929) repeated this using adduction and abduction of the two hands; Travis (1928) and Jasper (1932) used mirror tracing; Fagan (1931) and Jasper (1932) used simultaneous writing with both hands on a horizontal surface; and Van Riper (1935) employed simultaneous drawing of figures on a winged apparatus which permitted a quantitative measurement of laterality in terms of the angular displacement of the writing surface from the vertical. All of these studies indicated that the performance of a large number of stutterers resembled that of the left-handed or ambidextrous more than it did that shown by right-handers.

There are an impressive number of studies using similar procedures which lend doubt to the figures just mentioned. Daniels (1940) gave handedness and speech tests to 1,548 college students. Of the 34 left-handers, one was a stutterer; of the 138 who were ambidextrous, four stuttered. Putting it another way, he reported that stuttering was found in 1.1 per cent of the right-handed students, in 2.9 per cent of the ambidextrous, and in 2.9 per cent of the left-handers. Spadino (1941) matched 70 stuttering school children with 70 controls and applied a battery of tests including handedness, eyedness, and footedness. There were no significant differences on any of the tests. Van Dusen (1939) also gave a battery of tests to stutterers and nonstutterers and found no differences. Johnson and King (1942) replicated Van Riper's angle board study and, using a different method of scoring, found no laterality differences between stutterers and nonstutterers. The nonstutterers were unselected with respect to handedness. Pierce and Lipcon (1959), in a small sample, found no differences in handedness between their stutterers and their controls. Streifler and Gumpertz (1955) and Daskalov (1962) in a large sample of 850 stutterers found that the percentage of left-handedness in stutterers approximated that of the normal population. The same lack of differences in laterality between child stutterers and normal speakers was demonstrated by the research of Johnson (1959) and by Andrews and Harris (1964), who did no testing but only questioned the parents of their subjects.

Records, Heimbuch, and Kidd (1977) found no significant peripheral laterality differences in a population of 446 stutterers and their controls. They entitled their article "Handedness and Stuttering: A Dead Horse?" and the question seemed to be answered in the affirmative.

SHIFT OF HANDEDNESS

No one has shown that a shift of peripheral handedness can alter central cerebral dominance, and most of the research indicates that the old belief that such a shift can cause stuttering is far from being corroborated. The evidence supporting this belief comes from research which is fairly old. Haefner (1929) found that 24 per cent of 41 children who had been shifted stuttered. Oates (1929) reports an experiment in which 12 sub-normal right-handed children were shifted to the left hand; all of them stuttered after five months of such training, and the stuttering disappeared when the training ceased. Fagan (1931) reported that 27 per cent of his stutterers had had their handedness changed; Bryngelson (1935) and Bryngelson and Rutherford (1937) give shift figures ranging from 60 per cent to 70 per cent; Hirschberg (1965) reported that 25 per cent of his stutterers had been shifted.

Opposed is the research of Ojemann (1931) who shifted 23 pure left-handed children in writing and saw no stuttering appear. Daniels (1940) discovered that only 1 of 20 stutterers had been shifted. Among African stutterers, Aron (1958) found that only 2 per cent had been shifted in handedness. Daskalov (1962) mentions that none of 114 left-handed individuals began to stutter after being forced to work with the right hand. It should be a simple matter to dispose of this question by simply getting a large population of individuals who have been shifted at various ages and then determining the incidence of stuttering in this group and comparing it with that of a control group which has not been shifted. However, this research has not to our knowledge been performed and so once again we are left with ambiguity instead of ambilaterality.

A very common assertion in this connection has been that the forced shift of handedness when accomplished unpleasantly creates emotional conflicts and these are what causes the stuttering when it does occur. Although plausible, no one has demonstrated that this is true. We have in our files three case studies of boys who deliberately shifted their own handedness to become like their fathers or to become southpaw (left-handed) baseball pitchers and subsequently developed stuttering which then disappeared when they reluctantly went back to right-hand usage. In this connection we give a quotation from Bloodstein who is certainly no advocate of the cerebral dominance theory:

> It is difficult to read certain case reports of children who began to stutter after a shift of handedness, or to study accounts of certain adults who experienced fluency disturbances after enforced use of the nonpreferred hand without being impressed by the possibility that laterality is a factor in some cases (1959, p. 35).

So what can we conclude about this matter of peripheral sidedness in stutterers? It is that the hounds of research were barking up the wrong tree. No strong evidence exists that stutterers differ from normal speakers generally in terms of handedness nor that a forced shift in handedness early in life can precipitate the disorder in any consistent fashion. Peripheral sidedness and central laterality are not closely related. Most left-handed persons show the same left-cerebral dominance for speech that characterizes right-handed individuals so the question of stutterers' handedness is of little importance. What we need to know is whether stutterers show differences from nonstutterers in central rather than peripheral laterality.

DIFFERENCES IN CENTRAL LATERALITY

We begin with the study of R. K. Jones (1966) which we mentioned earlier. Jones, a neurosurgeon, was preparing to operate on four patients who had stuttered severely since childhood but who had recently developed brain pathology, and he had decided to use a new technique pioneered by Wada (1949). The technique consisted of injecting sodium amytol directly into first the right and then the left carotid arteries while the patient is conscious and talking. As Wada and Rasmussen (1960) demonstrated, when this drug is introduced into the system in this way, a temporary aphasia results, provided the artery serving the dominant hemisphere of the brain is the one injected. To his surprise, Jones found that all four of these stutterers developed transient aphasia when the drug was injected into *either* the right or left carotid arteries, thus indicating that they had a bilateral cortical control of speech, that there were "speech centers" in both hemispheres. Jones then performed his surgery on the damaged hemisphere and found that complete remission of stuttering took place in all his patients. After recovery, he administered the sodium amytol as before and discovered that now the exstutterers became aphasic only when one artery was injected (the one serving the nonoperated hemisphere). They no longer had cortical representation for speech in both hemispheres but only in one. Jones remarks that "the results on stammering of a one-sided operation for unrelated lesions in these four patients were quite startling and can only be explained by the view that stammering is associated with an interference by one hemisphere with the speech performance of the other."

These results were so striking that replication soon followed. In Australia Andrews, Quinn, and Sorby (1972), using the Wada technique, injected amytol into the carotid arteries of three stutterers. Two of them showed the normal left dominance; the third (who had suffered a head injury before beginning to stutter) had bilateral cortical representation for speech. A year later, Luessenhop, Boggs, Laborwit, and Walle (1973) also used the Wada procedure to determine dominance for speech in three stutterers and all three showed the usual left dominance. Once more, a promising lead had failed.

Another study by Guillaume, Mazars, and Mazars (1957) had reported a similar complete recovery from stuttering in an epileptic after surgical removal of an epileptogenic focus in the right temporal lobe. They write:

> During the operation, when we were starting the resection of the fusiform gyrus, we were astonished to hear the subject articulate with extraordinary ease and to express his surprise at no longer stuttering. Following this intervention, the patient was entirely cured of his epileptic attacks and his stammer.

Another related case study from Russia is provided by Shtremel (1963) in which a normal speaking adult began to stutter and showed aphasic symptoms at the age of 51. After surgical removal of a tumor ("as large as a Mandarin orange") the stuttering disappeared, although some aphasic difficulties remained.

The fact of cerebral dominance is indisputable. In the majority of people, including some of those who are left-handed, the left cerebral hemisphere appears to be the one dominant in the integration of speaking. Penfield and Rasmussen (1949) and Penfield and Roberts (1959) show that approximately two-thirds of left-handed persons have speech localized in the left hemisphere as have right-handed persons. According to Goodglass and Quadfasel (1964) about 60 per cent of left-handed aphasics had their pathology in the left hemisphere rather than in the right.

Benson and Geschwind (1968) review studies which show that there are anatomical asymmetries on the upper surface of the left temporal lobe which might be responsible for left hemisphere dominance, and they even suggest that some left-handedness might be the result of early lesions in the left hemisphere causing a shift to an unnatural right-brain dominance. According to Zangwill (1960) in early childhood, the usual left hemispheric dominance for speech does not seem to be fully developed or stabilized and if cerebral insults occur in one hemisphere, the other may assume the speech function. This has been shown rather clearly by Basser (1962). If the brain damage occurs before the onset of speech, it does not seem to matter whether the injury is in either the left or right hemispheres so far as the later acquisition of speech is concerned. After the onset of speech, however, and especially in adulthood, injuries to the left hemisphere disturb speech greatly. Damage to the right hemisphere does not. Nevertheless, using the Wada techniques, Branch, Milner, and Rasmussen (1964) and others have shown that in certain adult persons, usually the left-handed or ambidextrous, both cerebral hemispheres may contain integrating mechanisms for speech. Hécaen and de Ajuriaguerra (1963) and Zangwill (1960) feel that this hemispheric ambilaterality may be a hereditary trait.

Nevertheless some studies have shown the possibility that stutterers may be using the usually nondominant right hemisphere for linguistic tasks. Indeed, the modern concept seems to be that both hemispheres participate in processing auditory information and in the programming of motor responses but that generally the left hemisphere (irrespective of peripheral handedness) is the primary integrating center for nonstutterers and the right hemisphere for stutterers. Some of these researches, which we shall review later, have employed dichotic listening; others, auditory tracking, and still others have explored the presence or absence of alpha wave activity in the two hemispheres.

AUDITORY LATERALITY AS DETERMINED BY DICHOTIC LISTENING TESTS

Seeking a noninvasive and less dangerous method for determining cerebral dominance, several investigators have used dichotic listening techniques to demonstrate that when competing messages are presented simultaneously to the two ears, persons with left hemispheric cerebral dominance will be able to recall and perceive the one presented to the right (preferred) ear better than the message presented to the other ear. For those with right central dominance for speech the reverse is found; they, too, perceive verbal stimuli better when presented to the contralateral ear, showing left-ear dominance. The use of the Wada test has corroborated these findings. Other evidence comes from cerebral lesions.

Although each cochlea is represented bilaterally in the cortex, certain anatomical differences have been demonstrated which may account for this lateral dominance. Rosenzweig (1951) for example, administered clicks to a single ear of a cat and measured the resulting cortical potentials, concluding that "At the level of the auditory cortex . . . the population of cortical units representing the contralateral ear is larger than the population representing the ipsilateral ear."

Boone (1959) found that right hemiplegics, given tasks in which they listened with one ear or the other, made many more errors when listening with the left ear than did left hemiplegics with injuries in the right cortical hemispheres. Kimura (1961a) gave patients with known lesions in the right and left temporal lobes stimulation with two digits presented simultaneously to right and left ears. Those with lesions of the left temporal lobe had much poorer digit spans than those with lesions in the right temporal lobe. Bocca and Calearo (1963) and others have shown that tests of discrimination using distorted or interrupted speech as stimuli showed no binaural differences for normal subjects, but significantly depressed scores were found for patients when stimulated in the ear contralateral to the lesion.

Curry (1967) had 25 left-handed and 25 right-handed subjects perform three dichotic listening tasks, two verbal and one nonverbal. The mean right-ear score was higher than the left-ear score on the *verbal* tasks, but the left-ear score was higher for the nonverbal task, and this held true for both groups, although the difference approached significance only for the righthanders. Since other research has indicated that the central organization of verbalization seems to be located usually in the left hemisphere irrespective of peripheral handedness, this may not be too surprising. What might be more important is a study by Curry and Gregory (1967) in which 11 of 20 stutterers had higher left-ear scores on a dichotic listening task as compared to only 5 of the normal speaking controls. Moreover the size of the differences between right- and left-ear scores were significantly smaller for the stutterers. Nonverbal tasks showed no differences. The authors speculate that this may indicate less clear-cut cerebral dominance in the stutterers. Kimura (1961b; 1963; 1967), Bryden (1963), Dirks (1964), and Carr (1969) have all shown that when competitive verbal material is fed simultaneously to the two ears, a right-ear preference is shown by most speakers. Kimura feels that the "crossed auditory pathways are stronger than the uncrossed and that the dominant temporal lobe (the left one) is more important than the nondominant in the perception of spoken material (Kimura, 1961b, p. 171)."

Several other studies using the dichotic listening task soon followed the Curry and Gregory publication and some of them (Perrin and Eisenson 1970; Hinkle 1971; Brady and Berson 1975; and Sommers, Brady, and Moore 1975) showed that stutterers did not manifest the strong right-ear preferences demonstrated by their normal speaking controls. Instead, they either showed a left-ear advantage or a very weak and inconsistent right-ear preference. This led to the interpretation that stutterers seemed to lack the marked cerebral dominance of the left hemisphere so characteristic of most normal speakers.

Unfortunately for this new evidence of organicity, other studies quickly appeared which did not corroborate these findings. No significant differences in dichotic listening scores were found by Gruber and Powell (1974) for stuttering and nonstuttering children, and Quinn (1972), Slorach and Noehr (1973), Cerf and Prins (1974), Dorman and Porter (1975), and Sussman and MacNeilage (1975) found none for adults. We cannot account for the discrepancy between these two sets of researches except perhaps in terms of the population mix. It is possible that those who found differences may have had more "organic stutterers" in their groups of subjects. In any event, most of the studies have indicated a wide variability among subjects and the actual amount of ear advantage was not very large.

How can we resolve the conflict between these two sets of dichotic researches? One possible explanation is that the three studies that found differences between normals and stutterers in dichotic listening used linguistic stimuli (words), whereas those that found no differences used digits or nonmeaningful syllables. The other explanation, and perhaps of greater probability, is that there may be subgroups of stutterers with organic involvement that may be responsible for the lack of right-ear preference and that the experimental populations did not have the same proportions. In any event, we can only conclude that the hypothesis that stutterers as a group differ dichotically from nonstutterers in perceptual auditory laterality has not been entirely confirmed.

OTHER STUDIES OF CEREBRAL DOMINANCE

Another research by Sussman and MacNeilage (1975) approached the problem of auditory laterality in a different way. A separate tone was introduced into each earphone of the subject. One varied unpredictably in frequency, and the subject, by using his or her jaw or hand, controlled and tried to match the pitch of the variable target tone. The target tone was switched from one ear to the other to determine which one yielded the better tracking. Again we find that though there was some overlap, a substantial number of stutterers showed a left-ear advantage on the jaw tracking though not on hand tracking. Once more we get a hint that some but not all stutterers may have different auditory processing systems than those of normal speakers. Unfortunately Neilson and Neilson (1979) did not corroborate these findings.

Besides auditory tracking, there are several other approaches to the determining of central dominance for speech in stutterers and nonstutterers. Moore (1976) who used bilateral tachistoscopic procedures showed that a greater proportion of stutterers revealed left half-field preferences than did their controls, thus indicating a reversed cerebral dominance for the stutterers.

Tsunoda and Moriyama (1972) devised an ingenious technique for ascertaining lateral dominance in auditory perception. Their subjects had to tap out a pattern of sound stimuli fed into their ears, with both ears hearing the sound simultaneously, then later with one ear and then the other hearing the sound under delayed auditory feedback, a condition which disrupted the key tapping. The differing amount of disruption in terms of the loudness of the DAF served as the measure of lateral dominance.

Essentially the experiment revealed that a subgroup of stutterers showed the reversed dominance patterns characteristic of aphasics with unilateral temperal lobe lesions. The authors speculate that these stutterers may have had minimal brain damage.

Another attempt to determine whether stutterers show differences from nonstutterers in lateral dominance investigated the suppression of alpha wave activity during speech. It seems to be fairly well corroborated that in most males at least the left hemisphere shows a suppression of the alpha frequencies in the processing of linguistic material whereas the right hemisphere does not show this reduction (Galin and Ornstein 1975). In a preliminary investigation Moore and Lang (1977) found that stutterers showed a suppression of alpha activity in the right hemisphere whereas the nonstutterers showed it in the left. This was later corroborated by Moore and Haynes (1980). Zimmerman and Knott (1974) studied hemispheric shifts in slow potential brain wave activity. Just prior to speaking, most of their normal speakers showed larger shifts in the left hemisphere than in the right while their stutterers showed the opposite.

An interesting test of Travis's concept of a *margin* of cerebral dominance was provided by Ponsford, Brown, Marsh, and Travis (1975). Evoked EEG potentials from Wernicke's and Broca's area in the two cerebral hemispheres were obtained as stutterers and their controls said the word *fire* in two differing contexts of meaning. Differences between groups appeared that the authors interpreted as showing a lower margin of dominance for the stutterers.

One final study, a very old one which perhaps should not be forgotten, was done by Jasper (1932) who investigated the phi phenomenon in right-handed, left-handed, ambidextrous, and stuttering subjects. The phi phenomenon refers to the apparent movement between intermittent visual stimuli. When the light sources are placed in the midline, subjects perceive the light moving to the right or left, presumably reflecting lateral dominance of cerebral hemispheres. Stutterers perceived the shifting light much the same way as the ambidextrous subjects.

The continuing quest for evidence of organicity in studies of cerebral dominance is impressive but we can only conclude that at the present time the evidence is not too convincing. At best, it indicates only that some stutterers may show such organicity.

BRAIN DAMAGE

Another series of investigations have been concerned with the possibility that stutterers show evidence of brain damage, another indication of organicity. Some of these explored the etiology of stuttering as a result of aphasia, brain injury, or epilepsy. Others focused on brain wave abnormalities as revealed by electroencephalography.

There are many studies on brain damage as a factor in the etiology of stuttering. Much of it, however, consists of individual case studies, reports, or uncontrolled investigations. Moreover, just what sort of effect the brain damage has on the sequencing of speech is rarely if ever made clear. Nevertheless, the persistence of the idea that some organic or neurological substrate, possibly a result of brain damage, underlies at least some stuttering, requires that we examine this material.

In his survey of the early literature before 1900, Maas (1946) mentions case studies by Kussmaul, Cornil, Dejerine, and Pick in which stuttering began in adulthood as the result of injuries to the skull and brain. Froeschels (1919) described the case of a young soldier with aphasia and clonic-tonic stuttering brought on by an injury to the temporal lobe. Szondi (1932) used various neurological tests (and measurements of skull size!) and found that 20 per cent of his stutterers showed "signs" of organic damage. Peacher and Harris (1946) mention cases of stuttering in soldiers brought on by combat injuries to the head. Göllnitz (1955) found evidence of cerebral lesions in many young stutterers.

There are many accounts of stuttering onset occurring after head injuries in adults. Froeschels (1931) describes a man who began to stutter at the age of 68 after a stroke. He also reported two other aphasic cases in which the aphasia was followed by stuttering. Warren and Akert (1964) report the occurrence of stuttering following frontal lobe lobotomy or lobectomy. Abbott, Due, and Nosik (1943) give accounts of stuttering resulting from blast injuries. Some of these effects may possibly be similar to those produced by Brickner (1940) and Penfield and Rasmussen (1949) who stimulated the cortex electrically in conscious patients and were able to produce repetitions of sounds and syllables as well as phonatory arrest. Helm, Butler, and Canter (1980) describe a patient whose stuttering appeared after head trauma. Quinn and Andrews (1977) reported two cases whose stuttering appeared in adulthood due to cerebral injury and neurological disease.

STUTTERING IN APHASIA

The appearance of stuttering, or something closely resembling it, following a cerebral trauma that resulted in aphasia has been repeatedly observed. Some examples are those of Head (1926), Nielson (1942), Eisenson (1947), Granich (1947), and Wepman (1947). Arend, Handzel, and Weiss (1962) describe very carefully the changes in speech in two cases of aphasia; they note that stuttering increased and decreased along with the other aphasic symptoms. One of the most interesting case reports is that by McKnight (1936) in which the author, herself an aphasic, describes in detail the development of her stuttering difficulties. An impressive review of all the literature on aphasia and stuttering by Shtremel (1963) makes it very clear that stuttering may be one of the sequellae of aphasia. Shtremel also presents careful studies of three cases. Two of these developed speech dyspraxias and subsequently stuttering following head contusions. In the third case, the pathology was due to a cerebral tumor which, when removed, eliminated the stuttering. All of the lesions in these cases were in the left parietal lobe.

But is it really stuttering? There seem to be some differences. Often these aphasic stutterers do not show the usual adaptation effect and the loci are different. Often the stuttering is transient rather than persistent (Rosenfield 1972; Rosenbeck, Messert, Collins, and Wertz 1978). Farmer (1975) found more similarities than dissimilarities in aphasic and ordinary stuttering symptoms. The excellent review by Helm, Butler, and Cantner (1980) of acquired stuttering, however, lists seven differences, including the lack of anxiety and the absence of struggle, which seem to distinguish aphasic stuttering from the usual kind.

OTHER BRAIN DAMAGE

Stuttering has also been attributed to injuries or abnormalities in the functioning of *noncortical areas* of the brain. A much higher incidence of stuttering is reported by Palmer and Osborn (1938), and Rutherford (1944) for the cerebral palsied (in which extrapyramidal pathology is involved). Gerstmann and Schilder (1921) described the onset of stuttering after encephalitis. Goda (1961) gives a case study of a child whose stuttering appeared subsequent to spinal meningitis. Anton Schilling (1956) describes a case in which Rh damage to the brain stem resulted in chorea with severe stuttering appearing later. We could report several others from our own files. However, it was Seeman (1934) who first constructed a theory of the nature and cause of stuttering based on the malfunctioning of the subcortical areas of the brain-specifically that which serve the autonomic nervous system. His neurological theory of stuttering, one which is remarkably sophisticated, and, if its assumptions are correct, does explain the core behavior of stuttering and the way in which it is affected by emotion. In this early article he summarizes the research of others and presents evidence in 85 per cent of 260 stutterers that the respiratory and phonatory and other functions of the striopalladum were disturbed.

Generally speaking, Seeman believes that the sympathetic part of the autonomic nervous system becomes hyperactive, in part because of emotional stress or because of lack of inhibition from the cortex, and that this produces disturbances in all of the fundamental processes on which speech is based, that is, respiration, phonation, and sequencing. Sovak (1935) gave stutterers adrenalin which increases sympathetic arousal and found that his stutterers got worse, while pilocarpin, which activates the parasympathetic system, caused a reduction in stuttering. Seeman (1941) found that 235 stutterers had shorter phonation times and related this to heightened activity of the sympathetic nervous system. Sovak (1935) presented a series of cases of stutterers who seemed to show increased sympathetic irritability.

Sedlacek (1947–48) studied the solar and oculocardiac reflexes of 229 stutterers. These reflexes (which are set off by sudden pressure on the carotid sinus or solar plexus) cause differential changes in pulse rate according to the presumed irritability of the sympathetic or parasympathetic nervous system. Although Sedlacek found that some of the stutterers (13 per cent) showed normal responses, more of them (34 per cent) showed hyperactive sympathetic systems, and the remainder showed either vagotonic or ambivalent responses. The act of stuttering produced almost the same effect on the pulse as the punch to the solar plexus in 98 per cent of the cases.

Ataxia. This term refers to a difficulty in coordination produced by brain damage. It is often found in patients who have suffered cerebral insult. Usually it impairs the smooth movements of walking and other automatic motor activities but it can also affect voluntary activities as well.

Wyke (1974) has suggested that stuttering can be viewed as a phonatory ataxia resulting from mistimings in the voluntary presetting of the glottal musculatures and the involuntary compensatory reflex activities of those muscles.

Apraxia. Another disorder due to brain damage is apraxia. Its main characteristic is the inability to execute a movement voluntarily when the same movement can be performed automatically. For example, a patient with this disorder might be completely unable to protrude his tongue when asked to do so yet be able to lick some peanut butter off his upper lip without any trouble. The stutterer's inability to get started or to say an integrated word presents a similar picture since often when distracted or when singing he may have no difficulty. An excellent paper exploring the possibility that stuttering may reflect apraxia is that by Rosenbek (1980).

DISEASE SEQUELLAE

Berry (1938) surveyed the medical histories of 430 stutterers and 462 controls and found that the stutterers had significantly more diseases of the respiratory system and more convulsive disorders than the controls. Kanner (1942) reports stuttering as part of the sequellae of encephalitis and that in juvenile paresis, "There was a seemingly 'logoclonic' repetition of the same word or word fragment." Schilling's (1956) case, cited above in which stuttering developed out of chorea and a lesion in the striatum should be recalled here, too. Boland (1951) found more instrument births among 209 stutterers than occur in the general population. Opposed to these earlier studies are the more careful and later ones of Johnson (1959) and Andrews and Harris (1964), who found no differences either in birth injuries or diseases.

STUTTERING IN EPILEPSY

A greater incidence of stuttering among epileptics has also been reported but the evidence is not impressive. Harrison (1947) reported a large number of stutterers in an epileptic colony. In similar settings, however, Barbara (1946) found an incidence of 2.4 per cent and Wise, quoted in Freund (1955), found only 1.6 per cent. Streifler and Gumpertz (1955) report a stuttering incidence of 1 per cent among the epileptics seen in their neurological clinic. A particularly fascinating study is that by Guillame, Mazars, and Mazars (1957) in which three stuttering cases are described as having epileptic or convulsive symptoms. Surgery for the first case excised the focal cortical areas responsible for the epileptic discharges and the stuttering stopped. Anticonvulsant medication reduced the stuttering almost completely in the other two cases. In four stutterers, Jones (1966) found that a similar remission of stuttering occurred following brain surgery to remove brain tumors or other brain pathologies. West's (1958) speculations concerning pyknolepsy as the core of much stuttering have been challenged strongly by Hamre and Wingate (1967), who show clearly the basic differences between stuttering behaviors and those of the petit mal type sometimes called pyknolepsy.

MOTOR PERSEVERATION

Eisenson (1958) has described the tendency toward perseveration as one of the constitutional aspects of stuttering, relating it in part to the well-known finding that epileptics and other brain-damaged individuals show greater perseveration, both motorically and perceptually, than normals. We will review only the motoric research, since it is this which bears directly upon coordination. The question is whether stutterers, or definite subpopulations of stutterers, show more perseveration in motor activities than normals. Presumably, the greater the coordinative disability, the more difficult it will be to shift from one task to another.

Unfortunately, most of the tasks used in the research involved no speech sequencing, so that the definitive research still remains to be done. Eisenson (1937) compared 30 stutterers with their controls in their ability to change suddenly to a different task while copying letters and doing simple arithmetic problems. The stutterers perseverated longer than the normals. King (1961) tested the ability to alternate between writing and drawing activities (motor perseveration), and he also tested dispositional rigidity (for example, changing from capital to lower-case letters) in 82 stutterers and their controls. He found the stutterers more perseverative than the nonstutterers on most of the tests. Martin (1962), however, using other but similar copying and writing tests with 52 stutterers and 109 controls, found no differences of significance between them. Kapos and Standlee (1958) tested the ability to shift from one task to another in an electromaze and found no evidence of greater perseveration (behavioral rigidity) in 15 stutterers than in the controls. Wingate (1966), using another test of general behavioral rigidity on 12 stutterers and controls, found no differences. We conclude that the case for greater perseveration in stutterers has not been proven.

ELECTROENCEPHALOGRAPHIC ABNORMALITIES

A fairly substantial amount of research has dealt with the examination of electroencephalographic (EEG) records of stutterers. As is now well known, the brain as a whole produces rhythmical electrical discharges, beginning in the occipital areas of the cortex and sweeping forward into the other areas. At rest, an alpha rhythm of about eight to ten waves per second occurs, and these are large in amplitude. When the brain is stimulated, smaller and faster and more irregular waves occur. These can be picked up and recorded with amplification from electrodes placed on or in the scalp. EEG abnormalities are frequently shown in epilepsy, or other disorders due to brain damage or malfunctioning in the form of brief bursts of electrical potential (spikes), slow wave patterns, focal areas of abnormality, bilateral phase differences, and various forms of dysrhythmias.

Reports of abnormal EEGs must be considered with caution since about 10 to 15 per cent of presumably normal individuals show them, especially when triggered by overbreathing (hyperventilation) or by intermittent flashes of light (photic stimulation). Unfortunately, the techniques used in recording and in evaluating abnormality have varied from investigator to investigator. Some researchers used hyperventilation or photic stimulation; others did not. Some investigators recorded from one cortical hemisphere; others from both. Some used monopolar electrodes; others used bipolar ones. Although more EEG abnormalities seem to be found among the younger than the older subjects, the age of the stutterers was frequently disregarded. Far too often no control groups were used.

It should also be mentioned that the absence of EEG abnormality (when scalp electrodes are used) may not indicate the true state of affairs since Kiloh and Osselton (1961) report that intense epileptic discharges may be missed by surface or scalp electrodes but may be picked up by electrodes inserted only one millimeter below the cortical surface. In many of the studies, it is difficult to determine just what the criteria of abnormality are. Moreover visual inspection of EEG records may fail to reveal true differences which appear when autocorrelation or crosscorrelation techniques are applied. Finally, the authors' interpretations of their data often leave the seeker of the truth completely baffled. With these considerations in mind we now report the experiments roughly in the order in which they were published.

Travis and Knott (1936) found no major differences in EEGs between their 17 stutterers and 19 controls in silence or speech. Two of their cases, however, showed spikes which occurred after the moments of stuttering. Travis and Malamud (1937) compared EEGs of normal speakers, stutterers, and schizophrenics and found no major differences. Freestone (1942) compared 20 adult stutterers with their controls. The stutterers showed larger waves during stuttering than during fluent speech and more waves in free speech than in silence. The shift from silence to speech in terms of interruption to the alpha waves was more marked in the normals. Freestone attributed these findings to the stutterers' tendency to undergo states of reduced consciousness.

Lindsley (1940) examined the EEGs of 65 normal children and two severe stutterers, recording them from both hemispheres of the cortex. He found that, in the stutterers, periods of asynchronization between the EEG on the right and left hemisphere in the occipital and parietal areas and unilateral blockings or phase reversals preceded almost every recorded stuttering episode. Rheinberger, Karlin, and Berman (1943) found no differences in EEGs between a very small sample of stutterers and controls. Douglass (1943) compared the EEGs of 20 stutterers and normal speakers and found no differences between stuttering and fluent speech in the stutterers, but he did find some unilateral blocking of the alpha rhythm in silence which did not appear in the normals. His findings were corroborated by Knott and Tjossem (1943) with a similar group of subjects. Scarborough (1943), recording from only the left hemisphere, found no differences between stutterers and normals.

Luchsinger and Landolt (1951), in the first of many European studies, compared the EEGs of stutterers and clutterers and found that almost 90 per cent of the latter group showed abnormalities but that the stutterers generally had normal encephalograms. Dew (1952) recorded the EEGs of stutterers awake and asleep, and reported that stutterers showed fewer alpha waves in sleep. Landolt and Luchsinger (1954) and Luchsinger and Landolt (1951) found that there were many more abnormal EEGs in clutterers than in stutterers and more in stutterer-clutterers (96 per cent) than in "pure" stutterers. In this last group only 2 of 21 had atypical EEGs. Streifler and Gumpertz (1955), however, could not find any such marked differences between their stutterers and clutterers. In about 35 per cent of both their groups, pathological EEG records were obtained, and the authors reported that of 100 normal speakers, only 15 per cent had similar EEG abnormalities. Murphy (1952) examined the EEGs of 30 male adult stutterers and their controls under conditions of rest, and during frustration and recovery in a listening task, and measured the amount of alpha wave activity from both hemispheres. No differences appeared in silence, both groups showing synchronous alpha waves in both hemispheres. However, the stuttering group showed greater interhemispheric differences in reactivity to frustration, and they were slower to recover normal EEG displays. Bente, Schönhärl, and Krump (1956) report that 59 per cent of their German stutterers showed EEG abnormalities. Busse and Clark (1957) found only 3 of 27 stuttering children with EEG abnormalities. Knott, Correll, and Shepherd (1959), using photic stimulation, found no EEG differences between stutterers and nonstutterers, although one group of stutterers showed the kind of EEG activity characteristic of high anxiety subjects. Pierce and Lipcon (1959) compared the EEG recordings of 36 stuttering naval recruits with their controls and found no differences. Graham and Brumlik (1961), using hyperventilation and sleep, reported more EEG abnormality in their stutterers than in their controls and also that the five of their more severe stutterers showed the greatest EEG abnormalities. Schilling (1960) found a correlation of abnormal EEG activity with diaphragmatic tremors and abnormalities during silence in children who stuttered. In another study, Schilling (1962), found that 31 per cent of a large number of stutterers had definitely abnormal electroencephalograms, and 27 per cent borderline abnormalities. Five per cent of them showed spikes although none were manifest epileptics. Moravek and Langova (1962) found more EEG abnormalities in clutterers than in stutterers and more in stutterers than in normal speakers.

Langova and Moravek (1964) found abnormal encephalograms in 16 per cent of stutterers, 39 per cent of stutterer-clutterers, and 50 per cent of "pure" clutterers. Schönhärl and Bente (1960) analyzed 400 EEG records of stutterers. Of these, 54 per cent showed dysrhythmias or spike disturbances. They found that the younger stutterers, aged 5 to 12, showed more generalized abnormalities. This age difference, indicating that younger stutterers (9 to 10 years) have more EEG abnormalities than older ones (11 to 15 years), has also been demonstrated by Fritzell, Peterson, and Sellden (1964) in Sweden. They found too that stutterers as a group have fewer normal electroencephalograms than their controls. Sutu, Mironescu, Cocinschi, Tirziu, and Miscoia (1964) showed that the EEG abnormalities in young stutterers were present before they developed avoidance, struggle, or neurotic behaviors. Hirschberg (1965), in Hungary, found that 60 per cent of 91 stutterers had abnormal EEGs. Negative EEGs were found for only 36 cases. EEGs characteristic of seizures were found in 15 subjects. Cali, Pisani, and Tagliareni (1965) procured EEG records from 58 Italian stutterers ages 3 to 16. Among them they found only 16 normal tracings. Of the 42 abnormal records, most again were found in the younger age groups. Six of these had focal asymmetries and dysrhythmias of the epileptic type although the children were not epileptic.

In Austria, Schmoigl and Ladisch (1967), excluding all cases in which a cluttering component seemed present, found abnormal EEGs in 70 per cent of 50 stutterers. Six per cent had spikes in their recordings. In the United States, Fox (1966) compared 13 adult stutterers with their matched controls during normal speech, simulated stuttering, and silence with eyes opened and when closed. She found no major differences. However, Sayles (1966), in a very careful investigation using hyperventilation, intermittent photic stimulation, and sleep with 23 stutterers and their controls found highly significant differences between the groups in amount of EEG abnormalities. Thirty per cent of his stutterers showed EEG abnormalities as compared with only 8 per cent of the normal speakers. Stromsta (1964) compared bilateral EEG recordings of 15 adult stutterers and their controls using both autocorrelation and cross-correlation. No differences appeared when autocorrelation was employed, but the two groups could be significantly differentiated by cross-correlation. The normal speakers showed more synchrony in the alpha rhythms in the two sides of the cortex than the stutterers.

The most extensive investigation of brain wave abnormalities was done in Germany by Siegert, Daute, Klust, Kunze, and Muller (1974). A total of 477 stutterers, aged 5 to 14 years were examined and their EEGs recorded and analyzed. Seven per cent showed borderline abnormalities and 6 per cent were definitely pathological. When all these EEG researches are viewed dispassionately it seems impossible to reconcile their different findings to be certain that most stutterers show this kind of organicity, but again it also seems evident that a minority of them do.

BIOCHEMICAL FACTORS

A number of researchers have investigated the biochemistry of stutterers, primarily the composition of the blood, urine, and saliva. The rationale for these studies has usually been that these secretions, which are controlled primarily by the autonomic nervous system, might reveal an organic pathology or malfunctioning of that system which could make the person more prone to stutter. To cite but one example, stuttering is characterized by excessive tension and clonic and tonic behaviors. So also is *tetany*, a calciometabolic imbalance that results in hyperirritability of neuromuscular activity causing clonic and tonic spasms. Tetany may also be latent, appearing only under stress. Kopp (1934), in his biochemical study of blood composition in stutterers, interpreted his data as supporting the concept of stuttering as a form of latent tetany. Shackson (1936) interprets the results of his electromyographic study of muscular contraction in stuttering as also indicating a possible latent tetany. Various European authors such as Fremel, (1913) have also held this view. Also the study by B. Weiss (1967) supports the hypothesis that some stutterers show a latent tetany. Employing electromyographic recordings of muscle excitability with hyperventilation and compression, she found evidence of the same changes usually found in latent tetany in a significant proportion of her 78 stutterers. They had normal serum calcium levels however.

Tetany, latent or otherwise, is caused by a deficiency of calcium in the blood. Such deficiencies have been attributed to heredity, to improper diet, or to a malfunction of the parathyroid glands, which monitor the blood serum balance between diffusable calcium and the plasma proteins.* Most of the research, however, does not seem to substantiate the belief of Hogewind (1940) and others that a calcium deficit exists in stutterers. If anything, serum calcium levels are slightly higher in stutterers than in normal speakers, as Hill (1944a) in his excellent review of biochemical factors in stuttering has made very clear. Almost all the research he cites indicates that stutterers show normal or higher calcium levels, and it has long been known that muscular activity and emotional upheaval can elevate these. Thus any differences may be the results of the stutterer's fear and struggle. Oblique support for Hill's position is also found in the study by Chapin and Kessler (1950), who found that 100 stutterers had fewer dental caries than the controls. If the stutterer has a blood calcium deficit, their teeth, according to these authors, should reflect that deficit. Further studies seem to substantiate this negative conclusion. Brown and Shulman (1940) measured the intermuscular tension of stutterers and normal speakers during silence and found no differences that might indicate a latent tetany. Johnson, Stearns, and Warweg (1933) found no deficiencies in serum calcium or blood sugar in their stutterers, but no

---

* In this connection, several writers, notably Knight Dunlap (1934), have stressed the importance of a diet rich in meat as part of the treatment of stuttering. In a Czechoslovakian journal, Weissova and Handzel (1962) present a detailed description of a familial, and probably hereditary insufficiency of the parathyroid glands in a father and three sons, all of whom stuttered and showed the usual signs of tetany. In view of the sex ratio in the incidence of stuttering it is interesting that in women the parathyroids are 20 per cent larger than in men. Certain relationships between thyroid and parathyroid glandular activity exist but are not as yet thoroughly understood. There are several reports of stuttering having been precipitated by thyroid medication and terminated when the medication was discontinued (Gordon 1928; Cabanas 1954) and we have had two cases whose stuttering improved remarkably under parahormone therapy. It should be noted that more parathyroid hormone is secreted when blood calcium falls below normal limits.

control group was used. Johnson, Young, Sahs, and Bedell (1959), using hyperventilation to precipitate signs of tetany, found no significant difference in the amount of stuttering shown by the stutterers during hyperventilation tetany, although their controls showed a slight increase in the number of disfluencies in this condition. In view of all these investigations, latent tetany must be regarded as an unsatisfactory explanation for stuttering, at least in the large majority of cases. Karlin, Karlin, and Gurren (1965) offer these other negative comments:

> The biochemical approach to stuttering was suggested by the fact that stuttering is characterized by tonic and clonic spasms. It was naturally believed that stuttering was therefore associated with latent tetany. Tetany is characterized by hyperirritability of the nervous system and is usually caused by a deficiency of calcium and Vitamin D. However, calcium and vitamin studies on stutterers fail to demonstrate abnormal blood levels. These studies seem to rule out tetany as a possible cause of stuttering. Furthermore, tetany usually occurs much earlier than stuttering and can develop at two months of age. This tendency for its early occurrence makes tetany a higher unlikely cause of stuttering (1965, pp. 101–2).

Dopamine and Haloperidol. There are several syndromes that are characterized by tremor and speech disturbances which seem to be due to too little or too much dopamine secretion in the brain. Among these are Parkinson's disease in which difficulty in getting speech started, cluttering, and compulsive repetitions of whole words or phrases are demonstrated. Parkinsonism is due to a dopamine deficiency and often responds to treatment by L-dopa. Another disorder precipitated by the same deficiency and responsive to the same medication is *dystonia* which is characterized by fixed postures. Difficulty in moving the articulatory and phonatory structures affects the prosody of speech as well as articulation (Darley, Aronson, and Brown 1975). In Huntington's Chorea (St. Vitus Dance), there seems to be an excess of dopamine and here, too, we find much disfluency which becomes worse if L-dopa is given. Finally, there is an odd disorder called the Gilles de la Tourette Syndrome whose etiology is not thoroughly understood but seems to involve dopamine secretion. Its victims have difficulty in producing phonation, and grunt or bark or utter compulsive obscenities as they struggle to speak. Since haloperidol, a drug which seems to counteract or inhibit excess dopamine, had been shown to be very successful in treating the Gilles de la Tourette syndrome, Wells and Malcolm (1971) tried it out on 36 stutterers and found a remarkable decrease in the severity of stuttering.

Other studies soon followed and most of them seem to corroborate this finding. Rosenberger, Wheelden, and Kalotkin (1976) found that the duration of stutterings but not their frequency decreased when haloperidol was given in a double blind experiment. Martin and Hershey (1975) provide a case report showing that haloperidol produced some real improvement in a therapy resistant client but they warn of the side effects of the medication. Rantala and Petri-Larma (1976), using haloperidol on

58 stutterers, found a significant reduction of severity but they concluded that the drug should only be used as an adjunct to regular speech therapy and psychotherapy. According to Murray, Kelly, Campbell, and Stefanik (1977), 11 of 18 patients benefited more from haloperidol than from the placebo, the reduction in struggle behavior being pronounced. They caution that the usefulness of the drug will be limited because of side effects, need for continuous medication and only partial success in eradication of symptoms. Burns, Brady, and Kuruvilla (1978) tried out haloperidol on twelve stutterers, nine of whom showed an average of 25 per cent stuttering in oral reading and 40 per cent in spontaneous speech. Three stutterers did not improve. These authors also administered apomorphine, a dopamine agonist, but this did not appear to have significant effects. Rosenberger (1980) gives a lucid presentation of our present knowledge about the dopamine system and its possible effects on stuttering.

Our review of these studies has not persuaded us that an organic cause of stuttering is to be found in the malfunctioning of the dompaminergic tracts in the brain.

CONCLUSIONS

As we review all this incredible mass of information it seems that organicity must play some part but only in some stutterers. Most of them do not have family histories of stuttering but almost a quarter of them do. Although most of them are indeed male, there are female stutterers, too, but the sex ratio cannot be attributed solely to cultural factors. With respect to differences in cerebral lateral dominance, again we find a minority (although still a substantial number) of stutterers who show differences from normal speakers. More stutterers than nonstutterers manifest brain wave irregularities but many of them do not. Brain damage has occasionally produced stuttering behaviors. Few biochemical differences are evident. Altogether, the case for organicity in stutterers has been only partially supported.

BIBLIOGRAPHY

Abbot, W. E., O. F. Due and W. A. Nosik, 1943.   Subdural hematoma and effusion as a result of blast injuries. *Journal of the American Medical Association* 121: 664–65; 739–41.

Abe, N. 1934.   Statistical observation of stutterers at the time of their draft in the Army. *Naval Surgeon Magazine* (Japan) 23: 232–34.

Andrews, G., and M. Harris. 1964.   *The syndrome of stuttering.* London. Heinemann.

Andrews G., P. T. Quinn, and W. A. Sorby, Stuttering: An investigation into cerebral dominance for speech. *Journal of Neurology, Neurosurgery and Psychiatry* 35: 414–18.

Appelt, A. 1911.   *The real cause of stammering and its permanent cure.* London: Methuen.

AREND, R., L. HANDZEL, AND B. WEISS. 1962. Dysphatic stuttering, *Folia Phoniatrica* 14: 55–66.

ARON, M. 1958. An investigation of the nature and incidence of stuttering among a Bantu group of school-going children. Masters thesis, University of the Witwatersrand, South Africa.

BALDAN, G. 1965. Study of the vestibular function in a group of stutterers: electronystagmographic researches. *De Therapia Vocis et Loquellae* 1: 349–51.

BALLARD, P. B. 1912. Sinistrality and speech. *Journal of Experimental Psychology* 1: 298–310.

BARBARA, D. A. 1946. A psychosomatic approach to the problem of stuttering in psychotics. *American Journal of Psychiatry* 103: 188–95.

BASSER, L. S. 1962. Hemiplegia of early onset and the faculty of speech with special reference to the effects of hemispherectomy. *Brain* 85: 427–60.

BELL, C. 1832. Philosophical transaction. II, *Archives of General Medicine* (2nd series).

BENSON, D. F. AND N. GESCHWIND. 1968. Cerebral dominance and its disturbances. *Pediatric Clinics of North America* 15: 759–69.

BENTE, D., E. SCHÖNHÄRL, AND J. KRUMP. 1956. Elektroencephalographische befunde bei stottereren und ihre bedeutung für die medikamentöse therapie. *Archive für Ohrenheilkunde* 169: 513–19.

BENTON, A. L. 1959. *Right-Left Discrimination and Finger Localization: Development and Pathology.* New York: Hoeber-Harper.

BERRY, M. F. 1938. A study of the medical histories of stuttering children. *Speech Monographs* 5: 97–114.

———. 1937. Twinning in stuttering families. *Human Biology* 9: 329–46.

BIGNARDI, F. AND L. SPETTOLI. 1955. Stuttering and contrasted left-handedness: clinical study. *Giornale de Psichiatria e di Neuropatologie* 133: 357–61.

BILTO, E. W. 1941. A comparative study of certain physical abilities of children with speech defects and children with normal speech. *Journal of Speech Disorders* 6: 187–203.

BLACKBURN, W. E. 1931. A study of voluntary movements of the diaphragm, tongue, lips, and jaw in stutterers and normal speakers. *Psychological Monographs* 41: 1–13.

BLOODSTEIN, O. 1959. A handbook on stuttering for professional workers. Chicago: National Society for Crippled Children and Adults.

BLUEMEL, C. S. 1913. *Stammering and Cognate Defects of Speech*, vol. 1. New York: Stechert.

BOCCA, E. AND C. CALEARO. 1963. Central hearing processes. In *Modern Developments in Audiology*, ed. J. Jerger. New York: Academic Press.

——— AND V. CASSINARI. 1954. A new method for testing hearing in temporal lobe tumours: preliminary report. *Acta Otolaryngologie* 44: 219–21.

BOLAND, J. L. 1951. Type of birth as related to stuttering. *Journal of Speech and Hearing Disorders* 16: 40–43.

BOLIN, B. J. 1953. Left-handedness and stuttering as signs diagnostic of epileptics. *Journal of Mental Science* 99: 483–88.

BOOME, E. J. AND M. A. RICHARDSON. 1932. *The Nature and Treatment of Stuttering.* New York: Dutton.

BOONE, D. R. 1959. Communication skills and intelligence in right and left hemiplegics. *Journal of Speech and Hearing Disorders* 24: 241–48.

BRADY, J. AND J. BERSON, Stuttering, dichotic listening and cerebral dominance. *Archives of General Psychiatry* 32: 1449–52.

BRANCH, C., B. MILNER, AND T. RASMUSSEN. 1964. Intercarotid sodium amytol for the lateralization of cerebral speech dominance. *Journal of Neurosurgery* 21: 399–405.

BRICKNER, R. M. 1940. A human cortical area producing repetitive phenomena when stimulated. *Journal of Neurophysiology* 3: 128–30.

BROWN, S. R. AND E. E. SHULMAN. 1940. Intramuscular pressure in stutterers and nonstutterers. *Speech Monographs* 7: 63–74.

BRUNO, G., V. CAMARDA, AND L. CURI. 1965. Contribution to the study of organic causal factors in the pathogenesis of stuttering. *Bolletino delle Malattie dell'Orecchio, della Gola, del Naso* 83: 753–58.

BRUNT, M. AND C. P. GOETZINGER. 1968. A study of three tests of central function with normal hearing subjects. *Cortex* 4: 288–97.

BRYANT, F. A. 1917. Influence of heredity in stuttering. *Journal of Heredity* 8: 46–47.

BRYDEN, M. P. 1963. Ear preference in auditory perception. *Journal of Experimental Psychology* 65: 103–5.

BRYNGELSON, B. 1934. The problem of sidedness and its relationship to stuttering. *Proceedings of the American Society for the Study of Disorders of Speech* 4: 63–70.

———. 1935. Sidedness as an etiological factor in stuttering. *Journal of Genetic Psychology* 47: 204–17.

———. 1940. A study of laterality of stutterers and normal speakers. *Journal of Social Psychology* 11: 151–55.

——— AND T. B. CLARK. 1933. Left-handedness and stuttering. *Journal of Heredity* 24: 387–90.

BRYNGELSON, E. AND B. RUTHERFORD. 1937. A comparative study of laterality of stutterers and nonstutterers. *Journal of Speech Disorders* 2: 15–16.

BURNS, D., J. P. BRADY AND K. KURUVILLA. 1978. The acute effect of haloperidol and apomorphine on the severity of stuttering. *Biological Psychiatry* 13: 255–64.

BUSSE, E. W. AND R. M. CLARK. 1957. The use of the encephalogram in diagnosing speech disorders in children. *Folia Phoniatrica* 9: 182–87.

CABANAS, R. 1951. Report on a particular case of stuttering. *Folia Phoniatrica* 3: 10–13.

———. 1954. Some findings in speech and voice therapy among the mentally retarded. *Folia Phoniatrica* 6: 34–37.

CALEARO, C. AND A. R. ANTONELLI. 1963. Cortical hearing tests and cerebral dominance. *Acta Oto-Laryngologica* 56: 17–26.

CALI, G., F. PISANI AND F. TAGLIARENI. 1965. Stuttering and electroencephalographic curves. *Clinical ORL* 17: 316–28.

CAPLAN, L. 1972. An investigation of some aspects of stuttering-like speech in adult dysphasic patients. *Journal South African Speech and Hearing Association* 19: 52–66.

CARR, B. M. 1969. Ear effect variables and order of report in dichotic listening. *Cortex* 5: 63–68.

CARTERETTE, E. C. (ed). 1966. *Brain Function*, vol. 3. Berkeley: Univ. of California Press.

CERF, A. AND D. PRINS. 1971. Stutterers' ear preference for dichotic syllables. Convention paper, ASHA, Las Vegas.

CHAPIN, A. B. AND H. E. KESSLER. 1950. Dental caries in individuals who stutter. *Dental Items of Interest* 72: 162–67.

CHWOROWSKY, C. R. 1952. A comparative study of diadochokinetic rates of stutterers and nonstutterers in speech related and nonspeech related movements. *Speech Monographs* 19: 192 (abstract).

CLAIBORNE, J. H. 1917. Stuttering relieved by reversal of manual dexterity. *New York Medical Journal* 105: 577–81; 619–21.

CLARK, M. M. 1957. *Left Handedness, Laterality Characteristics, and Their Educational Implications.* London: Univ. of London Press.

COOPER, E. B. 1972. Recovery from stuttering in a junior and senior high school population. *Journal of Speech and Hearing Research* 15: 632–38.

CROSS, H. M. 1936. The motor capacities of stutterers. *Archives of Speech* 1: 112–32.

CURRY, F. K. W. 1967. A comparison of left-handed and right-handed subjects on verbal and nonverbal dichotic listening tasks. *Cortex* 3: 343–51.

———. 1968. A comparison of the performances of a right hemispherectomized subject and 25 normals on four dichotic listening tasks. *Cortex* 4: 144–53.

——— AND H. H. GREGORY. 1967. A comparison of stutterers and nonstutterers on three dichotic listening tasks. Convention Address, ASHA.

DANIELS, E. M. 1940. An analysis of the relation between handedness and stuttering with special reference to the Orton-Travis theory of cerebral dominance. *Journal of Speech Disorders* 5: 309–26.

DARLEY, F. L., A. E. ARONSON AND J. R. BROWN. 1975. *Motor speech disorders.* Philadelphia: W. B. Saunders.

DASKALOV, D. D. 1962. On the problem of the basic principles and methods of prevention and treatment of stammering. *Zhurnal Nevropatologii i Psikhiatrii imeni S. S. Korsakova* 53: 1047–52.

DE AJURIAGUERRA, J. 1966. Speech disorders in childhood. In *Brain Function III*, ed. C. C. Carterette. Berkeley: Univ. of California Press.

———, R. DIATKINE, S. DE GOBINEAU AND M. STAMBAK. 1958. Le Bégaiement, *Presse Medicale* 66: 953–56.

DELACATO, C. 1963. *The Diagnosis and Treatment of Speech and Reading Problems.* Springfield, Ill.: Thomas.

DENHARDT, R. 1890. *Das stottern: eine Psychose.* Leipsig: Ernst Keil's Nachfolger.

DEW, R. 1952. Electroencephalographic study of stutterers during sleep. *Speech Monographs* 19: 192–93.

DIRKS, E. 1964. Perception of dichotic and monaural verbal material and cerebral dominance for speech. *Acta Otolaryngologica* 58: 73–80.

DORMAN, M. F. AND R. J. PORTER. 1975. Hemispheric lateralization for speech perception in stutterers. *Cortex* 11: 181–85.

DOUGLASS, L. C. 1943. A study of bilaterally recorded electroencephalograms of adult stutterers. *Journal of Experimental Psychology* 32: 247–65.

DUNLAP, K. 1934. Possible dietary predisposition to stammering. *Science N.S.* 80: 206.

EISENSON, J. 1947. Aphasics: observations and tentative conclusions. *Journal of Speech Disorders* 12: 290–92.

———. 1958. A perseverative theory of stuttering. In *Stuttering: A Symposium*, ed. J. Eisenson. New York: Harper.

————. 1937.   Some characteristics of the written speech of stutterers. *Journal of Genetic Psychology* 50: 457–58.

————. 1975.   Stuttering as a perseverative disorder. In *Stuttering: A Second Symposium*, ed. J. Eisenson. New York: Harper and Row.

———— AND E. PASTEL. 1936.   A study of the perseveratory tendency in stutterers. Quarterly Journal of Speech 22: 626–31.

EISENSON, J. AND C. N. WINSLOW. 1938.   The perseverating tendency in stutterers in a perceptual function. *Journal of Speech Disorders* 3: 195–98.

FAGAN, L. B. 1931.   Graphic stuttering. *Psychology Monographs* 43: 67–71.

————. 1931.   The relation of dextral training to the onset of stuttering. A report of cases. Quarterly Journal of Speech 17: 73–76.

FARMER, A. 1975.   Stuttering repetitions in aphasic and nonaphasic brain damaged adults. *Cortex* 11: 319–96.

FINK, W. H. AND B. BRYNGELSON. 1934.   The relation of strabismus to right or left handedness. *Transactions of the American Academy of Ophthomology and Otolaryngology* 9: 247–66.

FINKELSTEIN, P. AND S. E. WEISBERGER. 1954.   The motor proficiency of stutterers. *Journal of Speech and Hearing Disorders* 19: 52–57.

FOX, D. R. 1966.   Electroencephalographic analysis during stuttering and nonstuttering. *Journal of Speech and Hearing Research* 9: 488–97.

FREESTONE, N. W. 1942.   A brainwave interpretation of stuttering. *Quarterly Journal of Speech* 28: 466–70.

FREMEL, F. 1913.   Stottern und fazialsphammen. *Wien Medizinische Wochenschrift* 63: 2207–9.

FRESHEL, E. 1963.   In Stuttering in the left parietal lobe syndrome, by A. Kh. Stremel. *Zhurnal Nevropatologii i Psikhiatrii imeni S. S. Korsakova* 63: 828–32.

FREUND, H. 1966.   *Psychopathology and the problems of stuttering.* Springfield, Ill.: Thomas.

————. 1955.   Psychosis and stuttering. *Journal of Nervous and Mental Diseases* 122: 161–72.

————. 1952.   Studies in the interrelationship between stuttering and cluttering. *Folia Phoniatrica* 4: 146–68.

FRITZELL, B., I. PETERSON AND U. SELLDEN. 1965.   An EEG study of stuttering and nonstuttering school children. *De Therapia Vocis et Loquellae* 1: 343–46.

FROESCHELS, E. 1943a.   Pathology and therapy of stuttering. *Nervous Child* 2: 148–61.

————. 1915.   Stuttering and nystagmus. *Monatschrift für Ohrenheilkunde* 49: 161–67.

————. 1943b.   Survey of the early literature on stuttering, chiefly European. *Nervous Child* 2: 86–95.

————. 1919.   Die sprachärztliche therapie im Kriege III das stottern. *Monataschrift für Ohrenheilkunde* 53: 161–90.

————. 1964.   *Selected papers (1940–1964).* Amsterdam: North-Holland.

GALIN, D. AND R. ORNSTEIN. 1972.   Lateral specialization of cognitive mode: an EEG study. *Psychophysiology* 9: 412–18.

GARDNER, W. H. 1937.   The study of the pupillary reflex with special reference to stuttering. *Psychological Monographs* 49: 1–31.

GEDDA, L., L. BRANCONI AND G. BRUNO. 1960.   Su alcuni casi di balbuzie in coppie gemellari mono-e dizigotiche. *Acta Geneticae Medicae et Gemellologiae* 9: 407–26.

GERSTMANN, J. AND P. SCHILDER. 1921. Studien über bewegungstörungen über die typenextrapyramidaler pseudobulbar paralyse. *Zeitschrift für Neurologie und Psychiatrie* 79: 350–54.

GHENT, L. 1961. Development changes in tactual thresholds on dominant and nondominant sides. *Journal of Comparative Physiology and Psychology* 54: 670–73.

GIRONE, D. AND G. BRUNO. 1957. Some characteristics of the glycemic curve in stutterers. *Folia Phoniatrica* 9: 87–91.

GODA, S. 1961. Stuttering manifestations following spinal meningitis. *Journal of Speech and Hearing Disorders* 26: 392–93.

GÖLLNITZ, G. 1954. *Die bedeutung der frühkindlichen hirnschädigung für die kinderpsychiatrie.* Leipsig: Thieme.

———. 1955. Zusammenhänge zwischen stottern und frühkindlicher hirnschädigung. *Medecin Klinik* 50: 685–89.

GOODGLASS, H. AND F. A. QUADFASEL. 1964. Language laterality in left-handed aphasics. *Brain* 77: 521–48.

GORDON, M. B. 1928. Stammering produced by thyroid medication. *American Journal of Medical Science* 175: 360–65.

GRAF, O. I. 1955. Incidence of stuttering among twins. In *Stuttering in Children and Adults*, eds. W. Johnson and R. Lentenneger. Minneapolis: Univ. of Minnesota Press.

GRAHAM, J. K. 1958. A neurologic and electroencephalographic study of adult stutterers and matched normal speakers. Doctoral dissertation, Northwestern University.

——— AND J. BRUMLIK. 1961. Neurologic and encephalographic abnormalities in stuttering and matched nonstuttering adults. *ASHA* 3: 342 (abstract).

GRANICH, L. 1947. *Aphasia.* New York: Grune and Stratton.

GRAY, M. 1940. The X family: a clinical and laboratory study of a "stuttering" family. *Journal of Speech Disorders* 5: 343–48.

GRUBER, L. AND R. L. POWELL. 1974. Responses of stuttering and nonstuttering children to a dichotic listening task. *Perceptual and motor skills* 38: 203–04.

GUILLAUME, J., G. MAZARS, AND Y. MAZARS. 1957. Epileptic mediation in certain types of stammering. *Revue Neurologique* 99: 59–62.

GUNDERSON, H. 1949. A quantitative analysis of digital tremor in male stutterers. Doctoral dissertation, Teachers College, Columbia University.

GUTTSMANN, H. 1939. Erbbiologische, soziologische und organische faktoren die sprachstörungen begungstigen. *Archive für Sprach-Stimmheilkunde* 3: 133–36.

———, 1898. *Das stottern.* Frankfurt: J. Rosenheim.

———. 1937. Konstitution und sprachstörung. *Hippokrates* (Stuttgart) 8: 369–71.

HAASE, C. A. 1846. *Das Stottern: Oder Darstellung und Bleuchtung der Wichtigsten über Wesen, Ursache und Heilung, Desselben, Nebst Abhandlung des Hieronymus Mercurialis "De Balbutie" für Pädagogen und Medicin.* Berlin: Hirschwald.

HAEFNER, R. 1929. *The Educational Significance of Left-Handedness.* New York: Teachers College, Columbia University Press.

HAMILTON, P. G. 1940. The visual characteristics of stutterers during silent reading. Doctoral dissertation, Teachers College, Columbia University.

HAMRE, C. E. 1972. A comment on the possible organicity of stuttering. *British Journal of Disorders of Communication* 7: 148–50.

―――― AND M. E. WINGATE. 1967. Pyknolepsy and stuttering. *Quarterly Journal of Speech* 53: 374–77.

HARRISON, H. S. 1947. A study of the speech of sixty institutionalized epileptics. Masters thesis, Louisiana State University.

HEAD, H. 1926. *Aphasia and Kindred Disorders of Speech.* London: Macmillan.

HÉCAEN, H. 1962. Clinical symptomatology in right and left hemisphere lesions. In *Interhemispheric Relations and Cerebral Dominance,* ed. V. B. Mountcastle. Baltimore: Johns Hopkins Press.

―――― AND J. DE AJURIAGUERRA. 1963. *Les gauchers, préférance manuelle et dominance cérébrale.* Paris: Presses Universitaires de France.

HELM, N. A. AND R. B. BUTLER. 1980. Neurogenic acquired stuttering. *Journal of Fluency Disorders* 5: 269–79.

―――― AND D. F. BENSON. 1978. Acquired stuttering. *Neurology* 28: 1159–65.

HELM, N. A., R. B. BUTLER, AND G. J. CANTNER. 1980. Neurogenic acquired stuttering. *Journal of Fluency Disorders* 5: 269–79.

HERREN, R. Y. 1931. The effect of stuttering on voluntary movement. *Journal of Experimental Psychology* 14: 289–98.

――――. 1932. The relation of stuttering and alcohol to certain tremor rates. *Journal of Experimental Psychology* 15: 87–96.

HILL, H. 1944a. Stuttering I: A critical review and evaluation of biochemical investigations. *Journal of Speech Disorders* 9: 245–61.

――――. 1944b. Stuttering II: A review and integration of physiological data. *Journal of Speech Disorders* 9: 289–324.

HINKLE, W. G. 1971. A study of subgroups within the stuttering population. Doctoral dissertation, Purdue University.

HIRSCHBERG, J. 1965. Stuttering. *Orvosi Hetilap* 106: 780–84.

HOGEWIND, F. 1940. Medical treatment of stuttering. *Journal of Speech Disorders* 5: 203–8.

HOWIE, P. M. 1976. A twin investigation of the etiology of stuttering. Convention paper, ASHA, Houston.

HUNT, J. 1870. *Stammering and Stuttering, Their Nature and Treatment,* 7th ed. London: Longmans, Green.

INGEBRETSEN, E. 1936. Some experimental contributions to the psychology and psychopathology of stutterers. *American Journal of Orthopsychiatry* 6: 630–50.

JASPER, H. H. 1932. A laboratory study of diagnostic indices of bilateral neuromuscular organization in stutterers and normal speakers. *Psychological Monographs* 43: 172–74.

JOHNSON, W. 1959. *The Onset of Stuttering.* Minneapolis: Univ. of Minnesota Press.

――――, S. BROWN, J. CURTIS, C. EDNEY, AND J. KEASTER. 1967. *Speech Handicapped School Children,* 3d ed. New York: Harper and Row.

JOHNSON, W. AND A. KING. 1942. An angle board and hand usage study of stutterers and nonstutterers. *Journal of Experimental Psychology* 31: 293–311.

JOHNSON, W., G. STEARNS, AND E. WARWEG. 1933. Chemical factors and the stuttering spasm. *Quarterly Journal of Speech* 19: 409–15.

JOHNSON, W., M. A. YOUNG, A. L. SAHS, AND G. N. BEDELL. 1959. Effects of hyperventilation and tetany on the speech fluency of stutterers and nonstutterers. *Journal of Speech and Hearing Research* 2: 203–15.

JONES, R. K. 1967. Dyspraxic ambiphasia—a neurophysiologic theory of stammering. *Transactions American Neurological Association* 92: 197–201.

————. 1966. Observations on stammering after localized cerebral injury. *Journal of Neurology and Neurosurgery* 29: 192–95.

JOST, H. AND L. W. SONTAG. 1944. The genetic factor in autonomic nervous function. *Psychosomatic Medicine* 6: 308–10.

KAMIYAMA, A. 1967. *Handbook for the Study of Stuttering.* Tokyo: Kongo-Shupan.

KANNER, L. 1942. *Child Psychiatry.* Springfield, Ill.: Thomas.

KAPOS, E. AND L. S. STANDLEE. 1958. Behavioral rigidity in adult stutterers. *Journal of Speech and Hearing Research* 1: 294–96.

KARLIN, I. W. 1947. Psychosomatic theory of stuttering. *Journal of Speech Disorders* 12: 319–22.

————, D. B. KARLIN, AND L. GURREN. 1965. *Development and Diseases of Speech in Childhood.* Springfield, Ill.: Thomas.

KARLIN, I. W. AND A. E. SOBOL. 1940. A comparative study of the blood chemistry of stutterers and nonstutterers. *Speech Monographs* 7: 75–84.

KIDD, K. K. 1977. A genetic perspective on stuttering. *Journal of Fluency Disorders* 2: 259–69.

————, J. R. KIDD, AND M. A. RECORDS. 1978. The possible causes of the sex ratio in stuttering and its implications. *Journal of Fluency Disorders* 3: 13–23.

KIDD, K. K. AND M. A. RECORDS. 1979. Genetic methodologies for the study of speech. In *Neurogenics: Genetic Approaches to the Nervous System,* ed. N. Breakfield. New York: Elsevier.

KILOH, L. G. AND J. W. OSSELTON. 1961. *Clinical Electroencephalography.* London: Butterworth.

KIMURA, D. 1961a. Cerebral dominance and the perception of verbal stimuli. *Canadian Journal of Psychology* 15: 166–71.

————. 1967. Functional asymmetry of the brain in dichotic listening. *Cortex* 3: 163–78.

————. 1961b. Some effects of temporal lobe damage on auditory perception. *Canadian Journal of Psychology* 15: 156–65.

————. 1963. Speech lateralization in young children as determined by an auditory test. *Journal of Comparative Physiology and Psychology* 56: 899–902.

KING, P. T. 1961. Perseveration in stutterers and nonstutterers. *Journal of Speech and Hearing Research* 4: 346–57.

KISTLER, K. 1930. Linkshändigkeit und sprachstörungen. *Schweitz-Medizinische Wochenschrift* 11: 32–34.

KLINGBEIL, G. M. 1939. The historical background of the modern speech clinic. *Journal of Speech Disorders* 4: 115–32.

KNOTT, J. R., E. CORRELL, AND J. N. SHEPHERD. 1959. Frequency analysis of electroencephalograms of stutterers and nonstutterers. *Journal of Speech and Hearing Research* 2: 74–80.

KNOTT, J. R. AND T. D. TJOSSEM. 1943. Bilateral encephalograms from normal speakers and stutterers. *Journal of Experimental Psychology* 32: 357–62.

KOPP, G. A. 1934. Metabolic studies of stutterers: I. Biochemical study of blood composition. *Speech Monographs* 1: 117–32.

KOPP, H. 1936. Les troubles de la parole dans leur rapport avec les troubles de la motrice. *L'Evolution Psychiatrique* 2: 77–112.

————. 1946. Psychosomatic study of fifty stuttering children. III. Oseretsky tests. *American Journal of Orthopsychiatry* 16: 114–19.

————. 1942–43. The relationship of stuttering to motor disturbances. *Nervous Child* 2: 107–16.

Kussmaul, A. 1877. Die störungen der sprache. In *Cyclopaedia Medica*, ed. H. V. Ziemssen.

Landolt, H. and R. Luchsinger. 1954. Language disorder, stuttering, and chronic organic psychosyndrome; electroencephalographic results and studies of pathology of speech. *Deutsche Medizinische Wochenschrift* 79: 1012–15.

Langova, J. and M. Moravek. 1962. Experimental study on stuttering and stammering. *Casopis Lekaru Ceskych* 101: 297–300.

————. 1964. Some results of experimental examinations among stutterers and clutterers. *Folia Phoniatrica* 16: 290–96.

Larson, M. 1949. Representative 19th-century stuttering therapists. Masters thesis, University of Denver.

Launay, C. 1960. Troubles neurologiques dane le bégaiement. *Journal Franc. d'Otorhinolaryngologie* 9: 269–79.

Lenneberg, E. H. 1966. Speech development: its anatomical and physiological components. In *Brain Function III*, ed. E. C. Carterette. Berkeley: Univ. of California Press.

Lerbert, G. 1965. La dominance latérale. *Année Psychologie* 66: 411–38.

Lindsley, D. B. 1940. Bilateral differences in brain potentials from the two cerebral hemispheres in relation to laterality and stuttering. *Journal of Experimental Psychology* 26: 211–25.

Lovett, D. J. W. and L. I. M. Coleman. 1955. The psychophysics of communication. III. Discriminatory awareness in stutterers and its measurement by the critical flicker fusion threshold. *Archives of Neurology and Psychiatry* 74: 650–52.

Luchsinger, R. 1940. Die sprache und stimme von ein-und zweieiigen zwillingen in beziehung zur motorik und zum erbcharakter. *Archive Julius-Klaus-Stiftung* 15: 457–62.

————. 1959. Die vererbung von sprach-und stimmstörungen. *Folia Phoniatrica* 11: 17–64.

————. 1944. Biological studies on monozygotic and dizygotic twins relative to size and form of the larynx. *Archive Julius Klaus-Stiftung für Verergungsforschung* 19: 3–4.

————. 1943. Function of sympathetic nervous system as indicated by pupillary reactions in stutterers. *Schweizer Medizinische Wochenschrift* (July 10).

————. 1954. Gibt es organische bedingte stottererfalle? *Archive für Ohrenheilkunde* 165: 612–14.

————. 1959. Stottern. *Phonetica* 3: 183–89.

———— and G. E. Arnold. 1965. *Voice-speech-language*. Belmont, Cal.: Wadsworth.

Luchsinger, R. and H. Landholt. 1951. Electroencephalographische untersuchungen bei stotteren mit und ohne polterkomponente. *Folia Phoniatria* 3: 135–51.

Luessenhop, A. J., J. S. Boggs, L. J. Laborowit, and Walle. 1973. Cerebral dominance in stutterers determined by Wada testing. *Neurology* 23: 1190–92.

Maas, O. 1946. On the etiology of stuttering. *Journal of Mental Science* 92: 357–63.

MacKay, B. G. 1968. Metamorphosis of a critical interval: age linked changes in delay in auditory feedback that produces maximal disruption of speech. *Journal of the Acoustical Society of America* 43: 810–20.

MAKUEN, G. H. 1914. A study of 1000 cases of stammering with special reference to the etiology and treatment of the affection. *Therapeutic Gazette* 38: 385–90.

MARTIN, R. 1962. Stuttering and perseveration in children. *Journal of Speech and Hearing Research* 5: 332–39.

MARTIN, S. AND L. G. HERSHEY. 1975. The use of haloperidol in the management of stuttering: a case study. *Journal of Fluency Disorders* 1: 13–17.

MCKNIGHT, R. V. 1936. A self-analysis of a case of reading, writing, and speaking disability. *Archives of Speech* 1: 18–47.

MEYER, B. C. 1945. Psychosomatic aspects of stuttering. *Journal of Nervous and Mental Illness* 101: 127–57.

MOORE, W. J. 1976. Bilateral tachistoscopic word perception of stutterers and normal speakers. *Brain and Language* 3: 434–42.

MOORE, W. H. AND W. O. HAYNES. 1980. Alpha hemispheric asymmetry and stuttering: some support for a segmentation dysfunction hypothesis. *Journal of Speech and Hearing Research* 23: 229–47.

MOORE, W. H. AND M. LANG. 1977. Alpha symmetry over the right and left hemispheres of stutterers and control subjects preceding massed oral reading. *Perceptual and Motor Skills* 44: 223–30.

MORAVEK, M. AND J. LANGOVA. 1962. Some electrophysiological findings among stutterers. *Folia Phoniatrica* 14: 305–16.

MURPHY, A. T. 1952. An electroencephalographic study of frustration in stutterers. Doctoral dissertation, University of Southern California.

MURRAY, T. J., P. KELLY, L. CAMPBELL, AND K. STEFANIK. 1977. Haloperidol in the treatment of stuttering. *British Journal of Psychiatry* 130: 370–73.

MUSSAFIA, M. 1964. The role of heredity in language disorders. *Folia Phoniatrica* 16: 228–38.

MYGIND, H. 1898. Über die ursuchen des stotterns. *Archive für Laryngologie una Rhinologie* 8: 294–307.

NELSON, S. 1939. Personal contact as a factor in the transfer of stuttering. *Human Biology* 11: 393–401.

———, N. HUNTER, AND M. WALKER. 1945. Stuttering in twin types. *Journal of Speech Disorders* 10: 335–343.

NEILSON, M. AND P. NEILSON. 1979. Systems analysis of tracking performance in stutterers and normals. Convention paper, ASHA, Atlanta.

NIELSEN, J. M. 1942. Epitome of agnosia, apraxia, and aphasia with proposed physiologic-anatomic nomenclature. *Journal of Speech Disorders* 7: 105–41.

OATES, D. W. 1929. Left-handedness in relation to speech defects, intelligence and achievement. *Forum of Education* 7: 91–105.

OJEMANN, R. H. 1931. Studies in handedness; III. Relation of handedness to speech. *Journal of Educational Psychology* 22: 120–26.

ORTON, S. T. 1927. Studies in stuttering. *Archives of Neurology and Psychiatry* 18: 671–72.

———. 1937. *Reading, Writing, and Speech Problems in Childhood.* New York: Norton.

——— AND L. E. TRAVIS. 1929. Studies in stuttering; IV. Studies of action currents in stutterers. *Archives of Neurology and Psychiatry* 21: 61–68.

OTSUKI, H. 1958. Study on stuttering: statistical observations. *Otorhinolaryngology Clinic* 5: 1150–51.

PALMER, M. F. AND C. D. OSBORN. 1938. One thousand consecutive cases of speech defects. *Transactions of the Kansas Academy of Science* 4: 116.

PEACHER, W. C. AND W. E. HARRIS. 1946. Speech disorders in World War II: stuttering. *Journal of Speech Disorders* 11: 303–8.

PENFIELD, W. AND T. RASMUSSEN. 1949. Vocalization and arrest of speech. *Archives of Neurology and Psychiatry* 61: 21–27.

PENFIELD, W. AND L. ROBERTS. 1959. *Speech and brain mechanisms.* Princeton: Princeton Univ. Press.

PERRIN, K. L. AND J. EISENSON. 1970. An examination of ear preference for speech and non-speech stimuli in a stuttering population. Convention paper, ASHA, New York.

PFAÑDLER, U. 1952. Les vices de la parole dans l'optique du geneticien. *Problema Acta Phoniatrie et Logopedie* 1: 35–40.

PIERCE, C. M. AND H. H. LIPCON. 1959. Stuttering: Clinical and electroencephalographic findings, *Military Medicine* 12: 511–19.

PONSFORD, R. C., W. S. BROWN, J. MARSH, AND L. E. TRAVIS. 1979. Evoked potential correlates of cerebral dominance for speech perception in stutterers and nonstutterers, *E.E.G. Journal* 39: 434.

QUINAN, C. 1921. Sinistrality in relation to high blood pressure and defects of speech. *Archives of Internal Medicine* 27: 255–61.

———. 1938. Stammering and left handedness—a graphic study. *Journal of Experimental Psychology* 22: 90–96.

QUINN, P. T. 1972. Stuttering, cerbral dominance and the dichotic word test. *Medical Journal of Australia* 2: 639–43.

——— AND G. ANDREWS, 1977. Neurological stuttering—a clinical entity? *Journal of Neurology, Neurosurgery and Psychiatry* 40:: 669–701.

RANTALA, S. AND M. PETRI-LARMI. 1976. Haloperidol (Serenase) in the treatment of stuttering. *Folia Phoniatrica* 28: 354–61.

RECORDS, M. A., R. C. HEIMBUCH, AND K. K. KIDD. 1977. Handedness and stuttering: A Dead Horse? *Journal of Fluency Disorders* 2: 271–82.

RECORDS, M. A., K. K. KIDD, AND J. R. KIDD. 1976. Stuttering among relatives of stutterers, Convention paper, *ASHA*, Houston.

RHEINBERGER, M. B., W. I. KARLIN, AND A. B. BERMAN. 1943. Electroencephalographic and laterality studies of stuttering and nonstuttering children. *Nervous Child* 2: 117–33.

ROSENBEK, J. 1980. Apraxia of speech—relation to stuttering, *Journal of Fluency Disorders* 5: 233–54.

ROSENBECK, T. C., B. MESSERT, M. COLLINS, AND R. WERTZ. 1978. Stuttering following brain damage. *Brain and Language* 6: 82–96.

ROSENBERGER, P. B. 1980. Dopaminergic systems and speech fluency. *Journal of Fluency Disorders* 5: 255–68.

———, J. A. WHEELDEN, AND M. KALOTKIN. 1976. The effect of haloperidol on stuttering. *American Journal of Psychiatry* 131: 331–34.

ROSENFIELD, D. B. 1980. Cerebral dominance and stuttering. *Journal of Fluency Disorders* 5: 171–85.

————. 1972. Stuttering and cerebral ischemia. *New England Journal of Medicine* 287: 991.

ROSENZWEIG, M. R. 1951. Representations of the two ears at the auditory cortex. *American Journal of Physiology* 167: 147–58.

ROSSI, G. F. AND G. ROSADINI. 1967. Experimental analysis of cerebral dominance in man. In *Brain Mechanisms Underlying Speech and Language*, eds. C. H. Millikan and F. L. Darley. New York: Grune and Stratton.

RUTHERFORD, B. 1944. A comparative study of loudness, pitch, rate, rhythm, and quality of the speech of children handicapped by cerebral palsy. *Journal of Speech Disorders* 9: 263–71.

RYLANDER, G. 1948. Personality analysis before and after frontal lobotomy. *Publications of the Association for Nervous and Mental Diseases* 27: 691–705.

SACHS, M. W. 1924. Zur aetiologie des stotterns. *Klinische Wochenschrift* 37: 113–15.

SANDER, E. 1975. Untangling stuttering: a tour through the theory thicket. *ASHA* 17: 256–62.

SAYLES, D. G. 1966. Brain wave excitability, perseveration, and stuttering. Doctoral dissertation, University of Michigan.

————. 1971. Cortical excitability, perseveration and stuttering. *Journal of Speech and Hearing Research* 14: 462–75.

SCARBROUGH, H. E. 1943. A quantitative and qualitative analysis of the electroencephalograms of stutterers and nonstutterers. *Journal of Experimental Psychology* 32: 156–67.

SCHILLING, A. 1959. Electronystamographic findings as indication of central coordination defect in stutterers. *Archive für Ohren-Nasen- und Kehlkopfheilkunde Vereinigt mit Zeitschrift* 175: 457–61.

————. 1962. Organische faktoren bei der entstchung des stotterns. *HNO* 10: 149–53.

————. 1960. Radiokymograms of the diaphragm in stammerers. *Folia Phoniatrica* 12: 145–53.

————. 1956. Stottern bei Rhesus-bedingter stammhirnechädigung. *Archive Ohrenheilkunde* 169: 501.

———— AND W. KRÜGER. 1960. Untersuchungen über die motorik sprachgestörter kinder nach der motometrischen skala von Oseretsky-Göllnitz unter besonderer berücksichtingung dei frühkindlichen hirnschädigung. *HNO* 8: 205–9.

SCHILLING, R. AND A. SCHILLING. 1960. On the diagnosis of early childhood brain injuries in stutterers. *Aktuelle Probleme der Phoniatrie und Logopaedia; Supplementa ad Folia Phoniatrica* 1: 134–40.

SCHMOIGL, S. AND W. LADISCH. 1967. EEG investigation in stutterers. *Electroenceph. Clin. Neurophysiol.* 23: 184–85.

SCHÖNHÄRL, E. 1964. Age-connected changes in the structural picture of stuttering. *HNO* 12: 152–54.

———— AND D. BENTE. 1960. Veränderungen im EGG bei stottern. *Kongress, Gemeinrhaftstg. allg. Angew. Phonetik.*, Hamburg-Altona.

SCRIPTURE, E. W. 1909. Penmanship stuttering. *Journal of American Medical Association* 52: 1480–81.

SCRIPTURE, M. K. AND O. GLOGAU. 1916. Speech conflict as an etiological factor in stuttering. *Journal of Nervous and Mental Disorders* 43: 37–46.

SEDLACEK, C. 1947–48. Reactions of the autonomic nervous system in attacks of stuttering. *Folia Phoniatrica* 1: 97–103.

SEEMAN, M. 1966. Speech pathology in Czechoslovakia. In *Speech Pathology*, eds. R. W. Rieber and R. S. Brubaker. Philadelphia: Lippincott.

————. 1959. *Sprachstörungen bei Kindern*. Marhold: Halle-Saale.

————. 1947. Sur la régulation neurovegitative de la durée de la phonation. *Folia Phoniatrica* 1: 22–37.

————. 1937. The significance of twin pathology for the investigation of speech disorders. *Archive gesamte Phonetik*, Part II, 1: 88–92.

————. 1934. Über somatische befunde bei stottern. *Monatschrift für Ohrenheilkunde* 68: 895–912.

————. 1941. Untersuchungen über phonationsdauer bei stotterern. *Archive für Sprach- und Stimmphysiologie* 5: 211–13.

SELZER, C. A. 1933. Lateral dominance and visual fusion. *Harvard Monographs in Education*, No. 12. Cambridge, Mass.: Harvard Univ. Press.

SETH, G. 1934. An experimental study of the control of the mechanism of speech and in particular that of respiration in the stutterer. *British Journal of Psychology* 24: 375–88.

————. 1958. Psychomotor control in stammering and normal subjects: an experimental study. *British Journal of Psychology* 49: 139–43.

SHACKSON, R. 1936. An action current study of muscle contraction latency with special reference to latent tetany in stutterers. *Archives of Speech* 1: 87–111.

SHEEHAN, J. AND M. M. MARTYN. 1966. Spontaneous recovery from stuttering. *Journal of Speech and Hearing Research* 9: 121–35.

SHEEHAN, J. G. AND M. S. COSTLEY. 1977. A reexamination of the role of heredity in stuttering. *Journal of Speech and Hearing Disorders* 42: 47–59.

SHIRAIWA, T. AND J. KAWAKUBA. 1967. Study of the cause of stuttering. Abstract No. 185, in *A Handbook for the Study of Stuttering*, ed. G. Kamiyama. Tokyo: Japan.

SHTREMEL, A. K. 1963. Stuttering in left parietal lobe syndrome. *Zhurnal Nevropatologii i Psikhiatrii imeni S. S. Korsakova* 63: 828–32.

SIEGERT, E., K. H. DAUTE, E. KLUST, E. KUNZE AND G. MULLER. 1974. EEG, brain injury and stuttering. *Proceedings International Congress of Logpedics and Phoniatrics*, Interlaken.

SLORACH, N. AND B. NOEHR. 1973. Dichotic listening in stuttering and dyslalic children. *Cortex* 9: 295–300.

SMITH, A. AND C. W. BURKLAND. 1966. Dominant hemispherectomy: preliminary report on neuropsychological sequellae. *Science* 153: 1280–82.

SNYDER, M. A. 1958. Stuttering and coordination. *Logos* 1: 36–44.

SOMMERS, R. K., W. A. BRADY, AND W. R. MOORE. 1975. Dichotic ear preference of stuttering children and adults. *Perceptual and Motor Skills* 41: 931–38.

SOVAK, M. 1935. Das vegetative nervensystem bei stottern. *Monatschrift für Ohrenheilkunde* 69: 666–80.

SPADINO, E. J. 1941. *Writing and Laterality Characteristics of Stuttering Children*. New York: Teachers College, Columbia University Press.

SSIKORSKI, J. A. 1891. *Uber das Stottern*. Berlin: Hirschwald.

STIER, E. 1911. *Untersuchen über linkshändigkeit und die funktionellen differenzen der hirnhälften*. Jena: Fischer.

STREIFLER, M. AND F. GUMPERTZ. 1955. Cerebral potentials in stuttering and cluttering. *Confinia Neurologica* 15: 344–59.

STROMSTA, C. 1966. Role of bone conducted sidetone in stuttering. Terminal Progress Report, Grant NB 03541-02-03, U.S. Public Health Service.

———. 1964. EEG power spectra of stutterers and nonstutterers. *ASHA* 6: 418–419 (abstract).

STROTHER, C. R. AND L. S. KRIEGMAN. 1943. Diadochokinesis in stutterers and nonstutterers. *Journal of Speech Disorders* 8: 325–35.

———. 1944. Rhythmokinesis in stutterers and nonstutterers. *Journal of Speech Disorders* 9: 239–44.

STUTTE, H. 1960. Quellenmaterial zur kinderpsychiatrischen prävention. *Annals Crianca Portuguesa* 19: 415–33.

SUBIRANA, A. 1964. The relationship between handedness and language function. *International Journal of Neurology* 4: 215–34.

———, J. COROMINAS, R. PUNCERNAU, L. OLLER-DAURELLA, AND J. MONTEYS. 1952. Nueva contribucion al estudio de la dominancia cerebral. *Medicamenta* 10: 255–58.

SUSSMAN, H. M. AND P. F. MACNEILAGE. 1975. Hemispheric specialization for speech production and specialization in stutterers. *Neuropsychology*. 13: 19–26.

SUTU, A., D. MIRONESCU, R. COCINSCHI, O. TIRZIU, AND M. MISCOIA. 1964. Contributii clinice si electroencefalografice la studine patogenzei biblielii. *Pediatrica* 8: 39–40.

SWIFT, W. J., E. W. SWIFT, AND M. ARELLANO. 1975. Haloperidol as a treatment for adult stuttering. *Comprehensive Psychiatry* 16: 61–67.

SWIFT, W. B. 1932. Why visualization is the best method for stuttering. *Proceedings of the American Speech Correction Association* 2: 89–91.

SZONDI, L. 1932. Konstitutionanalyse von 100 stotterern. *Wien Medizinische Monatschrift* 82: 922–28.

TOMATIS, A. 1963. *L'Oreille et le language.* Paris: Éditions du Seuil.

———. 1954. Recherches sur la pathologie du bégaiement. *Journal Française ORL* 3: 384–90.

TRAVIS, L. E. 1928. A comparative study of the performances of stutterers and normal speakers in mirror tracing. *Psychological Monographs* 39: 45–51.

———. 1937. Brain potentials and the temporal course of consciousness. *Journal of Experimental Psychology* 21: 302–7.

———. 1934. Dissociation of the homologous muscle function in stuttering. *Archives of Neurology and Psychiatry* 31: 127–33.

———. 1927. Disintegration of breathing movements during stuttering. *Archives of Neurology and Psychiatry* 18: 673–90.

———. 1931. *Speech Pathology.* Englewood Cliffs, N.J.: Prentice-Hall.

——— AND R. Y. HERREN. 1929. Studies in stuttering: V. A study of simultaneous antitropic movement of the hands of stutterers. *Archives of Neurology and Psychiatry* 22: 487–94.

TRAVIS, L. E. AND J. R. KNOTT. 1936. Brain potentials from normal speakers and stutterers. *Journal of Psychology* 2: 137–50.

TRAVIS, L. E. AND D. B. LINDSLEY. 1933. An action current study of handedness in relation to stuttering. *Journal of Experimental Psychology* 16: 359–81.

TRAVIS, L. E. AND W. MALAMUD. 1937. Brain potentials from normal subjects, stutterers, and schizophrenic patients. *American Journal of Psychiatry* 93: 929–36.

TROMNER, E. 1929. *Das stottern, die sprachzwangneurose: II. Versammlung der deutschen gesellschaft für sprach-und stimmheilkunde.* Leipsig: Kabitzsch.

TSUNODA, T. AND H. MORIYAMA. 1972. Specific pattern of cerebral dominance for various sounds in adult stutterers. *Journal of Auditory Research* 12: 216–27.

TWITMEYER, E. B. 1930. Stammering in relation to hemato-respiratory factors. *Quarterly Journal of Speech* 16: 278–83.

VAN DANTZIG, B. 1939. Writing, typing, and speaking. *Journal of Speech Disorders* 4: 297–301.

VAN DUSEN, C. R. 1939. A laterality study of nonstutterers and stutterers. *Journal of Speech Disorders* 4: 261–65.

VAN RIPER, C. 1952. Report of stuttering on a musical instrument. *Journal of Speech and Hearing Disorders* 17: 433–34.

———. 1935. The quantitative measurement of laterality. *Journal of Experimental Psychology* 17: 327–32.

WADA, J. 1949. A new method for the determination of the side of cerebral dominance: a preliminary report on the intracarotid injection of sodium amytol in man. *Medical Biology* 14: 221–22.

——— AND T. RASMUSSEN. 1960. Intracarotid injection of sodium amytol for the lateralization of cerebral speech dominance. Experimental and clinical observations. *Journal of Neurosurgery* 17: 266–82.

WARREN, J. M. AND K. AKERT, (eds.) 1964. *The Frontal Cortex and Behavior.* New York: McGraw-Hill.

WEINSTEIN, E. A. 1964. Affections of speech with lesions of the nondominant hemisphere. In *Disorders of Communication,* eds. D. M. Rioch and E. A. Weinstein. Baltimore: Williams and Wilkins.

——— AND E. A. SERSEN. 1966. Tactual sensitivity as a function of handedness and laterality. *Journal of Comparative Physiology and Psychology* 54: 663–67.

WEISS, B. 1967. Neuromuscular excitability in stutterers. *Folia Phoniatrica* 19: 117–24.

WEISS, D. A. 1964. *Cluttering.* Englewood Cliffs, N.J.: Prentice-Hall.

———. 1950. Der zusammenhang zwischen poltern und stottern. *Polia Phoniatrica* 4: 252–62.

WEISSOVA, B. AND L. HANDZEL. 1962. Familial stuttering caused by parathyroid gland insufficiency. *Czechoslovakia Otolaryngologie* 11: 57–61.

WELLS, P. B. AND M. T. MALCOLM. 1971. Controlled trial of treatment of 36 stutterers. *British Journal of Psychiatry* 119: 603–4.

WEPMAN, J. M. 1939. Familial incidence in stammering. *Journal of Speech Disorders* 4: 199–204.

———. 1947. The organization of therapy for aphasia: I. The in-treatment center. *Journal of Speech Disorders* 12: 405–9.

WEST, R. 1958. An agnostic's speculations about stuttering. In *Stuttering: A Symposium,* ed. J. Eisenson. New York: Harper and Row.

———. 1943. The pathology of stuttering. *Nervous Child* 2: 96–106.

——— AND M. ANSBERRY. 1968. *The rehabilitation of speech.* New York: Harper.

WEST, R., S. NELSON, AND M. BERRY. 1939. The heredity of stuttering. *Quarterly Journal of Speech* 25: 23–30.

WEST, R. AND E. NUSBAUM. 1929. A motor test for dysphemia. *Quarterly Journal of Speech Education* 15: 469–79.

WESTPHAL, G. 1933.   An experimental study of certain motor abilities of stutterers. *Child Development* 4: 214–21.

WILLIAMS, D. E. 1955.   Masseter muscle action current potentials in stuttered and nonstuttered speech. *Journal of Speech and Hearing Disorders* 20: 242–61.

WINGATE, M. E. 1966.   Behavioral rigidity in stutterers. *Journal of Speech and Hearing Research* 19: 626–30.

WYKE, B. 1969.   Deux ex nachina vocis: an analysis of the laryngeal reflex mechanisms. *British Journal of Disorders of Communication* 4: 3–25.

————. 1970.   Neurological mechanisms in stammering: an hypothesis. *British Journal of Disorders of Communication* 5: 6–16.

————. 1974.   Phonatory reflex mechanisms and stammering. *Folia Phoniatrica* 26: 321–38.

YASTREBOVA, A. V. 1962.   *Peculiarities in the oral and written speech of stuttering pupils.* Moscow: Institute of Defectology.

ZALESKI, T. 1965.   Rhythmic skills in stuttering children. *De Therapia Vocis et Loquellae* 1: 371–72.

ZANGWILL, O. 1960.   Speech. In *Handbook of Physiology*, vol. 3, ed. J. Field. Washington, D.C.: American Physiological Society.

ZIMMERMAN, G. N. AND J. R. KNOTT. 1974.   Slow potentials of the brain related to speech processing in normal speakers and stutterers. *EEG Clinical Neurophysiology* 37: 599–609.

STUTTERING AS THE RESULT OF DISTURBED FEEDBACK

15

In this chapter we present the view that stutterers possess a defective monitoring system for speech. The basic theory is that ongoing sequential speech movements are controlled by a cybernetic system which depends upon feedback sensory information for the maintenance of error-free performance. When error occurs as detected by the matching of performance against a standard model, then the system automatically corrects for the defective output by searching for the appropriate output until it is achieved (Fairbanks, 1957). Stuttering behaviors are viewed as reflecting this corrective process, or as being due to the lack of a stable standard pattern of speech movements for the syllable or word, or to a perceptual disability on the input side in the processing of sensory information. Essentially, those who hold this point of view maintain that the automatic sequencing of motor speech operates as a closed loop system in which feedback, primarily auditory feedback, plays a very important role.*

Unfortunately, our current knowledge of how speech is programmed and controlled is far from satisfactory. The influence of Wiener's (1948) cybernetic theory has led to a number of hypothetical models, such as those by Fairbanks (1954) and Mysak (1966), which describe closed feedback loops as the essential monitoring system for speech. In Fairbanks's well-known model** we have an effector unit, a sensor unit, a storage unit, a comparator to match input information against the patterns contained

* Not all workers believe this to be true. Peterson and Shoup (1966) and others feel that an open loop explanation for speech production is more satisfactory.

** The Fairbanks model has been criticized as not taking into account the transmission times for the inflow of sensory information and the outgo of motor impulses. However, if the syllable or some feature thereof is the unit used in monitoring, this objection does not seem to be valid. The average duration of a syllable is about 130 milliseconds and the shortest time between the onset of a tone and its arrival in the cortex is about 10 milliseconds (Stromsta, 1959, p. 298).

in the storage component, and a mixer or controller regulating mechanism which alters the output so as to reduce future error signals. In trying to alter the output, the system may be thrown into oscillation or fixation if too much overload or too much distortion is present in the feedback.

Some controversy exists as to whether or not an on-going motor performance such as speech is monitored continuously or intermittently. The latter seems more tenable although possible neurological mechanisms for continuous monitoring, despite Lashley's (1951) objections, do apparently exist. In any event, motor speech seems to operate like an automatic or semiautomatic servosystem under ordinary conditions. However, since the timing of the simultaneous and successive bilateral musculatures involved in respiration, phonation, and articulation demand an almost incredible precision to produce integrated speech, it is not difficult to understand why distortions or overloads in the feedback signals could cause breakdowns.

Information about the speech output is returned to the central integrating mechanism through six auditory channels, via the right and left feedback routes from (1) airborne side-tone, (2) bone-conducted side-tone, and (3) tissue connected side-tone. Other feedback signals come from the kinesthetic-tactile-proprioceptive sensors on both sides of the body. Stromsta (1962) showed that the auditory feedback signals in these different channels arrive at markedly different times and that the temporal information-processing of speech output by the brain is very complex. Some central mechanisms for integrating all these feedback signals must be present, although their nature is not yet known.

From this cursory sketch, it should be evident that at least there are many possible sources of distortion in the feedback systems used to monitor speech. Asynchrony of feedback signals that arrive in the right and left cortical hemispheres may be involved; differential delays in bone-, tissue-, and air-conduction of a person's voice might create the distortion in auditory feedback which results in stuttering. These may have an organic basis and yet produce disruption only under stress as reflected in cybernetic noise. Transcerebral transit times, as Tomatis (1963) claims, may create a privately owned delayed auditory feedback system within the skull. Auditory feedback may interfere with proprioceptive feedback. All we are saying is that there is ample opportunity built into the system that we use in monitoring our speech for the kinds of signal distortion, interference, or overload which could lead to stuttering. In the succeeding sections of this chapter we will attempt to summarize what little basic information there is about how speech can be disrupted by altering its feedback, and we will try to show how these effects might have some pertinence to stuttering.

DELAYED AUDITORY FEEDBACK (DAF)

When delays are inserted into the return flow of information from the sensory end organs during the performance of serial activities of many kinds, those motor performances tend to be disrupted. Smith (1962) showed that manual tracking of a moving visual target was greatly impaired when a visual delay was introduced. Also an auditory delay in the sound of key tapping disrupts that activity (Chase and others 1961; Tsunoda and Moriyama 1972). Most dramatic, however, is the effect which occurs when auditory delays are introduced when a person is speaking. Normal speakers tend to show stutteringlike behaviors, and surprisingly, many stutterers become more fluent under DAF. Although the phenomenon had long been known, Lee (1951) and Black (1951) were the first to report that when a normal speaker's verbal output was fed back to his ears after a short delay of about one fifth of a second, marked breaks in fluency occurred. Lee called this effect the "artificial stutter." Individuals differ in their vulnerability to this delayed auditory feedback (DAF). Some subjects are relatively unaffected by DAF, while others show marked speech interference. Those who do experience disruption under DAF respond in different ways: sounds and syllables are repeated or prolonged; blocks in phonation are observed; changes in rate, pitch, and vocal intensity occur. Yates (1963b) explains these individual differences in this way:

> . . . whether or not an individual is highly susceptible to DAF . . . depends upon the degree to which he utilizes auditory feedback in monitoring his speech. Individuals who are highly dependent on auditory feedback will be subject to severe breakdown under DAF, while individuals who rely mainly upon bone-conducted or kinesthetic feedback will show less breakdown.

This reasoning has also been accepted by Cohen and Edwards (1965) and other authors.

DAF EFFECTS IN NORMAL SPEAKERS

Although the literature on DAF has become so voluminous as almost to defy review here, some of major findings for normal speakers under this condition can be summarized. DAF produces repetitions of syllables and prolongations of sounds (Black 1951; Lee 1951). Spectrographic analysis of speech under DAF shows a greater prolongation of the vowels (Rawnsley and Harris 1954) and of glides and continuant sounds (Coblenz and Agnello 1965). Delayed auditory feedback slows oral reading and speaking rate (Black 1951; Fairbanks 1955; Fairbanks and Guttman 1958).

These authors noted that the substitutions involved in the articulatory errors under DAF were unusual ones and occurred primarily on the stressed syllables. There were many omitted sounds, but the bulk of the errors were repetitive reduplications of sounds and syllables resembling stuttering. According to Beaumont and Foss (1957) there are marked individual differences in the way people react to DAF, and all authors have made similar observations. Some persons show pronounced emotional reactions as measured by the galvanic skin response and other methods, as Haywood (1963) has demonstrated. Others remain relatively unaffected. In some subjects, vocal intensity increases under DAF (Atkinson 1953; Spilka 1954). The fundamental pitch of the voice tends to rise (Fairbanks

1955). These effects may be due to the subject's attempt to cope with the disruption. Pitch variability decreases and the vibrato becomes uneven (Deutsch and Clarkson 1959). As a result of these disturbances the intelligibility of speech under delayed feedback becomes somewhat impaired (Atkinson 1953).

Subjects generally show little adaptation to DAF in repeated readings or at different intervals of delay (Atkinson 1953; Tiffany and Hanley 1956). However, when very prolonged exposure to DAF is administered, some temporary adaptation does seem to take place according to Winchester, Gibbons, and Krebs (1959) and Hanley, Tiffany, and Brungard (1958). This decrease in speech disturbance may not be true adaptation however. It may merely mean that the speakers by using certain strategies learn to "beat the machine." They do this by using very slow speaking or sudden shifts of pitch or loudness or sudden speech attempts timed by finger movements or other means. Goldiamond, Atkinson, and Bilger (1962) showed that when subjects were instructed not to listen to the DAF they could read more words per minute than when they were asked to listen to it. In this way attention to proprioceptive feedback probably creates a buffer against the DAF stimuli.

In some few individuals, prolonged exposure to DAF produced residual effects for some hours, but for most subjects, the speech returns to normal fluency as soon as the delay is terminated. Black (1955) found a residual disruption effect lasting about three minutes after the delay was turned off, and Tiffany and Hanley (1956) report that the behavior of those individuals severely affected by delayed feedback seems to persist for a while after the delay is ended. A description of these lingering effects from DAF is illustrated by the following quotation from their article:

> This subject (a normal speaker) had experienced increasing difficulty with the side-tone readings, particularly on one word—pony. Following the delayed side-tone readings, he continued to experience great difficulty with this word even though no side-tone delay was present. He exhibited stuttering-like symptoms as though the experimental readings had produced a kind of specific anxiety for this word. He not only appeared to be more nonfluent than before the side-tone experience but also appeared to show tension and avoidance behavior.

We too have found a few normal adult speakers who showed similar responses, but the effect seems to be more pronounced with certain young children. We have been reluctant to use DAF with children ever since we discovered these long-term effects. Goldfarb and Braunstein (1958), who tested 25 normal speaking children aged 8 to 10 years under a delayed feedback time of .16 seconds (which would probably not produce maximal disruption), found that there was great speech impairment under the delay. Since children probably have less stable motor configurations for their words than adults, we can understand why DAF might create some havoc. Chase (1958), who found that his subjects could repeat the sound /b/ faster under DAF than when delay was not present, speaks about the facilitating effect of DAF upon syllabic repetitions and gives this personal testimony: "Experimenting with his own vocal responses under delay, the writer has observed that although he does not usually repeat words or speech sounds under delay, once he *voluntarily* repeats various speech elements, it is difficult to stop. Other observers have reported the same experience." This compulsive characteristic of the DAF speech disruptions is commonly experienced by many otherwise normal speakers. Some become quite emotional. A slight relationship between personality characteristics and vulnerability to DAF has been reported by Spilka (1954) and Goldfarb and Braunstein (1958).

Sex differences. In view of the sex-ratio in the incidence of stuttering, it is interesting to note that several studies have found females less susceptible than males to disruption under DAF (Bachrach 1964; Mahaffey and Stromsta 1965; Timmons 1971). The last author felt that females showed more adaptation to the delay. Most of the research has demonstrated that females require longer delay times than males to manifest the disturbance in speech. Buxton (1969), however, found no sex differences in vulnerability to DAF.

Age differences. There seem to be differences in reaction to DAF which are related to the age of the speaker. Younger children seem to be more vulnerable to disruption but longer delay times are needed to produce the maximum effect (Mackay 1968; Buxton 1969). Figure 16 shows MacKay's

DELAY IN FEEDBACK
(seconds)

Figure 16. Frequency of repetitions (stutters) per syllable as a function of feedback delay for the three groups of subjects of different ages. (From MacKay, 1968, by permission.)

data. Buxton found that for children aged 4 to 9 the critical delay was 60 milliseconds (.60 second); for subjects 10 to 26 years it was 20 milliseconds, and for the aged (60 to 81) it was 40 milliseconds. Timmons and Boudreau (1978) also showed that younger children are more affected by longer delay times than by shorter ones. Siegel and others (1980) also found that younger children were more vulnerable to DAF than older individuals but their data did not confirm earlier findings that longer delay times with younger persons to produce DAF disruption were necessary.

CRITICAL DELAY TIMES
AND FEEDBACK INTENSITY

Individuals differ somewhat in terms of the delay interval required to produce the DAF effect, but the critical delay for most young male adults seems to range from 0.16 to 0.22 second with females showing a longer critical delay time. The best delay time for producing disruption and the intensity of the delayed signal are related, but the most pronounced effects are found when the delayed feedback is at least loud enough to mask the fundamental frequency of the bone-conducted side-tone—50 dB or more above threshold (Butler and Galloway 1957). Brubaker (1952) also showed that the sound pressure level of the DAF signal must be greater than that of the subject's own speech before disruption occurs. Since, as Butler and Galloway (1957) demonstrated, DAF has more disruptive effects at the higher levels of intensity, most investigators have used sound levels of 80 decibels or more for the delay. Binaural DAF produces more disturbance than monaural. Arends and Popplestone (1959) found that normal speakers with high verbal facility (as measured by verbal IQ on the Wechsler— a dubious criterion)—were able to resist the DAF better than those with low verbal IQs. Buxton (1969) reported that the faster a speaker's maximum rate of speech, the shorter the delay time that produces the most disruption. Also, rapid speakers in general were less affected by DAF at all delay intervals from .10 to .60 seconds. In this connection, MacKay (1968) also says, "The slower the subject's maximum rate, the higher his frequency of stuttering under DAF." By accelerating the feedback electronically so that one's speech is heard even more swiftly than normally, speech rate is improved and so is the fluency according to Peters (1954) and Davidson (1959).

SIMILARITIES OF DAF DISRUPTIONS
TO STUTTERING BEHAVIORS

The basic behaviors of stuttering, repetition of syllables and prolongations of sounds, have been found consistently in some normal speakers under delayed auditory feedback. It is also interesting that the spectrograms of repeated syllables of normal speakers under DAF show the same coarticulation defects found in stutterers (Rawnsley and Harris, 1954). If one can assume that the basic disturbance in normal speakers under DAF is temporal disruption in the programming of the motor sequences; that is, that the time order of events is disturbed, then as Black (1951) and others have suggested, the increase in intensity or pitch or the slowdown in rate may be considered to be secondary reactions to this core experience. Such reactions are commonly found also in young stutterers once they begin to react to their stuttering.

Some authors feel that DAF nonfluencies are not stuttering. Neelley (1961) compared the performances of a group of twenty-three stutterers with a similar group of normal speakers under a DAF time of 0.14 seconds delay at a level of 75 dB above threshold and again under normal nondelay conditions. He concluded that the DAF speech disruptions of normal speakers as judged by listeners were dissimilar from those of stutterers when stuttering.

The Neelley study has been widely accepted as evidence that DAF speech disruptions are completely different from those shown by stutterers and this is unfortunate. Yates (1963b) has pointed out two extremely important weaknesses in the study "which make Neelley's conclusions quite unacceptable." First of all, Neelley used only one delay time (.14) and one intensity level, and this delay time is not the one that usually produces breakdown of speech in normal adult speakers, but instead it is a delay time that often improves the speech of stutterers. Secondly, Neelley asked his listener judges to distinguish between samples of speech, some from stutterers *speaking under no delay* and some from normal speakers under DAF. His judges of course were able to tell that the samples were different and so Neelley concluded that DAF disruptions bore no resemblance to stuttering ones. Yates's (1963b) remarks in this connection seem quite pertinent:

> But these empirical findings are totally irrelevant to the issue whether speech behaviour under DÁF is determined by the same factors which maintain stammering behaviour. The two groups are in no way meaningfully comparable in these respects. The stammerers in the experiment had presumably spent many years adapting to, and working out ways of dealing with, their perceptual defect (assuming it to exist). The Ss with normal speech were being, on the contrary, subjected to DÁF for the first time. Hence, it is in no way surprising that the speech of Ss subjected to DÁF for the first time is different from that of long-standing stammerers. The problem concerning underlying mechanisms of stammering cannot in fact be resolved by the kind of experiment reported by Neelley. The problem can be solved only by a direct attack on the auditory monitoring skills of stammerers (1963b, p. 116).

Perhaps the most revealing research concerning whether or not the disruptions produced in normal speakers are similar to the stuttering was performed by Venkatagiri (1980b). He analyzed the different kinds of disfluency produced by nonstutterers under DAF and concluded that they were very similar to stuttering behaviors. Part word repetitions and prolongations were the types found most often; whole word and phrase repetitions were infrequent. He also showed that the loci, adaptation, and consistency effects were similar but as we have seen earlier these characteristics have been found in the disfluencies of normal speakers.

One study that might be interpreted as revealing a difference was done by Dorman, Freeman, and Borden (1976) who procured emg's of the laryngeal musculatures during DAF disruption in normal speakers. While they found evidence of the prolongations and tremors characteristic of stutterers they did not show the difficulty in initiating voice that some stutterers do. However, this difference might be explained in terms of the development of struggle reactions to disruption in stutterers; normal speakers presumably have not had this experience.

DO STUTTERERS BECOME
MORE FLUENT UNDER DAF?

Many stutterers become much more fluent under DAF. This surprising fact has been attested by many researchers and we will list only a few of them.

Let us review some of the major findings. Bohr (1963) in South Africa found that stutterers were more fluent under DAF; Zerneri (1966) found two groups among 102 stutterers, one of which (the primarily clonic ones) improved under DAF. Lotzmann (1961), in a German article, found that by varying the delay times until an optimal delay was reached, blockings of all kinds were reduced or completely eliminated. He mentions that the most favorable times for fluency were shorter than those normally used to produce the DAF effect, varying around a delay time of .05 seconds. Lotzmann showed that for 62 stutterers DAF reduced the frequency of stuttering at least by one-third, and that a delay of .05 seconds seemed to produce the greatest fluency. Nessel (1958) found that stutterers, unlike normal speakers, were generally unaffected by DAF in oral reading or were able to read faster and with fewer errors. Soderberg (1969) reports that his stutterers, especially the severe ones, showed a significant reduction in the frequency and duration of stuttering under DAF in both oral reading and spontaneous speech. Chase, Sutton, First, and Rubin (1961) also reported a marked improvement under DAF in one-third of their stutterers.

Later studies also show that some stutterers react to DAF by decreases in stuttering. Among them are those by Webster, Schumacher, and Lubker (1970), Hutchinson and Burke (1973), Burke (1975), Novak (1978), and Lechner (1979). When we remember that DAF usually increases disfluency in normal speakers, this decrease in stutterers seems even more significant.

Nevertheless, not all stutterers show this amelioration. Macioszek (1973) in West Germany found that the severity of stuttering was an important factor; the more severe the stutterer, the more he tended to be fluent under DAF. This has been shown by other workers too (Naylor 1953; Burke 1975). The milder stutterers, like normal speakers, tend to have more disruptions under DAF than do the severe ones.

It is of some interest that the amount of delay seems to play a part in lessening the frequency and severity of stuttering in those stutterers who do improve. Shorter delay times tend to make the stutterers more fluent (Webster, Schumacher, and Lubker 1970; Burke 1975; Timmons and Boudreau 1978). Preus (1981) found significant differences in the effects of different delay times on the amount of stuttering, a short delay (50 milliseconds) reduced stuttering markedly while a delay of 200 milliseconds increased it. His stutterers may have been the more severe ones. Novak (1978) found that 55 milliseconds delay was best for extended use. There seem to be many individual differences in the specific delay times which produce improvement in fluency. Those who have used DAF clinically have reported that it was necessary to determine these critical delay times for each individual stutterer.

Although most of the research has been done using oral reading, the DAF effect in improving fluency has also been demonstrated in such spontaneous speech as describing pictures or narrating. Burke (1975) found that spontaneous speech under DAF resulted in more fluency than when his subjects read orally but others have shown no differences. Adamczyk and Smolka in Poland (1976), using different delay times with thirty stutterers, found that very short delays (less than 0.10 seconds) produced a decrease in the severity of stuttering when it did occur but delay times longer than 0.20 seconds produced a slight increase in severity.

Although most of the researches demonstrating a decrease under DAF have used counts of molar moments of stuttering, we have some indication that certain types of stuttering behaviors decrease more than others. Hayden, Scott, and Addicott (1977), using only one delay time, found that the number of complete blockings decreased under DAF even though prolongations (mainly of the vowel) increased while the number of repetitions stayed about the same. Cohen and Edwards (1965), using a randomized application of DAF over a period of weeks found that their stutterers showed a decline in severity which was marked by an increase in repetitions and easy prolongations at the same time that their severe blockings and secondary reactions decreased.

Why DAF disrupts the speech of normal speakers and facilitates fluency in stutterers is a question that remains unanswered at the present time. All we have are hypotheses and speculations because the neurological mechanisms for organizing and executing the motor patterns of speech are not well known. Nor do we know exactly how auditory stimuli are processed or what part they play in the control of motor speech. We were born too soon.

Stromsta's explanation. One of the most interesting and comprehensive explanations of the DAF effect has been offered by Stromsta (1958). He holds that somewhere in the brain there must be some integrating mechanism which times the simultaneous and successive motor impulses so they are synchronized bilaterally. His research (Stromsta 1964) indicates that the temporal patterning of the bilateral alpha brain waves of stutterers differ from those of normal speakers. The alpha rhythms of stutterers require more precise timing of the incoming sensory and the outgoing motor impulses than do those of nonstutterers if those impulses are to be able to enter or exit the central control system at the appropriate instant. This is termed *gating* and stutterers are said to have narrower alpha excitability gates than do normal speakers, a difference which is thought to be constitutional.

The only way that the central integrating control system can know whether or not the appropriate motor impulses have been transmitted at the proper time is by examining the auditory or proprioceptive-tactile feedback and matching the output against the motor plans for syllables and words held in storage. If discrepancies appear, then the system shuts down and tries again and again until they are no longer evident. This blocking and hunting process constitutes the core feature of the stuttering or DAF disruptions.

Stromsta (1965) in a longitudinal study found that those children whose early repetitive stuttering or speech disruptions contained sudden blockages or arrests were still stuttering ten years later. Spectrograms of these repetitions lacked coarticulatory formants. Those children whose "stuttering" or speech disruptions did not show sudden arrests or the lack of transitional formants and maintained airflow throughout their repetions were speaking fluently and had overcome their disfluencies. This corroborated his belief that some basic difficulty in the central timing of the incoming or outgoing nervous impulses must exist. In still another study (Stromsta 1959) found that similar blockages of phonation could be produced in normal speakers by altering and distorting the auditory feedback. Moreover, he discovered that the speakers reacted to these stoppages by exhibiting many of the struggle reactions characteristic of severe stutterers.

In another study, Stromsta (1972) investigated various frequencies of bone-conducted side-tone to determine if there were differences between stutterers and nonstutterers in presumed arrival times in the two hemispheres. By adjustments of the phase and amplitude of the airborne signal while a tone was simultaneously driven through their upper teeth, Stromsta's subjects were able to cancel both tones until they were no longer heard. This procedure provides a measure of inter-ear phase disparity which in turn may reflect different arrival times in the two hemispheres for auditory information. At one of the frequencies tested (2000 Hz.), the stutterers showed interaural differences comparable to the feedback lags produced by DAF. The nonstutterers did not. Since the discrepancies between bone- and air-conducted feedback were smaller for normal speakers, the delay times would be too brief to cause disruption, whereas in the stutterers the discrepancies were large enough to produce the DAF effect and disrupt speech. Coupled with the information about the differences in alpha rhythms, we have here a possible explanation why some people stutter and why others do not. Loosely speaking, stutterers may have a built-in DAF apparatus in their heads.

Tomatis's theory. Another interesting explanation by Tomatis attributes stuttering to a perceptual disorder which also is produced by an auditory processing system with a built-in delayed auditory feedback. Briefly, Tomatis (1963) feels that stutterers monitor their speech with the ear opposite that which should be dominant, and that when this is true, the information (feedback) coming in from their vocal output must be shunted intracerebrally before it can be used. He feels that in stutterers there is a lag in transit time due to the stutterer using the wrong "directing" ear. This lag thus produces the same stuttering disruptions that are the result of delayed auditory feedback.

Tomatis (1963) stated that 90 per cent of his stutterers had a hearing loss in the ear which should have been their preferred or directing ear. He claimed that the dominant ear could be ascertained by masking one and then the other ear as the subject is talking. When the rate of speech slows down, it is the directing (dominant) ear that is being masked. To check this, he suggests delaying the feedback to the directing ear until speech slows down. The delay time then presumably equals the intercerebral transference time. Tomatis also claims that this dominant ear is usually on the same side as the dominant eye. Moreover he says that dominance can also be ascertained by masking each ear in turn and then observing changes in voice quality. Tomatis has also devised an "Electronic Ear" which he uses for the treatment of stuttering. Although he has not reported its construction, this device is evidently some sort of binaural hearing aid in which appropriate counter delays are built in. We have been unable to assess his research since its reporting leaves much to be desired.

Some oblique support for Tomatis's theory of stuttering is found in the research of Curry and Gregory (1967) mentioned earlier. Also, Asp (1965), using fifteen adult stutterers and their controls, found that the stutterers had significantly longer interaural localization times. He suggests that this time difference might be related to the same sort of fragmenting of speech produced by the delayed auditory feedback apparatus, and that perhaps Tomatis was correct. On the other hand Aimard, Plantier, and Wittlung (1966) challenged Tomatis's statement that the naturally dominant ear of stutterers was hypacusic. Only one of their fourteen stutterers showed such a unilateral loss. Also no lateral differences in central auditory perception on a dichotic phonetic integration test was demonstrated in this study. Stromsta (1966) somewhat supported the Tomatis method of discovering the presumably dominant ear. He, too, found that stutterers and normal speakers both showed significant differences in reading time when one ear was masked.

Why don't stutterers always stutter? If stutterers do possess a constitutional difference in the way they process auditory information, then why are they apparently fluent so much of the time? One answer is that they may only be perceptually fluent, that lying below the threshold of awareness are miniature timing lags and asynchronies insufficient to call attention to themselves or to produce obvious disruptions of speech (Zimmermann 1980). Another explanation has been proposed by Timmons and Boudreau (1972). They suggest that "under anxiety-producing conditions, when muscles tighten and the contour of the oral cavity changes," additional discrepancies and distortions of auditory feedback will occur, and these may be sufficient to trigger speech disruptions. Normal speakers have learned to tolerate and adapt to these discrepancies but stutterers have not.

THE UNANSWERED QUESTION

But why does DAF tend to disrupt fluency in normal speakers and facilitate it in stutterers? A possible answer is that the imposed delay creates the kind of situation in normal speakers which naturally occurs in stutterers. In contrast, when the DAF delay is added to the built-in delay of stutterers, the total delay may be too great to produce the usual disruption. Or perhaps stutterers have had more experience in coping with auditory delays than their normal speaking counterparts and so are more able to resist DAF. Perhaps they have learned not to listen to themselves because the experience is often so distressing. Some other explanations for improved fluency of stutterers under DAF have also been offered. Goldiamond (1965) felt that it occurred because the interference produced a novel way of talking, an explanation echoed later by Wingate (1970) who points to the marked changes in phonation which occur under DAF. Others have attributed the effect to the slower rate or the prolongation of the vowels which often accompany speaking under delayed auditory feedback, or to the increase in loudness which in some stutterers is very apparent.

Distraction, too, has been mentioned as the facilitating agent; for example, it is difficult to think much about the possibility of stuttering when being bombarded by echoes in one's speech. Zelniker (1971) showed that fewer disfluencies occurred in normal speakers under monaural DAF when they also listened to digits being fed into the other ear. Brandt and Wilde (1977), using a similar procedure, fed masking noise, metronome beats, and choral reading into one ear of stutterers while the other ear received DAF. All of these reduced disfluencies, perhaps because of distraction but most distractions lose effectiveness with prolonged use and the DAF effect does not show much adaptation. While all of these explanations may have some partial validity, we feel that it is also possible that the main reason many stutterers become more fluent under delayed auditory feedback is that they have learned to ignore the latter and try instead to monitor their speech through proprioception. We shall discuss this further in the last section of this chapter.

ALTERING FEEDBACK BY MASKING NOISE

If stuttering is caused by some essential difference in the manner by which speech is monitored auditorily, then we would expect that a loud masking noise would have some effect upon its frequency or severity. The research

generally shows that this is true. When stutterers can\
themselves speaking most of them become more fluent.

This effect has been known for a long time. Kern (\
beating of loud drums to produce the temporary deafening.\
using a 95 dB masking white noise, found that her stutter\
their stuttering by 83 per cent under this condition and tha\ ... of her
twenty-five subjects showed no stuttering at all. That the noise was not
just a distraction was suggested by the fact that the decrease did not occur
when the noise was not as loud (25 dB). Many other workers have
corroborated the reduction of stuttering under masking (Cherry and
Sayers 1956; Maraist and Hutton 1957; Bohr 1963; Conture 1974; Altrows
and Bryden 1977). There are only a few negative findings. One of them
by Hutchinson and Norris (1977) found no significant decrease in the
frequency of stuttering under masking noise when they spoke spontaneously although the same subjects did show a decrease during oral
reading. Others, however (Trotter and Lesch 1967; De War and Barnes
1976), have demonstrated that the masking effect is not confined to
reading. The normal disfluencies of nonstutterers also decrease under
masking (Silverman and Goodban 1972).

The decrease of stuttering under masking noise has been shown not
only for the molar moments of stuttering but also especially for sound and
syllable repetitions and for prolongations (Conture and Brayton 1975;
Altrows and Bryden 1977).

Certain changes in the manner of speaking occur under masking noise.
According to Lane and Tranel (1971) and Adams and Moore (1972), vocal
intensity increases (the Lombard effect). The stuttering subjects of Cherry
and Sayers (1956) and Parker and Christopherson (1963), however, were
able to speak *quietly* under loud noise and still showed reduced stuttering.
Vowel durations are also longer (Brayton and Conture 1978).

In stutterers, the fundamental frequency also tends to rise under
masking (Lechner 1979) but this pitch rise has long been known to occur
in normal speakers too (Atkinson 1952), probably as part of the Lombard
effect. Changes in the rate of speaking have also been noted but the
research is equivocal. Soderberg (1968) reported slower rates under
masking; Yairi (1976) found a faster rate under binaural masking but not
under monaural masking.

Continuous masking noise produces more decrease in stuttering than
does intermittent noise (Murray 1969; Burke 1969). Altrows and Bryden
(1977) using intermittent masking noise prior to, during, and after the
speech attempts found that only when it coincided with speech was the
masking noise effective. This finding conflicts with the report of Sutton
and Chase (1961).

In their early investigation, Cherry and Sayers (1956) used high- and
low-pass sound filters to see if there were differences perhaps due to the
elimination of feedback from bone conduction or the fundamental voice
frequency. They found that elimination of the low frequencies produced
more decrease in stuttering. Stromsta (1958) found less stuttering as the

se changed from 500 to 100Hz. However, May and Hackwood (1968) and Conture (1974) were unable to corroborate these findings.

Explanations for the masking effect. The first explanation attributes the improvement in the stutterer's fluency under masking noise to the by-passing of a disordered auditory processing system. By shutting off self-hearing, any defect or malfunctioning of this system could be prevented or partially prevented. Stromsta (1956, 1959, 1972), as we have seen earlier, suggested that the auditory processing systems of stutterers differ from those of normal speakers mainly because of discrepancies in the delays of bone-conducted and air-conducted sound, or interaural phase relationships. Tomatis (1963) claimed that stutterers monitor their speech with their nondominant ear and thereby create a lag in transit time between the two hemispheres sufficient to produce a disrupting effect resembling DAF. Finally, there are several authors who have attributed stuttering to malfunctioning of the middle-ear muscles. Since we have already discussed the views of Stromsta and Tomatis, let us now present the research concerning the third explanation.

Abnormal middle-ear reflexes. According to Metz (1946) and Salomon and Starr (1963), the stapedius muscle of the middle ear contracts just prior to phonation or concurrently with its onset to attenuate the hearing of one's own voice. It is viewed as a protective mechanism to prevent overloading. (Otherwise, a bullfrog might die of its own croak!) This stapedial reflex (sometimes termed the cochleo-recurrential reflex) can be classically conditioned (Djupeland 1964) and so stimuli associated with fear or stress can activate it, thus accounting for the intermittency of stuttering. Butler and Stanley (1966), Webster and Lubker (1968), Webster and Dorman (1970), and Webster (1974) have explained how stuttering might result from the malfunctioning of this middle-ear reflex, and they point to the masking-noise effect as supporting their auditory interference theory.

Masking noise, especially if intermittent, can activate and maintain the stapedial reflex (Kryter 1970). By doing so, it would prevent the unstable and varying changes in audition that a malfunctioning stapedius might otherwise set off, changes that could produce stuttering. Or so the speculation goes. Unfortunately perhaps, this explanation has had little support from the research. Shearer and Simmons (1965) found no differences in middle-ear impedance between stutterers and nonstutterers. Mangan (1977) found no differences in middle-ear muscle functioning between stutterers and normals. To our knowledge there is only one research that partly supports the hypothesis that stuttering may somehow be due to aberrant activity in the stapedial muscle. It was done by Horovitz and others (1978). The stutterers and controls did not differ in stapedial-reflex thresholds in a nonanxiety testing session but when anxiety was created, the stutterers showed threshold changes which the normals did not.

Our review has also shown that continuous masking is more effective in reducing stuttering than intermittent masking, and that when the noise is timed to occur just prior to vocalization the stuttering is not reduced. Both of these findings are contrary to the characteristics of the middle-ear reflex. This middle-ear auditory interference theory is ingeniously attractive but it certainly needs refinement and research support before it is at all acceptable.

Masking noise as an anxiety-reducer and as a distraction. In Shane's early study of masking noise (1955), she suggested that the marked decrease in stuttering under noise was due to the stutterer's being unable to hear his stutterings and therefore to a decrease in anxiety about them. Adams and Moore (1972) tested this assumption by getting palmar sweat measures while reading under a binaural 90 dB white noise. Their subjects showed no significant change in this measure of emotional arousal as the masking led to improved fluency.

Another explanation for the effect of masking is that the noise distracts the stutterer from the usual preoccupation with speech and stuttering. It diverts his attention from searching for cues indicative of approaching difficulty. If this were true, then we would expect that masking noise just prior to speech attempt would reduce stuttering more than if it were administered later but this has not been demonstrated. Also, intermittent masking should be more effective than continuous masking if the noise is merely a distractor. This, as we have seen, does not seem to be the case. Again, most distractors usually wear out with extended use since they lose their novelty and thereby their ability to command attention. Here the research is pretty clear. Trotter and Lesch (1967), Yairi (1976), and Altrows and Bryden (1977) have all shown that masking noise does not lose its effectiveness with prolonged use. One negative study by Garber and Martin (1974) has been reported. They found that the effectiveness of masking noise in reducing stuttering decreased when it was used over a longer period of time.

One final explanation for the masking effect was suggested by Wingate (1970), who speculated that the reduced stuttering was not due directly to any interference with auditory processing but instead indirectly to the different manner of talking which the masking seemed to produce, that is due to speaking more loudly or with a higher pitch or with longer vowel durations or at a slower rate.

Possibly related to the masking effect is the reported low incidence of stuttering among the deaf, a topic we have already discussed in an earlier chapter but some of which we might review briefly here. Backus (1938) found only six totally deaf stutterers in surveying 13,691 children in schools for the deaf. Albright and Malone (1942) in a similar study also failed to discover more than a handful of deaf stutterers in a large population of the hearing handicapped. We ourselves have one authenticated case of an adult male who had stuttered severely from infancy and who immediately stopped stuttering completely after an accident in which ompletely deafened. The cessation of stuttering occurred hours of the trauma and shortly after he began to speak.

c use of masking noise. Masking noise has also been used in stuttering therapy. In Russia, Derazne (1966) reported that as early as 1939 he had invented a portable masking device called the "D.C." (Derazne Correctophone) consisting of a low-pitched noise generator and earphones. At first this was carried in a knapsack, according to our information, but later miniaturized. Derazne writes:

> In looking over extended results in the treatment of stutterers, we confirmed the fact that it was possible for us to remove stuttering in the majority of our cases. In a small number of cases we noticed recurrences, but this happened as a result of repeated breakdowns of higher nervous function or of a repeated experience of fear, trauma, infectious disease, etc. Those stutterers who had suffered relapses were again treated with the D.C. but for a short period of time (2 or 3 weeks) and consequently resumed normal speech. Our methods did not give positive results in stuttering which was of an organic nature (1966, p. 616).

Parker and Christopherson (1963) designed a portable masker and reported that training in its use produced remarkable improvement in their three stuttering patients. Van Riper (1965) also designed a portable masker and reported a reduction in severity but less of a reduction in frequency in twenty-four of twenty-five stutterers when the masker was used intermittently. Difficulties in getting the stutterer to turn on the masker at the appropriate times were demonstrated. Murray (1969), in a careful study, found that masking noise reduced both the frequency and duration of stutterings, but his results showed clearly that continuous masking was more effective than random or intermittent masking when the noise was controlled either by the stutterer or experimenter. An article by Trotter and Lesch (1967) illustrates the effectiveness of the portable masker.

> Some speech pathologists have asked me if I thought the stutter-aid was another distraction device that would eventually become useless. I do not think so. In the two and one half years that I have worn the aid, I estimate that I have turned the aid on between 5000 to 6000 times. My stuttering blocks are shorter or absent as the result (1967, p. 272).

No reported carry-over was experienced. Perkins and Curlee (1969) had three stutterers compare portable masking units which presented either white noise or signal pulses (from 25 to 590 Hz). Both decreased stuttering, but the stutterers did not seem particularly enthusiastic about employing the devices. Little carry-over effect was observed.

De War and Barnes (1976) describe the use of the Edinburg masker, a device which uses a throat microphone to automatically trigger the masking noise. While the masker produced temporary decreases in stuttering, no transfer to general speech occurred even after twenty-two weeks of use. This lack of carry-over, along with the disinclination of stutterers to use the instruments, has been found by many of the clinicians who have attempted to use them in therapy.

COMPETING FEEDBACK CHANNELS

That stuttering usually has its onset during the years from two to four is not surprising when it is recalled that words are learned motor sequences and that they are first learned and habituated by acoustical matching of the child's output against a model presented by others. When the words are first learned, the auditory channel must be the one through which the essential information flows if the comparison of output with the interiorized model and the consequent reduction of error signals are to be accomplished. However, we need our ears for other important functions—for perceiving our own verbalized thoughts and the thoughts of others. It would be too burdensome if we always had to play our speech by ear—if we were eternally doomed to listen to each sound and syllable of each word to ensure its correctness. In our opinion, the human being, as he always does when overloaded, finds a shorter and easier way. In this case, he turns over the major responsibility for the monitoring of speech to another available information processing system—the kinesthetic-tactual-proprioceptive one—as soon as possible. This change we believe occurs as soon as the auditory system stops giving error signals; as soon as the motor sequences involved in word production seem to be able to be produced correctly without constant auditory scrutiny.

This possible turnover of control to proprioception cannot be viewed as a sudden flip-flop sort of process. The change probably takes place gradually and intermittently at first. For some time there may be some interference between the auditory and proprioceptive signals which could lead to broken words. Or there may be overload. As a child learns to communicate verbally, he must find it difficult to scan his listener visually, to make sure he keeps out phonemic mismatching, to reel off the appropriate motor sequences and to unfold the semantic content he intends. We should not be surprised then to find many children with a history of delayed speech beginning to stutter once they begin to talk—or, for that matter, to find most children being disfluent when they first begin to talk in sentences. Overloaded circuits oscillate and jam. Once the monitoring of the motoric sequencing of words can be turned over to proprioception, much of this overload is reduced. Auditory interference no longer has much impact. Some oblique evidence for these statements is found in the studies that show that young children are more vulnerable to DAF than are older ones (Mackay 1968; Siegel and others 1980).

In our opinion it seems tenable that normal speaking adults monitor their speech primarily by somesthesia (touch-kinesthesia-proprioception). We can speak fluently even when we are in the presence of loud masking noise. Adults who suddenly become deaf do not begin to stutter. Indeed, it takes a long time before they begin to show phonemic distortions in their speech and, even after these occur, the speech remains normally fluent. Normal speakers also remain fluent when distortion is introduced into the auditory signals by high-pass or low-pass filters. What is more illuminating in this regard is that delayed auditory feedback requires great amplification (enough to overcome any self-hearing) before it disrupts our speech. If the motoric sequencing of speech depended primarily upon auditory feedback, we would not expect these results. On the other hand, if the sequencing of speech is monitored primarily by somesthetic feedback, we can readily understand why they occur.

This switching from one sense modality to another in the control of sequential behaviors is not uncommon. We find much the same sort of thing occurring in handwriting where at first visual monitoring is mandatory as the child painstakingly traces his first words. As the motoric patterns become thoroughly learned, kinesthetic and proprioceptive controls take over. We eventually become able to write even in complete darkness though usually vision plays an accessory but subordinate role. Experiments with mirror tracing, where the visual feedback is reversed, show that kinesthesia can serve as a major control.

In speaking, as we have said, we need to use our eyes to scan our listener's reactions and our ears to discover what we are saying and what he may say in return. We do not think of all the words of a sentence first and then speak them later. Our messages unfold and we scan what we are saying in order to know whether or not we have expressed our intent. By turning over the major responsibility for the monitoring of our motor sequences to somasthesia, we doubtless facilitate the auditory scanning of the *meaning* of our messages. In this connection, Broadbent (1958) has offered a theory of perception which has much to offer here as we attempt to explain why some early stuttering tends to occur during the alleged shift from auditory to proprioceptive feedback control of spoken words. Broadbent views the nervous system as acting like a single communication channel of limited capacity. When the input to this channel overloads its capacity, some filtering process occurs so that only selected bits of information having features in common will be allowed to enter the system. If two or more messages with high information value are received through two different internal channels at the same time, the system may jam and the information will not be transmitted into the perceptual system in an orderly way. Although there must be some temporal parallelism in the bits of information being processed through proprioception and audition, it is probably inexact.

Most of the research (Travers 1964) seems to indicate that when information from more than one sense modality is provided simultaneously in the governing of a given activity, no advantage is gained and inhibitory interference tends to be the more probable result. We do not yet know where this selective filtering mechanism is located, but there are some indications that it resides in the reticular system (Hernandez-Péon, 1961). Moreover it appears that the blocking of one channel is rarely complete and that some information still gets through to the higher cortical center in attenuated form where again some central inhibitory mechanisms may selectively exclude certain kinds of sensory information (Hernandez-Péon, Scherrer, and Jouvet 1956).

If it is true, as Webster and Lubker (1968) and others hypothesize, that the disruption in timing which produces stuttering is due to distorted auditory feedback signals, then it would follow that masking should reduce stuttering. The need to disregard DAF signals (to beat the machine) would also stop the stutterer from continually listening to himself and thereby improve his fluency. He would be forced to do what all normal speakers probably do—control his speech primarily by proprioceptive-tactile feedback. By concentrating his attention on the feel of his speech musculatures, the stutterer can create barriers against any auditory interference or distortion which might be present.

From this point of view it is also possible to understand why stutterers seem to be able to speak more fluently while whispering and to be completely fluent when pantomiming speech. In the latter connection we found (in an unpublished study) that stutterers had no stuttering when giving commands by pantomime to skilled lip readers. Also the marked or complete reduction of stuttering produced by using an electrolarynx, a process which requires a high degree of conscious articulation in the pantomiming movements, seems to support this view (McKenzie 1955). Several reports are also available which indicate that laryngectomized stutterers who learn esophageal speech (where very careful articulation is mandatory and also probably some disregard of the acoustic features exists) do not show any stuttering when speaking in this way (Oldrey 1953; Irving and Webb 1961).

In any event, our previous review of the masking research has shown that a reduction in auditory feedback does produce a decrease in stuttering. But what happens when proprioceptive feedback is similarly prevented? Hutchinson and Ringel (1975) anesthetized the oral cavity through nerve block procedures that interrupted the *sensory* flow of impulses from this area. Under anesthesia, as opposed to a placebo injection or no injection, there was a marked increase in both the frequency and severity of stuttering, the major change occurring in prolongation behaviors. These two contrasting findings seem to indicate that stutterers may monitor their speech too much by self-hearing or self-listening and not enough by somosthesia. When forced by DAF or masking to rely on proprioception they become more fluent. Further support for this speculation is found in the increased fluency of stutterers under conditions of pantomimed or whispered speech or when using the electrolarynx.

We were born too soon to understand how the intermorphemic breaks in fluency we call stuttering are really produced, but it seems highly plausible that distortion in the total feedback signal system might possibly be responsible for them. The distortion may reside in the auditory signals alone and be introduced by bilateral phase differences between bone- and air-conducted side-tone, or in the interference produced by auditory and proprioceptive competition, or in overload, or in the central processing of the information. Any of these may disrupt the precise timing of antagonistic or bilateral sets of muscles and thereby produce stuttering. At the present time we just do not know what happens neurologically when broken words instead of integrated words are produced. Nevertheless, we feel very strongly that this area, which we are just beginning to explore, will teach us much about the essential nature of stuttering.

BIBLIOGRAPHY

ADAMCZYK, B. 1959. Use of instruments for the production of artificial feedback in the treatment of stuttering. *Folia Phoniatrica* 11: 216–18.

—— AND E. SMOLKA. 1976. Echo reverberation correlation by influence on stuttering. *Folia Phoniatrica* 28: 197.

ADAMS, M. R. AND J. HUTCHINSON. 1974. The effects of three levels of auditory masking on selected vocal characteristics and the frequency of disfluency of adult stutterers. *Journal of Speech and Hearing Research* 17: 682–688.

ADAMS, M. R. AND W. H. MOORE. 1972. The effects of auditory masking on the anxiety level, frequency of disfluency, and selected vocal characteristics of stutterers. *Journal of Speech and Hearing Research* 15: 572–78.

AIMARD, P., A. PLANTIER, AND M. WITTLUNG. 1966. Le Bégaiement: contribution de l'audition et de l'intégration phonétique," *Revue Laryngologie* 87: 254–56.

ALBRIGHT, M. A. AND J. Y. MALONE. 1942. The relation of hearing acuity to stammering. *Journal of Exceptional Children* 8: 186–90.

ALTROWS, I. AND M. P. BRYDEN. 1977. Temporal factors in the effects of masking noise on fluency of stutterers. *Journal of Communication Disorders* 11: 315–29.

ARENDS, C. J. AND J. A. POPPLESTONE. 1959. Verbal facility and delayed speech feedback. *Perceptual and Motor Skills* 9: 270.

ASP, C. W. 1965. An investigation of the localization of interaural stimulation by clicks and the reading times of stutterers and nonstutterers under monaural sidetone conditions, *De Therapia Vocis et Loquellae* 2: 353–55.

ATKINSON, C. J. 1953. Adaptation to delayed sidetone. *Journal of Speech and Hearing Disorders* 18: 386–91.

——. 1952. Vocal responses during controlled aural stimulation. *Journal of Speech and Hearing Disorders* 17: 419–26.

BACHRACH, D. L. 1964. Sex differences in reactions to delayed auditory feedback. *Perceptual Motor Skills* 19: 81–82.

BACKUS, O. 1938. Incidence of stuttering among the deaf. *Annals of Otology, Rhinology and Laryngology* 47: 632–35.

BARON, F. AND G. DELUMEAU. 1956. An etiology of stuttering. *Annals of Otology, Rhinology and Laryngology* 73: 962–64.

BARR, D. F. AND N. R. CARMEL. 1970. Stuttering inhibition with the high frequency narrow band masking noise. *Journal of Auditory Research* 10: 59–61.

BEAUMONT, J. AND B. FOSS. 1957. Individual differences in reacting to delayed auditory feedback. *British Journal of Psychology* 48: 85–89.

BLACK, J. W. 1951. The effect of delayed sidetone upon vocal rate and intensity. *Journal of Speech and Hearing Disorders* 16: 56–60.

——. 1955. Studies of delayed sidetone. *Contributi del Laboratorie di Psicologia, Nuova Sene.* Milano: Vita e Pensiero.

BOHR, J. W. F. 1963. The effects of electronic and other external control methods on stuttering: a review of some research techniques and suggestions for further research. *Journal of South African Logopedic Society* 10: 4–13.

BRANDT, D. E. AND C. G. WILDE. 1977. A technique for controlling speech disfluencies by delayed auditory feedback. *Journal of Fluency Disorders* 2: 149–56.

BRAYTON, E. R. AND E. G. CONTURE. 1978. Effects of noise and rhythmic stimulation on the speech of stutterers. *Journal of Speech and Hearing Research* 21: 285–94.

BROADBENT, D. E. 1962. Attention and the perception of speech. *Scientific American* 206: 143–51.

———. 1958. *Perception and Communication*. London: Pergamon Press.

BRUBAKER, R. 1952. An experimental investigation of speech disturbance as a function of the intensity of delayed auditory feedback. Doctoral dissertation, University of Illinois.

BURKE, B. D. 1969. Reduced auditory feedback and stuttering. *Behavior Research and Therapy* 7: 303–9.

———. 1975. Susceptibility to DAF and dependence on auditory or oral sensory feedback. *Journal of Communication Disorders* 8: 79–96.

———. 1975. Variables affecting initial reactions to delayed auditory feedback. *Journal of Communication Disorders* 8: 141–55.

BUTLER, R. A. AND F. T. GALLOWAY. 1957. Factoral analysis of the delayed speech feedback phenomenon. *Journal of the Acoustical Society of America* 29: 632–35.

BUTLER, R. R. AND P. E. STANLEY. 1966. The stuttering problem considered from an automatic control point of view. *Folia Phoniatrica* 18: 33–44.

BUXTON, L. F. 1969. An investigation of sex and age differences in speech behavior under delayed auditory feedback. Doctoral dissertation, Ohio State University.

CHASE, R. A. 1959. Comparison of the effects of delayed auditory feedback on speech and key tapping. *Science* 129: 903–4.

———. 1958. Effect of delayed auditory feedback on the repetition of speech sounds. *Journal of Speech and Hearing Disorders* 23: 583–90.

———. I. RAPIN, L. GILDEN, S. SUTTON, AND G. GUILFOYLE. 1961. Studies on sensory feedback II. Sensory feedback influences on key tapping motor tasks. *Quarterly Journal of Experimental Psychology* 13: 153–67.

CHASE, R. A., S. SUTTON, D. FIRST, AND J. RUBIN. 1961. A developmental study of changes in behavior under delayed auditory feedback. *Journal of Genetics and Psychology* 99: 101–12.

CHERRY, E. C. 1957. *On Human Communication*. New York: John Wiley and Sons.

——— AND B. M. SAYERS. 1956. Experiments upon the total inhibition of stammering by external control, and some clinical results. *Journal of Psychosomatic Research* 1: 233–46.

——— AND P. MARLAND. 1956. Some experiments on the total suppression of stammering; and a report on some clinical trials. *Bulletin of the British Psychological Society* 30: 43–44.

COBLENZ, H. AND J. G. AGNELLO. 1965. The effects of delayed auditory feedback on the manner of consonant production. Convention Address, ASHA.

COHEN, J. G. AND A. E. EDWARDS. 1965. The extraexperimental effects of random sidetones. *Proceedings of the Annual Convention of the American Psychological Association* 1: 211–12.

CONTURE, E. G. 1973.   The influence of noise on the stutterer's different disfluency types. Convention paper, ASHA, Detroit.

————. 1974.   Some effects of noise on the speaking behavior of stutterers. *Journal of Speech and Hearing Research* 17: 714–23.

CONTURE, E. G. AND E. R. BRAYTON. 1975.   The influence of noise on stutterers' different disfluency types. *Journal of Speech and Hearing Research* 18: 381–84.

CURLEE, R. F. AND W. H. PERKINS. 1973.   Effectiveness of a DAF conditioning program for adolescent and adult stutterers. *Behavior Research and Therapy* 2: 395–401.

CURRY, F. K. W. AND H. H. GREGORY. 1967.   A comparison of stutterers and nonstutterers on verbal and nonverbal dichotic listening tasks. Convention Address, ASHA.

DAVIDSON, G. O. 1959.   Sidetone delay and reading rate, articulation, and pitch. *Journal of Speech and Hearing Research* 2: 266–70.

DERAZNE, J. 1966.   Speech pathology in the U.S.S.R. In *Speech pathology*, eds. R. W. Rieber and R. S. Brubaker. Philadelphia: Lippincott.

DEUTCH, J. AND J. CLARKSON. 1959.   Musical feedback, *Scientific American* 200: 66.

DE WAR, A. AND H. E. BARNES. 1976.   Automatic triggering of automatic masking in stammering and cluttering. *British Journal of Disorders of Communication* 11: 19–26.

DJUPELAND, G. 1967.   *Contractions of the tympanic muscles in man.* Oslo: University of Oslo.

DORMAN, M. F., F. J. FREEMAN, AND G. J. BORDEN. 1976.   The effect of delayed auditory feedback on phonation: an electromyographic study. *Haskins Laboratories Status Report on Speech Research* pp. 45–56, 184–95.

FAIRBANKS, G. 1954.   Systematic research in experimental phonetics—I. A theory of the speech mechanism as a servomechanism. *Journal of Speech and Hearing Disorders* 19: 133–39.

————. 1955.   Selective vocal effects of delayed auditory feedback. *Journal of Speech and Hearing Disorders* 20: 142–53.

———— AND N. GUTTMAN. 1958.   Effects of delayed auditory feedback upon articulation. *Journal of Speech and Hearing Research* 1: 12–22.

FILLENBAUM, S. 1964.   Delayed auditory feedback with different delay times at each ear. *Journal of Speech and Hearing Research* 7: 369–71.

FRANKENBERGER, R. 1968.   Disruption of speech under delayed auditory feedback: a function of syllable duration and duration of delayed auditory feedback. Doctoral dissertation, Ohio University.

GARBER, S. AND R. E. MARTIN. 1974.   The effects of white noise on the frequency of stuttering. *Journal of Speech and Hearing Research* 17: 73–77.

————. 1977.   Effects of noise and increased vocal intensity on stuttering. *Journal of Speech and Hearing Research* 20: 233–40.

GARBER, S., G. SIEGEL, H. PICK, AND S. ALCORN. 1976.   The influence of selected masking noises on Lombard and sidetone amplification effects. *Journal of Speech and Hearing Research* 19: 525–75.

GIBNEY, N. J. 1973.   Delayed auditory feedback: changes in the volume intensity and the delay intervals as variables affecting the fluency of the stutterer's speech. *British Journal of Psychology* 69: 55–63.

GOLDFARB, W. AND P. BRAUNSTEIN. 1958.   Reactions to delayed auditory feedback in schizophrenic children. In *Psychopathology of Communication*, eds. P.H. Hock and J. Zubin. New York: Grune and Stratton.

GOLDIAMOND, I. 1965. Stuttering and fluency as manipulatable operant response classes. In *Research in Behavior Modification*, eds. L. Krasner and L. P. Ullman. New York: Holt.

———, C. J. ATKINSON, AND R. C. BILGER. 1962. Stabilization of behavior and prolonged exposure to delayed auditory feedback. *Science* 137: 437–38.

GROSS, C. M. 1964. A study of certain effects of local and topical anesthetics on the speech of stutterers. Masters thesis, Western Michigan University.

GROSS, M. S. AND S. N. NATHANSON. 1966. A study of the use of a DAF shaping procedure for adult stutterers. Convention Address, ASHA.

GRUBER, L. 1965. Sensory feedback and stuttering. *Journal of Speech and Hearing Disorders* 30: 373–80.

HAM, R. AND M. D. STEER. Certain effects of alterations in auditory feedback. *Folia Phoniatrica* 19: 53–62.

HANLEY, C. N., W. R. TIFFANY, AND J. M. BRUNGARD. 1958. Skin resistance changes accompanying the sidetone test for auditory malingering. *Journal of Speech and Hearing Research* 1: 286–93.

HARMS, M. AND J. MALONE. 1939. The relationship of hearing acuity to stammering. *Journal of Speech and Hearing Disorders* 4: 363–71.

HAYDEN, P. A. 1975. The effects of masking and pacing on stutterers' and nonstutterers' speech initiation times. Doctoral dissertation, Purdue University.

———, D. A. SCOTT, AND J. ADDICOTT. 1977. The effects of delayed auditory feedback on the overt behaviors of stutterers. *Journal of Fluency Disorders* 2: 235–46.

HAYWOOD, H. C. 1963. Differential effects of delayed auditory feedback on Palmar sweating, heart rate, and pulse pressure. *Journal of Speech and Hearing Research* 6: 181–86.

HERNANDEZ-PÉON, R. 1961. Reticular mechanisms of sensory control. In *Sensory Communication*, ed. W. A. Rosenblith. New York: Wiley.

———, H. SCHERRER, AND M. JOUVET. 1956. Modification of electric activity in cochlear nucleus during attention in unanesthetized cats. *Science* 123: 331–32.

HOROVITZ, L. J., S. B. JOHNSON, R. C. PEARLMAN, E. J. SHAFFER, AND D. HEDIN. 1978. Stapedial reflex and anxiety in fluent and disfluent speakers. *Journal of Speech and Hearing Research* 21: 762–67.

HUTCHINSON, J. M. AND K. W. BURKE. 1973. An investigation of the effects of temporal alterations in auditory feedback upon stutterers and clutterers. *Journal of Communication Disorders* 6: 193–205.

HUTCHINSON, J. M. AND G. M. NORRIS. 1977. The differential effect of three auditory stimuli on the frequency of stuttering behaviors. *Journal of Fluency Disorders* 2: 283–92.

HUTCHINSON, J. M. AND R. L. RINGEL. 1975. The effects of oral sensory deprivation on stuttering behavior. *Journal of Communication Disorders* 8: 249–58.

IRVING, R. W. AND M. W. WEBB. 1961. Teaching esophageal speech to a preoperative severe stutterer. *Annals of Otology, Rhinology and Laryngology* 40: 1069–80.

KARLOVICH, R. S. AND J. T. GRAHAM. 1966. Effects of pure tone synchronous and delayed auditory feedback on key tapping performance to a programmed visual stimulus. *Journal of Speech and Hearing Research* 9: 596–603.

KERN, S. 1931. Der einfluss des hörens auf das stottern. *Arch. Psychiat.* 97: 429–449.

KRYTER, K. D. 1970. *The effect of noise on man.* New York: Academic Press.

LANE, H. AND B. TRANEL. 1971. The Lombard sign and the role of hearing in speech. *Journal of Speech and Hearing Research* 14: 677–709.

LASHLEY, K. S. 1951. The problem of serial order in behavior. In *Cerebral Mechanisms in Behavior*, ed. L. A. Jeffress. New York: Wiley.

LECHNER, B. K. 1979. The effects of delayed auditory feedback and masking on the fundamental frequency of stutterers and nonstutterers. *Journal of Speech and Hearing Research* 22: 343–53.

LEE, B. S. 1951. Artificial stutter. *Journal of Speech and Hearing Disorders* 16: 53–55.

LOGUE, R. 1962. The effects of temporal alterations in auditory feedback upon the speech output of stutterers and nonstutterers. Masters thesis, Purdue University.

LOTZMANN, G. 1961. On the use of varied delay times in stammerers. *Folia Phoniatrica* 13: 276–310.

MACIOSZEK, G. 1973. On delayed auditory feedback in stuttering with various levels of stuttering severity. *Zeitschrift für Klinische Psychologie* 11: 278–99.

MACKAY, D. G. 1968. Metamorphosis of a critical interval: age-linked changes in the delay in auditory feedback that produces maximal disruption of speech. *Journal of the Acoustical Society of America* 19: 811–21.

————. 1967. To speak with an accent: effects of nasal distortion on stuttering under delayed auditory feedback. *Perceptual Psychophysics* 5: 183–88.

MACNEILAGE, P. F. 1970. Motor control of serial ordering of speech. *Psychological Review* 77: 182–96.

MAHAFFEY, R. B. AND C. STROMSTA. 1965. Effects of peak-clipped and center-clipped delayed sidetone. *ASHA* 7: 413–14.

————. 1965. The effects of auditory feedback as a function of frequency, intensity, time, and sex. *De Therapia Vocis et Loquellae* 2: 233–35.

MANGAN, J. E. 1977. Functional characteristics of the middle ear muscles of stutterers and nonstutterers. Doctoral dissertation, University of Iowa.

MARAIST, J. A. AND C. HUTTON. 1957. Effects of auditory masking upon the speech of stutterers. *Journal of Speech and Hearing Disorders* 22: 385–89.

MARTIN, H. 1963. Rehabilitation of the laryngectomee. *Cancer* July, p. 824.

MAY, A. E. AND A. HACKWOOD. 1968. Some effects of masking and eliminating low frequency feedback on the speech of stutterers. *Behaviour Research and Therapy* 6: 219–24.

MCCROSKEY, R. 1958. The relative contribution of auditory and tactile cues in certain aspects of speech. *Southern Speech Journal* 16: 86–90.

MCKENZIE, F. A. 1955. A stutterer's experience in using an electro-larynx. In *Stuttering in Children and Adults*, ed. W. Johnson. Minneapolis: Univ. of Minnesota Press.

METZ, O. 1946. The acoustic impedance measured in normal and pathological ears. *Acta Otolaryngology*, Supplement 63.

MURRAY, F. P. 1960. An investigation of variably induced white noise upon moments of stuttering. *Journal of Communication Disorders* 2: 109–14.

MYSAK, E. D. 1960. Servo theory and stuttering. *Journal of Speech and Hearing Disorders* 25: 188–95.

————. 1966. *Speech Pathology and Feedback Theory.* Springfield, Ill.: Thomas.

NAYLOR, R. V. 1953. A comparative study of methods of estimating the severity of stuttering. *Journal of Speech and Hearing Disorders* 18: 30–37.

NEELEY, J. N. 1961. A study of the speech behavior of stutterers and nonstutterers under normal and delayed auditory feedback. *Journal of Speech and Hearing Disorders, Monograph Supplement,* No. 7, 63–82.

NESSEL, E. 1958. Die verzögerte sprachrückkopplung (Lee Effect) bei Stottern, *Folia Phoniatrica* 10: 87–99.

NOVAK, A. 1978. The influence of delayed auditory feedback on stutterers, *Folia Phoniatrica* 30: 278–85.

OLDREY, M. 1953. *Speech Therapy: A Book of Readings,* ed. C. Van Riper. New York: Prentice-Hall.

PARKER, C. S. AND F. CHRISTOPHERSON. 1963. Electric aid in the treatment of stammer. *Medical Electronics and Biological Engineering* 1: 121–25.

PENFIELD, W. AND T. RASMUSSEN. 1949. Vocalization and arrest of speech. *Archives of Neurology and Psychiatry* 41: 21–27.

PERKINS, W. H. AND R. F. CURLEE. 1969. Clinical impressions of portable masking unit effects in stuttering. *Journal of Speech and Hearing Disorders* 34: 360–62.

PETERS, R. W. 1954. The effect of change in sidetone delay and level upon rate of oral reading of normal speakers. *Journal of Speech and Hearing Disorders* 19: 483–96.

PETERSON, G. E. AND J. E. SHOUP. 1966. A physiological theory of phonetics. *Journal of Speech and Hearing Research* 9: 5–67.

PREUS, A. 1981. *Attempts at identifying subgroups of stutterers.* Oslo: University of Oslo Press.

RAWNSLEY, A. F. AND J. D. HARRIS. 1954. Comparative analysis of normal speech and speech with delayed sidetone by means of sound spectrograms, Bureau of Medical Research. Project No. NM003-041.56.03.

SALOMON, G. AND A. STARR. 1963. Electromyography of middle ear muscles in man during motor activity. *Acta Otolaryngology* 39: 161–68.

SHANE, M. I. S. 1955. Effect on stuttering of alteration of auditory feedback. In *Stuttering in Children and Adults,* ed. W. Johnson. Minneapolis: Univ. of Minnesota Press.

SHEARER, W. M. AND F. B. SIMMONS. 1965. Middle ear activity during speech in normal speakers and stutterers. *Journal of Speech and Hearing Research* 8: 203–07.

SIEGEL, G. M., C. A. FEHST, S. R. GARBER, AND H. L. PICK. 1980. Delayed auditory feedback with children. *Journal of Speech and Hearing Research* 23: 802–13.

SIEGENTHALER, B. M. AND R. S. BRUBAKER. 1957. Suggested research in delayed auditory feedback. *Pennsylvania Speech Annual* 14: 24–31.

SILVERMAN, F. H. AND M. T. GOODBAN. 1972. The effect of auditory masking on the speech of normal speakers. *Journal of Speech and Hearing Research* 15: 543–46.

SMITH, K. U. 1962. *Delayed Sensory Feedback and Behavior.* Philadelphia: Sanders.

SODERBERG, G. A. 1969. Delayed auditory feedback and the speech of stutterers. *Journal of Speech and Hearing Disorders* 33: 20–29.

————. 1968. Delayed auditory feedback and stuttering. *Journal of Speech and Hearing Disorders* 33: 260–67.

SPILKA, B. 1954. Some vocal effects of different reading passages and time delays in speech feedback. *Journal of Speech and Hearing Disorders* 19: 33–47.

STARK, R. E. 1967. Effects of delayed auditory feedback upon a speech related task in stutterers. Convention Address, ASHA.

STEPHENS, S. G. 1975. Delayed auditory feedback: type of feedback as a variable affecting the fluency of stammerer's speech on a reading task. *Speech Perception* 21: 135–36.

STROMSTA, C. 1965. Averaged evoked responses of stutterers and nonstutterers as a function of interaural time relationships. Technical Report. National Institutes of Health, Project NB-03541-03.

———. 1962. Delays associated with certain sidetone pathways. *Journal of Acoustical Society of America* 34: 392–96.

———. 1964. EEG power spectra of stutterers and nonstutterers. *ASHA* 6: 418–19.

———. 1958. The effects of altering the fundamental frequency of masking on the speech performance of stutterers. Technical Report, National Institutes of Health, Project, B-1331.

———. 1972. Interaural phase disparity of stutterers and nonstutterers. *Journal of Speech and Hearing Research* 15: 771–80.

———. 1961. Interear phase disparity of bone-conducted sound energy in stutterers and nonstutterers. Technical Report, National Institutes of Health, Project B-1331-C2.

———. 1956. A methodology related to the determination of the phase angle of bone conducted speech sound energy of stutterers and nonstutterers. *Dissertation Abstracts* 16: 1738–39.

———. 1966. Role of bone-conducted sidetone in stuttering. Terminal Progress Report. Grant NB 03541-02-03 U.S. Public Health Service.

———. 1965. A spectrographic study of dysfluencies labeled as stuttering by parents. *De Therapia Vocis et Loquellae* 1: 317–20.

———. 1958. Stuttering: some evidence toward an organic etiology. Convention paper, *ASHA*, New York.

SUTTON, S. AND R. CHASE. 1961. White noise and stuttering. *Journal of Speech and Hearing Research* 4: 72.

TIFFANY, W. R. AND C. HANLEY. 1956. Adaptation to delayed sidetone. *Journal of Speech and Hearing Disorders*, 21: 164–72.

TIMMONS, B. A. 1971. Sex as a factor influencing sensitivity to delayed auditory feedback. *Perceptual and Motor Skills* 32: 824–26.

——— AND J. P. BOUDREAU. 1972. Auditory feedback as a major factor in stuttering. *Journal of Speech and Hearing Disorders* 37: 476–84.

———. 1978. Delayed auditory feedback and the speech of stuttering and nonstuttering children. *Perceptual and Motor Skills* 46: 551–555.

TOMATIS, A. 1963. *L'Oreille et le Langage.* Paris: Éditions du Seuil.

TRAVERS, R. M. W. 1964. *Research and Theory Related to Audio-visual Information Transmission.* Bureau of Educational Research, University of Utah.

TROTTER, W. D. AND M. M. LESCH. 1967. Personal experiences with a stutter-aid. *Journal of Speech and Hearing Disorders* 32: 270–72.

TSUNODA, T. AND H. MORIYAMA. 1972. Specific pattern of cerebral dominance for various sounds in adult stutterers. *Journal of Auditory Research* 12: 216–27.

VANNIER, J., R. SAUMONT, L. LABARRAQUE, AND R. HUSSON. 1954. Production experimentale des blocages synaptiques recurrentials par des stimulations auditives homorythmiques avec déphasages réglables. *Revue de Laryngologie,* Supplement I, Bordeau, February.

VAN RIPER, C. 1965. Clinical use of intermittent masking noise in stuttering therapy. *ASHA* 6: 381

VENKATAGIRI, H. S. 1980a. The core disruption under delayed auditory feedback: evidence from adaptation study. *Journal of Communication Disorders* 13: 365–72.

———. 1980b. The relevance of DAF-induced speech disruption to the understanding of stuttering. *Journal of Fluency Disorders* 5: 87–98.

WEBSTER, R. L. 1974. A behavioral analysis of stuttering: treatment and theory. In *Innovative Treatment Methods in Psychopathology,* eds. K. S. Calhoun, H. E. Adams, and K. E. Mitchell. New York: Wiley.

——— AND M. F. DORMAN. 1970. Decrease in stuttering frequency as a function of continuous and contingent forms of auditory masking. *Journal of Speech and Hearing Research* 13: 82–86.

——— AND R. B. LUBKER. 1968. Interrelationships among fluency producing variables in stuttered speech. *Journal of Speech and Hearing Research* 11: 754–66.

———. 1968. Masking of auditory feedback in stutterers' speech. *Journal of Speech and Hearing Research* 11: 219–23.

WEBSTER, R. L., S. J. SCHUMACHER, AND B. B. LUBKER. 1970. Changes in stuttering frequency as a function of various intervals of delayed auditory feedback. *Journal of Abnormal Psychology* 75: 45–49.

WIENER, N. 1948. *Cybernetics.* New York: Wiley.

———. 1960. *The Human Use of Human Beings.* Boston: Houghton-Mifflin.

WINCHESTER, R. A. AND E. W. GIBBONS. 1958. The effect of auditory masking upon oral reading rate. *Journal of Speech and Hearing Disorders* 23: 250–52.

———, E. W. GIBBONS, AND D. F. KREBS. 1959. Adaptation to sustained delayed sidetone. *Journal of Speech and Hearing Disorders* 24: 25–28.

WINGATE, M. E. 1970. Effect on stuttering of changes in audition. *Journal of Speech and Hearing Research* 13: 861–73.

YAIRI, E. 1976. Effects of binaural and monaural noise on stuttering. *Journal of Auditory Research* 16: 114–19.

YATES, A. J. 1963a. Delayed auditory feedback. *Psychological Bulletin* 60: 213–32.

———. 1963b. Recent empirical and theoretical approaches to the experimental manipulation of speech in normal speakers and stammerers. *Behavior Research and Therapy* 1: 95–119.

ZELNIKER, T. 1971. Perceptual attenuation of an irrelevant auditory verbal input as measured by an involuntary response in a selective attention task. *Journal of Experimental Psychology* 86: 52–56.

ZERNERI, L. 1966. Attempts to use delayed speech feedback in stuttering therapy. *Journal of Francais d' Oto-Rhino-Laryngologie et Chirurgie Maxilla-Faciale* 15: 415–18.

ZIMMERMANN, G. 1980. Articulatory dynamics of fluent utterances of stutterers and nonstutterers. *Journal of Speech and Hearing Research* 23: 95–107.

STUTTERING AS A DISORDER OF COORDINATION 16

Over a century ago Kussmaul (1877) called stuttering a spastic coordination neurosis, the symptoms of which reflected a breakdown in speech coordinations due to emotional stress. Since then many others have held the same view and recently we have seen a revived interest in this "discoordination hypothesis" as Perkins (1976) has termed it. The concept is attractive since even a cursory scrutiny of stuttering behaviors reveals a disruption in the motor patterning of speech. The basic questions to be answered however are these: Is the presumed discoordination found generally in all of the stutterer's motor activity or is it shown only in his speech? If the stutterer is poorly coordinated, why is he intermittently fluent so much of the time? Let us consider this last question first.

IS THE STUTTERER'S FLUENT SPEECH REALLY FLUENT?

Stutterers and their listeners would certainly answer the question affirmatively but we now have some evidence that they may not be correct. By turning away from the scrutiny of the characteristics of stuttered speech, investigators have now examined and analyzed the motor production of the stutterer's *nonstuttered* words and syllables and some interesting differences between the fluent utterances of stutterers and those of normal speakers have been discovered.

Articulatory lags and asynchronies. Zimmermann (1980), using high-speed cineradiography, studied the movements, positions, and timing of lip and jaw structures in the production of the isolated syllables /pap/, /mam/, and /bab/. Although these syllables were spoken by stutterers, only those

396

syllables that appeared to be spoken fluently were examined. Zimmermann discovered that, compared to the utterances of the same syllables by normal speakers, these "fluently" spoken syllables had marked differences. They showed longer durations of movement onset; the voice onsets were slower; and the stutterers took longer to attain peak velocity of the lip and jaw movements. Their transition times were longer and they held their postures longer. In addition, the stutterers manifested more asynchrony between lip and jaw movements than did the normal speakers. Though these hidden anomalies were not sufficient to produce any impression of stuttering in either the speaker or the listener, that is, the syllables seemed to be spoken fluently, they seemed to point to some basic difficulty in motor organization, timing, and control. If replicated and corroborated, this research is of the highest significance. If the perceptually fluent speech of stutterers is consistently underlain by such lags and asynchronies, one can see how tension, fear, or communicative stress might magnify them enough so that "overt" stuttering would emerge.*

Phonatory lags. Even before Zimmermann's research had appeared, there were other indications that the fluent speech of stutterers differed from that of nonstutterers. Agnello and Wingate (1971) found that stutterers were slower in terminating phonation in the production of perceptually fluent CV syllables. Other research revealed similar lags in the onset of the fluently uttered syllables of stutterers (Agnello, Wingate, and Wendell 1974; Agnello 1974). DiSimoni (1974) found that longer durations of consonants and vowels characterized the fluent speech of stutterers as compared with normal speakers. Hillman and Gilbert (1977), using ongoing speech instead of isolated syllables, corroborated these findings of time lags in the stutterers' fluent speech. They write:

> When VOT (voice onset time) values for stop consonants of similar place of articulation are compared between the stutterers and nonstutterers in the present study, it is clear that the lag in voicing is greater in the fluent speech of stutterers than nonstutterers. Breathing disturbances often exhibited by stutterers may account for the long VOT values observed in the fluent speech of stutterers. Such disturbances as shallow inhalations and shallow exhalations bring about reduced subglottal pressures and weak airflows which may be slow to start and may be of limited duration. The inability to generate adequate and steady subglottal pressures would also contribute to a delay in the onset of phonation and an increase in voice onset time. (1977, p. 611).

There are other studies which show that the voice onset times of stutterers are longer than those of nonstutterers. Metz, Conture, and Caruso (1979) and Hand and Luper (1980) also found such differences. One study by Cullinan and Springer (1980) did not find significantly slower voice onset times except with those stuttering children who also had articulatory and

---

* The implications for treatment are also apparent. Instead of trying to achieve a precarious zero level of stuttering, should we not seek to teach the stutterer how to cope with these lags and asychronies?

language problems. Taken as a whole, however, these researches seem to indicate that stutterers find it more difficult to coordinate the timing of phonation with lip and jaw opening. We must be cautious in our interpretation of these results. The differences are rather small—about 20 milliseconds and some stutterers do not show these lags. Nevertheless, we have here some evidence that stuttering may be the result of a basic coordination difficulty that is present even when they seem to be speaking fluently.

Duration of vowels. There is considerable evidence that the fluent speech of stutterers is characterized by longer durations of their vowels and longer transition times than compared with nonstutterers. This has been shown by Adams, Runyan, and Mallard (1975), DiSimoni (1974), Brayton and Conture (1978), Colcord and Adams (1979), Starkweather and Myers (1978), and Hand and Luper (1980). It is interesting that singing and DAF which promote fluency in the stutterer also tend to result in prolongations of the steady state of vowels. Vowel prolongation and slow transitions (the glide) have also been used therapeutically. Perhaps these prolongations give the stutterer more time to program into the vowel the necessary coarticulatory features. In any event, the fluent speech of stutterers seems to differ from that of normal speakers in this regard, too.

Reaction time studies. If these phonatory lags reflect a basic coordinative difficulty, then we should find stutterers slower to produce voice when a sudden signal is given. Certainly stutterers have often claimed to have difficulty "getting started" and we have previously discussed the many strategies and behaviors they use to begin an utterance. We have also seen that more stuttering occurs on the first words after a pause. Do stutterers differ from normal speakers in their vocal reaction times?

Most of the research has shown that stutterers are indeed slower in being able to produce voice or speech when a sudden signal is given, and, moreover, that this is not necessarily due to any overt stuttering that can be observed. Adams and Hayden (1976) required their subjects to say /a/ as soon as they heard a tone signal. The stutterers were significantly slower than their matched normal speaking controls. Hayden (1975) had previously shown that this also occurred when the same vowel initiated a phrase. Starkweather, Hirschman and Tannenbaum (1976), asked their subjects to produce a syllable as a response to a sudden flash of light, and demonstrated that the stutterers were again slower than nonstutterers in responding. Cross, Shadden, and Luper (1979) and Cross and Luper (1977) measured the response latency in producing isolated vowels to pure tone signals and their stutterers, too, were slower than the normal speaking controls. Prosek, Montgomery, Walden, and Schwartz (1979), using monosyllabic VC words and manual responses to visual and tonal signals, found that stutterers were slower than the normal speakers in the utterance of the words after a tone signal but that their manual reaction times did not differ. Reaction times to the visual signal did not differ either.

MacFarlane and Prins (1978), using neural response times, found that

Figure 17. Mean voice reaction times (VRT) for 5-year-old, 9-year-old, and adult stutterers and nonstutterers (sets combined). (From Cross and Luper, 1978, by permission.)

stutterers were slower in responding to auditory but not to visual signals in producing the syllables /pae/ and /bae/ and also in silently closing the lips. This sluggishness of stutterers in lip closure had also been discovered earlier by Stark and Pierce (1970). Kerr and Cooper (1976) showed that stutterers were slower in shifting from one phoneme to another, for example, from /a/ to /s/ and other voiced-voiceless combinations, than were nonstutterers.

In other words, in the fluent speech of stutterers there seem to be tiny delays in shifting from silence to speech or in shifting from one speech posture to another or even in terminating utterance once it has begun. Those delays do not appear in the fluent speech of nonstutterers. They may not last long enough to be perceived but they imply that a basic coordinative difficulty may underlie stuttering.

Airflow and air pressure differences in the stutterer's fluent speech. There is still another set of phenomena in the fluent speech of stutterers that seems to differ from the fluent speech of normal speakers. Agnello and Wingate (1971, 1972) discovered that the air pressure of stutterers within the mouth cavity was significantly higher than that shown by nonstutterers when single syllables were uttered *fluently*. This was later corroborated by Hutchinson (1975). The possible significance of this aberration is that blockage of airflow and phonation (two common characteristics of stuttering) can occur when supraglottal pressure exceeds the subglottal pressure.* As Adams (1974) remarked, "Had these (intraoral air) pressures been even larger, it is quite possible that the stutterer's airflow and phonation would have been impeded" (p. 41). The stutterers pronounced the syllables fluently and without any sign of overt stuttering but just a bit more oral cavity air pressure might have precipitated laryngeal blockages. That this might possibly be true was indicated by Agnello and Wingate (1972) and Hutchinson and Navarre (1977) who showed that, during *overt stuttering*, very high and sudden intraoral air pressures occur. If stutterers, as this research indicates, have somewhat elevated mouth cavity pressures in their "fluent" speech, and even greater pressures during overt stuttering, these can only be produced by momentarily constricting or partially blocking the airway with the tongue or lips or by increasing subglottal air pressure. Is this why many stutterers, when very relaxed, seem to stutter much less frequently or severely? In any event, these findings suggest that stutterers even when apparently fluent are not timing the respiratory musculatures in relation to the articulatory ones in the same way that normal speakers do.

Listener discrimination of stutterers' fluency from nonstutterers' fluency. Is it possible that the so-called fluent speech of stutterers might be distinguished from that of nonstutterers simply by listening to it carefully? Wendahl and Cole (1961) prepared taped segments in which the "actual" stutterings were removed by clipping and then paired them with similar segments from the speech of normal speakers. They found that judges could distinguish between them. However Young (1964) replicated the experiment and failed to corroborate the finding. According to Hotchkiss (1973) those of his listeners who could successfully discriminate the stutterer's fluency from the normal speaker's fluency did so by using syllable duration as the cue. The stutterers used longer ones. Love and Jeffress (1971) examined the fluent speech of both stutterers and nonstutterers and found that the former had a greater number of very short pauses (150 to 250 milliseconds). They say, "The stutterer's identification of his own fluent speech as stuttered may be due in part to brief pauses which he alone can detect" (p. 238). Even after adaptation trials which apparently eliminated all stuttering, "The stutterer continues to do something different from the normal even when he is not stuttering."

Another approach was used by Runyan and Adams (1978). They studied segments of "completely fluent" speech of "recovered" stutterers and then had a panel of judges try to distinguish them from matched segments of fluent speech from normal speakers. They found that their judges could indeed identify the fluent segments produced by the recovered stutterers from those of the normal speakers. But again there is one negative study to report. Few and Lingwall (1972) found their listeners

---

* Related to this is the finding of Adams, Runyan, and Mallard (1975) that stutterers, when speaking fluently, showed higher air-flow characteristics than normal speakers, as well as longer syllabic durations.

unable to distinguish between samples of fluency produced by stutterers from those of normal speakers.

Frequency of stuttering and rate of speaking. If stutterers have a motor coordination disability, then one would expect they would show less stuttering when speaking slowly. The research of Johnson and Rosen (1937) though it did not control for adaptation and other effects, demonstrated that stutterers had more trouble speaking at fast rates than at slower ones. Fransella and Beech (1965) found that their stutterers had less stuttering when reading slowly. Adams, Lewis, and Besozzi (1973) exposed single words at a rate of one per second and fifteen of their eighteen stutterers had less stuttering in this condition, a finding which might possibly have been due to the metronome effect.

Ingham, Martin, and Kuhl (1974) compared the stuttering frequencies of three stutterers when they spoke at rates 50 per cent greater and 50 per cent slower than their base-rates. One stutterer had more stuttering at the slow rate; another had less stuttering at the fast rate, so it is difficult to assess these results. Perkins, Bell, and Johnson (1979) had their stutterers achieve slower rates by deliberately prolonging their syllables. The frequency of stuttering declined dramatically in this condition though we cannot be sure that the effect was due solely to the slower "phone rate," or to the distracting novelty of this unusual way of speaking, or to the metronome effect. Another indication that slowing the rate of utterance promotes fluency is the use in some therapy programs of very slow speech to create a nucleus of nonstuttered speech which can then be reinforced. A representative report is that by Curlee and Perkins (1969). In general, those studies which showed less stuttering when the rate of utterance is slowed seem to support the view that stutterers may have a disability in coordination.

Complexity of the speech coordinations. Besides the speed of response, the complexity of response is also a factor in coordination. More simple coordinations such as those involved in lifting a finger are usually less demanding of coordinative ability than those which involve the manipulation of many structures simultaneously and successively. The movements required in speech production are very complex since respiration, phonation, and articulation must be integrated. One way of determining whether stutterers possess some kind of a coordinative disability is to see if they stutter less when one or more of these components is omitted.

Perkins, Rudas, Johnson, and Bell (1976) instructed their stutterers to read using only lipped (pantomimed speech), whispered speech, and vocalized speech. The pantomimed speech showed very little stuttering, whispered speech a bit more, and vocalized speech the most stutterings. Commodore and Cooper (1978) found only a few stutterings in pantomimed speech. The more complex the coordinations involved, the more likely it was that stuttering would occur. Brenner, Perkins, and Soderberg (1972) had their stutterers read silently, then silently but with pantomimed speech, then when whispering, and finally when reading aloud. Only the trial in which the stutterers read the passage aloud was there a significant decrease in stuttering due to the adaptation effect. When using the electrolarynx, neither phonation nor respiration is required and McKenzie (1955) found that stutterers did not stutter when speaking with this device. We also have a report by Beck (1956) of a stutterer who stopped stuttering after his larynx was removed and he had to use esophageal speech.* In summary, it seems tenable that when the complexity of the synergetic coordinations increases, the stuttering also tends to increase. This again points to the role of a disability or coordinative difficulty as a major factor in stuttering.

DISCOORDINATION DURING OVERT STUTTERING

Thus far we have been presenting the evidence indicating that mistimings and other anomalies of coordination exist in the perceptually fluent speech of stutterers. Now let us examine the overt stuttering itself. Again we find time lags in initiating movements, inappropriate functioning of various musculatures and a lack of synchronization of respiration, voice, and articulation.

Respiratory abnormalities. The older research demonstrated that many coordinative anomalies were characteristic of adult stutterers during moments of stuttering. Fixations of the respiratory structures were noted by many of these early workers (Travis 1927; Fossler 1930; Murray 1932; Henrickson 1936). The normal reciprocal relationships between thoracic and abdominal contractions were found to be lacking in stutterers by Henrickson (1936) and others. Tremors in the respiratory musculatures were found by Trumper (1928) and Schilling (1960) during the act of stuttering. Initially these coordinative anomalies were even viewed as the cause of stuttering but later research (Hill 1944) showed that they were probably due to the effects of disruptive negative emotion.

Articulatory anomalies in coordination. Similar incoordinations indicate that disruptions in coordination have been shown to occur in the articulatory movements of the speech of stutterers. Tremors, co-contractions of antagonistic muscle groups, timing lags, and asynchronies have been demonstrated by the research of Gertner and Luper (1967), Fibiger (1971, 1977), and Zimmermann 1980b). Hutchinson and Watkin (1976) found delays in the onset of phonation after jaw movement, and Hutchinson (1975) showed that disruptions in airflow or voicing probably contributed to anomalies in oral air pressure. Zimkin (1968), using cinefluoroscopic studies of the lips, tongue, and pharynx, also found that during stuttering the movement of these structures showed evidence of timing lags and asychronies.

---

* However, we also have two other reports (Doms and Lissons 1973; Tuck 1979) describing laryngectomized clients who continued to stutter when employing alaryngeal speech.

Laryngeal discoordinations during stuttering. The same disruptions have also been demonstrated to occur in laryngeal functioning. In France, Chevrie-Muller (1963), using glottography, discovered clonic flutterings of the vocal folds during stuttering. Fujita (1966) filmed X-ray pictures of a Japanese stutterer which revealed irregular movements and asymmetric closures in the pharyngeal and laryngeal structures. Another Japanese film by Ushijima, Kamiyama, Hirose, and Niimi (1965), using fibroscopic photography of the larynx, discovered unusual constrictions and movements including closure of the ventricular folds during attempted phonation. Conture's excellent film revealed other evidences of abnormal laryngeal activity and these were described by Conture, Brewer, and McCall (1977). Among these abnormalities were disruptions in the normal reciprocal relationship between opposing muscle groups. Again, in Freeman's study (1979), we have more evidence that during stuttering agonist and antagonist muscular contractions often occur simultaneously rather than reciprocally, thereby producing fixations and oscillations (tremors?) which do not occur in nonstuttered speech. There seems to be little doubt that coordinative disruptions are shown in laryngeal functioning during stuttering.

Indeed some authors have felt that the basic mistiming and incoordination are located within the larynx alone. Schwartz (1974) even goes so far as to attribute stuttering to the malfunctioning of a single laryngeal muscle, the posterior crico-arytenoid, but his view has gained little acceptance. However, it seems unwise to attribute the core discoordination in stuttering to laryngeal functioning alone when it also appears in articulatory and respiratory functions, too. Perhaps the following quote

→ EMG of Orbicularis Oris

→ Integrated EMG of O. O.
→ Integrated EMG of Digastric

→ Voice channel

→ EMG of Digastric
(anterior belly)

Figure 18. EMG recording showing relationships between antagonistic muscle groups during a long repetitive stuttering on the word "peep." Subject displays a 7-per-second tremor in both lip and digastric musculatures. Extreme mandibular jerk preceded final utterance.

from Freeman (1979) offers the most reasonable conclusion:

> Most of the investigators, this author included, agree with Conture when he
> finds that present research does not support claims for laryngeal causation of
> stuttering, but that laryngeal behaviors are an important aspect of the disrupted
> peripheral speech physiology that characterized stuttering (1979, pp. 86–87).

Studies of diadochokinesis. Another way to measure the coordination ability
of stutterers is to ascertain the maximum rates at which a motor activity
or a syllable or series of syllables can be repeated. This is termed
diadochokinesis. With a few exceptions that will be mentioned, the research
has generally found that stutterers have slower diadochokinesis rates than
nonstutterers in producing silent movements of the articulators and in the
production of spoken syllables.

An early study by West and Nusbaum (1929) found stutterers to be
slower than normal speakers in jaw and eyebrow movements. Blackburn
(1931) reported that stutterers were markedly inferior to their controls in
the speed and regularity of voluntary movements of the tongue, lips, and
diaphragm but not in arm or hand movements. Seth (1934) and Cross
(1936), however, did not corroborate Blackburn's findings except for the
movements of the diaphragm. Hunsley (1937) investigated the effects of
increasing rate on the rhythmic patterning of jaw, lip, tongue, and
breathing movements. She found that her 23 stutterers were inferior to
their controls in performing these precise silent movement sequences at
all levels of rate, and that they showed clonic and tonic blockings.

There are, however, two negative reports. In studies similar to Hunsley's,
but using only 15 stutterers and different scoring procedures, Strother
and Kriegman (1943; 1944) found no differences of significance. Chworowsky (1952) used the Sylrater to get the diadochokinetic rates of ten
Iowa stutterers and their controls for puh, tuh, kuh, and hand tapping
under normal and frustration conditions, finding no differences.

More recently, Rickenberg (1956), in a careful study, procured diadochokinetic rates for nine different cv syllables representing lip, tongue
tip, and back-tongue coordinations. His 15 stutterers were significantly
inferior to their controls for all the syllables. He concludes: "With respect
to the rate at which one impulse can be shifted from one group of muscles
to its antagonistic group, stutterers are significantly slower than nonstutterers." Zaleski (1965), in Poland, provides the only careful study using a
respectable number of subjects—50 stutterers and their controls. Finger
tapping and utterance of "pa," "ta," and "ka" were performed while paced
metronomically at differing speeds. On both the finger tapping and speech
movements, stutterers were significantly ($p < .01$) inferior to the normal
speakers. We should also report here Travis's original study (1934), in
which he showed that discrepancies in the arrival times and patterning of
action currents in the peripheral bilateral musculatures of speech occurred
during stuttering but not during normal speech in stutterers, nor in the
speech of normal speakers. Williams (1955) performed a somewhat similar
study with different placement of electrodes and using single words and

faked stuttering. When instructed to fake stuttering, the normal speakers showed most of the same abnormalities as did the stutterers. These studies need further replication, but both of them can be said to demonstrate that the fine motor coordinations of speech in either "real" or simulated stuttering show disruptions.

After reviewing all these studies, it is difficult not to conclude that stutterers show coordinative deficiency in the timing of their speech musculatures. While there are three negative findings, both on very limited samples, most of the evidence supports the belief that many stutterers have difficulty in such timing.

ARE STUTTERERS POORLY COORDINATED GENERALLY?

Thus far we have been concerned with the information dealing with the coordination of the speech musculatures. Now let us see if stutterers also show coordinative difficulties in other kinds of motor activities. The research unfortunately has often been of poor quality. Small numbers of subjects have been used, often with no controls when the data were gathered, and unstandardized tests have been employed. We are tempted to ignore many of them for these reasons but since mention of their procedures may impel others to do a better job, we shall include most of them here.

Kasanin (1931) used a selection of tests from the Oseretsky and Kwinte batteries with 50 assorted stuttering children and reported them to have motor development considerably below their chronological age. Westphal (1933), using some unstandardized motor tests with 26 boys and their controls, found that the stutterers were not as efficient in eye-hand coordinations, strength, or manual manipulation. Bilto (1941) used the standardized Brace Motor Ability Tests, the Nielson-Couzens Jump-and-Reach Test, and a measure of eye-hand coordination, and found that more than two-thirds of the stutterers performed below the mean of the nonstutterers on all three, but concluded that no marked retardation in gross motor ability was present.

Kopp (1942–43) applied the Oseretsky and other tests to 450 stutterers and concluded that they showed marked motor disabilities. She gives detailed data on only 28 of these in an English article and it is impossible to evaluate them. Scrutiny of her French article (1936) shows that a large percentage of the stutterers, varying with the test items used, scored low on the Oseretsky tests. No control group was used. In a later study, Kopp (1946) analyzed the results of Oseretsky tests with 50 stuttering children and found retardation in terms of motor age levels especially in "synkinetic movements, in rhythm and coordination." Despert (1946) also reported motor delay in her stutterers.

In contrast, at Iowa, Finkelstein and Weisberger (1954) found that a small number (15) of stutterers were, if anything, better coordinated than their controls on a different form of the Oseretsky test. In Germany, Schilling and Krüger (1960) examined 300 children, those with normal speech, a group of stutterers, and a group of children with delayed speech, using the Göllnitz modification of the Oseretsky test. Obvious motor retardation (at least a two-year delay) was found in 5 per cent of the normals, in 18 per cent of the stutterers and in 41 per cent of children with delayed speech. Snyder (1958) gave a battery of test items, most of which came from the Minnesota Mechanical Ability test, using three equal groups of 20 stutterers but with varying degrees of severity and 25 controls, individuals with other types of speech disorders. The stutterers were found to be significantly inferior, and the more severe the stuttering, the more marked the lack of coordination.

In Japan, Shiraiwa and Kawakuba (1967) state that their 70 child stutterers had no deficiency in gross motor coordination but that difficulties in fine coordination were found in 60 per cent of their subjects. Launay (1960), in France, applied various psychomotor tests to stutterers and their controls and found no differences. Pierce and Lipcon (1959) found significantly more disparate arm movements while walking in their 36 subjects than in their controls. Delacato (1963) claimed that 10 of 18 of his stutterers could not cross-pattern in creeping smoothly and accurately.

We can only conclude that no definitive conclusions are possible at this time with regard to gross motor coordinations in stutterers. There are just too many discrepancies in the reported results of these studies to enable anyone to be sure.

OTHER FINE COORDINATIONS
NOT RELATED TO SPEECH

Seth (1934) found no differences in the speed of hand or foot movements in stutterers and normal speakers. Cross (1936) compared 31 right-handed and 11 left-handed normal speakers with 26 stutterers in unimanual (bulb-squeezing) and bimanual (spool packing) activities. There were no differences in the unimanual activities, but stutterers were inferior in the bimanual ones. Murray (1932) found more incoordinations in eye movements in the silent reading of 18 stutterers than in his controls and so did Moser (1938,) but Hamilton (1940) failed to corroborate this on a larger number (71) of stuttering children. In Italy, Baldan (1965) gave the Kwinte Motor Facial Test to 50 normals, 50 with strabismus, and 50 stutterers. Eighty-five per cent of the normal speakers performed normally for their age, but only 57 per cent of the stutterers and 45 per cent of the strabismus cases did so. Baldan also found a very high stuttering incidence of 17.5 per cent in the strabismic population, almost the same as that discovered 30 years earlier by Fink and Bryngelson (1934), who found that nine of 60 unselected strabismus cases were stutterers, an incidence of over 18 per cent.

Further evidence of incoordination in fine movements comes from investigations of nystagmus. Baldan (1965), used electronystagmography to investigate the vestibular reflexes of 60 Italian stutterers during silence but with eyes either open or closed. He found marked abnormality in the rhythm of the nystagmoid movements in 80 percent of his subjects. Two other electronystographic studies by Castellini, (1973) and by Langova, Moravek, Sroky and Svab (1962) also showed some evidence of coordinative disability in stutterers.

In breathing, Schilling (1960), using radiokymography, also found involuntary pathological movements in the diaphragm resembling those of chorea in 16 of 35 stuttering children while silent and at rest. Their histories and EEGs were said to have indicated early brain damage. Somewhat similar results were described by Shiraiwa and Kawakuba (1967).

Gunderson (1949) recorded the involuntary finger tremors of 75 male stutterers in silence, oral reading, silent reading, and extemporaneous speaking. She found more tremor irregularities in the speaking than in the silent situations, a result also reached by Herren (1931) in his study of voluntary rhythmic hand and foot movements.

"STUTTERING" IN OTHER COORDINATED ACTIVITIES

Stuttering or stutteringlike behaviors have been noted in other activities requiring precise sequential coordination. Denhardt, as early as 1890, described blocking movements and postures similar to stuttering in handwriting or in playing musical instruments. We also find that Yastrebova (1962) analyzed the correlation of abnormalities in the written and oral speech of stuttering school children, but it is difficult to assess the author's findings. Van Riper (1952) has reported a case of trumpet stuttering, and Froeschels (1943a) described piano and violin stuttering. Scripture (1909) described penmanship stuttering in some detail. Other cases in which written letters were involuntarily disrupted or pens were described as "stuck to the paper" have been cited by Ssikorski (1891), Eisenson (1937), Van Dantzig (1939), and Cabanas (1951).

We also have several carefully done studies of "graphic stuttering" by Fagan (1931), Roman (1959), and Thomas and Richter (1972) which show incoordination and mistiming of the movements involved in handwriting. In the last of these researches, judges who were trained in handwriting analysis were able to differentiate the written samples of stutterers from those penned by nonstutterers. Again, in an activity that demands precise sequential timing, the stutterers showed discoordination.

In summary it should be pointed out, of course, that merely attributing stuttering to coordinative disruptions does not by itself solve the ancient problem. We still must answer the question of why these coordinations are disrupted. Certainly we must go back further into the nervous system to learn what causes these aberrations, to discover perhaps the reasons for the mistiming of the speech musculatures. Does the stutterer possess a deficient neurological timer or are these mis- or discoordinations merely the result of classically conditioned emotional flooding? Even if either or both of these possibilities are partially true, a large share of the stutterer's overt speech abnormality can be attributed to learned coping or avoidance reactions. Nevertheless, any theory which seeks to explain all the features of stuttering must come to grips with the problem of discoordination.

BIBLIOGRAPHY

ADAMS, M. R. 1974. A physiologic and aerodynamic interpretation of fluent and stuttered speech. *Journal of Fluency Disorders* 1: 35–47.

—— AND P. HAYDEN. 1976. The ability of stutterers to initiate and terminate phonation during production of an isolated vowel. *Journal of Speech and Hearing Research* 19: 290–96.

ADAMS, M. R., J. LEWIS, AND T. BESOZZI. 1973. The effect of reduced reading rate on stuttering frequency. *Journal of Speech and Hearing Research* 16: 671–95.

ADAMS, M. R. AND R. REIS. 1971. The influence of the onset of phonation on the frequency of stuttering. *Journal of Speech and Hearing Research* 14: 639–644.

ADAMS, M. R., S. RIEMENSCHNEIDER, D. METZ, AND E. CONTURE. 1974. Voice onset and articulatory constriction requirements in a speech segment and their relation to the amount of stuttering adaptation. *Journal of Fluency Disorders* 1: 23–29.

ADAMS, M. R., C. RUNYAN, AND A. R. MALLARD. 1975. Air flow characteristics of the speech of stutterers and nonstutterers. *Journal of Fluency Disorders* 1: 3–12.

AGNELLO, J. 1974. Laryngeal and articulatory dynamics of disfluency interpreted within a vocal tract model. In *Vocal tract dynamics and fluency*, eds. M. Webster and L. Furst. New York: Speech and Hearing Institute.

—— AND M. E. WINGATE. 1971. Air pressure and formants of stutterers and nonstutterers. Convention paper, *ASHA*, Chicago.

——. 1972. Some acoustical and physiological aspects of stuttered speech. Convention paper, *ASHA*, San Francisco.

AGNELLO, J., M. E. WINGATE, AND L. MOULIN. 1970. Coarticulation patterns of stutterers and nonstutterers. *ASHA*. 13 Abstract.

AGNELLO, J., M. E. WINGATE, AND M. WENDELL. 1974. Voice onset and voice termination times of child and adult stutterers. *Journal of the Acoustical Society of America* 56: 362.

ALLSCHULER, S. L. 1980. Stuttering in an alaryngeal speaker: a case report. Convention paper, *ASHA*, Detroit.

BALDAN, G. 1965. Study of the vestibular function in a group of stutterers: electronystagmographic researches. *De Therapia Vocis et Loquellae* 1: 349–51.

BECK, J. 1956. La voix oesophagienne de replacement les laryngectomises. *Revue de Laryngologie, Otologie, Rhinologie* 77: 729–39.

BILTO, E. W. 1941. A comparative study of certain physical abilities of children with speech defects and children with normal speech. *Journal of Speech Disorders* 6: 187–203.

BLACKBURN, W. E. 1931. A study of the voluntary movements of the diaphragm, tongue, lips and jaw in stutterers and normal speakers. *Psychological Monographs* 41: 1–13.

BRAYTON, E. R. AND E. G. CONTURE. 1978. Effects of noise and rhythmic stimulation on the speech of stutterers. *Journal of Speech and Hearing Research* 21: 285–94.

BRENNER, N. C., W. H. PERKINS, AND G. A. SODERBERG. 1972. The effects of rehearsals on the frequency of stuttering. *Journal of Speech and Hearing Research* 15: 483–86.

BRUCE, M. C. AND M. R. ADAMS. 1978. Effects of two types of motor practice on stuttering. *Journal of Speech and Hearing Research* 21: 421–28.

CABANAS, R. 1951. Report on a particular case of stuttering. *Folia Phoniatrica* 3: 10–13.

CASTELLINI, V. 1973. Electronystagmographic studies in 30 cases of stammering. *Otorhinolaryngology Clinic,* University of Genoa, 15: 27–32.

CHEVRIE-MULLER, C. 1963. A study of laryngeal function in stutterers by the glottographic method. *Proceedings of the Vii Congress of the French Society for Voice and Speech.*

CHWOROWSKY, C. R. 1952. A comparative study of diadochokinetic rates of stutterers and nonstutterers in speech related and nonspeech related movements. *Speech Monographs* 19: 192.

COLCORD, R. D. AND M. R. ADAMS. 1979. Voicing durations and vocal SPL changes associated with stuttering reduction during singing. *Journal of Speech and Hearing Research* 22: 468–79.

COMMODORE, R. W. AND F. B. COOPER. 1978. Communicative stress and stuttering frequency during normal, whispered and articulation without phonation. *Journal of Fluency Disorders* 3: 1–12.

CONTURE, E. G. AND L. V. GOULD. 1980. The descent of the larynx during stuttering. Convention paper, *ASHA,* Detroit.

———, G. M. McCALL, AND D. W. BREWER. 1977. Laryngeal behavior during stuttering. *Journal of Speech and Hearing Research* 20: 661–68.

COOPER, M. H. AND G. D. ALLEN. 1977. Timing control accuracy in normal speakers and stutterers. *Journal of Speech and Hearing Research* 20: 55–71.

CROSS, D. E. AND H. L. LUPER. 1979. Voice reaction time of stuttering and nonstuttering children. *Journal of Fluency Disorders* 4: 661–68.

CROSS, D. E., B. B. SHADDEN, AND H. L. LUPER. 1979. Effects of stimulus ear presentation on the voice reaction times of adult stutterers and nonstutterers. *Journal of Fluency Disorders* 4: 45–58.

CROSS, H. M. 1936. The motor capacities of stutterers. *Archives of Speech* 1: 112–32.

CULLINAN, W. L. AND M. T. SPRINGER. 1980. Voice initiation and termination times in stuttering and nonstuttering children. *Journal of Speech and Hearing Research* 23: 344–60.

CURLEE, R. F. AND W. H. PERKINS. 1968. The effect of punishment of expectancy on the frequencies of subsequent expectancies and stuttering. *Journal of Speech and Hearing Research* 11: 787–95.

DE AJURIAGUERRA, J. 1966. Speech disorders in childhood. In *Brain Function III,* ed. C. Carterette. Berkeley: Univ. of California Press.

DELACATO, C. 1963. *The diagnosis and treatment of speech and reading problems.* Springfield, Ill.: Thomas.

DESPERT, J. L. 1946. Psychosomatic study of fifty stuttering children. *American Journal of Orthopsychiatry* 16: 100–13.

DINNAN, J. A., C. McGUINESS, AND L. PERRIN. 1970. Auditory feedback: stutterers versus nonstutterers. *Journal of Learning Disabilities* 3: 208–13.

DiSIMONI, F. 1974. Preliminary study of certain timing relationships in the speech of stutterers. *Journal of the Acoustical Society of America* 56: 697.

DOMS, M. AND D. LISSENS. 1973. Stuttering and the laryngectomee. In *Neurolinguistic Approaches to Stuttering*, eds. Y. Le Brun and R. Hoops. The Hague: Mouton.

EISENSON, J. 1937. Some characteristics of the written speech of stutterers. *Journal of Genetic Psychology* 50: 457–58.

FAGAN, L. B. 1931. Graphic stuttering. *Psychological Monographs* 43: 67–71.

FEW, L. R. AND J. B. LINGWALL. 1972. A further analysis of fluency within stuttered speech. *Journal of Speech and Hearing Research* 15: 356–63.

FIBIGER, S. 1971. Stuttering explained as a physiological tremor. *Speech Translations Laboratory. Quarterly Progress Report*. Speech Transmission Laboratory, Royal Institute of Technology, Stockholm.

———. 1972. Further discussion on "Stuttering explained as a physiological tremor." *Quarterly Progress and Status Report*, Speech Transmission Laboratory, Royal Institute of Technology, Stockholm.

———. 1977. Quantitative electromyographic evaluation of stuttering severity by means of description of the course of muscle activity in the lip-articulatory muscles in connection with labial stop consonants. *Proceedings XVII Congress of Logopedics and Phoniatrics*. Interlaken.

FINK, W. H. AND B. BRYNGELSON. 1934. The relation of strabismus to right or left handedness. *Transactions of the American Academy of Ophthalmology and Otolaryngology* 73–76.

FINKLESTEIN, P. AND S. E. WEISBERGER. 1954. The motor proficiency of stutterers. *Journal of Speech and Hearing Disorders* 19: 52–57.

FOSSLER, H. R. 1930. Disturbances in breathing during stuttering. *Psychological Monographs* 40: 1–32.

FRANSELLA, F. AND H. R. BEECH. 1965. Rhythm as a distractor in the modification of stuttering. *Behavior Research and Therapy* 3: 195–201.

FREEMAN, F. J. 1974. Fluency and phonation. In *Vocal Tract Dynamics and Disfluency*, eds. L. M. Webster and L. Furst. New York: Speech and Hearing Institute of New York.

———. 1979. Phonation in stuttering: a review of current research. *Journal of Fluency Disorders* 4: 77–89.

——— AND T. USHIJIMA. 1975. Laryngeal activity accompanying the moment of stuttering: a preliminary report of EMG investigations. *Journal of Fluency Disorders* 1: 36–39.

———. 1978. Laryngeal muscle activity during stuttering. *Journal of Speech and Hearing Research* 21: 538–62.

———. 1975. The stuttering larynx: an EMG fiberoptic study of laryngeal activity accompanying the moment of stuttering. *Haskins Laboratories Status Report on Speech Research*, SR-41. New Haven: Haskins Laboratories.

FUJITA, K. 1966. Pathophysiology of the larynx from the viewpoint of phonation. *Journal of the Japanese Society of Otolaryngology* 74: 459.

GAUTHERON, B., A. LIORZON, AND B. VALLANCIEN. 1973. The role of the larynx in stuttering. In *Neurolinguistic Approaches to Stuttering*, eds. Y. Le Brun and R. Hoops. The Hague: Mouton.

GERTNER, L. L. AND H. L. LUPER. 1967.   A cinefluorographic study of the duration and number of lingua-alveolar articulatory contacts and reading times of stutterers and nonstutterers. Convention paper, *ASHA*.

GUNDERSON, H. 1949.   A quantitative analysis of digital tremor in male stutterers. Doctoral dissertation, Columbia University.

HAMILTON, P. G. 1940.   The visual characteristics of stutterers during silent reading. Doctoral dissertation, Teachers College, Columbia University.

HAND, C. R. AND H. L. LUPER. 1980.   Durational characteristics of stutterers' and nonstutterers' fluent speech. *ASHA* 22: 709.

HAYDEN, P. A. 1975.   The effects of masking and pacing on stutterers' and nonstutterers' speech initiation times. Doctoral dissertation, Purdue University.

———, D. A. SCOTT, AND J. ADDICOTT. 1977.   The effects of delayed auditory feedback on the overt behaviors of stutterers. *Journal of Fluency Disorders* 2: 235–46.

HEALEY, E. C. 1979.   Comments on laryngeal behavior during stuttering. *Journal of Speech and Hearing Research* 22: 412–13.

———. 1980.   Fundamental frequency contours of stutterers' vowels following fluent stop consonant productions. *ASHA* 22: 709.

———, A. MALLARD, AND M. R. ADAMS. 1976.   Factors contributing to the reduction of stuttering during singing. *Journal of Speech and Hearing Research* 19: 475–80.

HENRICKSON, E. H. 1936.   Simultaneously recorded breathing and vocal disturbances of stutterers. *Archives of Speech* 1: 133–49.

HERREN, R. Y. 1931.   The effect of stuttering on voluntary movement. *Journal of Experimental Psychology* 14: 289–98.

HILL, H. 1944.   Stuttering II: a review and integration of physiological data. *Journal of Speech Disorders* 9: 289–324.

HILLMAN, R. E. AND H. H. GILBERT. 1977.   Voice onset time for voiceless stop consonants in the fluent reading of stutterers and nonstutterers. *Journal of the Acoustical Society of America* 61: 610–11.

HOTCHKISS, J. 1973.   Perceptual differences in the fluent speech of stutterers and nonstutterers. Doctoral dissertation, Purdue University.

HUNSLEY, Y. L. 1937.   Disintegration in the speech musculature of stutterers during the production of a nonvocal temporal pattern. *Psychological Monographs* 49: 32–49.

HUTCHINSON, J. M. 1975.   Aerodynamic patterns of stuttered speech. In *Vocal Tract Dynamics and Dysfluency*, eds. L. M. Webster and L. C. Furst. New York: Speech and Hearing Institute of New York.

———, P. N. DEPUTY, AND S. R. McGEE. 1980.   Phonatory onsets and stuttering frequency in children. Convention paper, *ASHA*, Detroit.

HUTCHINSON, J. M. AND B. M. NAVARRE. 1977.   The effect of metronome pacing on selected aerodynamic patterns of stuttered speech. *Journal of Fluency Disorders* 2: 189–204.

HUTCHINSON, J. M. AND K. L. WATKIN. 1976.   Jaw mechanics during release of the stuttering moment: some initial observations and interpretations. *Journal of Communication Disorders* 9: 269–79.

INGHAM, R. J., R. B. MARTIN, AND P. KUHL. 1974.   Modification and control of rate of speaking by stutterers, *Journal of Speech and Hearing Research* 17: 489–96.

JOHNSON, W. AND L. ROSEN. 1937.   Effects of certain changes in speech patterns upon the frequency of stuttering. *Journal of Speech Disorders* 2: 10–14.

KASANIN, H. R. I. 1931.   The motor development of children suffering from stammering. *American Journal of Diseases of Children* 44: 1123–25.

KERR, S. AND E. B. COOPER. 1976.   Phonatory adjustment times in stutterers and nonstutterers. Convention paper, *ASHA*, Houston.

KOPP, H. 1946.   Psychosomatic study of fifty stuttering children: III. Oseretsky Tests. *American Journal of Orthopsychiatry* 16: 114–19.

———. 1936.   Les troubles de la parole dans leur rapport avec les troubles de la motrice. *L'Evolution Psychiatrique* 2: 77–112.

———. 1942–43.   The relationship of stuttering to motor disturbances. *Nervous Child* 2: 107–16.

KUSSMAUL, A. 1877.   Die storungen der sprache. In *Cyclopaedia Medica*, ed. H. V. Ziemssen.

LANGOVA, J., M. MORAVEK, A. SROKY, AND L. SVAB. 1962.   Experimental study on stuttering and stammering. *Casopis Leharu Ceskych* 101: 297–300.

LAUNAY, C. 1960.   Troubles neurologiques dans le begaiement. *Journal Francais d'Otorhinolaryngologie* 9: 269–79.

LOVE, L. R. AND L. A. JEFFRESS. 1971.   Identification of brief pauses in the fluent speech of stutterers and nonstutterers. *Journal of Speech and Hearing Research* 14: 229–40.

MACKAY, D. G. 1970.   Errors in patterns of finger movements rapidly produced by stutterers and nonstutterers. Convention paper. *ASHA*, New York.

MANNING, W. H. AND K. J. COUFAL. 1976.   The frequency of disfluencies during phonatory transitions in stuttered and nonstuttered speech. *Journal of Communication Disorders* 9: 75–81.

McCLEAN, A. E. AND E. B. COOPER. 1978.   Electromyographic indications of laryngeal area activity during stuttering expectancy. *Journal of Fluency Disorders* 3: 205–19.

McFARLANE, S. J. AND D. PRINS. 1978.   Neural response time of stutterers and nonstutterers. *Journal of Speech and Hearing Research* 21: 768–78.

McKENZIE, F. A. 1955.   A stutterer's experience in using an electrolarynx. In *Stuttering in Children and Adults*, ed. W. Johnson. Minneapolis: University of Minnesota Press.

METZ, D. E., E. G. CONTURE, AND A. CARUSO. 1979.   Voice onset time, frication and aspiration during stutterers fluent speech. *Journal of Speech and Hearing Research* 22: 649–56.

MOSER, H. M. 1938.   A qualitative analysis of eye-movements during stuttering. *Journal of Speech Disorders* 3: 131–39.

MURRAY, E. 1932.   Disintegration of breathing and eye movements in stutterers during silent reading and reasoning. *Psychological Monographs* 43: 218–75.

PERKINS, W., J. RUDAS, L. JOHNSON, AND J. BELL. 1976.   Stuttering discoordination of phonation with articulation and respiration. *Journal of Speech and Hearing Research* 19: 509–22.

PIERCE, C. M. AND H. H. LIPCON. 1959.   Stuttering: clinical and electroencephalographic findings. *Military Medicine* 12: 5–19.

PROSEK, R. A., A. A. MONTGOMERY, V. E. WALDEN, AND D. M. SCHWARTZ. 1979.   Reaction time measures of stutterers and nonstutterers. *Journal of Fluency Disorders* 4: 269–79.

REIS, R. AND M. R. ADAMS. 1978.   Comments on the Adams and Reis observations revisited. *Journal of Fluency Disorders* 3: 299–302.

RICKENBERG, H. E. 1956. Diadochokinesis in stutterers and nonstutterers. *Journal of the Medical Society of New Jersey* 53: 324–25.

ROLAND, B. C. 1972. Eye movements of stutterers and nonstutterers during silent, oral and choral reading. *Perceptual and Motor Skills* 35: 297–98.

ROMAN, K. G. 1959. Handwriting and speech. *Logos* 2: 29–39.

RUNYAN, C. M. AND M. R. ADAMS. 1978. Perceptual study of the speech of successfully therapeutized stutterers. *Journal of Fluency Disorders* 3: 25–39.

—— AND R. A. PROSEK. 1980. Temporal characteristics of the fluent speech of stutterers. *ASHA* 22: 709–10.

SCHILLING, A. 1960. Roentgen-Zwerfell-Kymogranne bei stottern. *Folia Phoniatrica* 12: 145–53.

—— AND W. KRÜGER, 1960. Untersuchungen über die motorik sprachgestörter kinder nach der motometrischen skala von Oseretsky-Göllnitz unter besonderer berücksichtingung dei frühkindlichen hirnschädigung. *HNO* 8: 205–9.

SCHWARTZ, M. F. 1974. The core of the stuttering block. *Journal of Speech and Hearing Disorders*, 39: 169–77.

SCRIPTURE, E. W. 1909. Penmanship stuttering. *Journal of the American Medical Association* 52: 1480–81.

SETH, G. 1934. Psychomotor control in stammering and normal subjects: an experimental study. *British Journal of Psychology* 49: 139–43.

SHAFFER, G. 1940. Measures of jaw movement and phonation in nonstuttered and stuttered production of voiced and voiceless plosives. *Speech Monographs* 7: 85–92.

SHIRAIWA, T. AND J. KAWAKUBA. 1967. Study of the cause of stuttering. In *A Handbook for the Study of Stuttering*, ed. G. Kamiyama. Tokyo: Japan, Abstract No. 185.

SNYDER, M. A. 1958. Stuttering and coordination. *Logos* 1: 36–44.

SSIKORSKI, J. A. 1891. *Über das Stottern.* Berlin: Hirschwald.

STARK, R. E. AND B. R. PIERCE. 1970. Effects of delayed auditory feedback on a speech-related task in stutterers. *Journal of Speech and Hearing Disorders*, 13: 245–53.

STARKWEATHER, C. W., P. HIRSCHMAN, AND R. TANNENBAUM. 1976. Latency of vocalization onset: stutterers versus nonstutterers. *Journal of Speech and Hearing Research* 19: 481–92.

STARKWEATHER, C. W. AND N. MYERS. 1978. The intervocalic interval in stutterers and nonstutterers: a close analysis. Convention paper, *ASHA*.

STROTHER, C. R. AND L. S. KRIEGMAN. 1934. Diadochokinesis in stutterers and nonstutterers. *Journal of Speech Disorders* 8: 325–35.

——. 1944. Rhythmokinesis in stutterers and nonstutterers. *Journal of Speech Disorders* 9: 239–44.

THOMAS, B. AND J. RICHTER. 1972. Psychological inquiries regarding the handwriting of stutterers. *Psychiatrie, Neurologie und Medizinische Psychologie* 24: 201–9.

TRAVIS, L. E. 1927. Disintegration of breathing movements during stuttering. *Archives of Neurology and Psychiatry* 18: 673–90.

——. 1934. Dissociation of the homologous muscle function in stuttering. *Archives of Neurology and Psychiatry* 31: 127–33.

—— AND R. Y. HERREN. 1929. Studies in Stuttering: V. A study of simultaneous antitropic movement in the hands of stutterers. *Archives of Neurology and Psychiatry* 22: 487–94.

TRUMPER, M. 1928. A hematorespiratory study of 101 consecutive cases of stammering. Doctoral dissertation, University of Pennsylvania.

TUCK, A. E. 1979. An alaryngeal stutterer: a case history. *Journal of Fluency Disorders* 4: 239–43.

USHIJIMA, T., G. KAMIYAMA, H. HIROSE, AND S. NIIMI. 1965. Articulatory movements of the larynx during stuttering. Film. Tokyo: Research Institute of Logopedics and Phoniatrics.

VAN DANTZIG, B. 1939. Writing, typing and speaking. *Journal of speech Disorders* 4: 270–301.

VAN RIPER, C. 1952. Report of stuttering on a musical instrument. *Journal of Speech Disorders* 17: 433–34.

WATSON, B. C. AND P. J. ALPHONSO. 1980. Comparisons of LRT and VOT values between stutterers and nonstutterers. Convention paper. *ASHA*, Detroit.

WENDAHL, R. W. AND J. COLE. 1961. Identification of stuttering during relatively fluent speech. *Journal of Speech and Hearing Research* 4: 281–86.

WEST, R. AND E. NUSBAUM. 1929. A motor test for dysphemia. *Quarterly Journal of Speech Education* 15: 469–79.

WESTPHAL, G. 1933. An experimental study of certain motor abilities of stutterers. *Child Development* 4: 214–21.

WILLIAMS, D. E. 1955. Masseter muscle action current potentials in stuttered and nonstuttered speech. *Journal of Speech and Hearing Disorders* 20: 242–61.

WOLK, L. 1980. Vocal tract dynamics in a single stutterer. Convention paper, *ASHA*, Detroit.

YASTREBOVA, A. V. 1962. Peculiarities in the oral and written speech of stuttering pupils. Moscow: Institute of Defektology.

YOUNG, M. A. 1964. Identification of stutterers from recorded samples of their "fluent" speech. *Journal of Speech and Hearing Research* 7: 302–3.

ZALESKI, T. 1965. Rhythmic skills in stuttering children. *De Therapia Vocis et Loquellae* 1: 371–72.

ZIMKIN, N. I. 1968. *Mechanisms of Speech.* The Hague: Mouton.

ZIMMERMANN, G. N. 1980b. Articulatory behaviors associated with stuttering: a cinefluorographic analysis. *Journal of Speech and Hearing Research* 23: 108–21.

———. 1980a. Articulatory dynamics of fluent utterances of stutterers and nonstutterers. *Journal of Speech and Hearing Research* 23: 95–107.

———. 1980c. Stuttering: a disorder of movement. *Journal of Speech and Hearing Research* 23: 122–36.

THE NATURE OF STUTTERING
an attempted synthesis

17

Although we know the attempt will not be entirely successful, in this chapter we will try to outline an explanation for the nature of stuttering which will bring together most of the hard information we have about the disorder—and some of the soft. Actually, there is not enough information about the essential nature of stuttering to allow more than a general outline of its patterning. But if we must fail, let us fail forward! Others will mend and build upon the insecure foundations on which this precarious monument to human benightedness is so hesitantly erected.

We should like to suggest that stuttering be considered a disorder of timing. We feel that when a person stutters on a word, there is a temporal disruption of the simultaneous and successive programming of muscular movements required to produce one of the word's integrated sounds, or to emit one of its syllables appropriately or to accomplish the precise linking of sounds and syllables that constitutes its motor pattern. If we ignore for the moment the entire complex overlay of reactions to this experience, we find the essence of the disorder in this fracturing and disruption of the motor sequence of the word. The integrity of a spoken word demands great precision in the timing of its components. When, for any reason, that timing is awry and askew, a temporally distorted word is produced, and when this happens, the speaker has evinced a core stuttering behavior.

There are real advantages to this definition. It escapes much of the foggy confusion in which stuttering has been enveloped. In the future, the amount of temporal disruption might be measured objectively; the structures involved in the mistiming might be located; and, hopefully, the asynchrony might be traced to its origin.

If stuttering is considered a disorder of timing it is possible to synthesize most of the various points of view concerning the nature of the disorder.

Mistiming could be attributed to an organic proclivity, to emotional stress, or to a malfunctioning servo system. The huge overlay of the variable struggle and avoidance reactions to the experiencing of mistimed words as well as much of the overt and covert phenomenology of the disorder are explained best with the principles of learning and conditioning, for it is probable that stuttering grows and maintains itself largely through differential learning experiences. In short, most of the information we have about stuttering makes sense if its original or core behaviors are temporal disruptions of the motor patterns of words. In the beginning was the word—the broken word!

The weight of the research evidence assembled in our last chapters seem to support the notion that mistimings characterize stuttering. Lags and delays have been observed in the functioning of all of the speech musculatures not only during the overt stuttering act but even in the apparently fluent speech of stutterers. The asynchronies between lips, tongue, or jaws seem to occur because one or another of these structures fails to move when it should move. The basic synergies of voice, respiration, and articulation are disrupted because the normal timing relationships between them are changed by similar delays. More specifically, we find over and over again that co-contraction of agonist-antagonistic muscle groups occur in the speech system during the moment of stuttering. This means that the normal reciprocal functioning of antagonists does not occur; for example, when there is a delay in the relaxation of the abductor muscles as the abductor muscles contract, postural fixations and tremors are produced and these in turn create further delays.

At the present time we have no theory concerning the timing control of the movements involved in speech which has gained general acceptance. Lashley (1951) proposed an open loop explanation in which a central control neural assembly operating like a neural clock generated the syllabic pulses and subassemblies for motoric components thereof. Kozhevnikov and Chistovitch (1965) performed some anesthetization experiments and supported this view that, once the motor programs have been learned through the aid of sensory feedback, they can be executed independently of proprioception or audition. The implication of this position is that the mistimings in stuttering may be due to unstable central motor programs.

Is there some central deficiency in timing which might account for these peripheral lags and delays? Do the neural clocks of stutterers stutter, too? We have only a few researches that remotely support such an hypothesis. Ringel and Minifee (1966) found that stutterers, especially the severe ones, had significantly lower protensity scores than normal speakers, protensity being measured as the accuracy of being able to judge an elapsed interval of ten seconds. Cooper and Allen (1977) asked their subjects to repeat sentences, paragraphs, nursery rhymes, and finger-tapping patterns in the same way over and over again (80 trials), and they then measured the variability in the time it took them to do these activities. Stutterers were more variable than the nonstutterers and the authors suggest that the neural clocks of stutterers may be less accurate and that they might have basic timing deficiencies. However, these two researches are hardly sufficient to support the hypothesis that the cause of the peripheral mistimings and delays are due to the central processing of motor programs.

In contrast, the large number of studies we have reviewed in our chapter concerning disturbed feedback tend to attribute the lags and mistimings to disruptions or anomalies in the return flow of information from the periphery. Continuous (or intermittent) sampling of the state of the auditory or spatial targets is felt to provide the basis for control in a closed loop system. When aberrant signals are received by the central motor program center, the output is interrupted and then varied until appropriate feedback has been achieved.

If we are to understand the nature of stuttering, we cannot be content with merely noting that such delays and mistimings do take place. Where is the source and what is the cause of these peripheral lags in motor functioning? Here, unfortunately, we enter the dark jungle of the unknown in the land of speculation. The exact nature of the central motor program or motor plan for even a simple limb movement is still not fully understood, and our knowledge about the motor programs for speech production is even more unsatisfactory.

WHAT CAUSES THE MISTIMINGS?

One of the most interesting speculations about the source of the motor delays in stutterers has been provided by Stromsta (1964). Let us review it again. Based upon his study of the power spectra of the bilateral alpha waves of stutterers and nonstutterers, he discovered that the latter were more "broadly tuned" than those of the stutterers. The bilateral potentials that were time-locked were concentrated at 10Hz in the stutterers, whereas those of nonstutterers showed a more uniform distribution within the alpha range (8 to 13Hz). In broad tuning, there are more brain cells being in a state of excitability or reactivity for a longer time period and hence the processing of incoming or outgoing neural events is more efficient than it would be in an individual whose time-locked bilateral alpha waves show evidence of narrow tuning. Since reaction times have been shown to be dependent upon the phase of the alpha rhythms, we may have here an explanation for the mistimings and delays that characterize stuttering.

Another explanation for the mistimings in the speech of stutterers has attributed them to the use of the right hemisphere for the processing of auditory information and motor output. According to Moore and Lang (1977) and Moore and Haynes (1980), this hemisphere, unlike the left hemisphere, seems to be less efficient in processing of segmental events such as those of speech. They write, "The use of a nonsegmental processor in dealing with segmental information at a linguistic-motor planning level may well result in a disruption of such programming which is seen behaviorally as stuttering" (p. 242).

Still another view holds that the mistimings and delays in speech are due to delays and distortions in the feedback systems governing speech. In Chapter 15 we have reviewed this material and find no need to summarize it again here. Basically, the position is that interruptions and delays in the motor programming of speech in stutterers are due to delays in the input signals. Since the central motor programs are probably organized in relation to their auditory targets (Abbs and Sussman 1971), disruptions or distortions in the incoming auditory information could be expected to disturb motor outputs.

Another explanation has been offered by Zimmermann (1980). His preliminary model attributed disfluent behaviors to asynchronies in timing of the synergies of respiration, phonation, and articulation. He writes:

> It is suggested that the speech structures operate within certain ranges of variability in terms of their movement parameters and interarticulator temporal and spatial relations. This variability may be influenced by emotional, perceptual and/or physiological events. When the "normal" ranges are exceeded, the afferent nerve impulses generated alter the gains of associated brain stem reflexes. Altering of the reflex gains throws the articulatory system out of balance and a breakdown in behavior occurs, often manifested as oscillations and static positioning (1980, p. 122).

Although the preceding quotation refers only to the articulatory system, Zimmermann (1980, p. 130) also applies the same explanation to laryngeal and respiratory functioning as well. This view is somewhat similar to that of Wyke (1974) who suggested that these may be two distinct varieties of stuttering, one in which abnormally slow presetting of the laryngeal and respiratory musculatures occurred, and the other in which various laryngeal and articulatory reflex systems disorganized this presetting.

Finally, on a less esoteric level, we find explanations for the mistimings based upon the interference effects due to competition between stuttering motor patterns and normal motor patterns. Frick writes,

> ... a major factor which acts to elicit stuttering is a deficit in the motor plan of the stutterer. By deficit in motor plan is meant that the stutterer, when experiencing fear or anticipation of stuttering, does not, or is unable to plan the sequence of motor acts necessary to utter the word or phrase or longer unit envisioned by the stutterer (1970, p. 1).

Frick feels that, under expectancy, the stutterer does not really try to say the word as a whole but only the feared first sound and so fails to achieve the necessary coarticulatory features of that sound or syllable and therefore will block, repeat, or prolong. Other authors (Van Riper, 1973) have suggested that abnormal preparatory sets may be conditioned to certain features of words and that these may interfere with the normal sets or motor programs even before utterance is attempted.

THE RHYTHM EFFECT

Other evidence for the view that stuttering is a disorder of timing comes from the many studies as well as clinical observations showing that the stutterer's fluency is enhanced if he times his utterance to the beat of a regular rhythm. This rhythm or metronomic effect has long been known and the history of the treatment of stuttering is filled with accounts of therapists using chanted, rhythmic utterance to facilitate fluency. So far as we can ascertain, it was Thewall, a British physician, in 1764 who first publicly advocated rhythmic speech controls for stutterers although Columbat de L'Isère (1831) is usually credited with the discovery of metronomic speech. It is interesting to read Columbat's rationale for his use of rhythmic speech in the treatment of stuttering:

> It has always been observed that stuttering ceases as though by magic when the afflicted person sings or recites words to musical or poetic rhythms. But no one has tried to explain this phenomenon. . . . Two causes, one the result of the other, may account for the stutterer's fluency in singing. The first is that, since he is able to impose the muscial or poetic rhythm upon his speech, the movements of his vocal organs must therefore move with greater accuracy and regularity. The second is that the stutterer by constantly concentrating upon the metrical beat modifies the cerebral excitations so that they proceed more slowly and more orderly (1831, p. 55).

The first *research* to demonstrate the effect was performed by Johnson and Rosen (1937). They asked 18 stutterers to read in various ways and found that uttering the words in a regular and rhythmic fashion produced by far the fewest stutterings. This was corroborated by Barber (1939) and by Bloodstein (1950). Van Dantzig (1940) showed that when stutterers were asked to time each syllable with a tapping of the finger, they immediately became fluent. In a second study, Barber (1940) used regular visual, auditory, and tactual stimuli to time the speech attempt on consecutively spoken words and found that all of them were equally effective in reducing stuttering. However, she also showed that when the timing stimulus was initiated too fast, more stuttering occurred. Meyer and Mair (1963) demonstrated in two stutterers that when they timed their words with a regularly beating device they became completely fluent but that when the beats were irregular and unpredictable, no reduction in stuttering was obtained. Fransella and Beech (1965) similarly showed that the number of stutterings produced when speaking in unison with a *rhythmic* metronomic timer was greatly reduced but that an arhythmic metronome had little effect. Fransella (1967) asked her stutterers to perform the additional task of writing numbers while reading aloud to the rhythmic beat of a metronome and concluded that the rhythmic effect could not be viewed merely as a distraction. In their book, Beech and Fransella (1968) describe another experiment which has significance for our view that stuttering is a disorder of timing. They write:

> Twenty stutterers served as their own controls in the experiment which involved a comparison of the difficulty experienced in reading words which were exposed on a screen for varying lengths of time. For half the words used, the point in time at which they were to be spoken was clearly indicated, while for the other words the utterance was required by unspecified moments during their exposure. The results confirmed the hypothesis, indicating that some means of enabling subjects to determine the moment at which an utterance should occur serves to facilitate fluency.

Probing further, Hutchinson and Navarre (1977) studied the effects of metronomic pacing on the aerodynamic patterns of the speech of stutterers and nonstutterers. They found that the

> . . . metronome signal not only slows the overall reading rate but increases the duration of initial phonetic elements in each utterance. Therefore the stutterer has not only the time afforded by the overall reduction in reading rate but also the prolonged time period of the initial phoneme to monitor, control, and adjust the vocal tract events, thereby reducing the possibility of stuttering (1977, p. 203).

They felt that the additional time taken to produce the initial consonants allowed the stutterer to achieve better synchronization of his motor commands. Not all of the metronomic studies show that speech rate is slowed under this condition. Barber's (1940) stutterers showed a marked decrease in stuttering even when the metronome was set at 184 beats per minute. Hanna and Morris (1977) found the metronomic effect to be independent of speech rate.

Other authors have also noted the fluency enhancing effect of metronomic speaking and have used it in their therapy programs. Greenberg (1970) employed it with young stutterers and found that the metronome reduced stutterings whether or not they were instructed to pace their speaking with its beat. This result might therefore be interpreted as being due to distraction but Silverman and Trotter (1974) and Trotter (1976) showed that extended use of a miniaturized metronome continued to reduce disfluencies even after periods as long as two years. Berman and Brady (1973), in a questionnaire study of 28 clinicians who had used the device, found that 73 per cent of the stutterers showed improvement in fluency.

Finally, Andrews and Harris (1964) report the results of lengthy training in syllable timed speech. Immediate fluency was usually obtained after a few trials, but the permanent carry-over into normal communication was unsatisfactory, probably because normal speaking is not regularly rhythmical. Children responded better than adults. Brandon and Harris (1967) claim that 18 of their 28 stutterers who received intensive training in syllable tapped speech showed a 60-per cent improvement after 18 months. This is hardly spectacular. Wohl (1968) gives a favorable evaluation to the use of an electric metronomic device by stutterers and several such devices have been patented and are presently for sale. In more recent articles in Australian journals, Andrews (1965, 1967) expresses dissatisfaction with syllable timed speech as the sole method of therapy because of the relapse problem. Most stutterers are simply not willing to speak in this unnatural way for any length of time, although a few of them may use a measured form of utterance to tide them over emergencies.

Nevertheless, the rhythm effect has important implications for a theory of stuttering. In our opinion rhythm works because it facilitates the timing of motoric patterns which are prone to asynchrony. The metronomic beat may drive the central mechanism responsible for programming the sound and syllabic coordinations. It may open the reticular or cortical gates with predictable regularity. It has been suggested by Andrews and Harris (1964) that the interval of silence between each timed word or syllable is long enough to overcome any built-in delay which might be operating within the servo system. It is also possible that each word's motor configuration has a dominant feature about which all the other movements are integrated and that this one serves as a surrogate for the whole sequence. If so, the beat of an accessory timing device coinciding with this feature (whether it be the breath pulse or a jaw movement acting as a prime mover) may thus facilitate the production of a nonfractured word. Most complex motor skills, such as a golf swing, involve such a dominant feature which times the integration of the whole sequence. All these remarks are, of course, the sheerest speculation. We do not know how or why the use of an accessory timing device helps to integrate the motor patterning of a word. We merely know that it does.

THE STUTTERER'S TIMING DEVICES

The stutterer knows this, too. Many of his most abnormal behaviors can be regarded as timing devices. He jerks his head or jaw; he protrudes his lips or tongue; he makes a sudden abdominal contraction; he produces a sudden surge of tension in some part of the speech mechanism. Examined closely, they are found to be ballistic movements usually used to time the moment of speech attempt or to effect a release from postponement or fixation. The use of a wide variety of "starters" has long been noted in the phenomenology of stuttering. A case could be made for the position that even the syllabic repetitions so characteristic of stuttering are searching behaviors which seek the precise timing required to utter a unified word.

It is also interesting to consider the common tendency of stutterers to postpone the speech attempt on feared words and to use that pause for tiny covert rehearsals of the motor patterns involved (Van Riper, 1936). Time gaining behaviors are very frequently manifested by stutterers and they are very vulnerable to time pressure. They stutter more frequently when required to speak swiftly (Johnson and Rosen 1937; Beech and Fransella 1968). Stutterers often find that if they can postpone long enough on a feared word, it may be spoken fluently. One explanation for this is that stutterers through covert rehearsal may finally discover the timing they need, and that when they are deprived of that opportunity for rehearsal, they have little opportunity to search for the timing.

THERAPEUTIC TIMING PROCEDURES

In addition to the use of metronomic speech, other workers have employed other methods to improve the motor timing of stutterers. In Germany, Fernau-Horn (1960) trained her stutterers to synchronize deliberately the breathing, vocalization, and articulation components of their utterances (ablauf training). Svend Smith (1955) sought to improve the basic timing abilities of his stutterers by having them master intricate patterns of chanted syllables. Tugova (1968) describes some of the Russian methods to improve the coordination and rhythmic abilities of preschool children. In the early years of our clinical practice, we ourselves sought to improve the timing abilities of stutterers directly as witness this quotation:

> Included in our rhythmic training was an apparatus we devised from an old phonograph, which carried discs with make and break contacts so that various temporal patterns of clicks could be produced and repeated at different speeds. This was connected with a clock counter and with a device which the stutterer held in or against his mouth so that he could jawbite or tongue thrust. If his jaw bite were made absolutely in unison with the clicks produced by the phonograph's contact discs, the counter was activated. If the stutterer's timing was off, the counter did not count. We thus had an apparatus which we could use to train the stutterer in rhythmokinesis. The stutterers called this the rhythm machine, and tried to improve their scores within a certain time limit and at different speeds. Some of them made gains which seemed to us almost incredible and these gains seemed to be reflected in improved fluency. Others, however, who made little gains in rhythm scores also improved in fluency. We used this for several years but finally discarded it. There was magic in it and suggestion, and we wanted to minimize both. (Van Riper 1958, p. 291).

A few other timing facilitating methods may be described, including Froeschels's breath-chewing technique which perhaps owed its usefulness to the strong jaw movements with which the sounds and syllables and words are attempted concurrently. Travis and Bryngelson's recommendation of simultaneous talking-and-writing therapy in which the stutterer makes the speech attempt in unison with the dominant stroke of the letter that initiates the written word is another case in point. Also, the use of voluntary stuttering in which the first syllable of the word is deliberately repeated several times before the word is actually attempted seems to be based upon timing and so, too, does Johnson's "bounce." Many of the breathing and vocalization rituals used in treating stutterers may also be viewed as timing devices for integrating the basic synergies of sound production.

CHORAL OR UNISON SPEECH

One of the curious features about the disorder is that most, but not all, stutterers find a marked decrease in stuttering when they read or speak the same words in unison with another speaker. Choral reading and unison speaking have been used for centuries to help stutterers achieve a precarious fluency, one that shows little carry-over, however. This fluency facilitator has been investigated by many workers. Johnson and Rosen (1937) attributed it to the imposed rhythm of the model's speech,

Barber (1939) to distraction, and Eisenson and Wells (1942) to reduced meaningfulness (propositionality). Lee (1951) felt that the decrease in stuttering in unison speaking was due to the stutterer being given a nondistorted feedback signal at the moment he was organizing the motor plan for the word. Some support for this belief was given by Barr and Carmel (1970) who showed that stutterers could immediately release themselves from their blockings if another speaker spoke the word on which they were having difficulty. Pattie and Knight (1944), who showed that stutterers read as well in unison over the telephone as in the presence of the model speaker, explained the effect as due to pacing.

The last explanation appears to us to be most convincing, though perhaps the other (with the additional factor of masking) may also play a part. As the stutterer utters his or her words in unison with the other speaker, the latter's utterance may serve as a timing signal. At any rate, the effect is dramatic. Many very severe stutterers can read in unison with another speaker with almost complete fluency, sometimes even when reading a foreign language they do not understand, and even when the model reads very softly. We have repeatedly demonstrated that the stutterer does not even have to say the exact words spoken by the model. The stutterer becomes more fluent when the latter merely speaks only the vowels of the words in the passage. Cherry and Sayers (1956) showed that when reversed speech or gibberish were fed into the stutterer's ears, he became more fluent when speaking concurrently. These findings make us cautious in attributing the decrease in stuttering under choral conditions to pace setting but it is possible that the stutterer may still be able to time enough speech attempts with the syllabic pluses of the model to facilitate timing.

Wingate (1969, 1976) has been critical of the pacing explanation for the decrease in stuttering during choral reading, claiming that under this condition stutterers modify their vocalization, slow down their speech rate by prolonging syllable durations and increase its loudness and that these are what produce the fluency. Attempts to test this position have resulted in equivocal results. Ingham and Carroll (1977) and Ingham and Packman (1979) found that some stutterers did change their manner of speaking according to Wingate's prediction but that others did not. Adams and Ramig (1980) found no increase in vocal sound pressure level (loudness) in choral reading and that stutterers decreased their syllabic vowel durations. In Poland, Adamczyck, Kuniszyk-Jozkowiak, and Sadowska (1976) showed that only a slight decrease in rate occurred in choral reading, hardly enough to account for the sudden decrease in stuttering. Hanley (1980) examined the "fluent" speech of stutterers produced by choral reading and found no significant differences in rate or loudness. He did find that his cinefluoroscopic pictures showed that the jaw duty cycle, synchrony of jaw and tongue tip onsets, and peak velocity of jaw closing movements were consistently related to the fluency enhancement under choral reading. This may be interpreted to support the view that the stutterer's timing improves when speaking in unison.

SHADOWING

Stutterers can often repeat fluently a word after another speaker has said it. Again there may be many reasons for this, but it is possible that the integrated utterance of the model may provide the timing model the stutterer needs. At any rate, we have a few studies showing that "shadowing," the technique in which the stutterer replicates automatically and immediately what the model speaker is saying, creates a marked or total elimination of stuttering. Colin Cherry in his book on *Human Communication* (1957) describes shadowing as follows:

> A tape recording is made of a reading from a passage of prose and played through headphones to a listener; the listener is instructed to repeat what he hears concurrently, in a subdued or whispered voice. He is then listening and speaking at the same time, but this is found to be an extremely simple task. His spoken repetition tends to be in irregular detached phrases and, with most people and most texts, is given in a singularly emotionless voice as though intoning. It seems as though he is unable to copy the emotional content of the words he hears and, since he is following so close upon the heels of these words, he is unable to see far enough ahead to create his own emotional content. He mouths the words like an automaton and extracts little semantic content, if any. If questioned subsequently, he can say little about the text, especially if it is at all "deep" or difficult. He cannot, for example, act upon a complicated set of instructions if he receives them under such conditions. He is almost in the situation of a parrot which has been taught to speak and can say "Wipe your feet!" or "Go to hell!" without having thoughts of dirty shoes or of damnation (1957, p. 279).

Cherry and Sayers (1956) reported an intensive investigation of the effects of masking noise on stuttering which included a further study of shadowing. They found that when stutterers shadowed the speech of another speaker they had nearly normal fluency. Cherry and Marland (1956) also found an almost total "suppression" of stuttering and suggested that the technique be used more widely in therapy. Walton and Black (1958) applied the method to telephone conversation with some success though this later comment by a subject who participated in the experiment may indicate some of the difficulty in carry-over most clinicians have discovered when using shadowing:

> When I came to the hospital I was extremely skeptical of success . . . but on discharge I am quite convinced that I have gotten into a healthier and better method of speech. I am certain that my general level has been maintained at its peak . . . I am still apprehensive about the telephone, but I no longer consider it an unsurmountable difficulty. I am convinced that I can get over it and that my telephone conversation can be brought up to my conversational level.

Kelham and McHale (1966) report striking success using intensive shadowing therapy with 28 stutterers, most of whom were children.

Finally, Sergeant (1961) trained subjects in "concurrent repetition" of stimulus words. He showed that their fluency and intelligibility improved, but that slower rates of stimulus presentation were needed and also that those subjects who had a better rhythmic sense profited the most from the shadowing. As in unison speaking, the improvement in fluency brought on by shadowing may be explained in many ways, but the pace-setting characteristic of the procedure should not be ignored.

SINGING

Most stutterers show none of the broken words they usually do when singing, although some of them, including the author, have occasionally experienced some minor difficulty. It is always surprising to the lay listener to discover the stutterer singing perfectly the same words that a moment previously he was unable to utter without great struggle. Nadoleczny (1927) and Witt (1925) showed that less than 10 per cent of their cases showed any stuttering while singing. Fletcher (1928), Johnson and Rosen (1937), Bloodstein (1950) and Klemm (1966) also found fluency when the stutterer sang.

Investigating the effect of singing more closely, Healey, Mallard, and Adams (1976) found that when shifting from reading to singing both the stutterers and nonstutterers lengthened the duration of their vocalizations as expected and that the stutterers stuttered less while singing. Colcord and Adams (1979) found the same result.

Wingate (1969) makes a pertinent comment about the phenomenon. He points out that unlike metronomic speech it is not the regularity of the rhythmic beats in singing which accounts for the fluency but some other factor involving time and intonation:

> The influence of singing has been interpreted as a special instance of the effect of rhythm. However, it is questionable whether the effect of singing can be explained adequately in this way. Although a meter of some kind does underlie song, the beat is frequently not clearly evident and the words of the song often do not have a close correspondence to the melody, which expresses the meter. Also, most songs do not have a simple redundant pattern; the tune varies, and many times a syllable may extend beyond one beat of the "time" (meter) or a beat may contain more than one syllable. However—and this is probably of critical significance—syllabic units do correspond to the musical notes. It seems likely that the salutary effect of singing might also be accounted for in terms more fundamental than that it contains a rhythm. Again, we can invoke the interpretation introduced earlier as providing what seems to be a more cogent explanation: in singing, a person intentionally emphasizes vocalization to express a pattern of stresses centering on the syllable nuclei (1969, p. 678).

We agree with Wingate but would emphasize the timing factor inherent in the "pattern of stresses centering on the syllabic nuclei," and the correspondence of the timing of syllables with the musical notes.

PROSODY

In another article Wingate (1966) showed that stuttering adaptation might be explained in part by the practice effect from repeatedly making the same transitional articulatory and phonatory coordinations. This practice effect could be attributed to improvement in timing the motor coordinations involved in the articulatory or the phonatory features of the transitions. Agnello (1966) showed that stutterers had substantial difficulty in producing the complicated transitions required in speaking tongue twisters. Besozzi and Adams (1969) added further support to this position when they found in effect that significantly more adaptation occurred when passages were always read orally than when some of the readings were read silently.

Brenner, Perkins, and Soderberg (1972) found that oral rehearsals of sentences significantly reduced stuttering. Frank and Bloodstein (1971) concluded that the decrease in stuttering in repeated adaptation readings resulted from the rehearsal of motor plans. As we have seen in our chapter on Loci and Adaptation, unfamiliar words, which have had less motor practice, tend to be stuttered upon more frequently than familiar words. Indirect as this evidence is, it still points another finger in the direction of stuttering as a disorder characterized by motor mistiming.

It is very difficult to evaluate the degree of support all of this scattered and often indirectly focused research lends to the position that stuttering is a disorder of disrupted timing. It has revealed that the possibility for temporal disruption certainly exists. It has shown that normal speakers' fluency may be disrupted by altering the time relationships of feedback. The imposition of procedures which facilitate the timing of sounds and syllables and words cause the stutterer to become *suddenly* very fluent. Nevertheless we can only conclude that our position is very far from being proven. At the present time it constitutes only a provocative hypothesis, but one which should generate some important research. Although evidence for the hypothesis is far from satisfactory, the same statement could be made about stuttering as a neurosis, as a product of learning, as the effect of organicity, or as the reflection of servo system instability. Perhaps the major contribution of this view of stuttering is its ability to explain some of the basic phenomena and to synthesize the other concepts of its nature. To this we now address ourselves.

THE POSSIBILITY FOR MISTIMING

The motoric configuration which produces a given word is so complex as to defy detailed description. Over 70 muscles may be involved and each of these must get its appropriate nervous impulses at the required moment in the sequence if the word is to be spoken without disruption. Respiration, phonation, and articulation must be coordinated with amazing precision and each of these component systems requires the reciprocal contraction-relaxation of antagonistic muscle groups. Bilateral synchronization is also necessary since the musculatures involved are located on both the right and left sides of the body. Moreover, in order to achieve successful integration and a smooth flow of unfolding speech sounds, the motor correlates of the component phonemes (the propemes or articulemes) must be preprogrammed so as to provide the necessary coarticulation. In the utterance of a word, the phonemes do not resemble beads on a string or even the links of a chain. Each phoneme is modified by its antecedents and by its consequents as spectrographic analysis shows. They must be blended sequentially. Even as the allophone of /s/ in the word *see* differs spectrographically from the allophone of /s/ in the word *sue*, so also do the motoric equivalents (the distinctive articulatory gestures or allopropes) of these two sounds differ from each other. The postures of the tongue and lips are altered to permit more effective transitions. All of these activities occur in time, the temporal constraints being in milliseconds. If this description of the motoric configurations involved in the production of a word seems unduly elaborate, it is not so at all, but instead it is woefully sketchy. Our purpose has been merely to demonstrate that the possibility for fracturing exists, to show that the mistiming of these simultaneous and successive motor activities could produce a broken word, that is, cause it to be spoken stutteringly.

THE SYNERGIES OF UTTERANCE

If it seems incredible, in view of this complexity of coordination, that any of us could ever speak a word fluently, we should remember that some of the necessary coordinations are inborn and that we have been spending most of our waking hours perfecting the others. We do not need to be taught how to inhale or to exhale or to produce voice any more than a dog has to learn how to bark, although we may need to discover how to modify these functions to provide the repertoire of sounds we need for effective communication. Long before the child has uttered his first word, he has not only mastered the basic synergistic coordination of respiration, voice, and articulation to produce a wide variety of vowellike sounds, but also in his babbling he has acquired the ability to produce syllables of many kinds and to repeat them. That these building blocks of motor speech are unfolded and evolved rather than learned seems very plausible, for even deaf babies show them.

This is not to say that all the vowels or all the syllables in our repertoire are unlearned and merely the product of maturation. The author first produced the Swedish vowel /ø/ at the age of 60 and he had to *learn* how to do so, but the basic coordinations which produced his early vowels before he was a year old served as models which he could modify to make that strange sound. He did not have to learn to coordinate the basic synergies of breathing and phonation; he did have to explore new movements of the tongue and lips.

HOW THE MOTORIC PATTERNS
OF WORDS ARE LEARNED

In much the same fashion, children mast⌣ the intricate coordinations involved in producing their first words. They begin with the coordinations they already have and modify them until a recognizable word is emitted. This does not mean that they additively produce a series of phonemic segments like cockleshells all in a row. Instead the child tries the word as a whole, seeking from the first a unified motor sequence, and modifying each successive approximation until the entire acoustic product becomes communicatively acceptable. In so doing, he uses motor patterns he has used before. As the reduplicative nature of the baby's first words (Mama, bye-bye, Daddy), and as a motoric analysis of any of his first approximations will demonstrate, the learning of a new word is a shaping process. At first, there may be only vocalization with appropriate intonation or syllabification. For the new word "Santa Claus" the child may only be able to coordinate a sequence of vowels (æ:a) but the æ is usually nasalized and accented. Then the following series of progressive approximations may occur, but not hout temporary regressions:

$$\tilde{æ}{:}a \rightarrow æn\partial {:}a \rightarrow \tilde{æ}nt\partial \, ta \rightarrow ænt\partial \, ka \rightarrow tæn\partial \, t\partial \rightarrow$$
$$sæn\partial \, ka \rightarrow sænt\partial \, kaz \rightarrow sænt\partial \, kl\mathupsilon z$$

THE ROLE OF FEEDBACK
IN ACQUIRING NEW WORDS

This shaping process requires feedback. Auditory feedback is particularly important in the learning of a new word, since the child must vary his motor patterns until their product matches the model presented to his ears by his parents. There are many difficulties to be overcome in this shaping, matching process. The auditory model must be discriminated in terms of its distinctive features and held in memory storage so that comparison can take place. The child must be able to discriminate the acoustic variations in his own speech output, and to recognize whether they are coming closer to the model or moving away from it. This is complicated by the fact that he hears himself not only by airborne side-tone but also by bone and tissue transmission of sound all mixed together in a most complicated pattern. Thus, even when the word sounds like the model to others, the child himself hears it somewhat differently. Nevertheless, when the parents indicate that the child has produced the word acceptably, this distorted auditory configuration comes to serve as the internalized template of the word. As this is being achieved, the child also comes to discriminate the major features of contact, posture, and movement which characterize the motor sequences of the model, and in this manner the correlated kinesthetic-tactile-proprioceptive feedback also becomes patterned. When it does, the child can be said to have learned how to say the word. The child now can whisper it or even mouth it in pantomime. The motoric patterning of the word has become stabilized enough to enable him to use it at will.

STABILITY OF THE MOTOR SEQUENCES OF WORDS

If stuttering consists essentially of broken motor sequences involved in the production of a word, as we have maintained, then some discussion of the stability of these particular motor patterns should be useful. We are not surprised to find the onset of stuttering occurring very early in life in most of our cases. The motor plans for the coordinations required to produce are complex, and there are thousands of words the child must learn. We recognize his early fumbling, stumbling efforts to integrate his speech as natural consequences of the learning process. Parents rarely become concerned when they hear broken words at this time. Stuttering is seldom diagnosed as a disorder when the child is still in the one-word sentence stage of development, even when gaps, repetitions, and prolongations are present. At this time we expect his motor sequences to show some instability. In addition, the amount of interference to communication probably is less apparent when a child has difficulty in emitting a single word than if that word were embedded in a sentence.

STABILITY AS A FUNCTION OF PRACTICE

The stability of a motor sequence, as the research on motor skills demonstrates, depends mainly on three factors: its history of usage (the practice effect), its complexity, and the effectiveness of the feedback systems used to monitor it. Children always show more broken words than adults, but even adults will falter frequently when saying unfamiliar or foreign words that they have not said before. Children who are delayed in speech acquisition often go through a period of stuttering before they achieve the fluent use of language. We might state as another general principle that, at least in children, the more often a word has been correctly spoken in the past the more stable it will be and the less it will tend to be stuttered. Conversely, for all stutterers of any age the more often a word has been spoken stutteringly in the past, the more likely it is to be spoken brokenly in the future. In the latter instance, conditioned disruption may also play a part. In any event, even in children who show no awareness of their stuttering, the general principle holds that the stability of the motor pattern of a word depends in part on practice.

STABILITY AS A FUNCTION OF THE COMPLEXITY
OF COORDINATION

Secondly, most of what we know about motor learning suggests that the more complex the word's coordinative pattern, the more difficult it will be to stabilize. The basic research on this is still to be done and it may be difficult to do. We would predict that if positional effects are controlled, that is, if the first words of sentences are disregarded, more stuttering will occur on polysyllabic words than on monosyllabic ones and on those whose transitional junctures are more complex than on those words in which they are not. About the only evidence we have is that adult stutterers seem to have more hesitation phenomena on longer than on shorter words when the position of the word in the sentence is eliminated as a factor. They have more trouble with tongue twisters. The old example of the word "statistics" as a problem in integration even for normal speakers is also a case in point. To state it generally, *the more complex the motor sequence, the more unstable it tends to be.*

THE ROLE OF FEEDBACK IN STABILITY

Probably of greater importance is the role of feedback. It is difficult to walk smoothly in the dark. When vision is added to proprioception in the monitoring of this complex motor activity, the coordinations of walking are much better integrated. Yet the blind can learn to walk smoothly, although even then they probably stumble more than those with sight. In speaking, we also have two major feedback systems, the auditory and the proprioceptive,* to help us speak fluently. When either is impaired (for example, by DAF or by deep anesthesia of the articulatory areas), we speak with more difficulty.

In speaking, we rely to some degree both on auditory and proprioceptive feedback systems. The young child probably needs the auditory feedback to maintain the integrity of his motor patterns of speech more than the adult does. As MacKay (1968) and Buxton (1968) have shown rather clearly, younger children are more affected by DAF than older ones or adults. This is probably to be expected since the child's first words were learned primarily by listening to himself and others, and by matching his output against the acoustic models provided by others. At first the child still needs ears to assist his mouth if he hopes to speak fluently. But speech can be monitored by proprioception alone once the motor patterns have become stabilized. We can speak fluently even in the presence of loud

---

* In this discussion we shall frequently use the words *proprioceptive* and *proprioception* more loosely and generally than their correct usage would require. We include in these terms not only proprioception but the correlated tactile and kinesthetic features. To have eternally to spell out the whole array whenever we must describe this form of somesthetic feedback seems too awkward.

masking noise, and the person who becomes deaf does no
The fact that we can pantomime a word without vocali
that auditory feedback is not essential to the production o
the proprioceptive motor patterns have become well inte
reasonable therefore to conclude that when a person o
sequential movements of a word without the aid of self-hea ...g, the motor
pattern of that word has become fairly well stabilized.

A corollary to this might be that the more distortion there is in the
auditory feedback the more likely it will be that some stuttering will occur.
Unlike adults, whose motor patterns are stabilized enough to let them
hear what they are saying rather than how they are saying it, children are
doubtless much more vulnerable to auditory feedback distortion. This is
probably why children have more broken words. The possibility for such
distortion seems almost to have been built into the auditory feedback
system. The multiplicity of auditory feedback channels makes disruption
likely. Perhaps this is why most of us switch as swiftly as we can to
proprioception as the major monitor of speech, and use our self-hearing
instead as an accessory control system. As we have made clear in Chapter
14 a strong case can be made that stuttering is the result of auditory
interference in the servo system. Let us tentatively submit therefore
another principle: *the more stable the motor sequence of a word, the more feedback
distortion it can undergo before it becomes disrupted.* Even under DAF, not all
words show breakage or changes in the programming of the sequential
movements. This is why no stutterer stutters on every word he utters. The
motor patterns of some words are more stable than others.

THE STABILITY HIERARCHY

Thus far we have been speaking primarily of broken words, of the
disrupted motor sequence patterns at the word level. But there are
integrated configurations of sequential movements both within the word
and beyond it. Words are made up of syllables and sounds, but our usual
utterances are composed of words, phrases, and sentences. Thus there
exists at least five levels at which fluency breaks may occur: at the level of
the sound, the syllable, the word, the phrase, and the sentence. As motor
configurations, however, these levels differ in their vulnerability to disruption and fracturing. To put it another way, they differ in stability, and
the hierarchy of stability may be represented from *greatest to least* stability
in terms of the following order: sounds, syllables, words, phrases, and
sentences.

The stability of the motor integrations at any of these levels probably
reflects the past history of usage. Sounds are more stable than syllables,
syllables than words, and words than phrases, because they simply have
been used more frequently. The total number of phonemic motor patterns
are fewer than all the available number of syllables. Thus inevitably they

used more often. Again there are fewer syllables in one's repertoire than there are words, and so the motor patterns of syllables get practiced more often than words do. Also since there are many fewer words than all the different phrases, or sentences which can be assembled, the words must have a longer past history of motor integration (and thus motoric stability) than that for phrases. Phrases have simply occurred less frequently.* The point we are making is that the motor patterns of speech differ in stability and resistance to disruption according to their history of usage and their level of segmental integration.

STABILITY AS RELATED TO SPEECH DEVELOPMENT

The Stability of Sounds

Now let us consider this in another way—in terms of the development of speech. The first motor speech patterns to be integrated seem to be the vowel sounds. They appear first as the cries and the cooing comfort sounds of the baby. As any parent knows, they are thoroughly practiced—especially in the dark hours of the night. The basic respiratory, laryngeal, and articulatory coordinations involved in these cries and early sounds are probably patterned in time inherently. Differentiation soon occurs, however, and the baby learns very early to phonate and articulate on exhalation rather than on inhalation and so on. For some time, the primitive sounds of crying and cooing comprise the bulk of the infant's utterance. Sounds are motorically simple compared to cv, vc, or cvc syllables, since little transitional or coarticulation phenomena are required in their production. Decerebrate animals and humans alike are able to produce sounds. The vowel sounds especially seem to be organized around the archetypal breath group. They have strong acoustic power and doubtless activate the first servo responses of the auditory system. In the life history of the individual, these sounds have the longest usage.

Since vowel sounds are probably the most highly integrated, the most basic of the elementary coordinations involved in speaking, they are the most stable of all the motor patterns used in speech and accordingly they are the most resistant to disruption. It has even been suggested that they are laid down in the cortex or its substructures as reverberatory circuits, deeply engrained in the functioning of the central nervous system. Since the temporal patterns of simultaneous and successive muscular contractions found in vowel utterance seem to be more stable, perhaps this is why less stuttering seems to occur on words beginning with vowels.

---

* Certain phrases such as "bread and butter" or sentences such as "How are you?" have also had similar overlearnings so that they may become as motorically stable as single words. They too can become unitary motor automatisms almost like single words, and their integrations are so stable as even to resist the disruptions of aphasia.

Stability of Syllables

The next most stable motor configuration of speech is that of the syllable, and it characterizes the babbling stage of speech development. That it exists as an integrated and basic motor pattern is demonstrated by the fact all babies babble syllabically. Like the sound, the syllable too can be evoked by electrical stimulation of the cortex. There is some evidence that the syllable, too, may be represented cortically or subcortically by some sort of reverberatory pattern. Penfield and Rasmussen (1949), for example, found that a syllable such as "te" would be repeated and continue involuntarily until the electrical stimulation was turned off. Chase (1958) found that syllable repetition can be facilitated by recycling the delayed feedback at appropriate delays. Syllabic repetition often appears under DAF when words, phrases, and sentences are disrupted. Many of the first words of infants are reiterative, composed of repeated syllables. Also, the diadochokinesis of the same syllable is faster than that of different syllables. Sonograms also show that syllables are unitary configurations, not mere successions of discrete sounds. They are closely conjoined and coarticulated so as to comprise highly integrated patterns. It is also perhaps of some interest here to observe that aphasics who cannot say a polysyllabic word can often tap out the number of syllables which comprise it or produce a jargon word of the same number of syllables.*

HOW SYLLABLES ARE INTEGRATED

Syllables, as Stetson (1951) and others have shown, occur as entities. They can be distinguished not only through auditory perception but also by examining the variations in air pressure and airflow. They can be distinguished both electromyographically as well as sonographically. Syllables seem to be timed by a sudden breath pulse produced by the contraction of the respiratory muscles. This sudden respiratory contraction may serve as the basic signal in the proprioceptive feedback system controlling the timing of the syllables as a whole. Hardy (1967) simultaneously recorded respiratory muscle action potentials and speech signals and concluded that there was strong evidence of "syllabic pulses by both thoracic and abdominal muscles." Hoshiko (1960) showed electromyographically that the single vowel /a/ or the syllable "pup" both at slow and rapid rates were initiated by a precisely timed sequence of musculature contractions, always in the following order: internal intercostals, rectus abdominis, and the external intercostals. Again we see how important the time relationships must be in syllable production.

* We suspect that even among syllables there are differences in the ability of their motor patterns and that the stability hierarchy (from most stability to least) is represented by the following order: v, vc, cv, and cvc. Certainly the relative frequencies of stuttering on these different types of syllables seems to indicate that this is plausible, but again the basic research is still to be done.

However, it is also possible that a specific lip, jaw, or tongue movement may also function as the surrogate for timing the entire array of simultaneous and successive muscular contractions that comprise the motor pattern of the entire syllable. Lashley (1951) long ago made the observation that there simply was not sufficient transit time to permit the return flow of impulses from the peripheral muscles to serve as feedback signals in the sequencing of the movements needed to speak a word. Lenneberg (1967) makes the same point. However, if one motor gesture may serve as the representative of the whole sequence, we can understand how syllables and words can be monitored by servocontrol.*

The utterance of a syllable demands a series of transitional movements, each one affected by its predecessor and by its successor. They must occur in a precise and definite temporal order. These syllabic sequences are wholes, like the expert fingering of a musical phrase in piano playing. Each movement flows into the next. The expert pianist often uses a head movement, assumes a complex wrist posture or uses some other way of integrating the sequence of flying fingers. The timing of the successive movements is not done deliberately or individually, but by timing the sequence as a whole. The pianist's nod or gesture or postural change seems to serve as the feedback representative of the entire series of finger movements. It too is a part of the entire motor sequence, but it is the controlling feature. When it is right, the entire sequence flows smoothly. When it is wrong, the sequence is spoiled. We do not know enough about these bits of behavior which serve as the integrating surrogates or prime movers of motor sequences, but we know that they must occur.

Like piano playing, but infinitely more complex, speech too consists of motor sequences. The production of a word or syllable requires motor patterns some of which resemble chords, timed simultaneously; while others follow themselves in time like the notes of a melody. The timing is of the essence, even as it is in piano playing, or swinging a golf club.

The motor integration of a syllable requires coarticulation. Innumerable sonographic studies have demonstrated that separate phonemes are not chained together serially to comprise a syllable, but that a fusion of components occurs instead. The work of Liberman (1967) and his colleagues of the Haskins group show that the initial consonant of a cv syllable, for example, affects the transition frequencies in the second formant of the succeeding vowel. Moreover, the particular vowel within that syllable also affects the production of the initial consonant. Some preliminary motor "instructions" must therefore have been decided upon before the syllable is uttered. To cite but two of the studies, Daniloff and Moll (1968) demonstrated that coarticulation of lip protrusion may occur and extend over as many as three preceding consonants in a sequence prior to the production of a vowel, as exemplified by such a word as "screw." And MacNeilage and De Clerk (1969), in a more elaborate

---

* An alternative explanation views sequential motor patterns as governed by motor commands which are programmed prior to attempt and which obviate the necessity for feedback. See S. W. Keele, "Movement Control in Skilled Motor Performance," *Psychological Bulletin 70* (1968):387–403.

investigation using cinefluorograms and electromyograms, found that the motor control of a later syllabic component was partially influenced by the characteristics of the preceding one, and that the reverse influence also occurred. The programming of sequential speech must demand an exactitude of timing which seems almost incomprehensible. That the stutterer fails in this timing of coarticulation is evidenced by the studies of Stromsta (1965) and Agnello and Buxton (1966). It is also of interest in this connection that Rawnsley and Harris (1954) found that normal speakers under delayed auditory feedback showed the same lack of normal formant transitions in their repeated syllables. One of the puzzling features about stuttering is its marked reduction during pantomimed speech or whispering. While this could be accounted for on the basis of a simplified synergy (the absence of voice and/or airflow) we may have a clue in the work of Schwartz (1967) who found that the average duration of syllables in whispering was significantly longer than when they were vocalized. Perhaps more time was available to permit synchronization in this case.

We feel that the most important feedback signal in the integration of a word is probably the accented syllable of that word. If that syllable is produced correctly, then the word will be integrated. Stutterers stutter less on unaccented syllables. Why do stutterers repeat the accented syllables over and over again? It is our belief that the syllables that are repeated are not the appropriate ones, not the proper syllables that fit the word wholes. Note how often the repeated syllables end in the schwa or neutral vowel. Stutterers say "Kuh-Kuh-Kuh-Katy." *Kuh* will never make a Katy. The syllable must be repeated and revised until it carries the transitional components that fit the word pattern. Searchingly the stutterers keep repeating it until by chance, or the decline of anxiety or expectation or for other reasons, they finally produce the *Ka* that belongs to Katy. Note the speed of the syllabic repetition, the instant recoil which often occurs. These stuttering syllabic repetitions are usually not produced at the same tempo as the syllables of the stutterer's nonstuttered speech. They are usually faster, jerkier. Often they are accompanied by other movements that add nothing to the possibility that the word can be spoken as a whole. They become invested *with tension* and this itself must create an abnormal feedback. If words are integrated in their motor sequences by some motoric feature of the dominant syllable, that syllable, that syllabic motor configuration must be normal, not abnormal, if it is to be spoken normally. If it isn't, then the syllable must be said again and again. When this occurs, a reverberatory oscillation is often created which subsides only when the stutterer feels that the needed timing of coarticulation has been achieved.

The stability of the motor patterns that comprise a syllable are of far reaching importance in stuttering. Their integrity determines whether the person will speak with broken words. Usually they are very well integrated, almost as solidly as the vowel sounds. Yet they, too, are vulnerable to disruption, especially by auditory interference if the speaker relies too much on self-hearing for the control of speech, and not enough on touch, kinesthesia, and proprioception. Syllables can be broken or temporarily distorted. When they are, the person will speak stutteringly.

THE MOTOR INTEGRATION OF WORDS

As the syllable seems to be on a unitary level of coordinative integration somewhat less stable than that of the sound, so also the word seems to be less stable than the syllable. Let us offer some commentary on the integration of whole words.

Following the babbling stage, the child enters the one-word sentence stage. To recapitulate, he now speaks in motor sequences which require the combination of sounds and syllables into larger units. He remains in this stage for some time before learning to combine these word units into phrases and sentences. During this period, the motor patterns of these single words are practiced repeatedly and are strongly reinforced through communicative facilitation and social rewards. Their sequences of muscular contractions are programmed in time and are monitored both proprioceptively and acoustically by servo processes. That they are units is shown by the pauses and other hesitation phenomena which occur much more often at morphemic boundaries than within the word. In normal speakers there are fewer part-word repetitions or pauses than whole-word repetitions, and more pauses occur before or after the utterance of a word than within its boundaries.

Words become unitary configurations of acoustic and proprioceptive sequences. They are mastered by a series of approximations. The child may omit the final sound at first, or use an incorrect initial sound, but eventually he learns the pattern of movements necessary to produce the unit which his listeners require for communicative interchange. The unitary nature of words is demonstrated by the fact that words can be predicted by the forward guessing devised by Shannon (1951), in which successively presented sounds in the sequence increasingly facilitate the recognition of the target word. Aphasics can often say a single word when they cannot use it in a meaningful phrase or sentence. Meaningful words can be spoken at faster diadochokinetic rates than nonsense words composed of the same sounds and syllables. The specific sequences of motor activities that comprise an individual word are practiced so often in the course of a person's life history that they finally become highly automatic and unitary.

THE MOTOR CONFIGURATIONS
OF SUPRA-MORPHEMIC SEGMENTS

With few exceptions, the motor patterns for phrases and sentences are not learned as are those for words, nor do they evolve through maturation as the configurations of sounds and syllables do. Although they, too, form unitary wholes, as shown by the modification of prior words by later ones as well as by the location of pauses and other hesitation phenomena, their bonding is less strong. One almost has to memorize a series of sentences before he can eliminate all the breaks from them. Normal speech is full of fluency breaks of one kind of another. We are not surprised to find that normal speech is full of disfluencies at the morphemic, phrase, or sentence boundaries. These supra-morphemic segments demand motor configurations that have rarely been repeated often enough to permit stabilization. They are generated rather than learned. They unfold as a result of constant decision making. This is why society rarely labels fluency breaks at morpheme, phrase, or sentence boundaries as stuttering. We expect some faltering in spontaneous verbal formulation. It seems quite normal to hesitate occasionally in the linking of words to form phrases, or phrases to form sentences, but a different situation exists when breaks occur too often *within* words. We expect the particular motor sequence which creates a word to be integrated, to be rather stable. When we find a speaker with broken words, with too many syllabic repetitions, or one who struggles to utter a sound, we sense abnormality and call it stuttering. It is for this reason that Wendell Johnson's valiant attempt to equate all kinds of disfluencies failed to be convincing even before the research demonstrated that he was wrong.

EFFECTS OF STRESS

We should like to offer the proposition that *the greater the stress, the more likely it is that the sequencing of speech will be disrupted at a more basic level of integration.* Thus, under mild degrees of stress (communicative, emotional, or cybernetic) we will find hesitation phenomena breaking up the smooth flow of the sentence. More stress will disrupt the phrasing, still more the motor patterning of the word; and it usually takes a great deal of stress to break up the integration of the syllable or sound. Although this principle seems to hold generally, it must be modified by consideration of the timing of the stress. If the impact of the stress is vividly sensed within the boundaries of one of these five motor segments, that segment will be the one disrupted. For example, when a neophyte public speaker becomes overwhelmed by emotion at the moment he begins to speak, he may not even be able to phonate. Or, if he feels the full impact of his emotional storm during the utterance of a phrase, he may not be able to finish his sentence. If a speaker experiences important listener loss and senses it keenly while he is in the middle of uttering a long word, he may repeat preceding words or the syllables of that particular word. Since all the motor patterns of speech are ordered in time, the timing of the stress is bound to play some part in determining which motor patterns will be disrupted. We wish to emphasize however that in the adult normal speaker it takes a lot of stress, and stress that is focused directly at the time the sound, syllable, or word is being produced, before these latter motor units are disrupted.

Under the same amount and impact of stress, children, whose motor patterns are less stable than adults, show more fracturing and disruption at the three more basic levels of integration than adults. As a consequence, they speak stutteringly more often. Moreover, they are probably not only more vulnerable but also more often subjected to communicative stress than adults. They have not yet developed the tolerance for listener interruption or listener loss or other communicative pressures which most of us develop as we grow older. And they probably are interrupted more and disregarded more when they are trying to talk. They are punished too often for what they have to say. Uncertainty whether to speak or to continue speaking abounds. They have not learned to keep their emotions within limits. They are entangled in many conflicts, most of which involve speaking.

Young children are also still in the process of mastering the language—its structure, its rules. They must still cope with perfecting their articulation. Their auditory memory spans are short. Often they forget what they began to say and do not remember what they have already said. Their vocabulary is often inadequate for the coding of the messages they ache to transmit and have understood. Young children have word-finding difficulties. The models of adult speech—so fast, so fluent, so complex—which they try to emulate, are often beyond their formulative capacities or motor abilities. More importantly, this is the period in their lives when children must switch their automatic controls of motor speech from acoustic monitoring to proprioceptive monitoring because they now have to listen to the thoughts they are expressing rather than to the sounds they are uttering.

This account of the stress to which young children are constantly exposed in trying to integrate their speech is far from comprehensive. Surely there is sufficient stress to account for the prevalence of disfluent speech in childhood and for the onset of stuttering without having to blame it always on a pregenital neurosis or upon anal and oral fixations. Considered simply as a problem in motor learning and coordination, one would expect more disfluency to occur in children. We would expect the more basic integrations involved in sound, syllable, and word production to be disrupted by such stress. Indeed, we would be astonished if stuttering usually began in adulthood. We are therefore not surprised to find the onset of the disorder occurring during these early years of overload.

HOW SPEECH IS DISRUPTED BY STRESS

The supra-morphemic (phrase and sentence) sequences are probably monitored by *auditory* and *visual* feedback primarily. We listen to what we say in order to determine whether or not we are saying what we wish to say. We watch our listener to see if he is comprehending the message we are sending and to ascertain the reaction to it. Our attention is focused on the coding and decoding of content rather than in scrutinizing our coordinations. When error signals appear in either the auditory or the visual feedback circuit, we begin to hunt and search for revisions which will produce the communication we intended. Most of the hesitation phenomena which characterize the normal speaker occur as reactions to failures in message sending. Many of them are filibuster reactions. They gain time so that the speaker may revise his output. They are signals to the listener not to interrupt; the speaker is still speaking even if an interruption in communicative flow is apparent. Some of these pauses are filled; some are unfilled. We halt silently for a moment or, more commonly, we say "ah" or "um" or repeat previous words and phrases until the revision we need is forthcoming. We hesitate in order to formulate.

To equate these supra-morphemic breaks in fluency with the infra-morphemic ones does not strike us as reasonable. They are of different kinds, the first being formulative, the other coordinative. They are apparently controlled by different feedbacks. Phrase and sentence integration requires auditory scanning for appropriate meaningfulness and visual scanning of the listener to see if the decoding process is effective and to ascertain the listener's reaction to the message. The fluency breaks that occur *within* sounds, syllables, or words are responses to the processing of bits of information concerning the tactual, positional, and movement features of the motor output. They are responses to haptic, kinesthetic, or proprioceptive error signals.

What are the options open to a speaker when he realizes that the message he is sending is not getting across, or is evoking listener responses that he does not seek? He may continue the defective verbalizations anyway until the end of the sentence and then say more sentences until error signals no longer return. This is probably what extremely fluent normal speakers do. But most of us stop when we get the error signal and use a filled or unfilled pause to go back to the boundary of an earlier encoding unit and begin to revise our utterance. We can go ahead, stop, or repeat but eventually we must alter our output if we want to get our message across. If we stop, we stop at one of the boundaries of the encoding units. We seldom stop in the middle of a word when we get a bad listener response or realize that we are saying the wrong word. We stop *after* that wrong word and then we say the new word, the different phrase or the changed sentence. In hesitating due to formulative difficulty, if we repeat, we do not repeat sounds or syllables, but the meaningful units of words or phrases. Our search is for meaning.

As we have said, however, there are times when a normal speaker under great stress will break a word. This occurs especially when that stress is pinpointed so that it is felt within the morphemic boundaries as when the speaker is saying a single word or the key word of an unacceptable sentence. For example, we have seen normal speakers start to say a vulgar word, realize suddenly that it is completely unacceptable, and then block. Or they may prolong the first sound or repeat the first syllable or part of the syllable ("Shih-shih-"). The stereotype of the suitor begging his beloved to "mm-mare-marry me" is another example. Approach-avoidance conflicts and other kinds of severe emotional stress tend to affect the basic level of integration, the motoric ones, more than they do the upper or formulative ones. Mahl (1957) has shown that filled pauses (*ah*'s and repetition of words and phrases) do not occur as often in the stress of psychiatric interviews as they do in ordinary speaking, while the hesitation phenomena he calls *non-ah*'s (the syllabic repetitions and the "stutterings") occur more often under profound emotion. Communicative stress tends to disrupt the upper integrative levels—phrasing and sentencing—while emotional and cybernetic stresses may disrupt the basic motor patterns of the sound, syllable, or word.

EFFECTS OF EMOTIONAL STRESS ON MOTORIC INTEGRATION IN THE PRODUCTION OF SOUND

We do not know the exact mechanism by which emotional stress disrupts motor coordination but that it can do so seems indisputable. When speech becomes hesitant under emotion we suspect that it is in part because the basic synergies involved in the coordination of respiration, phonation, and articulation become disturbed. The precise timing of the simultaneous and successive muscular contractions required for such a basic performance as sound production suffers alteration. That sound will not be forthcoming until the timing is straightened out.

Consider the effect of emotion on just the respiratory component. Emotional states profoundly affect breathing as well as heart beat and other functions. The amplitude of respiration, its rate, and the ratio of inspiration to expiration vary enough under negative emotion to allow these features to be used in polygraphic lie detection. Startle produces the short sudden gasp which can interrupt any other respiratory activity. We automatically hold our breath when danger threatens. The synchronization of abdominal and thoracic musculatures is also affected by emotion. Tremors of the diaphragm (flutter) have often been noted. Respiratory activity becomes dominated by the autonomic nervous system in states of emotional stress, and it is easy to understand why Seeman (1959) could attribute the core behaviors of stuttering to imbalanced functioning of the sympathetic and parasympathetic systems, or why Hill (1945) could view stuttering as basically composed of the physiological startle reaction. This does not, of course, mean that bad breathing habits are the cause of stuttering. We are not so naïve as to hold that ancient belief. We are saying merely that emotion can affect breathing so drastically that the basic synergy of respiration, phonation, and articulation may be momentarily disrupted enough to make it hard to utter a sound *at the precise instant* when it should be spoken. Recently, Sears and Davis (1968) have shown very clearly that the variations in respiration required for the changes in phonatory loading which constantly occur during speech are "anticipated by an appropriately phased activation of both intercostal fusimotor and alpha motoneurones." Since the timing of these nervous impulses must be amazingly precise, it is not hard to see that emotional stress could disrupt it.

EFFECT OF STRESS ON PHONATION

Phonation too may feel the influence of emotion quite apart from its relationship to respiration. In physiologic startle the laryngeal valve is suddenly and tightly closed by the contraction of both the true and often the ventricular vocal folds. Milder emotional states are often reflected in laryngeal tension (globus hystericus). Many of the hyperfunctional voice disorders, such as spastic dysphonia, reflect the common observation that phonation may be impaired by negative emotion. The delicate balancing of antagonistic muscle groups required for phonation can be altered by emotionally induced changes in muscular tension. If it is often difficult to speak under profound emotional stress, the reason may lie in the breakdown of either respiration or phonation or in the disruption of their synchronization.

In this connection, the work of Moravek and Langova (1968) is intriguing. They say:

> We regard the prephonational or initial tonus as the key to the problem of stuttering. By this tonus we mean that phase of speech in which the patient starts to form the voice and where the majority of the phonation muscles are in action, but where the corresponding vocal effect is not achieved. In order to overcome this speech block the stutterer increases his muscular effort but the situation does not improve; in fact it deteriorates.

Wyke (1974) also has stressed the importance of the prephonatory tuning of the laryngeal musculatures in accounting for the disordered laryngeal coordinations that occur in stuttering, and Abbs (1973) has shown how the gamma motor system can control the timing of jaw movement. The importance of this prephonational tonus—which is probably due to inappropriate gamma innervation of the muscle spindles—has also been stressed by Chevrie-Muller (1963) as accounting for some of the aberrant vocal fold activity shown in the glottograms of her stutterers. Long ago, Bryngelson (1932) found similarly minute vocal disturbances just prior to speech attempts which resulted in stuttering.

ARTICULATION: EFFECTS OF STRESS

Similar disturbances of timing may also be involved in articulation. The Japanese workers Hirose, Kiritani, and Shibata (1968) have shown, for example, that before a vowel sound is phonated, the articulatory muscles responsible for its cavity formation receive their motor impulses about one tenth of a second prior to the onset of phonation. This occurs even while the antecedent sound is being produced and it is independent of rate. While the effects of emotionally produced tension on the timing of articulatory movements have not, to our knowledge, been studied intensively, it seems plausible that such tension could produce some difficulty in utterance. The inability to produce a sound, in some instances, may be the result of the simultaneous contraction of antagonistic muscles, muscles paired functionally in such a way that one set relaxes as its opposing set contracts. Heightened tonus may impede the relaxation of the reciprocal muscle groups. In such a case normal movement may be impossible. Fixations may occur and tremors may appear in the structures being activated so that the fixation is prolonged even further. We find these tremors frequently in our EMG recordings of stuttering moments. Before any muscle contracts, it is placed in readiness by a heightening of tonus. We cock our muscle guns before we pull their triggers, but too much tension may cause the muscles to contract too soon, or too late, or it may cause the antagonists to fail in relaxing enough. Much of the effect of emotional stress on speech is probably caused by the mistiming produced by inappropriate changes in muscle tonus of the antagonistic muscle groups.

EFFECTS OF STRESS ON THE INTEGRATION OF SYLLABLES

As we have seen, the motor patterning of the syllable requires not only the synergic coordinations of the vowel sounds which comprise its nucleus, but also a very precise timing of the preparatory articulatory postures needed for coarticulation. Here again emotionally induced changes in tonus could disrupt the reciprocal timing of antagonistic muscles. Moreover, if the motor pattern of the syllable is integrated around or triggered by a breath pulse as Stetson (1951) claimed, the disturbed breathing produced by negative emotion may delay or distort that pulse and so wreck the syllable's timing. And certainly, since the vowel of the syllable depends on phonation, any unnecessary laryngeal closures brought on by emotion could impair syllabic production.

In short, it is not difficult to see that emotional stress might produce alterations in the basic motor patterning of the sound and the syllable and hence to produce the broken words we have called stuttering.

CYBERNETIC STRESS

As we have seen, the motor sequencing of speech is operated and controlled automatically by a most complex servo system. Like all self-regulating systems whose smooth functioning depends on feedback, trouble can occur in the servo system governing speech when the system is subjected to overload, or when the signal-to-noise ratio is too low, or for several other reasons. The fact that speech is monitored by scanning information coming in at the same time from several channels (proprioception, auditory, visual) creates a situation which can produce system instability. Time pressure may place exorbitant demands on the system's capacity to process and correct error signals. The possibility of a built-in distortion in auditory feedback of stutterers has been stressed by Stromsta (1956) and others. Mysak (1960) writes,

> ... many stutterers appear to possess over-correcting (underdamped) auditory monitoring systems. Such an oversensitive monitoring channel may feed back tonal flow signals which are so small that they would ordinarily be disregarded. This excessive backflow of inconsequential error-signals overactivates the corrector device and hence speech automaticaticity is disturbed.

Overloaded servo systems tend to go into oscillation or fixation. They may overshoot or undershoot in their attempt to change the output to correct for error. The motoric patterns which serve as the models in the comparator may themselves be indistinct (as in attempting unfamiliar or foreign words, or as experienced by young children still learning the language), and therefore the cybernetic "hunting" may continue even after the motor targets have been hit. Moreover, confirmed stutterers may have competing models against which the feedback is compared: both a stuttering model for the word and the normal speech model. Under fear, only the motor pattern of stuttering may become dominant, and then the regulator will determine that the speech output will conform to its abnormal structure. Multiple feedback loops afford the possibility of instability. Moreover, emotion, too, can flood the feedback systems with cybernetic noise, with "static," and thereby interfere with the motor integration of speech.

REACTIONS TO DISRUPTIONS OF MOTOR PATTERNING

It is interesting to observe that most of us react to any break in fluency by trying to reintegrate the sequencing at a lower level. Thus those of us who are highly "sentence-minded" (and stutterers are not, as Beebe [1957] has shown) respond to a formulative disruption by repeating the preceding phrase and only then finishing the sentence. Rarely does such a speaker respond by merely continuing after a formulative gap. He must reintegrate, make the entire communicative sequence a whole again. We find a similar situation when a person momentarily loses the crucial word of a phrase as in "It's a . . ." "It's a . . ." "It's a chameleon." He doesn't usually say, "It's a . . . . chameleon" (unless he uses some accessory vocalization as a substitute for the rephrasing). Similarly, if speech is fractured at the word level, most of us respond to the gap by syllabic repetition and we say the word as a whole before we continue. We don't say "Sta . . . stas . . . sta . . ." and then add "tistics." We say the word as a unit before proceeding further. But this characteristic return to more basic levels of integration fails when speech is broken at the level of the syllable. There is no place to go, no lower level, for the characteristic motor features of the phonemes which comprise the syllable overlap each other because of transitional juncturing.

Few normal speakers ever attempt to integrate the syllabic motor sequence by regressing to the sound level. They simply continue to repeat the syllable, varying it slightly, or they pause and make a new attempt on the word as a whole. In the early development of the disorder, the stutterer usually shows this same reaction. Stutterers repeat syllables when their words are broken. Only later do they begin to try to break the syllable into its illusory motor components, shattering the unitary sequence in the attempt to put the word together again. And then, of course, they get into real trouble, trying to integrate breathing, voice, and articulation voluntarily when the complexity of timing demands automaticity. Again, when they find they cannot integrate the syllable or sound, stutterers try to go even further back—to breathe differently; to make a sound, any sound; to move their lips or tongue or jaws voluntarily. The more they fractionate motor sequences, the farther away they get from the integrations needed and the more frustration and panic they experience. Then struggle and avoidance behaviors arise. It is interesting, in this connection, to find that Stromsta's (1959) normal speakers, when their phonation was suddenly arrested by introducing distortion and interaural phase shifts into their auditory feedback, responded with struggle, heightened tonus, and breathing irregularities very similar to those shown by severe stutterers. All these behaviors seem to be searching behaviors. They were the subjects' attempts (often random) to find the motor patterns needed to produce sound. The stutterer responds in much the same way when speech is broken at subsyllabic levels.

HOW STUTTERERS CREATE THEIR OWN STRESS AND MOTOR DISRUPTIONS

In our description of its phenomenology we have shown how stuttering, through its generation of fear, shame, and other negative emotional states, tends to produce its own precipitants. When this negative emotion becomes conditioned to verbal or situational cues, the perception of those cues itself creates sufficient stress to disrupt the motor sequencing involved in word production. Here we wish to call attention especially to the way the stutterer's perceptions of approaching difficulty contribute to the fracturing of words. First of all there is the stutterer's well-known tendency to fear certain phonemes. Rarely, if ever, do stutterers fear specific syllables, although the integration of the initial or accented syllable probably presents their major problem.

The result of this perception of "hard" or "Jonah" sounds is that they attempt to utter sounds, not syllables, thereby contributing to the fractionization of the normal motor sequences. Whole words become perceived abnormally, and the initial sound is usually perceived as the dominant feature of its configuration. As models, these abnormal motor sets compete with the normal ones in the feedback monitoring of utterance, and too often they win. Expecting broken words, stutterers listen for them and of course find them. Expecting repeated syllables, they use the schwa vowel in them and so spoil the word. By assuming abnormal trigger postures prior to the speech attempt, they introduce enough interference in the backflow of proprioceptive information to make integration difficult. Anticipating difficulty in phonating, they rehearse the very behaviors which make phonation impossible—the single and multiple closures of the airway. They even try to speak while holding their breath or gasping. They not only assume articulatory postures which are abnormal, they often alter the tonus of the antagonistic muscle groups so greatly that tremors are almost bound to be triggered by any attempt to shift from one posture to the next. The stutterer attempts sudden movements rather than smooth ones; he jerks rather than shifts. All of these perceptual and motor responses to the expectancy of stuttering make it more likely that disruption of the motor patterns of words will occur.

INDIVIDUAL DIFFERENCES

Why do some individuals show so many fractured words that they can be said to have the disorder of stuttering? We once hoped that we could identify a single cause of the disruption, but we have unsuccessfully chased that will-of-the-wisp over the hills and far away and in our old age we grow tired. There seem to be just too many different reasons for the breakdown of motoric speech to hope that we will ever find a simple and elegant one-factor explanation for stuttering. Instead we feel that there are multiple factors which probably determine whether or not a person will tend to have too many broken words. Certain of these factors may be absent or insignificant in their impact on a given individual while other factors may be potent enough to wreck his fluency. The timing of the simultaneous and sequential muscular contractions and relaxations which produce an integrated word can be affected by any one or any combination of these influences.

Perhaps some day we will have the technology to measure and compute a composite value which will represent the risk of stuttering. If so, we would probably assign different weights to each of the following factors and doubtless add others to the list: familial incidence; sex; brain damage; abnormal EEGs; bilateral coordination ability; interaural phase differences; intercerebral asynchronies and delays; tremor proneness. If we can dream a little longer we would also measure the individual's proneness toward the various forms of negative emotion, especially anxiety, guilt, and frustration, and his buffering ability to tolerate them. Into the matrix we could also insert measures of facility in free association, verbal intelligence, word-finding ability, and sentence-mindedness. We would include data reflecting the person's vulnerability to a range of delayed auditory feedback times, or some other index of his reliance on proprioceptive versus auditory feedback in the monitoring of speech. We would need data on both the maximal and habitual syllabic rates and the protensity scores to feed into our evaluative computer. Finally, we would need values for the amount, foci, and kind of communicative stress to which he is subjected

past history of fractured words, the amount of abnormal
ǝtion of word configurations, and perhaps some index of early
ǝvelopment.

The point we are making, of course, is that human beings will differ
one from the other on this monstrous collage of factors. Each one of them
would have his own unique profile and composite score. The degree of
deviance from the norms for each of these items when summated according
to some esoteric formula would indicate the probability of disrupted words
in that person's utterance. If we had such composite scores we could
probably pick out those persons who were already stuttering and identify
those children who would be likely to develop the disorder—without even
seeing them or listening to them. Perhaps some day we shall have such a
technology, but we shall not wait for that time with bated breath. There
is work to be done in the vineyard and we must use the tools of today.

SUMMARY

Let us see how well this view of stuttering fits the known facts about
stuttering. First of all, does it have any value in explaining why stuttering
is found universally among the human population? All human beings
speak, and all speaking requires the production of motoric sequences
which must be precisely timed. The normal distribution in motoric facility
would produce certain individuals who should have some difficulty in
accomplishing that timing. All humans are subject to communicative and
emotional stress. Surely there should be some whose motoric configurations
in time would show disruption. Why should only about one in one hundred
stutter? Perhaps this figure represents the extreme end of the normal
distribution in coordinative ability or stress vulnerability. Why does stuttering usually tend to have its onset in early childhood? All motor
configurations at this time are less stable. Those involved in word production have had little practice. A shift from auditory to proprioceptive
feedback in the monitoring of speech probably occurs at this time. Why
should stuttering appear more frequently in certain family strains? Athletic
ability seems to show much the same familial pattern. Perhaps the
neurological organization for timing bilateral sequential movements may
be hereditarily determined in some persons. Why should more males
stutter than females? All we can offer here is the research indicating that
females seem to require longer delays in auditory feedback before their
speech becomes disrupted and they seem to be less vulnerable to delays
(or to stress?) than males. Myelinization of the nerve tracts in the brain
seems to occur more swiftly in females. Why do we find the extensive
evidence of organicity in stutterers which we reported in Chapter 14?
Perhaps because the brain mechanisms for timing sequential movements
are indeed faulty in some stutterers.

Why do the behaviors common to all stutterers and those found most
frequently in the beginning stutterer consist of syllabic repetitions or
prolongations of sounds or silent articulatory postures or phonatory arrest?

These are the natural consequences of mistiming. When a motoric sequence is mistimed or interrupted, prolongation or repetition or cessation are about the only responses available. What else?

Why does stuttering show such variability in the adult or confirmed stutterer? The experience of excessively interrupted speech is unpleasant both to the speaker and to the listener. Different stutterers learn to respond in different ways to the experience or fear of broken speech. Those reactions which minimize the social penalties or reduce the frustration will be maintained and automatized. Much of the stutterer's struggle reactions began as searching behaviors seeking the proper timing for reintegration of broken words. They persist because they were followed by utterance. The most powerful reinforcer in the maintenance of stuttering is communicative consummation.

Why do some stutterers become neurotic though most of them do not? Why do stutterers develop self-concepts in which stuttering plays a major role? Why not?

Why does the stutterer usually show the same loci for stutterings that are found for the disfluencies of normal speakers? The same communicative stresses felt by the latter are also felt by the stutterer; they simply add an extra stress to an already overburdened timing system, but, by so doing, they determine the locus of the stuttering. The major exception—that stutterers have more trouble on the first words of utterances—simply reflects the stutterer's reduced ability to time his synergies or it reflects his fear of displaying his impediment. Why does he stutter more on accented syllables? Because these may be the features which serve as the basic feedback signals for the whole motoric sequence of the word. These above all must be timed appropriately.

Why do different stutterers have different feared words and situations? Because of differential learning experiences. Why do stutterers in general speak better when they are alone? Less communicative stress on the timing mechanism. Why do they stutter more to authority figures? More fear of penalty. Why do they stutter more under time pressure and when required to speak very swiftly? Because they have poor timing mechanisms. Why do they have more trouble when confessing guilt or shame? Emotional stress tends to disrupt all motor sequences. Why can they speak better when speaking in unison or shadowing? Because accessory timing signals are thereby provided. Why do so many of them speak better under masking or DAF? Because most of the mistiming probably has its origin in the processing of auditory feedback from their speech. Both masking and DAF shift the monitoring of motoric sequencing to proprioception.

As we contemplate this cursory summary of our assemblage of the pieces of the puzzle of stuttering, we are miserable. Let us confess it: We have failed. Our attempt to provide an adequate synthesis is far from satisfactory. Yet it is our impression that dimly we see the contours of the pattern of stuttering well enough to know that someone someday shall somehow manage to fit all of its pieces together. *Morituri te salutamus!* To him our salute! So we end this book with some of the feeling that Moses (also a stutterer) must have experienced when at the end of his days he was taken up on the mountain for a brief glimpse of the promised land, a land he knew he would never enter, but one which the children of his companions assuredly would make their own. Selah!

BIBLIOGRAPHY

ABBS, J. 1973. The influence of the gamma motor system on jaw movements during speech: a theoretical formulation and some preliminary observations. *Journal of Speech and Hearing Research* 16: 197–200.

ABBS, J. H. AND H. M. SUSSMAN. 1971. Neurophysiological feature detection and speech perception: a discussion of theoretical implications. *Journal of Speech and Hearing Research* 14: 23–36.

ADAMCZYK, B., W. KUNISZYK, AND E. SADOWSKA. 1976. Correction effect in chorus reading by stuttering people. *Proceeding International Congress of Logopedics and Phoniatrics*, Interlaken.

ADAMS, M. R. AND J. C. HOTCHKISS. 1973. Some reactions and responses of stutterers to a miniaturized metronome and metronome conditioned therapy. *Behavior Therapy* 4: 565–69.

ADAMS, M. R., J. LEWIS, AND T. BESOZZI. 1973. The effect of reduced reading rate on stuttering frequency. *Journal of Speech and Hearing Research* 16: 671–75.

ADAMS, M. R. AND P. RAMIG. 1980. Vocal characteristics of normal speakers and stutterers during choral reading. *Journal of Speech and Hearing Research* 23: 457–70.

AGNELLO, J. G. 1966. Some acoustic and pause characteristics of nonfluencies in the speech of stutterers. Technical Report, National Institute of Mental Health, Grant No. 11067-01.

—— AND M. A. BUXTON. 1966. Effects of resonance and time on stutterers' and nonstutterers' speech under delayed auditory feedback. National Institute of Mental Health, H.E.W. Project No. 11067-01.

AGNELLO, J. G. AND H. GOEHL. 1965. Spectographical patterns of disfluencies in the speech of stutterers. Convention address, ASHA.

AGNELLO, J. G. AND H. C. KAGAN. 1966. Delayed auditory feedback and its effect on the manner of speech production. Final Report, National Institute of Mental Health, Grant No. 11067-01.

ANDREWS, G. 1967. Stuttering: theoretical and therapeutic considerations: II syllable timed speech, group psychotherapy, and recovery from stuttering. *Australian Psychologist* 1: 64.

——. 1965. The nature of stuttering. *Journal Australian College of Speech Therapists* 15: 6–15.

—— AND M. HARRIS. 1964. *The Syndrome of Stuttering*. London: Heinemann.

BARBER, V. A. 1940. Studies in the psychology of stuttering: XV chorus reading as a distraction in stuttering. *Journal of Speech Disorders* 4: 371–83.

——. 1940. Rhythm as a distraction in stuttering. *Journal of Speech Disorders* 5: 29–42.

BARR, D. F. AND N. R. CARMEL. 1970. Stuttering inhibition with live voice interventions and masking noise, *Journal of Auditory Research* 10: 50–61.

BEEBE, H. 1957. Sentence mindedness. *Folia Phoniatrica* 9: 44–48.

BEECH, H. R. AND F. FRANSELLA. 1968. *Research and Experiment in Stuttering.* New York: Pergamon.

BERMAN, P. A. AND J. P. BRADY. 1973. Miniaturized metronomes in the treatment of stuttering: a survey of clinicians' experience. *Journal of Behavior Therapy and Experimental Psychiatry* 4: 117–19.

BESOZZI, T. E. AND M. R. ADAMS. 1969. The influence of prosody on stuttering adaptation. *Journal of Speech and Hearing Research* 12: 818–24.

BLOODSTEIN, O. 1950. Hypothetic conditions under which stuttering is reduced or absent. *Journal of Speech and Hearing Disorders* 15: 142–53.

———— AND C. N. BRADY. 1972. Behavior therapy of stuttering. *Folia Phoniatrica* 24: 355–59.

BRADY, J. D. 1971. Metronome conditioned speech retraining for stuttering. *Behavior Therapy* 2: 129–50.

BRANDON, S. AND M. HARRIS. 1967. Stammering—an experimental treatment programme using syllable timed speech. *British Journal of Disorders of Communication* 2: 64–68.

BRAYTON, E. R. AND E. G. CONTURE. 1978. Effects of noise and rhythmic stimulation on the speech of stutterers. *Journal of Speech and Hearing Research* 21: 285–94.

BRENNER, N. C., W. H. PERKINS, AND G. A. SODERBERG. 1972. The effects of rehearsals on the frequency of stuttering. *Journal of Speech and Hearing Research* 15: 483–86.

BRYNGELSON, B. 1932. A phonophotographic analysis of the vocal disturbances in stuttering. *Psychological Monographs* 43: 1–30.

BUXTON, L. F. 1968. *An investigation of sex and age differences in speech behaviors under delayed auditory feedback.* Doctoral dissertation, Ohio State University.

CHASE, R. A. 1958. Effect of delayed auditory feedback on the repetition of speech sounds. *Journal of Speech and Hearing Disorders* 23: 583–90.

CHERRY, E. C. 1957. *On Human Communication.* New York: Wiley.

———— AND P. MARLAND. 1956. Some experiments on the total suppression of stammering; and a report on some clinical trials. *Bulletin of the British Psychological Society* 30: 43–44.

———— AND B. M. SAYERS. 1956. Experiments upon the total inhibition of stammering by external control, and some clinical results. *Journal of Psychosomatic Research* 1: 233–46.

CHEVRIE-MULLER, C. 1963. A study of laryngeal function in stutterers by the glottographic method. *Proceedings, VII Congress of the French Society of Medicine for Voice and Speech, Paris.*

COLCORD, R. D. AND M. R. ADAMS. 1979. Voicing duration and vocal SPL changes associated with stuttering reduction during singing. *Journal of Speech and Hearing Research* 22: 468–79.

COLUMBAT DE L'ISERE, M. 1831. *Du begaiement et de tous les autres vices de la parole traites par des nouvelles methodes.* 2d ed.

COOPER, M. H. AND G. D. ALLEN. 1977. Timing control accuracy in normal speakers and stutterers. *Journal of Speech and Hearing Research* 20: 55–71.

DANILOFF, R. AND K. MOLL. 1968. Coarticulation of lip rounding. *Journal of Speech and Hearing Research* 11: 707–21.

EISENSON, J. AND C. WELLS. 1942. A study of the influence of communicative responsibility in a choral speech situation for stutterers. *Journal of Speech Disorders* 7: 259–62.

FERNAU-HORN, H. 1960. *Die Sprechneurosen*. Stuttgart: Hippokrakes Verlag.

FLETCHER, J. M. 1928. *The Problem of Stuttering*. New York: Longmans, Green.

FRANK, A. AND O. BLOODSTEIN. 1971. Frequency of stuttering following repeated unison readings. *Journal of Speech and Hearing Research* 14: 519–24.

FRANSELLA, F. 1967. Rhythm as a distractor in the modification of stuttering. *Behaviour Research and Therapy* 5: 253–55.

———— AND H. R. BEECH. 1965. An experimental analysis of the effect of rhythm on the speech of stutterers. *Behavior Research and Therapy* 3: 195–201.

FRICK, J. V. 1970. *Motor planning techniques for the treatment of stuttering*. University Park, PA: Pennsylvania State University Speech Clinic.

GOLDMAN-EISLER, F. 1967. Sequential temporal patterns and cognitive processes in speech. *Language and Speech* 10: 131–40.

GRAY, K. C. AND D. E. WILLIAMS. 1969. Anticipation and stuttering: a pupillographic study. *Journal of Speech and Hearing Research* 12: 833–39.

GREENBERG, J. B. 1970. The effect of a metronome on the speech of young stutterers. *Behavior Therapy* 1: 240–44.

HANLEY, J. M. 1980. The effects of fluency enhancement on articulation in stutterers: A Cinefluorographic Investigation. Doctoral dissertation, University of Iowa.

HANNA, R. AND S. MORRIS. 1977. Stuttering, speech rate and the metronome effect. *Perceptual and Motor Skills* 44: 452–54.

HARDY, J. C. 1967. Electromyographic evidence of syllabic pulses in respiratory muscles. Convention paper, ASHA.

HEALEY, C., A. MALLARD, AND M. R. ADAMS. 1976. Factors contributing to the reduction of stuttering during singing. *Journal of Speech and Hearing Research* 19: 475–80.

HILL, H. 1945. An interbehavioral analysis of several aspects of stuttering. *Journal of Speech Disorders* 32: 289–316.

HIROSE, H., S. KIRITANI, AND S. SHIBATA. 1968. An electromyographic study of articulatory movements. *Logopedics and Phoniatrics*, Annual Bulletin No. 2, University of Tokyo.

HOLGATE, D. AND G. ANDREWS. 1966. The use of syllable-timed speech and group psychotherapy in the treatment of adult stutterers. *Journal of Australian College of Speech Therapists* 16: 36–40.

HOSHIKO, M. S. 1960. Sequence of action of breathing muscles during speech. *Journal of Speech and Hearing Research* 3: 291–97.

HUTCHINSON, J. M. AND B. M. NAVARRE. 1977. The effect of metronome pacing on selected aerodynamic patterns of stuttered speech. *Journal of Fluency Disorders* 2: 189–204.

INGHAM, R. J. AND P. J. CAROLL. 1977. Listener judgments of differences in stutterers non-stuttered speech during chorus and non-chorus reading conditions. *Journal of Speech and Hearing Research* 20: 293–302.

INGHAM, R. J., R. B. MARTIN, AND P. KUHL. 1974. Modification and control of rate of speaking by stutterers. *Journal of Speech and Hearing Research* 17: 489–96.

INGHAM, R. J. AND A. PACKMAN. 1979. A further evaluation of the speech of stutterers during chorus and nonchorus reading conditions. *Journal of Speech and Hearing Research* 22: 784–93.

JOHNSON, W. 1944. Some fundamental objectives in special education. *Journal of Exceptional Children* 10: 115–16.

―――― AND L. ROSEN. 1937. Effects of certain changes in speech patterns upon the frequency of stuttering. *Journal of Speech Disorders* 2: 101–4.

JONES, R. K. 1966. Observations on stammering after localized cerebral injury. *Journal of Neurology and Neurosurgery* 29: 192–95.

KELHAM, R. AND A. McHALE. 1966. The application of learning theory to the treatment of stammering. *British Journal of Disorders of Communication* 1: 114–18.

KLEMM, M. 1966. In *Psychopathology and the Problems of Stuttering*, ed. H. Freund, Springfield, IL: C. C. Thomas.

KOZHEVNIKOV, V. AND L. CHISTOVITCH. 1965. Speech: articulation and perception. *Joint Publications Research Service Translation* 30: 543.

LASHLEY, K. S. 1951. The problem of serial order in behavior. In *Cerebral Mechanisms in Behavior*, ed. L. L. Jeffress. New York: Wiley.

LEE, B. S. 1951. Artificial stutter. *Journal of Speech and Hearing Disorders* 16: 53–55.

LENNEBERG, E. H. 1967. *Biological Foundations of Language*. New York: Wiley.

LIEBERMAN, P. 1967. *Intonation, Perception and Language*. Research Monograph 38, Cambridge: M.I.T. Press.

LINDSLEY, D. 1940. Bilateral differences in brain potentials from the two hemispheres in relation to laterality and stuttering. *Journal of Experimental Psychology* 26: 211–25.

MACKAY, D. G. 1968. Metamorphosis of a critical interval: age linked changes in delay in auditory feedback that produces maximal disruption of speech. *Journal of the Acoustical Society of America* 43: 810–20.

MACNEILAGE, P. F. AND J. L. DE CLERK. 1969. On the motor control of coarticulation in CVC monosyllables. *Journal of the Acoustical Society of America* 55: 1217–33.

MAHL, G. 1957. Disturbances and silences in the patient's speech in psychotherapy. *Journal of Abnormal Social Psychology* 52: 3–32.

MAHL, G. F. AND G. SCHULTZE. 1964. Psychological research in the extra linguistic area. In *Approaches to Semiotics*, ed. T. A. Sebeok. The Hague: Mouton.

METZ, O. 1946. The acoustic impedance measured in normal and pathological ears. *Acta Otolaryngologica*, Supplement 63.

MEYER, V. AND J. M. M. MAIR. 1963. A new technique to control stammering: a preliminary report. *Behaviour Research and Therapy* 1: 251–54.

MOORE, W. H. AND M. K. LANG. 1977. Alpha symmetry over the right and left hemispheres of stutterers and control subjects preceding massed oral readings: a preliminary investigation. *Perceptual and Motor Skills* 44: 223–30.

MOORE, W. H. AND M. K. LANG. 1977. Alpha symmetry over the right and left hemispheres of stutterers and control subjects preceding massed oral readings: a preliminary investigation. *Perceptual and Motor Skills* 44: 223–30.

MORAVEK, M. AND J. LANGOVA. 1968. Patofyziologie zachvatu kojtavsti. *Cas. Lek. Cesk.* 107: 536–38.

MYSAK, E. D. 1960. Servo theory and stuttering. *Journal of Speech and Hearing Disorders* 25: 188–95.

NADOLECZNY, M. 1927. Stuttering as a manifestation of a spastic coordination neurosis. *Archive für Psychiatrie* 82: 235–46.

PATTIE, F. A. AND B. B. KNIGHT. 1944. Why does the speech of stutterers improve in chorus reading? *Journal of Abnormal and Social Psychology* 39: 362–67.

PENFIELD, W. AND T. RASMUSSEN. 1949. Vocalization and arrest of speech. *Archives of Neurology and Psychiatry* 61: 21–27.

RAWNSLEY, A. AND J. HARRIS. 1954. Comparative analysis of normal speech and speech with delayed sidetone by means of sound spectrograms. *United States Navy Medical Research Laboratory Report* Project Number NM-003-041.56.03, No. 248.

RINGEL, R. L. AND F. D. MINIFEE. 1966. Protensity estimates of stutterers and nonstutterers. *Journal of Speech and Hearing Research* 9: 284–96.

SALOMON, G. AND A. STARR. 1963. Electromyography of middle ear muscles in man during motor activities. *Acta Neurologica Scandinavia* 39: 161–68.

SCHWARTZ, M. F. 1967. Syllable duration in oral and whispered reading. *Journal of Acoustical Society of America* 41: 1367–69.

SEARS, T. A. AND J. N. DAVIS. 1968. The control of respiratory muscles during voluntary breathing. *Annals of the New York Academy of Sciences* 155: 183–90.

SEEMAN, M. 1959. *Sprachstörungen bei kindern.* Marhold: Halle-Saale.

SERGEANT, R. L. 1961. Concurrent repetition of a continuous flow of words. *Journal of Speech and Hearing Research* 4: 373–80.

SHANNON, C. E. 1951. Prediction and entropy of printed English. *Bell System Technical Journal* 30: 50–64.

———— AND W. WEAVER. 1954. *The Mathematical Theory of Communication.* Urbana, IL: University of Illinois Press.

SILVERMAN, F. H. AND W. D. TROTTER. 1974. Does the effect of pacing speech with a miniature metronome on stuttering wear off? *Perceptual and Motor Skills* 39: 429–30.

SMITH, K. U., M. MYSZIEWSKI, M. MERGEN, AND J. KOEHLER. 1963. Computer systems control of delayed auditory feedback. *Perceptual Motor Skills* 17: 343–54.

SMITH, S. 1955. The pedagogic treatment of stuttering. *Nordisk Larebog for Talepedagoger.* Copenhagen: Rosenkilde og Baggers Verlag.

STETSON, R. H. 1951. *Motor Phonetics.* Amsterdam: North Holland.

STROMSTA, C. 1956. A methodology related to the determination of the phase angle of bone-conducted speech sound energy of stutterers and nonstutterers. Doctoral dissertation, Ohio State University.

————. 1965. Averaged evoked responses of stutterers and nonstutterers as a function of interaural time relationships. Technical Report. National Institutes of Health, Project NB-03541-03.

————. 1962. Delays associated with certain sidetone pathways. *Journal of Acoustical Society of America* 34: 392–96.

————. 1964. EEG power spectra of stutterers and nonstutterers. *ASHA* 6: 418–19.

————. 1959. Experimental blockage of phonation by distorted sidetone. *Journal of Speech and Hearing Research* 2: 286–301.

SUSSMAN, H. M. 1980. Methodological problems in evaluating lip/jaw reciprocity as an index of motor equivalence. *Journal of Speech and Hearing Research* 23: 699–702.

———— AND P. F. MACNEILAGE. 1975. Hemispheric specialization for speech production and perception in stutterers. *Neuropsychologia* 13: 19–26.

TROTTER, W. D. 1976. Long-term impact of a miniature metronome on stuttering: an interim report. *Perceptual and Motor Skills* 42: 1322.

TUGOVA, N. A. 1968. On exercises in rhythm with stuttering children. *Spesial 'naya Shkola* (Institute of Defektology), Moscow, No. 6, 78–82.

VAN DANTZIG, M. 1940. Syllable tapping: a new method for the help of stammerers. *Journal of Speech Disorders* 5: 127–33.

VAN RIPER, C. 1958. Experiments in stuttering therapy. In *Stuttering: A Symposium,* ed. J. Eisenson. New York: Harper and Row.

———. 1936. Study of the thoracic breathing of stutterers during expectancy and occurrence of stuttering spasma. *Journal of Speech Disorders* 1: 61–72.

———. 1973. *The treatment of stuttering.* Englewood Cliffs, N.J.: Prentice-Hall.

WALTON, D. AND D. A. BLACK. 1958. The application of learning theory to the treatment of stammering. *Journal of Psychosomatic Research* 3: 170–79.

WINGATE, M. E. 1969. Sound and pattern in "artificial" fluency. *Journal of Speech and Hearing Research* 12: 677–86.

———. 1976. *Stuttering: Theory and Treatment.* New York: Irvington-Wiley.

———. 1967. Slurvian Skill of Stutterers. *Journal of Speech and Hearing Research* 10: 844–48.

———. 1966. Stuttering adaptation and learning, II. Adequacy of learning principles in the interpretation of stuttering. *Journal of Speech and Hearing Disorders* 31: 211–18.

WITT, M. 1925. Statistische erhebungen über den einfluss des singens und flüstern auf stottern. *Vox* 5: 41–43.

WOHL, M. T. 1968. The electric metronome—an evaluative study. *British Journal of Disorders of Communication* 3: 89–98.

WYKE, B. 1974. Phonatory reflex mechanisma and stammering. *Folia Phoniatrica* 26: 321–38.

ZALESKI, T. 1965. Rhythmic skills in stuttering children. *De Therapia Vocis et Loquellae* 1: 371–72.

ZIMMERMANN, G. N. 1980. Articulatory behavior associated with stuttering: a cineradiographic analysis. *Journal of Speech and Hearing Disorders* 23: 108–21.

———. 1980. Stuttering: a disorder of movement. *Journal of Speech and Hearing Disorders* 33: 122–36.

AUTHOR INDEX

455

456

460

463

SUBJECT INDEX